The Role of Child Life Specialists in Community Settings

Genevieve Lowry
Bank Street College of Education, USA

Lindsey Murphy
Missouri State University, USA

Cara Smith
Missouri State University, USA

A volume in the Advances in Psychology, Mental Health, and Behavioral Studies (APMHBS) Book Series

IGI Global
PUBLISHER of TIMELY KNOWLEDGE

Published in the United States of America by
IGI Global
Information Science Reference (an imprint of IGI Global)
701 E. Chocolate Avenue
Hershey PA, USA 17033
Tel: 717-533-8845
Fax: 717-533-8661
E-mail: cust@igi-global.com
Web site: http://www.igi-global.com

Library of Congress Cataloging-in-Publication Data

Names: Lowry, Genevieve, DATE- editor. | Murphy, Lindsey, DATE- editor. | Smith, Cara, DATE- editor.
Title: The role of child life specialists in community settings / Genevieve Lowry, Lindsey Murphy, and Cara Smith, editor.
Description: Hershey PA : Medical Information Science Reference, [2022] | Includes bibliographical references and index. | Summary: "This book will help organizations visualize how a CCLS could fit within their psychosocial support team, benefiting the organization while furthering the reach of the CCLSs in helping children, youth and families cope with the stresses and challenges they face"-- Provided by publisher.
Identifiers: LCCN 2022015526 (print) | LCCN 2022015527 (ebook) | ISBN 9781668450970 (hardcover) | ISBN 9781668470589 (softcover) | ISBN 9781668450987 (ebook)
Subjects: MESH: Psychology, Child--methods | Allied Health Personnel--standards | Social Support | Psychosocial Intervention--methods | Child Health Services--organization & administration | Vulnerable Populations
Classification: LCC BF721 (print) | LCC BF721 (ebook) | NLM WS 105 | DDC 155.4--dc23/eng/20220510
LC record available at https://lccn.loc.gov/2022015526
LC ebook record available at https://lccn.loc.gov/2022015527

This book is published in the IGI Global book series Advances in Psychology, Mental Health, and Behavioral Studies (APMHBS) (ISSN: 2475-6660; eISSN: 2475-6679)

British Cataloguing in Publication Data
A Cataloguing in Publication record for this book is available from the British Library.

For electronic access to this publication, please contact: eresources@igi-global.com.

Advances in Psychology, Mental Health, and Behavioral Studies (APMHBS) Book Series

Harish C. Chandan
Argosy University, USA
Bryan Christiansen
Southern New Hampshire University, USA

ISSN:2475-6660
EISSN:2475-6679

Mission

The complexity of the human mind has puzzled researchers and physicians for centuries. While widely studied, the brain still remains largely misunderstood.

The **Advances in Psychology, Mental Health, and Behavioral Studies (APMHBS)** book series presents comprehensive research publications focusing on topics relating to the human psyche, cognition, psychiatric care, mental and developmental disorders, as well as human behavior and interaction. Featuring diverse and innovative research, publications within APMHBS are ideally designed for use by mental health professionals, academicians, researchers, and upper-level students..

Coverage

- Neurological Disorders
- Trauma & Stress
- Human Behavior
- Emotional Health
- Anxiety
- Human Interaction
- Counseling & Therapy
- Developmental Disorders
- Psychiatry
- Mental Health & Disorders

IGI Global is currently accepting manuscripts for publication within this series. To submit a proposal for a volume in this series, please contact our Acquisition Editors at Acquisitions@igi-global.com or visit: http://www.igi global.com/publish/.

The Advances in Psychology, Mental Health, and Behavioral Studies (APMHBS) Book Series (ISSN 2475-6660) is published by IGI Global, 701 E. Chocolate Avenue, Hershey, PA 17033-1240, USA, www.igi-global.com. This series is composed of titles available for purchase individually; each title is edited to be contextually exclusive from any other title within the series. For pricing and ordering information please visit http://www.igi-global.com/book-series/advances-psychology-mental-health-behavioral/110200. Postmaster: Send all address changes to above address.

Titles in this Series

For a list of additional titles in this series, please visit: www.igi-global.com/book-series

Latinx Mental Health From Surviving to Thriving
Edward A. Delgado-Romero (University of Georgia, USA)
Medical Information Science Reference • © 2023 • 335pp • H/C (ISBN: 9781668449011) • US $305.00

Handbook of Research on Play Specialism Strategies to Prevent Pediatric Hospitalization Trauma
Giulia Perasso (University of Milano-Bicocca, Italy) and Yagmur Ozturk (University of Trento, Rovereto, Italy)
Medical Information Science Reference • © 2023 • 400pp • H/C (ISBN: 9781668450680) • US $425.00

Counseling Strategies for Children and Families Impacted by Incarceration
Kenya Johns (Geneva College, USA)
Medical Information Science Reference • © 2022 • 365pp • H/C (ISBN: 9781799892090) • US $295.00

The Reproduction and Maintenance of Inequalities in Interpersonal Relationships
Tyler Ross Flockhart (Viterbo University, USA) Abigail Reiter (University of North Carolina at Pembroke, USA) and Matthew R. Hassett (University of North Carolina at Pembroke, USA)
Information Science Reference • © 2022 • 332pp • H/C (ISBN: 9781668441282) • US $215.00

Applying Mind Genomics to Social Sciences
Howard Moskowitz (Moskowitz Jacobs, Inc., USA) Arthur Kover (Fordham Business Schools, USA) and Petraq Papajorgji (European University of Tirana, Albania)
Information Science Reference • © 2022 • 281pp • H/C (ISBN: 9781799884095) • US $215.00

Developing, Delivering, and Sustaining School Counseling Practices Through a Culturally Affirming Lens
Sarah N. Brant-Rajahn (Messiah University, USA) Eva M. Gibson (Austin Peay State University, USA) and Mariama Cook Sandifer (Columbus State University, USA)
Information Science Reference • © 2022 • 383pp • H/C (ISBN: 9781799895145) • US $215.00

The Impact of the COVID-19 Pandemic on Child, Adolescent, and Adult Development
Nava R. Silton (Marymount Manhattan College, USA)
Information Science Reference • © 2022 • 262pp • H/C (ISBN: 9781668434840) • US $195.00

IGI Global
PUBLISHER of TIMELY KNOWLEDGE

701 East Chocolate Avenue, Hershey, PA 17033, USA
Tel: 717-533-8845 x100 • Fax: 717-533-8661
E-Mail: cust@igi-global.com • www.igi-global.com

Table of Contents

Detailed Table of Contents

child life specialists can contribute to simulations for children and youth, parents and caregivers, child life students and professionals, and interprofessional teams.

Organ, tissue, and eye donation is an essential component of healthcare necessary to save and enhance the lives of others. The decision to honor a loved one's designation, or consent to donation on the behalf of an eligible donor, is a choice fraught with a multitude of competing factors which may provide stress among family decision-makers, and the bereavement journey does not end once recovery is completed. Certified Child Life Specialists are expertly equipped with the knowledge, skills, and abilities to effectively and compassionately offer donation opportunities during potentially traumatizing or crisis-laden situations as family services coordinators. As indispensable members of any organ procurement organization, family services coordinators collaborate with clinical recovery coordinators, hospital services individuals, and hospital critical care teams to ensure families are poised to make well-informed decisions, honor their loved one in a uniquely profound and rare way, and provide ongoing bereavement and grief support to families experiencing the loss of a loved one.

This chapter explores the emerging field of child life specialists' (CLS) role in hospital and community-based palliative and hospice care services. Relying heavily on their knowledge of child development, play, family systems, and grief to support patients and families through the trajectory of one's illness, child life specialists can adapt their skills to provide support in this environment. A CLS cannot change what is happening medically but can promote positive experiences for children involved to mitigate the potential trauma, ideally resulting in more positive psychosocial outcomes. Goals of care for CLSs in these settings can include developmentally appropriate education about a diagnosis, treatment plan, physical changes, prognosis, or end of life; various forms of play and therapeutic interventions for processing and the expression of feelings or emotions; memory-making; legacy building; anticipatory grief support; promoting opportunities to say goodbye; funeral or memorial preparation and advocacy for involvement; and bereavement support.

Section 2
Settings

Child life specialists in schools help students, school staff, and families function more cohesively, advocating for the needs of each individual while continuing to prioritize child development. This chapter will outline the student and staff needs that child life specialists are uniquely suited to meet while also giving an overview of interventions, supports, roles, and coping strategies that can be led by a child life specialist within the school setting. Throughout this chapter, one will see how easily a child life specialist can integrate into existing systems or propose a new position within the school environment.

This chapter focuses on the role of the child life specialist working with families affected by incarceration. Children and families are at increased risk due to trauma exacerbated by arrests, incarceration, and re-entry. This chapter will focus on the ways a child life specialist working in jails, prisons, detention centers, and in communities with schools, non-profits, and faith-based organizations can provide developmentally appropriate explanations, preparation, play, expressive arts, and coping, facilitating opportunities that foster relationships and understanding while promoting resilience.

Child life specialists working with law enforcement are valuable in providing direct support and timely intervention in the community. This chapter discusses the implementation of a child life specialist in the role of a victim services provider including practical applications of interventions and opportunities for further consideration. With additional training on law enforcement basics and criminal justice processes, child life specialists have the expertise necessary to bridge the gap between law enforcement and victims of crime. This chapter also introduces the positive impact of employing Certified Child Life Specialists in the police athletic league setting. It illustrates the importance of the role of child life working in the urban community setting with youth and police officers to help normalize the environment, encourage positive coping techniques, and support and advocate for youth and families' psychosocial needs.

The nature of a visit to a child advocacy center (CAC) following an allegation of child abuse has the potential to be challenging for children and their non-offending caregiver for a variety of reasons. Within a CAC, Certified Child Life Specialists are able to call upon their unique skill set to support children throughout the many elements of a forensic evaluation process. In an effort to reduce anxiety, enhance coping, and provide developmentally appropriate play and education opportunities for children in this setting, child life specialists serve as integral members of the multidisciplinary team (MDT). In their active role, child life specialists are able to collaborate with community MDT members to creatively and effectively support children throughout the forensic evaluation process. The need for child life involvement in CACs and during the investigative forensic evaluation process is highly valuable when reflecting on the benefit and overall experience for children and their families.

Child life specialists have been supporting children and families in disaster relief settings for years. It is imperative to understand the needs of children affected by disasters and continue to integrate child life services to best support the psychological and emotional outcomes of children and families. This chapter will define disasters and the disaster management cycle, overview key factors in assessing children's needs related to disasters, identify how child life services are utilized during each phase of disaster relief, and identify future opportunities for child life services in disaster relief.

As the child life profession extends beyond the hospital setting, new opportunities unfold to utilize the profession's strengths of empowering children and families through stressful life experiences. This chapter proposes that therapeutic photography is a fitting and effective tool to be used in any child life setting to promote well-being and describes Through Their Eyes, a child life practice centered on therapeutic photography in a non-traditional setting in South Africa. Differentiations are made between therapeutic photography and phototherapy and therapeutic photography is expounded. The underpinning framework of therapeutic photography with a child life scope of practice is outlined and the therapeutic photography program, Through Their Eyes, is explained. Outcomes give evidence of the ways therapeutic photography programs can connect us to ourselves and to each other, strengthening sense of self, relationships, and family function.

This chapter focuses on using the child life competencies to support transgender/gender expansive children and their families. The chapter highlights challenges families face and addresses the important support they need, helping families identify coping skills and model peer interactions related to gender identity. Additionally, it is intended to provide child life specialists with foundational knowledge about gender identity which will guide and influence their work when they support children who are transgender or gender expansive.

A Certified Child Life Specialist (CCLS) has the knowledge, skills, and clinical training that is essential to work in the field of infant adoption. Child Life Specialists working as infant adoption specialists promote emotional support, education, and coping for the biological parent(s) and families who want to adopt a child. Using the competencies to ground the work, Child Life Specialists focus on the therapeutic relationship, attachment, and bonding while also understanding grief and loss experienced by the biological parent(s). This chapter also examines how socioeconomics, varying cultures, ethnicities, and trauma histories can affect the adoption process.

Many seasoned child life specialists begin to think about expanding their role to serve different pediatric populations and/or settings. This chapter will focus on child life specialists building and sustaining a private practice within the community. Topics will include the need for service, executing a business plan, building community partnerships, and staying within the ethical and professional boundaries as a Certified Child Life Specialist. Additionally, case studies that describe assessments, preparation, developmental explanations, interventions, expressive arts, and play are included. Examples of business documents to help guide child life specialists interested in starting a private practice within their community are also included.

Preface

INTRODUCTION

The Role of Child Life Specialists in Community Settings was written to highlight the work of child life specialists in roles within community settings. Using the Child Life Competencies as the foundation for child life work in the community provides the rationale that child life specialists bring value to the community setting and the children and families they support. Additionally, the book assists other professionals in understanding the value and role a child life specialist brings to their organizations and communities.

According to the Association of Child Life Professionals, "in both healthcare and community settings, Certified Child Life Specialists help infants, children, youth and families cope with the stress and uncertainty of acute and chronic illness, injury, trauma, disability, loss and bereavement. They provide evidence-based, developmentally and psychologically appropriate interventions including therapeutic play, preparation for procedures, and education to reduce fear, anxiety, and pain (ACLP, 2022a)." At the very foundation of child life practice is the Child Life Core Competencies which include (ACLP, 2022b):

- Assess the developmental and psychosocial needs of infants, children, youth, and families
- Initiate and maintain meaningful and therapeutic relationships with infants, children, youth, and families
- Provide opportunities for play for infants, children, youth, and families
- Provide a safe, therapeutic and healing environment for infants, children, youth, and families
- Support infants, children, youth, and families in coping with stressful events
- Provide teaching, specific to the population served, including psychological preparation for potentially stressful experiences, with infants, children, youth, and families
- Practice within the scope of professional and personal knowledge and skill base
- Continuously engage in self-reflective professional child life practice
- Function as a member of the service team
- Represent and communicate child life practice and psychosocial issues of infants, children, youth, and families to others
- Supervise child life students and volunteers
- Integrate clinical evidence and fundamental child life knowledge into professional decision- making
- Develop and evaluate child life services
- Implement child life services within the structure and culture of the work environment

It is clear that none of these competencies are situated strictly in healthcare or the medical field, child life specialists competencies are rooted in services, not specific to the setting or population served. The Domains of Child Life Services include (Boles et al., 2020):

Figure 1. The six domains of child life services

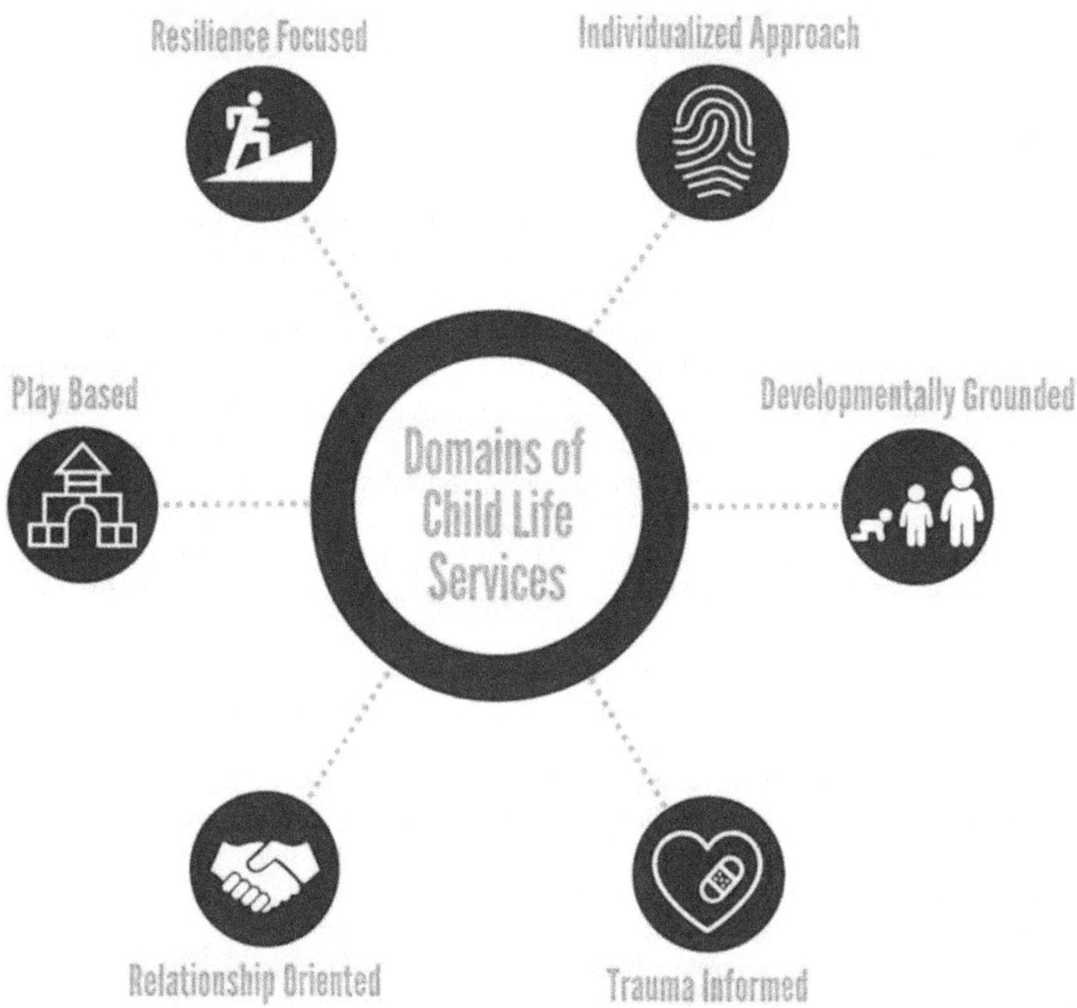

Authors describe how they use their child life competencies within the domains of child life services in each of the community settings or their work with diverse populations. This book provides a framework that allows the reader to envision themselves in these roles or include a child life specialist in their organization by clearly delineating the connections to child life practice. Authors also considered the future areas of potential growth within their setting.

The Role of Child Life Specialists in Community Settings builds on the book *Child Life Beyond the Hospital* (Hicks, 2008). At the time *Child Life Beyond the Hospital* was written, many CCLS were just beginning to recognize a need within the community for child life skills and expertise. The roles highlighted in the original book have continued to grow and provided the springboard to look at how child life practice has continued to expand and evolve. The editors of that book challenged readers to "let your imagination run free as you explore the possibilities (Hicks, 2008, p.V)." In *The Role of Child Life Specialists in Community Settings,* we celebrate the enormous growth that has taken place in community settings since the publication of that book as we hear from child life specialists who turned their imagination into reality.

This book contains the experiences of those CCLSs working in community settings who responded to a call for chapters and as such the chapters will reflect the individual's experiences and writing styles. We acknowledge there is much more work currently being done than what is included in this book, such as foster care, refugees, court systems, homelessness, military and many more. We hope that this book is an inspiration for continued expansion into services being provided to children and families in even more diverse settings.

It was important to the editors of the book that Certified Child Life Specialists were qualified for the roles and responsibilities of these positions without additional degrees or licensure. While some authors were not CCLSs at the time of publication, all authors at one point held CCLS certification. Those authors not currently certified disclosed barriers to maintaining certification in their community roles and therefore were still included. In addition and similarly to traditional healthcare settings where unit specific knowledge is sought, authors also discuss setting and population specific additional training that has been completed to further benefit their child life services in these diverse settings.

Currently, many child life specialists who practice in community settings operate under a different job title. While this initial entrance into these settings has supported the field's expansion through roles and titles familiar and budgeted to community organizations, there is high risk for the value of child life services to dissolve and become unrecognized as this integration continues. It is imperative that as Certified Child Life Specialists continue to integrate into their communities, their services are recognized as "child life" services. Throughout the book authors use either Certified Child Life Specialist, child life specialist or use the title of the role they are fulfilling. In all circumstances, the goal is to recognize that although we hope these positions will someday use the title of Certified Child Life Specialist, currently many do not. That does not negate the competencies demonstrated within these settings as those of a Certified Child Life Specialist.

THE EVOLUTION OF THE TITLE

The original working title of this book was *The Role of Child Life Specialists in Nontraditional Settings.*

The editors of the book had multiple discussions about the definition of nontraditional. In the child life profession nontraditional has historically been defined as work outside of the hospital walls but within mostly medical frameworks. CCLSs sought positions in home care, hospice, and working with children of adult patients in both hospital and nonprofit settings. These moves into the community expanded the reach of the child life specialist and were the beginning of a movement to broaden the professional scope of practice to include community settings. Historically, these positions were referred to as nontraditional, this implies that child life specialists working in community settings are the exception. The needs of children and families in communities necessitates that child life services become the standard of care in all settings. Therefore, the book title was changed to *The Role of Child Life Specialists in Community Settings*.

The Role of the Child Life Specialist in Community Settings highlights the work of child life specialists providing child life services to children and families in their communities, while staying grounded in the pillars of child life. The pillars of child life are applicable to any setting where children and youth are dealing with stress and challenge.

Pillars of Child Life

Table 1. Pillars of child life

Preparation	What unknowns will the child encounter? Are there unfamiliar experiences or transitions happening? (e.g., transitions in care or setting, unknown environments, changes in family structures)
Developmental Explanations	What concepts need to be defined, explained, or scaffolded? (e.g., addiction, prison, evacuation, shelter)
Expressive Arts	How can expressive arts support children and families' emotional responses and understanding?
Coping	What stressors are children encountering? How can we support regulation?
Play	How can play support a child and family experiencing stress? Where can play be integrated?

OVERVIEW OF CHAPTERS

The book is organized into four sections: healthcare, settings, populations, and frameworks. A brief description of each of the chapters follows:

Section 1: Healthcare

This section on healthcare focuses on innovative roles that have expanded child life services within healthcare settings. The role of child life services within research, simulation, organ procurement, and palliative care and hospice are explored.

- **Research:** The role of child life specialists as members of the research team within a hospital is explored. Concrete tools and suggestions for implementing the role successfully are provided.
- **Simulation:** Overview of simulation concepts and methods, while exploring the intersection of simulation with child life practice and identifying ways that child life specialists contribute to simulations for children and youth, parents and caregivers, and professionals.
- **Organ, Tissue, and Eye Procurement:** Child life specialists collaborate with a multidisciplinary team that supports families to make well-informed decisions, honor their loved one, and provide ongoing bereavement and grief support to families experiencing the loss of a loved one.
- **Palliative Care and Hospice**: Focusing on collaborations in care, transitions, and memory and legacy work this chapter provides insight into the growth of the role of the child life specialist in palliative care and hospice.

Section 2: Settings

Chapters that examine settings evaluate and examine child life work within a particular environment. These settings include school, prison, law enforcement, child advocacy center, disaster relief, and therapeutic photography.

- **School:** This chapter explores the role of child life specialists in school settings, beyond supporting healthcare transitions, to further include interventions, supports, roles, and coping strategies that can be led by a child life specialist.
- **Prison:** This chapter examines the role of a CCLS working with those affected by incarceration. The chapter discusses preparation for visitation, coping with re-entry and reunification, and the importance of play for building relationships. In addition, it also includes a feature of a child life specialist working with mothers and their children through various changes and transitions due to incarceration related to addiction.
- **Law Enforcement:** Two child life specialists roles are explored within law enforcement. Practical applications and interventions are provided.
- **Child Advocacy Center:** The work of a child life specialist working in a Child Advocacy Center supporting forensic interviews is explored.
- **Disaster Relief:** This chapter defines disaster and the disaster management cycle, overviews key factors in assessing children's needs related to disasters, identifies how child life services are used during each phase of disaster relief, and identifies future opportunities for child life services in disaster relief.
- **Therapeutic Photography:** This chapter explores therapeutic photography as a child life practice that is a fitting and effective tool to be used in any child life setting to promote well-being. The underpinning framework of therapeutic photography with a child life scope of practice is outlined. Outcomes give evidence of the ways therapeutic photography programs can connect individuals to self and other, strengthening sense of self, relationships, and family function.

Section 3: Populations

The Population section discusses application of child life services with diverse populations. Populations discussed include disability, behavioral health, human trafficking, transgender, and adoption.

- **Disability:** This chapter discusses current definitions and adapting child life interventions to support children with disabilities and their transitions in care.
- **Behavioral Health:** The purpose of this chapter is to discuss the developmental and behavioral needs of children and adolescents with mental health concerns and to demonstrate how child life services can be used in a variety of settings both in and out of healthcare.
- **Human Trafficking:** Describes the work of a Certified Child Life Specialist within a nonprofit aftercare organization in India dedicated to the physical, psychological, and educational support of women who have experienced trafficking.
- **Transgender or Gender Expansive:** This chapter will focus on using the competencies of a child life specialist to support children that are transgender, or gender expansive, and their families.

- **Adoption:** This chapter explores the unique needs of the adoption triad (biological parents, adoptive parents, and child) and the child life services that support their needs throughout the adoption journey.

Section 4: Frameworks

Finally, the Frameworks section provides ideas for how child life services may be structured in these community settings. Examples include private practice, virtual platforms, and nonprofits.

- **Private Practice:** This chapter will focus on child life specialists building and sustaining a private practice within the community. Topics include the need for service, executing a business plan, building community partnerships, and staying within the ethical and professional boundaries as a Certified Child Life Specialist.
- **Virtual Platforms:** The chapter examines how social media, podcasts, and telehealth are used to provide child life services and education to children, families, and professionals.
- **Nonprofits:** Guides the reader through the development and growth of a community-based nonprofit organization with a sustainable approach to the initial core values. The intention of this chapter serves as an informed roadmap for child life clinicians interested in pursuing the development of their own nonprofit.

As the profession continues to evolve the hope is this book pushes the field to assess, critically think, and evaluate the process in place to become a Certified Child Life Specialist in any setting, not just healthcare. Currently, the Association of Child Life Professionals Child Life Practice in Community Settings Position Statement (ACLP, 2022b), recommends that child life specialists working in community settings have a minimum of 6000 hours in healthcare settings. In addition, child life certification requires that students complete a 600 hour internship under a Certified Child Life Specialist in healthcare settings (ACLP, 2022c). Recommendations and requirements continuing to be centralized in healthcare create a barrier to expanding the role of child life in community settings. In order to prepare child life specialists for community settings, certification, clinical training (i.e., practicums and internships), and academic requirements should be centralized on evaluating child life competency which can be taught, trained, and assessed in any setting. In so doing, this supports opportunities to create more diverse and equitable entry into the child life field.

It has been an honor to hold space for the experiences of the authors you will read in this book. Our excitement for the contribution of Certified Child Life Specialists to helping children and families build resiliency in all areas of life has increased as we have worked with the authors of these chapters. Our hope is that one day child life specialists and their communities embrace the child life role in all settings where children and families face challenges.

Genevieve Lowry
Bank Street College of Education, USA

Lindsey Murphy
Missouri State University, USA

Cara Smith
Missouri State University, USA

REFERENCES

Association of Child Life Professionals. (2022a). *About Child Life*. https://www.childlife.org/the-child-life-profession

Association of Child Life Professionals. (2022b). *ACLP Official Documents*. https://www.childlife.org/the-child-life-profession/official-documents

Association of Child Life Professionals. (2022c). *Child Life Professional Certification Candidate Manual*. Association of Child Life Professionals. https://www.childlife.org/docs/default-source/certification/candidate-manual.pdf?sfvrsn=34

Boles, J. C., Fraser, C., Bennett, K., Jones, M., Dunbar, J., Woodburn, A., Gill, M., Duplechain, A., Munn, E., & Hoskins, K. (2020). *The value of Certified Child Life Specialists: Direct and downstream optimization of pediatric patient and family outcomes* (Full report). https://www.childlife.org/docs/default-source/the-child-life-profession/value-of-cclss-full-report.pdf?sfvrsn=5e238d4d_2

Hicks, M. (Ed.). (2008). *Child Life Beyond the Hospital*. Child Life Council.

Acknowledgment

Gathering the authors for this book together for the first time was indescribable. The energy was palpable, the excitement contagious, and the awe of the work that had been done overwhelming. To be in a space with other innovators, adventurers, and enthusiasts, all who had found ways to bring child life services to spaces, children, and families where it once didn't exist was invigorating. Their passion and commitment to pave the way into their communities and think outside the box is what allowed this book to be written. We want to thank all the authors for sharing their work and practice, their dedication to children and families, and their commitment to expanding the child life profession to reach children and families in diverse settings. We also want to thank the myriad of reviewers who provided their expertise to make each chapter stronger.

We continue to be inspired by the pioneers in the field who recognized a need in children's healthcare to seek a solution that pushed the boundaries of people's expectations of hospitalized children. They saw play as a right that not only supported a child's ability to cope with new experiences but also to heal. We were influenced by *The Pips in Child Life: Early Play Programs in Hospitals*, which so beautifully captured the essence of how the child life field began, and *Child Life Beyond the Hospital*, which was the first to recognize our application of child life services outside of healthcare. These works gave us permission to dream and consider "what could child life practice look like in community settings?"

We would like to thank our own families and friends who endured our fretting, listened to our processing, and supported us through long hours of writing, editing, and zoom calls. Without their support and belief in us, we would not have been able to edit this book. Lastly, we are eternally grateful to the children and families we have met while on our own journeys, for they are the true innovators of child life in community settings.

Section 1
Healthcare

Chapter 1
Research

Sarah Daniels
St. Jude Children's Research Hospital, USA

Shawn Brasher
St. Jude Children's Research Hospital, USA

ABSTRACT

Although the value of research has long since been acknowledged in the child life profession, limited resources exist that prescribe concrete steps for child life leaders to take which promote research in daily work efforts. Whether working on research part-time or full-time, it is important that child life specialists take on research activities as part of their job responsibilities. With options to work fully remote or to have boots on the ground, the impact of a child life research specialist reaches patients and families; professionals and students; the academic, psychosocial, and biomedical scholarly communities; and beyond. Throughout this chapter, readers will obtain justification and inspiration for the proposal of this unique position into their own programs. Further, this chapter will offer concrete tools and suggestions for implementing this role successfully.

INTRODUCTION

Child life specialists have many skills that are transferable from the hospital setting to other non-traditional environments. With an ability to understand children's responses to stress and to provide developmentally appropriate interventions, child life specialists are prepared to directly support children and families in any environment. Those who work in the child life profession acquire numerous additional skills that fulfill other job responsibilities outside of their direct clinical care. For instance, they may chair or participate on multidisciplinary committees, and contribute to institutional strategic planning, event organizing, student supervision, and more. Indeed, the roles of a child life specialist even within the hospital setting are ever-evolving, with unlimited potential.

This chapter encourages a new meaning of the phrase non-traditional as it applies to the child life specialist profession. Rather than describing how to apply the child life role to new settings outside of a hospital or medical clinic, this chapter reflects one example of how a child life specialist within the

DOI: 10.4018/978-1-6684-5097-0.ch001

hospital setting can take on a full-time role as a researcher. Although the hospital setting is traditional, the child life research specialist role is anything but typical of the child life profession. Fortunately, child life specialists have many qualities that enhance those of a researcher. When compassion and creativity are paired with a spirit for inquiry, we can best serve patients and families and contribute to remarkable growth in the child life profession.

BACKGROUND

Research is a formal process of inquiry, which aims to discover new information. There are several different types of research activities. The two most common approaches to doing original research are through the use of quantitative or qualitative methodologies. Quantitative research is an investigation aimed at discovering new truths about reality, testing hypotheses against theories, and measuring relationships between variables (Daniels et al., 2021a). Quantitative methodology is often characterized by its investigation of numbers as data and through its statistical analysis (Daniels et al., 2021a). Qualitative research explores, understands, or deconstructs the experiences of people, places, or things (Daniels et al., 2021a). Qualitative methodology commonly utilizes interview, observation, or document review for data collection and is characterized by its use of content, narrative, and thematic coding (Daniels et al., 2021a).

In addition to research, there are several other ways to engage in formal inquiry. For instance, evidence-based practice, quality improvement, and program evaluation are other forms of inquiry that involve examining practices or programs with the goal of improving those practices. Evidence-based practice (EBP) strives to solve problems in the health care setting by integrating an examination of current evidence on the topic, patient perspective and values, and clinical expertise (Sackett et al., 1996). EBP is used to meet standards of care and to inform clinical decision-making (Daniels et al., 2021a). Quality improvement (QI) projects are cycles of evaluation and intervention aimed at improving patient care, feasibility, and safety in an organization (Shirey et al., 2011). Program evaluation is a method of synthesizing information to look at the efficacy of programs and policies (Chen, 2015). Each of these distinct inquiry formats provide guidance for researchers to make improvements grounded in evidence.

For the child life profession to thrive and emerge as a field of inquiry, all child life specialists must embrace the importance of knowledge generation and acquisition. We must critically evaluate our foundation and build an evidence base that is not only grounded in research about children's development or psychology. Child life is its own unique profession, and each day child life programs are introducing new practices that we anecdotally know improve children's and families' experiences in stressful situations. It is more important now than ever to study and to document this work so that it can continue to be built upon.

UNCOVERING THE CHILD LIFE SPECIALISTS' ROLE IN RESEARCH

The role of scholarly inquiry and research is evident in the inception and growth of the child life profession (Sisk & Daniels, 2021). Consider first the preliminary works of Emma Plank, known anecdotally as the 'mother of child life' and for her creation of the first child life program for Cleveland's City Hospital in the 1950s (Case Western Reserve University, 2022). Emma Plank's efforts to address children's psychosocial needs, in addition to their physical ones, sought to improve the quality of children's medical experiences. In 1962 she authored *Working With Children in Hospitals,* a book that drew attention to the importance of play and the impact of illness and hospitalization on child development. These efforts exemplify the process of evaluating current practices, implementing improvements, and documenting findings- all characteristics of research (Sisk & Daniels, 2021). Emma Plank was a change agent in the future landscape of children's health care.

Fortunately, Emma Plank was just one of many early child life professionals who saw the value of research for improving health care experiences for children and families and for growing the child life profession. *The Pips of Child Life: Early Play Programs in Hospitals* and *The Pips of Child Life: The Middle Years of Play Programs in Hospitals* (Turner & Brown 2014, 2016) document several other influential individuals who contributed to child life's field of inquiry following the early years of child life work (Sisk & Daniels, 2021). As child life became a more established profession in the hospital setting, work was done in the 1980s to observe and evaluate programs (see Wolfer et al. 1988 and Gaynard et al. 1989). All of these foundational efforts highlighted the important roles of research and scholarly inquiry in the establishment of the child life profession.

Attention toward research related to child life theory and practice is also seen in professional publications put out by the Association of Child Life Professionals (ACLP), including the *ACLP Bulletin,* which contains newsletter content, and the *Child Life Focus,* which publishes research-related content. Dating back to 2003, the *ACLP Bulletin* featured a recurring column titled 'research review' which summarized and evaluated relevant research (Morehouse, 2003). Steps to improve child life specialists' research literacy were written in a later issue, including tips for critically understanding evidence presented in journal articles and translating that understanding to clinical practice (Farrokhi & Maytum, 2005). Calls to incorporate research in the academic preparation of future child life specialists and to prioritize research-related work among current professionals appeared a few years later. The piece, titled *But Is It a Field?,* questioned the role of research in the child life *profession* and the ability for child life to emerge as a *field of inquiry* (Thayer, 2007). The *ACLP Bulletin* and the *Child Life Focus* continue to publish pieces that emphasize the value of research to guarantee career longevity in child life, even recommending including research responsibilities in child life specialists' job descriptions (Boles, 2011). Other articles described concrete steps for child life specialists to become feasibly involved in evidence-based practice initiatives (Staab, 2012).

In recent years, several other major accomplishments have been achieved that honor the importance of research in child life. The publication of *The Value of Certified Child Life Specialists: Direct and Downstream Optimization of Pediatric Patient and Family Outcomes* (2020) expertly synthesized evidence-based outcomes of child life work efforts thereby indicating five key value drivers of child life services (Boles et al., 2020). The introduction of *The Journal of Child Life: Psychosocial Theory and Practice* in 2020 formalized a place to publish peer-reviewed psychosocial research related to child life professionals' work. In 2021 the textbook *Research Methods for Child Life Specialists* was published for use in academic preparation and in professional practice, allowing child life professionals to directly connect research methods to their clinical interests (Daniels et al., 2021a).

Now, child life scholars can reflect on these early recommendations and document the progress the child life profession has made to "nurture the growth of child life as a true field of inquiry" (Sisk & Cantrell, 2021). Importantly, research is valued in ACLP's mission, strategic plans, child life competencies and code of professional ethics, certification requirements, academic endorsement standards, internship accreditation, curriculum module requirements, and ACLP/Child Life Council (CLC) evidence-based practice statements (Sisk & Cantrell, 2021). The ACLP also demonstrates its endorsement of research through giving its annual student and professional research awards, through the development and oversight of the child life research fellows program, through the investment in and use of the child life professional data center (CLPDC), and more. While there is much progress to celebrate, there is also much work to be done to advance child life research involvement at the individual and organizational levels.

EXPANDING THE CHILD LIFE SPECIALISTS' ROLE IN RESEARCH

Over the past 20 years, the presence of child life content in peer-reviewed journal articles has grown (Boles et al., 2021). Brief mentions of the child life profession are the largest contributor to this presence, with a much smaller number of peer-reviewed articles featuring child life specialists and child life work as the focus of studies (Boles et al., 2021). Mentions of child life specialists in articles increase general awareness of the profession. But further documentation of evidence examining work performed by child life specialists is necessary. Until child life specialists' presence in research improves, the profession will feel limitations on the progress that can be made in practice.

One way to become involved in research activities is to join a multidisciplinary team of researchers. Indeed, many disciplines related to child life, like nursing and psychology, are involved in research activities as a part of their key job functions. If child life specialists are available to collaborate on a project, they have a seat at the table to influence the way child life is represented in a future publication of the work that is done. This step is one that any child life specialist can take by seeking out information on what research studies are ongoing at their institution. If a study is being done that aligns with child life assessment or intervention, simply sharing perspectives can carry significant weight.

Opportunities for child life specialists to design important objectives for a study through a child life lens are uncommon. More often, child life specialists are used as resources for carrying out study procedures and interventions. Indeed, articles with child life content published in the past 20 years most commonly focus on preparation and procedural support (Boles et al., 2021). It is equally important to increase child life involvement in research about other relevant topics, such as play or family support. Further, while it is important to demonstrate the efficacy of child life services, the participation of child life specialists in research projects should extend beyond the role of study personnel. This growth should include child life specialists' involvement in the dissemination of study findings. Currently, the percentage of child life specialists authoring research publications is steady over time (Boles et al., 2021). It is suggested that ongoing training may help prepare child life specialists to feel confident about their ability to contribute to all facets of research (Boles et al., 2021). In the next section, readers will gain concrete examples of child life work that connect with different phases of research.

IMPROVING CHILDREN'S RESEARCH EXPERIENCES

Children with special health care and social-emotional needs are often participants in clinical and psychosocial research. Because children are considered a vulnerable research population, certain safeguards are in place to ensure ethical research conduct with minors (Wittenberg & Cantrell, 2021). For instance, children under 18 years are required to have parental permission and to provide assent before participating in research (Wittenberg & Cantrell, 2021). But even when a study is deemed ethical for involving children as participants, it does not mean that it is enjoyable.

Some work explores children's perspectives about participating in research (Barned et al., 2018; Staphorst et al., 2015). Children perceive both benefits and burdens to research participation. For instance, children may acknowledge the value of helping others and receiving incentives, but also feel a sense of obligation to participate in research studies (Barned et al., 2018). Children report challenging physical and emotional experiences while participating in research, whether due to the study intervention itself (i.e., receiving a needle stick) or due to the research participation (i.e., boredom) (Staphorst et al., 2015). Fortunately, researchers have also asked children to describe what strategies would help them feel more comfortable with research procedures. Among the suggestions, children say that developmentally appropriate information and providing distractions would help improve research experiences (Staphorst et al., 2015). Child life specialists are already some of the professionals who provide these types of interventions to children, so involving them in the research process is one way to ensure child-friendly approaches to researching children's experiences. Indeed, it is the researcher's responsibility to consider children's perspectives and to utilize practices that protect children as research participants (Boles & Daniels, 2019).

Each research study is different and there are several steps involved in carrying out a successful research study (Daniels et al., 2021a). A research study begins with developing a concept and ends with sharing what is learned with others. On a basic level, there are four key phases of the research process (see Figure 1). The first phase of the research process is to conceptualize a study design. This part includes selecting the methodology, creating or identifying relevant measures, and outlining the steps of the research procedure. After a study has been designed, researchers begin recruiting participants and collecting data. This is often one of the lengthiest parts of the research process. Once data is collected, researchers can organize and analyze the information that they collected. During analysis, researchers begin to make sense of what they learned throughout the study and focus on connecting their findings to practice and to scholarly literature. The final phase of the research process is dissemination when researchers share their findings with a broader audience. Each key phase of the research process can be connected to aspects of the work child life specialists perform each day.

Figure 1. Four key phases of the research process

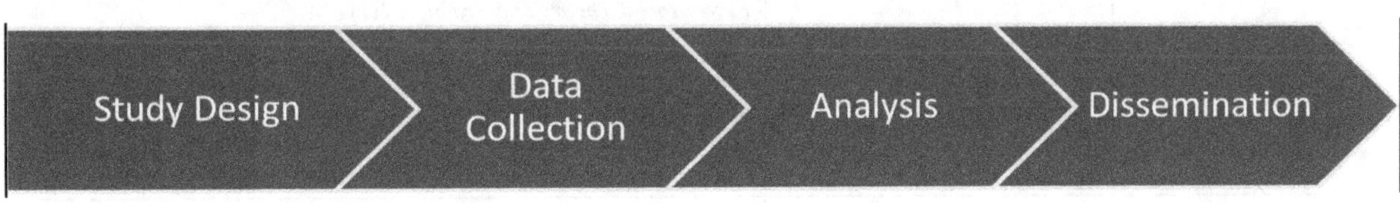

Study Design and Intervention Planning

Most research studies begin with an idea. As clinicians, we may encounter experiences that make us think about something in a new way. We may feel moved to encourage patients and families to share their stories, or we may want to learn more about whether an intervention we tried with one patient could help many other patients. If we observe a stressful experience, we are often motivated to consider ways to improve that situation in the future. Our curiosities grow with our experiences. Once we supervise a student, we may become interested in the best teaching methods for adult learners. If a facility dog joins our team, we want to learn the best ways to incorporate them into child life interventions. To answer these questions, we may benchmark with other programs, investigate what is published in the literature, attend conference presentations, and talk with coworkers. Another way to learn more about these questions is to research them.

The clinical skill that most informs study design is intervention planning. When child life specialists identify a need for child life services and begin to plan an intervention, they need to gather all the necessary information and tools to carry out that plan. For example, if a consult comes through for procedure preparation, a child life specialist does not simply go to that patient and do the same standard preparation they would do for anyone. First, they identify the context for the intervention. Where will the intervention take place? Then, they identify the target audience for the intervention, such as the patient, the sibling, or the family. They collect all the necessary supplies and consider the right time to deliver the intervention. There is no one-size fits all intervention to meet a given need. Instead, each intervention is meant to be tailored to the patient and family who needs it.

This same process is true for research. There is not a single approach to research that can address all questions. Some research questions are better addressed through surveys and questionnaires while others are better addressed through interviews or focus groups. The context for a research study might be the hospital setting or the academic setting. The participants could be patients and families or child life professionals. The key to designing a meaningful research study is to be as creative with the study design as you might be with an intervention. There is indeed some level of structure; you will always have your toolbox of methods. But each research question is unique, and the goals of a study will drive the design. See Table 1 below for some examples of different research designs in child life projects that have been published in recent years.

Table 1. Various study designs in recent child life research

Study Design	Method	Reference
Quantitative, Observational	Case-control	Claridge, A.M., Hajec, L.P., Montgomery, L.P., Knapp, B.M. (2020). Child and parent psychosocial experiences of hospitalization: An examination of the role of child life specialists. *The Journal of Child Life, Psychosocial Theory and Practice, 1*(1).
Quantitative, Experimental	Randomized controlled trial (RCT)	Coleman, D.N., Hurley, M.L., March, K.S., Schommer, K.W., Curry, A.M., Gordon, M.D., & Hagan, J.L. (2021). Virtual reality as a form of interactive distraction for pediatric patients receiving immediate hypersensitivity skin tests: A randomized controlled trial. *The Journal of Child Life, Psychosocial Theory and Practice, 2*(2).
Exploratory	Systematic Review	Kara, M., Foster, S., & Cantrell, K. (2022). Racial disparities in the provision of pediatric psychosocial end-of-life services: A systematic review. *Journal of Palliative Medicine.*
Qualitative, Phenomenological	Interview/Observation	Walker, K., & Lippard, C. (2021). Adolescent cancer survivors' oncology camp experience. *The Journal of Child Life, Psychosocial Theory and Practice, 2*(2).

Data Collection, Play, and Therapeutic Relationships

The next phase where child life specialists can incorporate their clinical skills into the research process is within data collection. Before you can collect data, you have to recruit participants. Recruiting participants requires an ability to explain the purpose of research in a way that the participant can understand. When working with children, child life specialists can use their skills to adapt instructions in child-friendly language and to address any misconceptions that children may have about what it means to participate in research.

When collecting data from participants, it is important to be thoughtful about the procedures of the study and about the methods used to gather information. One burden that children report related to research is the time it takes to participate in research (Staphorst et al., 2015). Being sensitive to children's routines and schedules is important when designing research procedures. Consider ways to collect data while a child is already at the institution, rather than asking them to complete additional tasks earlier or later in the day.

Additionally, using child-centered methods can encourage engagement in research. While parent reports can be insightful about revealing how parents perceive their children's experiences, there are also times when learning directly from children about their thoughts and emotions reveals something new. Some typical methods of data collection may be boring for children, like completing lengthy questionnaires. Some other studies done by child life specialists offer more playful methods to engage youth, like interpreting children's drawings, observing children's play experiences, and interviewing adolescents themselves to investigate their experiences (Boles & Winsor, 2019; Burns-Nader, 2016; Daniels et al., 2021b). Regardless of the method selected for data collection, researchers should take time to build therapeutic relationships with participants just as they do in clinical practice. Developing trust and communication between a researcher and a participant means creating a non-threatening environment. Just like play, research with children should be voluntary and fun.

Data Analysis and Developmental Assessment

Data analysis is the research skill that most child life specialists may feel unprepared to do independently. True, there are some analytical skills that require more academic preparation to learn. Simply identifying what type of statistical or qualitative analysis one should use with the data takes practice. Consider a quantitative study where the intent is to compare differences in anxiety levels between groups of participants who either received a stress-reducing intervention or did not receive that intervention. Depending on the type of data collected, this may require a chi-square test, a t-test, or even an ANOVA. Knowing how to score the measures used to collect the data and how to run the analyses can be challenging even for experienced researchers. Next, consider a qualitative study where the intent is to describe the lived experiences of parents caring for children with chronic illness. If focus groups or interviews were conducted, the data could be represented through narrative analysis, thematic analysis, or content analysis. For more information about data analysis, child life specialists can refer to research methods textbooks, and resources (see Daniels et al., 2021a).

Fortunately, when working as a part of a research team, consider working with other individuals who have more experience in a given area. As more child life specialists and students become involved in research, the immediate community will be resourceful. Many departments work with biostatisticians to perform the initial analyses of a study. One part of data analysis is either computing outcomes or coding, depending on your study's methodology. Another main part of data analysis is the actual interpretation of those results. Oftentimes, the results of a study may be unexpected or surprising. The researcher is required to think outside of their original expectations and contemplate what other factors may be at play. Child life specialists can use their skills in developmental assessment to draw meaningful conclusions about the results of a study. In developmental assessment, child life specialists are always thinking about several different aspects that affect one experience. For instance, child life specialists do not just assess a child's temperament, but also family dynamics, past experiences, engagement with others, and more. By reflecting on theories of child growth and development, child life specialists can best understand the many factors that contextualize information learned through research. Being able to think broadly is a strength that profoundly informs analysis.

Dissemination and Advocacy

A main purpose of engaging in research is to generate new knowledge. But many researchers reflect on the question, who then has access to that knowledge? Historically in medicine and in academia, dissemination of research findings happens within professional and scholarly publications which have limited and like-minded audiences. When disseminating the findings of a study it is important not to lose sight of the purpose of research, which is to make knowledge accessible to people who will translate that knowledge into practice. This does not mean only sharing information with health care professionals but also making information accessible to people in the community.

Child life specialists are constantly advocating on behalf of patients, families, themselves, and the profession. One way to translate this advocacy in practice to the research process is to be thoughtful about dissemination. Dissemination can occur on several different types of platforms, such as publication, presentation, or online (Burns-Nader et al., 2021). Some platforms will make more of an impact than others, depending on the goals of the study. For example, in a study about adolescent and young adult (AYA) perspectives about social media use during treatment for cancer, child life specialists learned how AYA social media habits and experiences correspond to aspects of psychosocial development and adjustment to hospitalization (Daniels et al., 2021b). The child life authors of this study wished to share the findings with a broad audience of health care professionals via journal publication. But most importantly, the child life specialists wanted to share tools for other child life professionals to use which would enhance their clinical practice in a way that honored these patients' stories.

In addition to publishing their findings, the child life authors of this study created a presentation to give at a child life regional conference. In this format, the child life specialists were able to dive deeper into the findings of the study and provide concrete handouts about how to incorporate questions about social media use into developmental assessments done with AYA patients (Daniels & Toohey, 2019). In sharing these resources that were created based on what they had learned, the child life specialists felt confident that their research findings would indeed translate to improved AYA assessment practices in many other hospitals.

Another avenue for dissemination lies within education. The courses that child life students take to prepare for entering the profession should be informed with evidence-based information. Researchers can disseminate findings to students by offering to guest lecture for a course related to their topic of interest and reviewing current evidence on that topic. Professors can review their syllabi to ensure that research studies are represented in their required and supplementary readings. University faculty will be involved in research as a part of their job responsibilities. Graduate students may be able to assist on research projects and share findings alongside the research team. Indeed, dissemination via education pathways ensures that child life students enter the profession prepared to advocate with information grounded in current evidence.

In truth, there are many ways child life skills underlie all of the phases of research. One could demonstrate how developmental assessment also plays a role in study design, or how advocacy plays a role in analysis. The purpose of this section is not to limit the scope of a child life researcher to these parts of the research process, but to reveal some of the ways that child life specialists are already prepared to translate their clinical skills to research.

JOB RESPONSIBILITIES

There are several key job functions that a child life research specialist can perform. It is important that this position be flexible to meet the needs of the organization employing the research specialist. A research project often requires months to years of work to complete, and there are ebbs and flows to the research process. At times, a project will require several hours of work each week. In other periods of time the project time requirements will slow down. During these periods child life research specialists can focus work efforts on staff engagement, student mentorship, and multidisciplinary networking.

Project Management

A child life research specialist should be responsible for managing research, evidence-based practice, and quality improvement projects related to child life theory and practice. The management of such projects should span from conceptualization through implementation, data collection, analysis, and dissemination. Refer to Figure 1 to see the four key phases of the research process. In the first phase, research design, the project's lead investigator will draft a research protocol. A research protocol is a document that describes the key features of a study. The protocol will include sections about study rationale, research questions and objectives, participant recruitment and targeted accrual, data collection methods and management, a proposed analytic strategy, and a discussion of the risks and benefits of the study. Once completed, the protocol will be reviewed by an Institutional Review Board (IRB). The purpose of the IRB is to determine whether the project is ethical and feasible. Once approval to complete the study is received, the researcher moves on to the next phase of the project, which is data collection. In this phase, the researcher will deliver intervention and assessment measures, surveys, conduct interviews, or collect data in an alternate method outlined in the study design. Once all data is collected, the researcher works to analyze the data and summarize the study's findings. Finally, the project is shared with others in publications and presentations.

Projects carried out by the child life research specialist should not be limited to studies that evaluate the efficacy of child life interventions. They should also critically examine outdated child development theory, explore developmental impacts of illness and trauma, study racial disparities in health care and in education, address staffing concerns, evaluate programming, examine professional engagement and burnout, student achievement barriers, and more. This ensures that the relevance of the work done by the child life research specialist benefits a broad audience and re-invests in several facets of the child life profession.

There are many ways to do research. Child life specialists bring creativity and individualization to all clinical interventions. The same approach should be used when designing research studies. It might not always be feasible to design a study that is prospective- meaning, collecting data from future participants. Another option is to utilize data that has already been collected- or do retrospective research. Because child life specialists document their work in the electronic medical record, data is essentially collected all the time. Consider research questions that can be explored using information that is already documented in the medical record. This type of study is still important and can shed light on the work that child life specialists do each day. In Table 2, you can see some examples of the different types of studies that the child life research specialist authoring this chapter has worked on or has planned to work on in the future.

Table 2. Example range of research projects and collaborators

Study Description	Collaborating Disciplines	Study Design	Study Measures
Multi-site study exploring a radiation therapy compatible audio-visual system allowing children to watch streaming video during treatment with goals of reducing the daily need for anesthesia through immersion in video.	Radiation Oncology	Quantitative	Questionnaires
Retrospective decedent cohort study describing the associations that exist between race and ethnicity and the provision of legacy and bereavement services by child life specialists at the end-of-life.	Palliative Care	Quantitative	Data abstraction from the medical record
Mixed methods quality improvement project investigating the informational needs and preferences contributing toward the development and implementation of a web-based educational platform for AYA with cancer.	Medical outreach Patient education	Convergent Mixed Methods	Focus groups Survey
Exploratory mixed methods study of the social experiences of adolescents and young adults with cancer during and after active therapy in a pediatric hospital setting.	Psychology	Exploratory Mixed Methods	Questionnaires Photo-elicited interview
Exploratory study evaluating the role of a child life play-based preparation on parent satisfaction and feasibility to use photobiomodulation therapy for prevention of oral mucositis in children and adolescents undergoing hematopoietic cell transplant.	Nursing Research	Quantitative	Survey
Retrospective study reviewing patient participation in mock MRI practice session(s) and imaging from scans completed without sedation.	Radiology	Quantitative	Data abstraction from medical record
Quality improvement project examining child life job engagement, organizational climate, peer and manager social support, role conflict, health care provider perceptions, and caregiver satisfaction throughout the implementation of a new service model within a pediatric hospital.	Child Life	Quality Improvement	Questionnaires Survey
Cross-sectional, convergent mixed methods study evaluating factors of career longevity and burnout among pre-professional and professional child life specialists.	Child Life	Explanatory Sequential Mixed Methods	Questionnaires Survey Interview
Retrospective qualitative analysis of adolescent and young adult oncology patients' perspectives on social media use during treatment.	Psychology Educational Psychology	Qualitative	Interview
Cross-sectional evaluation of adolescent and young adult medical and psychosocial needs and services during treatment for cancer using a formal assessment tool.	Oncology Psychology	Quantitative	Questionnaires
Phase II randomized controlled clinical trial evaluating the efficacy of virtual reality technology when added to standard pain management for patients with sickle cell disease experiencing acute pain crisis in the ambulatory care setting.	Anesthesiology Hematology	Quantitative	Survey

To fully maximize the benefits a program can gain from a full-time child life research specialist, other work efforts should supplement such project-related activities. For instance, assisting in searching and applying for grants that optimize departmental needs (including funding for resources, projects, staffing, etc.). An additional responsibility is to engage in scholarly writing and review of scientific and academic literature. The child life specialist may become involved in peer-reviewing manuscripts related to children's development and needs in traumatic experiences. Engaging in this type of work promotes ongoing evaluation of the scope and quality of current evidence related to child life theory and practice.

Promote Research Literacy and Participation

Beyond project management work efforts, there are also several opportunities to promote research literacy within a child life or multidisciplinary team. Creating resources, providing writing support, and raising awareness about newly published research are essential job functions of a child life research specialist. Even when child life specialists in patient-facing or management roles are not performing research themselves, they should remain actively involved in accessing research that supports or broadens their clinical approaches. The language used to describe research processes is unfamiliar for many people and can be a barrier to seeking out and understanding original studies. Resources that may be helpful in navigating this barrier include handouts that describe important terminology related to research design, methodology, analysis, and dissemination. Many child life specialists have an interest in attending and presenting at academic or professional conferences. Writing an abstract for a conference presentation can be intimidating to professionals with unfamiliarity navigating the search for and critical selection of quality and innovative evidence that supports their ideas. The child life research specialist can offer support and guidance through obtaining relevant articles and editing writing projects.

A primary way to promote familiarity with research is to host a recurring journal club. Journal clubs are non-threatening spaces where professional peers can come together to discuss publications that relate to their practices. Journal clubs are a method of engaging in evidence-based practice. They enhance critical thinking, increase research awareness, open an opportunity to debate perspectives, and close a gap in translating theory to practice (Honey & Baker, 2011). Anyone can start a journal club, and it is an easy way to begin engaging with research. That being said, there are limited resources that describe the process of journal clubs in health professional practice (see van Diggele et al., 2018).

When selecting an article for a journal club, it is not necessary to select an article authored by a child life specialist or specifically related to child life practice. Other topics to consider are projects related to child development, family dynamics, education interventions, stress and anxiety, trauma and resilience, cultural considerations, coping and adjustment, the impact of hospitalization and illness, the role of play or music, student and staff development, interdisciplinary care, end-of-life care, and more. A strong ar-

Table 3. Tips for Facilitating Journal Club

- Share the article with your team at least one week before meeting to allow for adequate time to review.
- Encourage your team to attend journal club even if they have not had a chance to read the article. There will not be a pop quiz!
- Consider inviting members of the multidisciplinary team to join the discussion.
- Begin journal club by providing a 10-minute description of the article. You should review:
  - o Background (brief)
    - Study purpose/aim(s)
    - Study setting
    - Any hypotheses reported by the authors
  - o Methods
    - Data collection procedures (i.e., participant recruitment)
    - Sample size/characteristics
    - Measures or tools used for data collection (i.e., questionnaires, interviews)
- consider whether the measures were validated before the study or constructed by the authors for the study
  - o Analysis (brief)
    - Steps performed to analyze the data
  - o Results
    - What did the authors learn?
  - o Conclusion
    - What are the implications of these findings?
    - How will these findings translate to child life practice?
  - o Overall evaluation of the article
    - What is the quality of this project and article? Are there any limitations that are important to highlight?
- Open discussion with a broad question. Consider asking, "what stands out to you about this article?"
- Include a few more specific questions for the group to discuss. Consider asking, "do you think the methods for data collection were appropriate to meet the goals of this study?"
- Allow time between members to discuss with one another. This is not a presentation or a question-and-answer format session. Silence is okay. It may feel comfortable to say, "I'll give everyone a minute to think about that question before sharing my own thoughts."
- Allow your peers to share questions that occurred to them when reviewing the article.
- Have fun! You are not expected to be an expert. Everyone is learning together.

ticle will thoroughly describe the methods and analytical strategy of a study alongside the background and discussion of results. See Table 3 for more tips on facilitating a journal club in your workplace.

Provide Research Mentorship to Staff and Students

The child life research specialist should play a role in supporting practicum and internship students who express interest in becoming more involved in research participation. In principle 12 of the Child Life Code of Ethics, child life specialists are given the responsibility to provide mentorship and training of professional values (Child Life Certification Commission [CLCC], 2020). Research is a value of the child life profession, but there is only one academic course required related to research to prepare for certification ("Becoming Certified", 2022). This requirement marks progress but may leave many individuals who learn best through hands-on experience unprepared to engage in research once they are practicing clinicians.

Many students are increasingly interested in research. Although a research methods course is required for certification, several students feel intimidated by research while learning about it in the classroom. Learning about research in a more immersive and hands-on setting can encourage motivation and connection to the subject. By having a child life research specialist on the team, it is possible to include seminars focusing on research and ethics for students to see firsthand the possibilities of participating in research in their future careers.

An especially unique opportunity is to offer a child life internship rotation focused on research. One program trialed this possibility by providing a 3-week research rotation to a child life intern who expressed interest. In the first week, the intern engaged in education related to research methods and learned about the ongoing projects in the child life program. In the second and third weeks, the child life intern had an opportunity to propose a final internship project of drafting a research proposal. The intern was able to network with multidisciplinary team members engaged in research projects throughout the institution, assisted with data management for ongoing projects, and gained deeper experience in scientific writing. This is a unique opportunity for child life students who are interested in strengthening both clinical and research skills during their internship, making them competitive candidates as they transition into the profession. See below for impressions from a former child life intern who was able to have this experience:

As a previous mentee of the child life research specialist, I had the opportunity to learn how this team member collaborates with interdisciplinary departments, integrates child development and patient perspectives into projects, and serves their child life department through quality improvement measures. The child life research specialist enhanced my perspective on integrating evidence-based practices directly into psychosocial care, as well as on collaborating with various team members in discussing, creating, and implementing quality research projects. This opportunity helped grow my confidence and understanding of how a child life specialist can be an essential member of a research project, and this knowledge is a solid foundation to start and continue my efforts in participating in research beneficial to the child life community. This internship rotation with the child life research specialist inspired my passion for continuing to seek out research opportunities that will positively impact the care and support provided to children and families facing stressful situations in the hospital environment. - Katie Lowe, MS, CCLS

In addition to student support, the child life research specialist can provide mentorship to child life staff who want to propose their own study or who want to become a member of a study team. Research is an effort that requires collaboration. The child life research specialist can take on responsibilities such as writing study protocols, managing data, and more while other child life specialists can participate by assisting with recruitment or by providing the study intervention. This type of partnership can help staff become familiar with the research process while only taking on some of the responsibilities. Once comfortable and interested in proposing their own study, the child life research specialist can advise other staff on designs, data collection procedures, analysis, and more.

Engage in Multidisciplinary and Professional Networking

Underlying these responsibilities is the foundational need for the child life research specialist to connect with the multidisciplinary team within the institution and to also engage in external research endeavors. Within the institution, the child life research specialist should aim to participate on research councils and in labs, to serve on ethics boards, and to review patient-facing data collection materials for developmental appropriateness. It is also important to network with researchers in settings that may align with child life research aims, like with peers in psychology, nursing research, palliative care, or radiology. Finally, the child life research specialist should remain an active participant in the ACLP research activities, such as joining a committee, serving on the *Journal of Child Life: Psychosocial Theory and Practice* editorial review board, applying to join the research fellows, and submitting work for annual conferences and research awards.

Job Qualifications

Given the range of responsibilities set out for a child life research specialist, the candidate for this position must have specific skills that relate both to a researcher and to a child life specialist. The child life research specialist should be proficient in academic and scholarly writing. Having prior publication and presentation experience is important for demonstrating the ability to navigate dissemination independently. Prior experience participating in research design and analysis is also necessary. The individual interested in this role should be able to demonstrate the ability to conduct original research independently, including knowledge of research ethics, methodology, and statistical and qualitative analysis. Academic preparation beyond an undergraduate degree is needed for this type of experience. Highly qualified candidates will also show exemplary skills related to communication strategies, project management and delegation, creativity, and persistence.

Depending on the institution, the length of time to get a job description approved may vary. See Figure 2 later in the chapter for an example timeline. Contacting human resources is usually the first step as they can provide comparable positions in the institution. For instance, job descriptions for clinical faculty in psychosocial professions, data scientists, and research associates can provide insight into which job responsibilities to include. If such descriptions are available, it can save time rather than having to seek input from those people outside of your organization.

When writing the job description, one must be careful not to write with only one person in mind. For example, an organization may be better to state master's required, PhD preferred, to allow for broader recruitment of candidates. While a PhD guarantees exposure to the research process, many master's programs offer candidates opportunities to perform research within a lab. If your organization has a clinical ladder in place, at a minimum this position should be the highest level. Candidates for this position typically have leadership experience that can help them provide effective communication to research committees and ethics councils, the institutional review board (IRB), and various manager groups (i.e., child life, psychosocial services or behavioral health, nursing, senior leaders, and hospital administration).

INVESTING IN THE FUTURE OF CHILD LIFE THROUGH RESEARCH

Many child life programs already feel understaffed. To justify a full-time position for a role that does not provide direct clinical care, reflect on the information that has been shared thus far. To begin building a case for the child life research specialist position, acknowledge the lack of space for this research to occur in the already established careers of child life practitioners and child life academicians. Then, consider the benefits that will occur by building opportunities for individuals, teams, and organizations to engage and use research. Even with strong justifications, it is important to prepare for the challenges you may face. Lastly, get buy-in from key personnel that will help support the transition as your department adjusts to the addition of a child life research specialists.

Identify the Gaps

Although some research opportunity exists for child life specialists, there are several barriers that hinder child life academicians and child life practitioners from achieving success alone. Recall that child life practitioners may have opportunities to become involved in study procedures but are often left out of the other phases of research. Even if those practitioners were provided the chance to collaborate on a research study from the initial idea, many child life specialists have limited clinical coverage that would allow them to step away and fully devote time to a research project. Child life academicians may have more time allocated for research as part of their job functions, but they face limitations as well. It can be challenging for child life academicians to connect with clinical sites necessary for data collection.

It is evident that child life academicians and child life practitioners rely on one another. Independently, they are unable to accomplish as much as they can together. A child life research specialist has access to a clinical population as well as to the academic landscape and skills needed to conduct research from start to finish. A key function of the child life research specialist is to bridge these relationships within their community and to bolster research opportunities on both sides.

When working together, child life practitioners and academicians can better approach gaps in research. Many topics are yet to be researched in child life. Consider the chapters within this text from simulation to law enforcement, there are many areas for investigation. As child life continues to expand into non-traditional areas, research can support a shift in the body of evidence from research focusing mostly in a hospital setting to other settings.

Consider the Benefits

Keep in mind the achievements that will happen with the creation of this position. There are benefits that will surface at the individual, team, institutional, and professional levels. Child life teams constantly seek to evaluate what is important and reprioritize efforts in a way that meets new goals. Child life specialists, managers, and directors do this regularly to ensure they provide the highest level of patient care. A child life research specialist position can benefit the team, institution, and profession by demonstrating the necessity for programs to grow. Growth will lead to a more robust job market for emerging professionals. Already, programs are encouraged to use resources provided by the ACLP such as the professional data center and the staffing calculator. Indeed, data is an important source of information that can help advocate for increased staffing. For instance, some research exists which connects the provision of child life services to a reduction in health-care costs (Grissom et al., 2016). Increasing research in child life ensures data is used in ways that not only highlight patient outcomes but also show the financial value of our services.

Many who enter helping professions feel their potential is limited at some point, with little room for mobility. Those in leadership positions should take time to ask staff what brings them joy and where they find passion. Doing so often takes time but is crucial in enhancing job satisfaction. Investing in a child life research position as a leader demonstrates support for professional development and the reward of specialized talent among individuals. This type of recognition and professional opportunity will retain child life specialists with skills in a clinically focused role, whereas currently many child life specialists with advanced expertise in research methods are situated in academic positions. Another benefit of such a position is the flexibility it offers qualified candidates. For instance, once research relationships are established within an institution and partnerships are made on-site, the research specialist may have the flexibility to perform many of their job functions remotely. By creating space for child life specialists to merge their child life scope of practice with other unique skill sets, like expertise in research and writing, the profession is sure to improve retention and longevity.

Advocating for staff takes bold leadership. Wisdom should be sought by the leader on when and how to support staff career goals. It is not something that can be done alone, but together with those you trust.

Just because someone states something is a passion does not mean it has to happen immediately; it is something that should continue to discuss over time. Waiting often allows time for those in leadership to truly process and evaluate how the staff's passion fits into the larger institutional and professional pictures. Many institutions call for increased research involvement as part of their strategic planning. Staffing a child life research specialist embeds a member of a child life program in that planning goal, increasing the likelihood that research aims associated with child life content are brought to focus. This involvement will start a wave of impact, such that the research being done can inspire growth within the institution while also broadening the evidence base that will promote longevity of the greater child life profession. To accomplish this rigorous research agenda, work efforts must be dedicated to studying the scope of child life work.

Prepare to Address Threats

Progress can only follow change. Once the decision is made to move in the direction of having a research position, it is important not to be distracted by criticism. It is equally as important to not be distracted by other tempting opportunities that are presented around the same time. For example, a new staffing opportunity could lead to an organization including a facility dog position, a special events coordinator, or a student coordinator. One hospital's clinical director often challenges those under his leadership with this question: "What are you willing to stop doing to start doing something else?" This impossible question requires the acknowledgment that each of these positions indeed adds value to a child life program but cannot all be advanced at one time. The value of a child life research specialist position is likely unseen as immediately as the others. Follow through is important and will help in understanding the value long-term.

Aside from considering threats that may occur at the job proposal level, one should also consider the potential barriers a child life research specialist may encounter once established. For example, the individual interested should know their institution's IRB process, funding availability, and access to statistical software. It is likely that there will be many resources already in place for individuals who perform research but securing access to those resources requires planning. Stay encouraged and do not let fear of setbacks get in the way of advocating for the child life research specialist position.

Get Buy-In from Key People

Buy-in from key people at all levels in an institution is essential. First and foremost, a child life specialist is needed who has the passion to incorporate research into their practice at this level. Second, the managers and director of the child life program need to be on board to face the potential challenges while supporting other staff. In addition to the support most central to this position, additional support will be needed at higher levels of administration. Seeking input from department chairs and chiefs of neighboring service lines can inform key ways for obtaining buy-in from senior leaders.

Many child life specialists state they are interested in research but have not been prepared to do so independently. Having a child life specialist who has been trained in advanced research methods and who has some level of experience can help influence the director's decision to begin to reprioritize the department. Some directors may be fortunate to request new positions. Others may need to restructure the delivery of care to allow a current staff member to take on research activities. Take time to brainstorm with the child life specialist who is interested, the director, and with other staff to determine ways to alleviate the burden of increased patient care on the rest of the team as the role of the child life research specialist begins. During that discussion, action plans and strategies can begin to be formed. Excitement will begin to flow as staff understand the purpose of this position as it relates to current child life practices. For instance, child life specialists are trained to identify problems and quickly come up with solutions to best serve patients and families. Child life programs must also learn the importance of equally discussing problems and solutions that will help the profession grow and expand through research practices.

Table 4. Perspectives from research peers about the child life research specialist's role

Key Personnel	Statement of Support
Child Life Colleague	*The role of the child life research specialist is not only beneficial but essential to our child life department. Our child life research specialist has unique and specialized skills in conducting quality research which enhances the services our child life department provides at our institution and the field of child life as a whole. As a child life specialist who is also interested in research, having a specialist dedicated to research creates opportunities for our department to collaborate with other disciplines on different projects. Further, it makes me hopeful for the continued growth of research in child life. This position carries so much potential to positively impact the lives of the patients and families the child life community serves each and every day. – Tori Hinton, MS, CCLS*
Psychologist	*As a psychologist who has worked closely with a Child Life Research Specialist, I can only espouse the benefits of such a position and collaboration opportunity. The inclusion of a CLRS on my research team has strengthened my current research studies. Specifically, the CLRS brings her perspective as a child life specialist to the development of research projects as well as analyses of completed data, providing a unique perspective on the day-to-day clinical lives of our patient population that helps to bring life to research data. Further, her knowledge of theory and research methods has been particularly helpful and in many ways complements and extends my own expertise. My goal with my research team is to build a team with complementary expertise and perspective; the inclusion of a CLRS has truly rounded out our group. – Tori Willard, PhD*
Chief of Psychosocial Services	*I have found the role of the child life research specialist to be incredibly valuable, not only to our Child Life department but to our broader Psychosocial Services department as well. Most child life specialists and other psychosocial providers spend the majority of their time delivering services to patients and families. This leaves very little time for planning or executing research or quality improvement projects. Having a dedicated child life research specialist ensures that the specialist designing and completing research studies has the right knowledge and expertise to effectively evaluate processes. It also allows for the time and effort necessary to devote to important evaluation and dissemination of best practices and facilitates cross-departmental collaboration in a way that helps us best meet the psychosocial needs of patients and families. – Valerie Crabtree, PhD*

Assemble Strategies for Success

The recommendations above will help create space for proposing a research specialist position into a child life program. Once that position becomes a reality, departments will need to transition focus onto actions that will set the position up for success from the beginning. Start by benchmarking with other child life programs. Consider whether other hospitals have research opportunities. Will this position help the child life program stand out, increasing the opportunity to attract unique talent and retain exceptional staff? Also, consider how disciplines like child life incorporate research staff into their programs. These examples can help shape the proposal for this type of position. After laying some groundwork, use the four tips listed below to ensure a successful launch of the position and to support long-term value.

Embed in Current Institutional Drivers

Successful child life programs do not work within a silo. Instead, they work closely with other departments in their community or institution. Collaboration ensures shared decision-making and mutual respect while each discipline strives to achieve new goals. Such goals are often outlined in strategic plans. Most institutions develop strategic plans every three to five years, and departments within the organization often develop their strategic plan. It is important to have alignment between the organization and the departmental strategic plan. When research is shown as an important driver in a hospital or other organization, leaders of child life programs should take the opportunity to prioritize it as a goal for their team. These markers are grounding points to justify the proposal of protected research time for current staff, and eventually for the proposal of a research position.

Start Small, Dream Big

When research is embedded in an institution's strategic plan, it becomes clear that all programs within that organization need to prioritize efforts that support research. Staff who are interested in research can begin to think of one-to-five-year strategies. A good place to start is to focus on obtaining 8-16 hours of research time per week in the first year. During that time, other staff in the child life program can adjust to providing coverage in the clinic, taking on 15-20% of that child life specialist's patient load each week. By the end of a five-year plan, the team will have had time to brainstorm together on the best ways to meet all direct patient care needs while also prioritizing research as a focal point of the work effort. See Figure 2 below for a timeline of how one child life program grew a full-time child life research specialist position over three years.

Figure 2. Child life research specialists position timeline

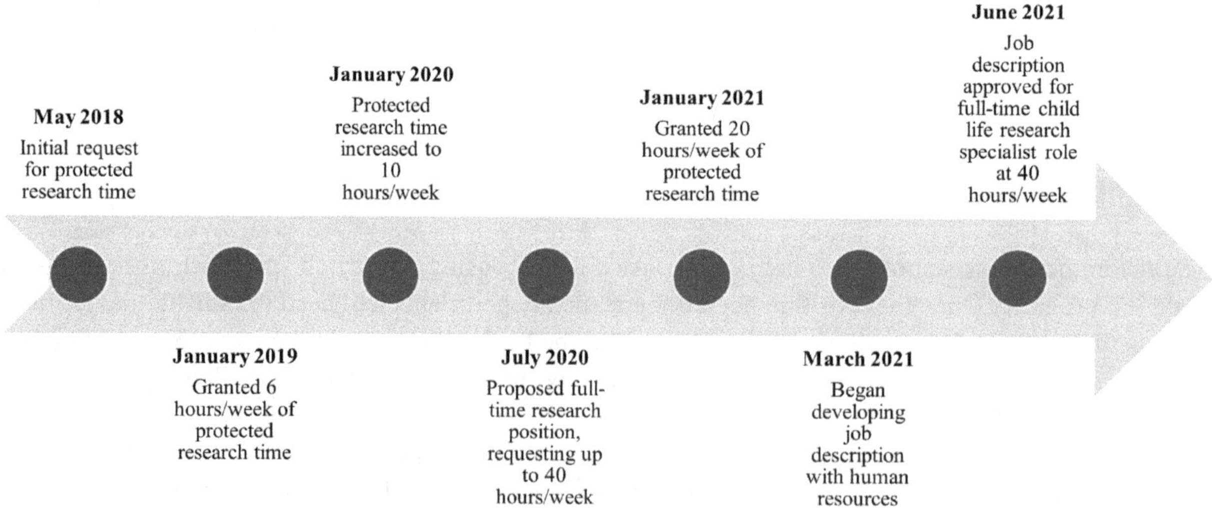

Be sure to ask the child life specialist taking on research in your program to document the amount of work effort for each project that they contribute toward. Having a clear picture of how much time it takes to meet with research study teams, contribute to committees, prepare research proposals, perform data collection and analyses, and work on manuscripts and presentations can be useful when conceptualizing the feasibility of a research workload.

Build a Research Community

If the demand for child life participation in research is low, starting small can at least allow the child life specialist time to network with research faculty at the institution or to build relationships with academicians in their community. Once those types of relationships are established, the child life specialist doing research within the organization will begin to build new opportunities. When starting a new research position it is essential to lean on experienced colleagues who are active in the research networks at the institution. This creates space for the child life specialist to assess potential areas for collaboration on existing projects and to learn which faculty may support new study ideas in the future.

When demand for child life participation in research is limited, do not hold back from prioritizing a research role on your team. Child life specialists can engage in research by looking at national data sets, creating and distributing surveys to professionals, and partnering on projects within their community. In the meantime, they can immerse themselves in relevant scientific literature and in devoting time to supporting other research initiatives, like creating staff and student educational content.

Cultivate Strategic Foresight

The success of this position depends upon the mapping of future impact and growth. The value of a child life research specialist is revealed over time. Significant planning is needed at first to establish a realistic workload. As projects come to an end, the child life research specialist must continue to transform the role to meet the needs of the program by proposing new projects, growing new relationships, and developing new content that benefits the child life community. Therefore, when proposing this position into a child life program it is important to not only consider what types of projects the child life research specialist can engage in now but to also consider what realistically lies ahead.

The vision for a child life research specialist role is young. Once this role is established and adopted, new opportunities can emerge. For instance, just as some programs employ child life assistants or have child life fellowships, perhaps there is an opportunity for a child life research fellowship following a clinical internship. As the child life profession welcomes individuals with different skills, we must accept people who are just as passionate about investing in patients, families, and students as they are about researching and documenting the growth of the profession overall.

CONCLUSION

It is exciting to see the child life profession expand to new settings and embrace non-traditional roles. For years, child life specialists have been involved in research and many are valuing research as a key job function. Just like other medical practitioners and academicians, child life specialists must perform research to not only sustain the work they do but to advance it forward. However, there continue to be limitations that set child life specialists back from being able to engage fully in research activities. This chapter serves as a guideline to demonstrate the value and feasibility of creating a child life research specialist role. Child life students, professionals, and leaders are encouraged to take inspiration from this case example and create similar positions on their teams. Further, readers should consider aspects from the other chapters in this text to inspire projects examining the unique roles of child life specialists in non-traditional settings.

The authors of this chapter would like to acknowledge the many child life researchers who came first and engaged in research despite facing barriers of having a lack of protected time. This foundational work changed lives, expanded possibilities, and paved the way for a full-time child life research position to hold meaning and value at an organizational and professional level.

REFERENCES

Association of Child Life Professionals. (2022, July 18). *Becoming certified: Academic requirements.* https://www.childlife.org/certification/becoming-certified

Barned, C., Dobson, J., Stintzi, A., Mack, D., & O'Doherty, K. C. (2018). Children's perspectives on the benefits and burdens of research participation. *AJOB Empirical Bioethics*, *9*(1), 19–28. doi:10.1080/23294515.2018.1430709 PMID:29369013

Boles, J. (2011, Fall). Creating a Culture of Research. *Child Life Bulletin.* https://www.childlife.org/docs/default-source/Publications/Bulletin/fall2011final.pdf?sfvrsn=2

Boles, J., Fraser, C., Bennett, K., Jones, M., Dunbar, J., Woodburn, A., Gill, M. A., Duplechain, A., Munn, E. K., & Hoskins, K. (2020). *The Value of Certified Child Life Specialists: Direct Downstream Optimization of Pediatric Patient and Family Outcomes.* Association of Child Life Professionals. https://www.childlife.org/the-child-life-profession/value-proposition-statement

Boles, J., Turner, J., Rights, J., & Lu, R. (2021). Empirical evolution of child life. *The Journal of Child Life: Psychosocial Theory and Practice*, *2*(1), 4–14.

Boles, J. C., & Daniels, S. R. (2019). Researching the experiences of children and youth with cancer: Considerations for practice. *Children (Basel, Switzerland)*, *6*(8), 93–104. doi:10.3390/children6080093 PMID:31426332

Boles, J. C., & Winsor, D. L. (2019). "My school is where my friends are": Interpreting the drawings of children with cancer. *Journal of Research in Childhood Education*, *33*(2), 225–241. doi:10.1080/02568543.2019.1577771

Burns-Nader, S. (2016). Examining children's healthcare experiences through drawings. *Early Child Development and Care*, *187*(11), 1809–1818. doi:10.1080/03004430.2016.1192616

Burns-Nader, S., Daniels, S., & Boles, J. (2021). Disseminating your study. In S. Daniels, S. Burns-Nader, & J. Boles (Eds.), *Research methods for child life specialists* (pp. 271–306). Cambridge Scholars Publishing.

Case Western Reserve University. (2022). Plank, emma nuschi. In *The Encyclopedia of Cleveland History*. https://case.edu/ech/articles/p/plank-emma-nuschi

Chen, H. T. (2015). *Practical Program Evaluation: Theory-Driven Evaluation and the Integrated Evaluation Perspective* (2nd ed.). SAGE Publications, Inc.

Child Life Certification Commission. (2020). *Child Life Code of Ethics*. Retrieved April 16, 2022, from https://www.childlife.org/docs/default-source/certification/child-life-code-of-ethics.pdf?sfvrsn=2

Claridge, A. M., Hajec, L. P., Montgomery, L. P., & Knapp, B. M. (2020). Child and parent psychosocial experiences of hospitalization: An examination of the role of child life specialists. The Journal of Child Life, Psychosocial. *Theory into Practice*, *1*(1).

Coleman, D. N., Hurley, M. L., March, K. S., Schommer, K. W., Curry, A. M., Gordon, M. D., & Hagan, J. L. (2021). Virtual reality as a form of interactive distraction for pediatric patients receiving immediate hypersensitivity skin tests: A randomized controlled trial. The Journal of Child Life, Psychosocial. *Theory into Practice*, *2*(2).

Daniels, S., Burns-Nader, S., & Boles, J. (Eds.). (2021a). Research methods for child life specialists (edited collection). Cambridge Scholars Publishing.

Daniels, S., & Toohey, S. J. (2019, September). *"Don't put your phone down!" Child life practice and the online worlds of hospitalized teens* [Conferences session]. 2nd Annual Southeastern Association of Child Life Professionals Regional Conference, Nashville, TN, United States.

Daniels, S. R., Yang, C., Toohey, S. J., & Willard, V. W. (2021b). Perspectives on social media from adolescents and young adults with cancer. *Journal of Pediatric Oncology Nursing*, *38*(4), 225–232. doi:10.1177/1043454221992319 PMID:33729902

Farrokhi, F., & Maytum, S. (2005, Winter). Why Research? *Child Life Bulletin*. https://www.childlife.org/docs/default-source/Publications/Bulletin/winter-2005-bulletin---final.pdf?sfvrsn=2

Gaynard, L., Hausslem, E., & Demarsh, J. P. (1989). Child life specialists: Report of an observational study. *Children's Health Care*, *18*(2), 75–81. doi:10.120715326888chc1802_3 PMID:10292919

Grissom, S., Boles, J., Bailey, K., Cantrell, K., Kennedy, A., Sykes, A., & Mandrell, B. N. (2016). Play-based procedural preparation and support intervention for cranial radiation. *Supportive Care in Cancer*, *24*(6), 2421–2427. doi:10.100700520-015-3040-y PMID:26634562

Honey, C. P., & Baker, J. A. (2011). Exploring the impact of journal clubs: A systematic review. *Nurse Education Today*, *31*(8), 825–831. doi:10.1016/j.nedt.2010.12.020 PMID:21247668

Kara, M., Foster, S., & Cantrell, K. (2022). Racial disparities in the provision of pediatric psychosocial end-of-life services: A systematic review. *Journal of Palliative Medicine*, *25*(10), 1510–1517. doi:10.1089/jpm.2021.0476 PMID:35588290

Morehouse, K. (2003, Spring). Research review: Children's psychological responses after critical illness and exposure to invasive technology. *Child Life Bulletin*. https://www.childlife.org/docs/default-source/Publications/Bulletin/2003---spring-bulletin.pdf?sfvrsn=69debe4d_2

Sackett, D., Rosenberg, W. C., Gray, J. A. M., Haynes, R. B., & Richardson, W. S. (1996). Evidence-based medicine: What it is and what it isn't. *BMJ (Clinical Research Ed.)*, *312*(7023), 71–72. doi:10.1136/bmj.312.7023.71 PMID:8555924

Shirey, M. R., Hauck, S. L., Embree, J. L., Kinner, T. J., Schaar, G. L., Phillips, L. A., Ashby, S. R., Sweny, C. F., & McCool, I. A. (2011). Showcasing differences between quality improvement, evidence-based practice, and research. *Journal of Continuing Education in Nursing*, *42*(2), 57–68. doi:10.3928/00220124-20100701-01 PMID:20672761

Sisk, C., & Cantrell, K. (2021, Spring). How far have we come? *Child Life Bulletin.* https://www.childlife.org/membership/aclp-bulletin/spring-2021-table-of-contents/how-far-have-we-come

Sisk, C., & Daniels, S. (2021). Introduction. In S. Daniels, S. Burns-Nader, & J. Boles (Eds.), *Research methods for child life specialists* (pp. 1–11). Cambridge Scholars Publishing.

Staab, J. (2012, Winter). Unveiling a standard for knowledge translation: An evidence-based practice model for the child life profession. *Child Life Bulletin.* https://www.childlife.org/docs/default-source/Publications/Bulletin/clcbulletinwinter2012.pdf?sfvrsn

Staphorst, M. S., Hunfeld, J. A., van de Vathorst, S., Passchier, J., & van Goudoever, J. B. (2015). Children's self-reported discomforts as participants in clinical research. *Social Science & Medicine*, *142*, 154–162. doi:10.1016/j.socscimed.2015.08.019 PMID:26310591

Thayer, P. (2007, Summer). But is it a field? *Child Life Bulletin.* https://www.childlife.org/docs/default-source/Publications/Bulletin/summer-2007-bulletin---final.pdf

Turner, J., & Brown, C. (Eds.). (2014). *The Pips of Child Life: Early Play Programs in Hospitals*. Kendall Hunt Publishing.

Turner, J., & Brown, C. (Eds.). (2016). *The Pips of Child Life: The Middle Years of Play Programs in Hospitals*. Kendall Hunt Publishing.

vanDiggele, C., Burgess, A., & Mellis, C. (2018). Journal clubs in health professional practice. *The Clinical Teacher*, *16*(1), 13–18. PMID:29436113

Walker, K., & Lippard, C. (2021). Adolescent cancer survivors' oncology camp experience. The Journal of Child Life, Psychosocial. *Theory into Practice*, *2*(2).

Wittenberg, B., & Cantrell, K. (2021). Ethical research conduct. In S. Daniels, S. Burns-Nader, & J. Boles (Eds.), *Research methods for child life specialists* (pp. 91–125). Cambridge Scholars Publishing.

Wolfer, J., Gaynard, L., Goldberger, J., Laidley, L., & Thompson, R. (1988). An experimental evaluation of a model child life program. *Children's Health Care*, *16*(4), 244–254. doi:10.120715326888chc1604_1 PMID:10286751

KEY TERMS AND DEFINITIONS

Dissemination: The process of sharing findings and can occur on several different types of platforms, such as publication, presentation, or online.

Evidence-Based Practice: Strives to solve problems in the health care setting by integrating an examination of current evidence on the topic, patient perspective and values, and clinical expertise.

Program Evaluation: A method of synthesizing information to look at the efficacy of programs and policies.

Qualitative Research: Explores, understands, or deconstructs the experiences of people, places, or things.

Quality Improvement: Projects that are cycles of evaluation and intervention aimed at improving patient care, feasibility, and safety in an organization.

Quantitative Research: An investigation aimed at discovering new truths about reality, testing hypotheses against theories, and measuring relationships between variables.

Research: The systematic and formal investigation into a problem with a goal of arriving at new ideas or discoveries.

Chapter 2
Simulation

Hilary Woodward
NewYork-Presbyterian Morgan Stanley Children's Hospital at Columbia University Irving Medical Center, USA

ABSTRACT

Simulation helps learners conceptualize and apply knowledge through experiential learning and shared reflection. Children and families, as well as professionals who work with these populations, can benefit from simulation-based education. Child life specialists' skills in interprofessional collaboration, developmentally appropriate language and preparation, child- and family-centered care, and emotional safety provide them with a solid foundation as simulation educators and facilitators. By developing their knowledge of the learning theories underpinning simulation as well as scenario design, simulation environments and modalities, psychological safety, and debriefing, child life specialists can incorporate simulation into their roles. This chapter provides an overview of simulation concepts and methods while exploring the intersection of simulation with child life practice. The chapter also identifies ways that child life specialists can contribute to simulations for children and youth, parents and caregivers, child life students and professionals, and interprofessional teams.

INTRODUCTION

Child life professionals frequently incorporate experiential learning for children, youth, and families into their clinical work. Children and youth learn from developmentally-appropriate play and exploration, and parents and caregivers may increase their own understanding of their children's experiences by participating in these common child life interventions with them. But what if there are ways to elevate experiential learning further? What if developmental theory and learning theory can be combined to optimize the experiential learning opportunities offered to learners across the lifespan? Simulation-based education offers such innovations.

Simulation is "a technique - not a technology - to replace or amplify real experiences with guided experiences that evoke or replicate substantial aspects of the real world in a fully interactive manner" (Gaba, 2004, p. i2). It is widely used for educating healthcare professionals, and increasingly, for educating children, youth, and families. Child life specialists already possess many of the competencies of an

DOI: 10.4018/978-1-6684-5097-0.ch002

effective simulation educator and facilitator, including the commitment to reflective practice, ability to assess a learner's needs and design developmentally appropriate interventions in response, proficiency with learner-centered communication skills, and ability to build trust and rapport while supporting healthy responses to stressful events (Association of Child Life Professionals, 2019). This overlap introduces invaluable opportunities for child life specialists to incorporate simulation into their practice (either in healthcare or elsewhere) and contribute to the growth of simulation education and science.

This chapter will:

- Examine child life involvement in simulation-based education and opportunities for future growth
- Introduce foundational elements of simulation, including learning theories, scenario development, simulation environments and modalities, psychological safety, and debriefing
- Connect simulation methodology and the Child Life Competencies, identifying areas of overlap
- Evaluate the value that child life specialists bring to simulation-based education, as well as the value that simulation brings to child life practice

BACKGROUND

Simulation is distinct from other forms of education and preparation due to its focus on experiential learning coupled with *debriefing* (guided reflection that supports integrating learning into action) in environments constructed to establish and maintain *psychological safety* (the sense that the environment is favorable to interpersonal risk-taking) (Edmondson, 1999; Rudolph et al., 2014; Sawyer et al., 2016). Facilitators coordinate the simulation scenario and lead the debrief. The facilitators may also lead a *prebrief* before a simulation to orient the learners and help them know what to expect.

Simulation-based education can be adapted to a wide variety of environments and learner needs. This flexibility makes simulation a valuable learning tool for children, youth, and adults alike. Incorporating simulation into child life practice is a progression of the profession's commitment to "identify teaching techniques for use with individuals of diverse developmental levels and learning needs" (Association of Child Life Professionals, 2019, p. 4). By offering opportunities to learn through simulation, child life specialists can meet a greater range of needs within the populations they serve.

Furthermore, child life specialists must "identify adult learning needs" (Association of Child Life Professionals, 2019, p. 6) and offer safe, responsive, and effective educational opportunities for child life learners, including child life students and interns. Simulation is an essential modality to use with child life learners. When used with learners from medical and nursing professions, simulation-based education can improve the learners' competence and confidence, as well as diagnostic and treatment processes (Auerbach et al., 2016; Lateef, 2010; Moslehi et al., 2022; Theilen et al., 2017). Such improvements help optimize patients' physical safety. Child life specialists advocate for the emotional safety of children and families to be valued and addressed alongside physical safety (Association of Child Life Professionals, 2019; Gordon, 2021). Therefore, it is ethical for child life specialists to use simulation when teaching child life learners to navigate encounters in which children and families are emotionally vulnerable. This use of simulation-based education protects children and families while upholding child life specialists' accountability for the training and supervision of others (Association of Child Life Professionals, 2020).

Child life specialists are obligated to teach not only child life learners, but to educate learners from other professions by sharing knowledge of the psychosocial needs of children, youth, and families (Association of Child Life Professionals, 2019). Simulation is an effective method for interprofessional education, and the Child Life Competencies urge child life specialists to learn and use effective educational methods. Child life specialists must "describe and integrate the basic concepts of…teaching methods appropriate to subject matter and audience" and "demonstrate effective advocacy for child life practice and psychosocial issues" (Association of Child Life Professionals, 2019, p. 6).

While simulation can be incorporated into any child life specialist's role, child life specialists can also work effectively in simulation-specific roles within simulation programs and centers. Simulation centers staffed by interprofessional and interdisciplinary teams of coordinators, technicians, researchers, and educators develop and facilitate simulations for healthcare settings, universities, and community partners. These centers are built with spaces that can replicate different environments, often with one-way mirrors for facilitators to observe simulations (as shown in Figure 1) (Lateef, 2010). Simulation centers are frequently affiliated with hospitals, and these affiliations can allow patients, families, and healthcare professionals to access simulation-based education.

Simulation programs are located around the world; the directory of the Society for Simulation in Healthcare (SSH) lists more than 800 simulation centers internationally (SSH, n.d.a). Professionals working in simulation connect and collaborate through organizations such as SSH, International Pediatric Simulation Society (IPSS), and International Network for Simulation-based Pediatric Innovation, Research & Education (INSPIRE), which foster shared knowledge and multi-center research (Cheng et al., 2018; Ramachandra et al., 2020). Additional organizations, such as Pediatric Simulation Training and Research Society (PediSTARS) in India and Netzwerk Kindersimulation in German-speaking countries, advance simulation practice within their regions and share findings with the global simulation community (Ramachandra et al., 2020; Shetty & Nadkarni, 2016; Wagner et al., 2021).

This chapter explores the integration of child life and simulation-based education for different populations of learners: children and youth, parents and caregivers, child life students and professionals, and interprofessional teams. Child life specialists who facilitate simulations for any of these populations should develop their knowledge of foundational concepts in simulation, including learning theories, scenario design, simulation environments and modalities, debriefing frameworks and approaches, and strategies for establishing psychological safety. This chapter provides a brief introductory overview of these foundational topics, as well as ways that child life specialists can contribute to global priorities for the advancement of simulation education and science.

SIMULATION FOR CHILDREN AND YOUTH

Simulation-based education can help children and youth prepare for healthcare encounters, including medical procedures. The inclusion of realistic experiences and opportunities for active participation and rehearsal may make simulation-based preparations more effective than commonly used pediatric preparation modalities, such as photo books, videos, or hospital tours (Potthoff et al., 2021). Simulation can give pediatric patients direct experience with some of the sensory input they will encounter during a procedure (for example, the sights and sounds of MRI or the smell and feel of EEG leads on the scalp) while allowing them to simultaneously rehearse (and then through debriefing, refine) a coping plan. By adjusting the simulation environment, materials, pace, and debriefing approach, these simulations can meet the needs of children and youth with a range of developmental abilities (Woodward et al., 2018).

Simulation-based education can also support children and youth in gaining developmentally appropriate autonomy in managing their health at home, at school, and elsewhere in the community. For example, simulation can help children and adolescents with chronic conditions respond to urgent personal medical needs, such as an anaphylactic reaction or a dangerously high or low reading on a glucose monitor (Diaz et al., 2016). Simulation allows the young learner to practice identifying an urgent need, using psychomotor skills to address the need (such as injecting epinephrine in response to anaphylaxis), and navigating the social situation to get help (directing an adult or peer to assist as needed).

Children and adolescents who have a sibling, parent, or caregiver with a potentially serious health condition may benefit from simulation to practice responding if their loved one experiences a medical emergency. As with other forms of preparation, simulation can enhance the child's sense of autonomy and control while increasing their understanding (and addressing any misconceptions) in developmentally appropriate ways. Facilitators can use debriefing to support young learners in both processing their emotions and synthesizing their learning. This application of simulation can promote resilience in both the child and the family.

The benefits of simulation-based education for children and youth extend to contexts outside healthcare. For instance, consider how active shooter drills in elementary, middle, and high schools could be reimagined utilizing simulation methodology. A simulation could be facilitated in the classroom to support the young learners in meeting objectives targeting both physical safety and coping needs. Before the simulation, prebriefing could help establish psychological safety by offering developmentally appropriate information about what to expect. Debriefing after the simulation could allow opportunities for emotional expression, discussion of the experience, and identification of learning points to apply to future scenarios. This approach is trauma-informed and can be adjusted to the developmental and psychosocial needs of different learners. Child life specialists working in schools, or in simulation centers collaborating with schools, could take a lead role in designing and facilitating such a simulation.

Child life specialists have contributed to the development and implementation of simulations for preparation before proton radiation therapy, spinal fusion surgery, MRI, and EEG. These simulation-based preparations may include in person experiences (for example, visiting a mock operating room or MRI scanner), distance simulations (in which the patient visits the mock operating room or MRI scanner via video chat platform), and/or screen-based simulations such as explorations of procedure spaces or simulation of the procedure itself using virtual reality (Galvez et al., 2019; Mednick et al., 2021; Potthoff et al., 2021; Stunden et al., 2021; Woodward et al., 2018). When designing and facilitating these simulations, child life specialists apply their assessment skills to:

- Identify children and youth who can benefit from simulation-based education
- Collaborate with children, youth, families, and professionals to understand the learning needs of identified individuals and/or groups of learners
- Continuously monitor the responses of children and youth during the simulation and the debrief, adjusting or pausing the experience in real-time as needed

Additionally, child life specialists use their intervention skills to:

- Involve children and youth in identifying their own learning needs and goals

- Apply knowledge of child development to design simulations that suit the cognitive, emotional, and physical needs and abilities of individuals and/or groups of young learners, including those with disabilities
- Incorporate identification and rehearsal of potential coping strategies into the simulation
- Prebrief and debrief learners
- Ensure the use of developmentally appropriate language and pacing when facilitating the prebrief, simulation, and debrief

SIMULATION FOR PARENTS AND CAREGIVERS

Caring for a child with complex medical needs at home, school, and in the community can be daunting for parents and caregivers. Simulation can help parents and caregivers develop the technical, cognitive, and behavioral skills to care for their child's medical needs and respond to emergencies that may occur outside the healthcare setting. Simulations for parents and caregivers should be designed and facilitated by collaborative teams with collective expertise in medical management, simulation and debriefing, and patient- and family-centered care (Diaz et al., 2016). Child life specialists contribute proficiency with the latter and can develop their skill sets to include additional knowledge of simulation and debriefing. Child life specialists are also skilled at interprofessional collaboration (Association of Child Life Professionals, 2019); just as child life specialists work with physicians, nurses, and respiratory therapists on patient care, they work with these professionals to co-design, co-facilitate, and co-debrief simulations for parents and caregivers. The medical professional teaches the technical and procedural skills that parents and caregivers need, while the child life professional brings expertise in the psychosocial dynamics inherent to providing such care.

Child life specialists have collaborated on simulations for parents and caregivers of children with a range of medical needs, such as tracheostomies, ventricular assist devices, and home parenteral nutrition (Amar-Dolan et al., 2020; Mednick et al., 2021; Raphael et al., 2021). As described by Diaz et al. (2016), essential elements of such simulations include the identification of relevant learning objectives (developed collaboratively between simulation facilitators and parent/caregiver learners), appropriate choice of simulation modalities and materials, prebriefing before the simulation to enhance psychological safety and clarify what to expect, and debriefing after the simulation to help parent/caregiver learners process their emotions while reflecting and learning from the experience. Each of those elements should be responsive to the family's unique needs, including the parent's/caregiver's schedule, learning style, stress level, and emotional needs (Diaz et al., 2016). Child life specialists provide vital input to the development of simulation curricula that incorporates each of these elements (Mednick et al., 2021).

When contributing to simulations for parents and caregivers, child life specialists use their assessment skills to:

- Identify parents and caregivers who can benefit from simulation-based education
- Understand the family's strengths, challenges, stress adaptations, and preferred coping techniques, and adapt simulations for each family accordingly
- Identify families who may benefit from additional resources within or outside the simulation curriculum, such as peer support

Child life specialists use their intervention skills to:

- Apply knowledge of family systems theories when co-designing and co-facilitating simulations
- Incorporate familiar environmental elements (for example, arrange a space in the simulation center to approximate a room in the family's home or at the child's school)
- Co-debrief parent and caregiver learners following the simulation

SIMULATION FOR CHILD LIFE STUDENTS AND PROFESSIONALS

Simulation can provide professional development for child life learners at all stages of experience and training: student, intern, newly certified professional, and seasoned professional. Simulation-based education can help students and interns master foundational skills (such as introducing child life services in different contexts or discussing developmentally appropriate responses to hospitalization with parents and caregivers) and allow professionals to develop and maintain advanced, potentially specialized skills (such as preparations for patients participating in new clinical trials). Child life learners at all stages may use simulation to practice skills that can feel challenging, including discussions of new diagnoses or end-of-life issues with families, or working with patients and families who are upset or angry (Crnjak et al., 2021; Rudder et al., 2019; Woodward & Patterson, 2020).

Simulations for child life learners may be conducted with individuals, pairs, or groups. In pairs or groups, the learners can work through the scenario together or by using a "fishbowl" style in which they take turns engaging in the scenario and watching other learners engage (Rudder et al., 2019; Vora et al., 2021). Alternately, child life learners may participate in simulations alongside learners from other psychosocial professions (such as social workers and chaplains) and/or alongside physician and nurse learners. This structure allows the child life learner to provide psychosocial support in tandem with another professional while being mindful of each profession's scope of practice and areas of expertise. As a result, the child life learner can both improve their skills and increase their knowledge of the other professional's role (Rudder et al., 2019; Patterson, 2020).

SIMULATION FOR INTERPROFESSIONAL TEAMS

Interprofessional simulations for healthcare teams allow groups of learners to work on medical management (including cognitive and technical skills), communication (with colleagues and with the patient and family), and teamwork skills (such as role delineation and mutual support). These simulations have been identified as an important educational approach for supporting improvements in the emotional safety of patients and families (Gordon, 2021). Simultaneously, the value that child life specialists bring to medical education is increasingly recognized (Pillai, 2020). By facilitating simulation-based education for interprofessional healthcare teams, child life specialists can drive advances in the provision of emotionally safe care by all members of the team.

A "blended" model of simulation for interprofessional teams, which includes medical, interprofessional teamwork, and patient-centered learning objectives in the same scenario, can increase learner engagement. For example, a simulation in which an adolescent with end-stage metastatic cancer presents to the emergency department with pain and respiratory distress may include the following objectives:

- **Medical:** Manage patient's pain and respiratory distress per palliative care opioid escalation guidelines
- **Interprofessional teamwork:** Mobilize palliative care and psychosocial teams within the first five minutes, utilizing frequent case summaries to promote a shared mental model
- **Patient-centered:** Ascertain and acknowledge patient's and family's goals of care, utilizing closed-loop communication, eye contact, and adjustments in tone and volume of voice (Woodward et al., 2017)

When requiring learners to consider the psychosocial and emotional needs of patients and families alongside their medical needs, simulation activates the affective learning domain and may improve the retention of content knowledge (Demaria et al., 2010; Woodward et al., 2017). Importantly, the blended model frames attention to the patient's and family's psychosocial and emotional needs as a vital aspect (rather than an extraneous aspect) of the overall care provided. As a result, the model promotes emotional safety and allows all interprofessional learners to improve their skills in this area (Woodward et al., 2017; Woodward & Ching, 2020).

Further, the blended model creates opportunities for child life learners (and learners from other psychosocial disciplines) to participate in interprofessional simulations alongside physicians, nurses, and additional medical team members. This engagement allows child life specialists and other psychosocial professionals to improve both their patient care and teamwork skills (Woodward & Ching, 2020; Woodward et al., 2017; Woodward et al., 2018). The latter skill set is particularly essential for child life specialists working in fast-paced, team-based care situations, such as resuscitations and traumas (Woodward & Ching, 2020).

The blended model translates effectively to mass casualty incident and disaster simulations, as the psychosocial and emotional needs of children and families are vital to address during such events (Cicero & Weiner, 2016; Woodward & Ching, 2020). For instance, learners from an emergency department team may engage in a simulation of an influx of patients and families following a mass shooting at a shopping mall. During the simulation, the learners must collaborate to address the medical, psychosocial, and emotional needs of the patients and families while applying best practices in mass casualty triage and allocation of resources. Emergency and disaster management agencies may also simulate mass casualty events in which pediatric patients arrive unaccompanied, such as a school bus crash or bombing. The learners can practice meeting the children's needs while also facilitating victim identification and family reunification processes.

Child life specialists can lead the integration of simulation-based education in training for professionals outside healthcare. Teachers, school administrators, camp counselors, daycare providers, police officers, foster care and adoption workers, behavioral support personnel, and personal care attendants for individuals with disabilities are some of the myriad professionals who can benefit from simulation to help them navigate challenging situations with children, youth, and families in safe, supportive, and developmentally appropriate ways. For example, simulation can be used to help police officers practice responding to an adolescent with autism who is experiencing a mental health crisis or to help teachers practice talking with students about the serious illness or death of a classmate. Child life specialists can both advocate for these professionals to have access to simulation-based education and contribute to the design and facilitation of such simulations.

FOUNDATIONS OF SIMULATION

Learning Theories

Simulation is rooted in learning theories that support the value of experiential, reflective opportunities. For example, Bloom's revised taxonomy names six levels of a cognitive learning hierarchy. From lowest to highest, the levels are:

- Remember
- Understand
- Apply
- Analyze
- Evaluate
- Create (Adams, 2015; Orgill & Nolan, 2021)

The higher levels of the hierarchy represent "deeper learning and transfer of knowledge and skills to a greater variety of tasks and contexts" (Adams, 2015, p. 152). Simulation is conducive to the application of knowledge, and simulation curricula may be designed to support learners in analyzing, evaluating, and creating. Debriefing the simulation provides further opportunity for engagement within the higher levels of the hierarchy.

For example, consider a simulation in which child life learners practice using a new assessment tool with a patient and family. During the simulation, the learners will apply their knowledge of the tool and evaluate its use, making adjustments in real-time as they interact with the simulated patient and family. Then, during the debrief, the learners can discuss those adjustments and engage in further evaluation, determining if they will make additional changes when using the tool in the future.

In addition to the cognitive domain, Bloom's taxonomy names two other learning domains: affective (emotional) & psychomotor. Simulations can be designed to support learners in engaging all three domains. For this reason, simulation is particularly important when teaching healthcare-related knowledge and skills, as healthcare encounters often require patients, families, and professionals to engage each domain (Adams, 2015; Orgill & Nolan, 2021).

Furthermore, Kolb's experiential learning cycle names four stages: concrete experience, reflective observation, abstract conceptualization, and active experimentation (Kolb & Kolb, 2009). Simulation-based education supports learners in moving through these stages. The simulation scenario provides an opportunity for active experimentation, and debriefing creates space for reflective observation. The combination of simulation and debriefing then allows learners to move toward abstract conceptualization of learning points (Sawyer et al., 2016).

Scenario Design

Simulation scenarios are designed by facilitators in advance, with instructions and guidance about how the simulation will unfold. To engage the learners during the simulation, facilitators must consider what action(s) will be taken, by who, and when. Each of these actions should serve the purpose of the simulation; what knowledge and skills should the learners apply, analyze, and/or evaluate during the simulation, and how can the design of the scenario support them in doing so?

The design of a simulation scenario begins with thoughtful selection and construction of learning objectives. Facilitators may identify goals (what they hope the learners will learn) from which they develop objectives (what the learners should be able to do after engaging in the simulation) (Harrington & Simon, 2021). Objectives can be created not only with the facilitators' goals and perceptions in mind but with learners' input on their own goals (Diaz et al., 2016).

Facilitators should verify that all simulation objectives are SMART: Specific, Measurable, Attainable, Relevant & Timely (Harrington & Simon, 2021). The use of SMART format helps ensure that the chosen objectives can feasibly be achieved by the intended learners during the simulation. When finalizing each objective, facilitators should check that there is clarity about what the objectives are and how it will be determined if the learners meet the objectives.

Learners engage in simulation by activating all three of the learning domains listed in Bloom's revised taxonomy: cognitive, affective, and psychomotor. As a result, objectives can (and should) encompass all applicable domains. Consider a simulation designed to help child life student learners practice preparing a pediatric patient for IV placement. Objectives may include:

- **Cognitive:** Describe steps of IV placement using correct sequence and developmentally appropriate language
- **Affective:** Validate patient's stated feelings and facilitate discussion of potential coping techniques
- **Psychomotor:** Use medical materials and a cloth doll to demonstrate IV placement for the patient

After the objectives are determined, facilitators construct the simulation scenario so that the learners can meet the objectives. The details and progression of the scenario should heighten learners' attention, interest, and arousal, without creating significant anxiety. As the Yerkes-Dodson Law illustrates, learner performance peaks when this state of optimal arousal is achieved (Yerkes & Dodson, 1908). Facilitators may consider Vygotsky's zone of proximal development; how must the simulation be structured so that learners engage in the space between what they can do independently and what they can do only with support (Rudolph et al., 2014)? Simulations should challenge learners, but not trick them or place them in scenarios far beyond their level of knowledge and skill.

The planned details of scenario progression may include timing cues (indicating how long the scenario will be and which elements will be introduced when), instructions and scripts for *standardized patients* (individuals who are trained to portray patients in the simulation) and *embedded participants* (individuals who are trained to play roles other than patients), and/or guidance for use of technology (Boyer & Mitchell, 2021). For example, if a high-fidelity manikin is used, when will the technician make the manikin speak, cry, moan, or show changes in vital signs? The use of if/then statements may be helpful: IF the learners take a particular action, THEN what should the standardized patient (or embedded participants, technicians, etc.) do?

Facilitators should consider how their inevitable assumptions and implicit biases may impact scenario construction. For example, if a standardized patient or embedded participant is portraying an identity that differs from that of the facilitator, are their scripted actions authentic to that identity rather than rooted in stereotypes? Assembling a facilitator team in which a range of personal and professional identities are represented can help mitigate biases, as can working with youth and family partners and community experts. When working with a diverse team, facilitators should be mindful of the potential emotional tax on collaborators and remember that one individual cannot speak for an entire group (Sagalowsky et al., 2020; Sagalowsky et al., 2021a; Vora et al., 2021).

Designing Pediatric Patient- and Family-Focused Simulations for Professionals

When designing simulations for professionals who work with youth and families, scenarios can be co-created with youth and family partners to develop pediatric patient-focused and family-focused simulations (Sagalowsky et al., 2020). This co-creation helps ensure that objectives and scenario details align with the authentic experiences and wishes of youth and families, as opposed to facilitators' perceptions of their experiences and wishes (Nestel & Kneebone, 2010; Sagalowsky et al., 2020). Because child life specialists "demonstrate the ability to partner with patients and families and share their unique perspectives in educating others on…psychosocial issues" (Association of Child Life Professionals, 2019, p. 6), they are excellent partners in the creation of pediatric patient- and family-focused simulations.

For example, when creating a pediatric patient- and family-focused simulation in which a medical student learner interacts with an adolescent standardized patient, communication objective(s) can be co-created with adolescents who have had prior real-life experiences as patients. A child life specialist can facilitate focus groups in which the adolescent advisors discuss the scenario and share which communication approaches and strategies they most want their providers to use. The child life specialist can then adapt the adolescent advisors' feedback into patient-centered communication objectives for the medical student learners.

There are innumerable potential objectives for this type of pediatric patient- and family-focused simulation. Some possibilities include that the medical student learners will:

- Offer opportunities for the adolescent to ask and answer questions (rather than just the parent/caregiver)
- Narrate the physical examination
- Explain the diagnosis to the adolescent patient using developmentally appropriate language
- Maintain the patient's privacy throughout the encounter, including the use of draping during the physical examination (Sagalowsky et al., 2020)

After the objectives are chosen, patient and family advisors may contribute to the development of scenario details and progression. Patients and families can coach standardized patients and/or embedded participants before the simulation to ensure that portrayals are as authentic as possible. They can also give feedback on the simulation environment, offering suggestions to improve the *fidelity* (or realism) of the simulation (Sagalowsky et al., 2020).

Simulation Environments and Modalities

Simulation facilitators select the environment for their scenario based on objectives, learner needs, and available resources. Simulations conducted in person may be facilitated in a simulation center (or other designated learning space) or *in situ* (in the actual environment in which the learners are most likely to use the skills, rather than in a replicated environment). For example, an in situ simulation for healthcare professionals would occur in their typical patient care area (exam room, trauma bay, operating room, etc.), while an in situ simulation for parents and caregivers could occur in their home, in their child's school, or in another community setting which their family frequents. Conducting the simulation in situ can improve the physical and functional fidelity, allowing learners to more easily suspend disbelief and identify the relevance of the scenario (Maa et al., 2016).

Facilitators may choose for learners to interact with humans (standardized patients and/or embedded participants) during the simulation, with other materials or technologies, or with a combination of modalities. Scenario objectives guide this choice. For instance, if the learning objectives target communication skills, the use of embedded participants and/or standardized patients may be important. If the objectives target psychomotor skills, facilitators may use manikins or other materials to allow learners to practice those skills.

In some cases, screen-based simulation may be facilitators' and learners' preferred modality. Screen-based simulation can replicate a range of environments while increasing the accessibility of simulation, since learners may participate from any location in which the applicable screen-based technology (computer, tablet, smartphone, or virtual reality headset) can be used. Screen-based simulation also allows a high volume of learners to participate over a long period since a screen-based program can be replicated across multiple devices and embedded participants, standardized patients, and other materials do not need to be available. However, the development of a screen-based simulation requires support from technology professionals, and the creation of a screen-based simulation may initially be expensive and time-consuming. Screen-based simulations may also lack the psychomotor input needed to fully conceptualize some learning points (Chang et al., 2016).

Tabletop simulation is useful for situations that are environmentally expansive and/or systemically complex. This simulation modality may be particularly helpful when the learning objectives target skills related to the management of mass casualty incidents and disasters (Cicero & Weiner, 2016). For example, tabletop simulation can help child life learners practice allocating resources for psychosocial support as a mass casualty incident progresses. Child life learners navigate the tabletop simulation similarly to a board game, manipulating cards that represent different needs and available resources during the mass casualty incident (Woodward & Ching, 2020).

Simulations may be conducted with all participants (learners, facilitators, technicians, standardized patients, and/or embedded participants) in the same physical location, or the scenario may be designed and conducted as a *distance simulation* with participants in different locations. Various technologies, including video chat platforms and remote controls, can support learners' participation in distance simulation (Society for Simulation in Healthcare, n.d.b). The use of distance simulation can help increase accessibility and inclusivity of simulation-based education.

Psychological Safety

All simulation participants must feel safe to take risks and secure that their input will be heard and respected. This sense of psychological safety is essential in all aspects of simulation and debriefing. When learners feel psychologically safe, they are more willing to reflect, make mistakes, and challenge themselves (Rudolph et al., 2014).

Child life specialists may already be familiar with emotional safety, or the "intentional, interdisciplinary practice to promote resiliency, healing, and trust for pediatric patients and their families during medical experiences" (Gordon, 2021, p. 5). Although psychological safety is a distinct and separate concept, child life specialists can apply some of the skills they use to foster emotional safety for children and families to the creation of psychologically safe environments for simulation. Assessment of the needs of each learner (and/or group of learners) and adaptation to those needs is necessary to establish and maintain psychological safety in simulation, as it is to establish and maintain emotional safety.

Simulation facilitators must consider: what actions should be taken to create and maintain psychological safety for simulation participants with varying personal identities (considering culture, race, religion, gender identity, sexual orientation, disability, etc.)? How might implicit power dynamics threaten psychological safety? For example, do real or perceived hierarchies negatively impact psychological safety when working with interprofessional groups (i.e. a healthcare team of physicians, nurses, and child life specialists), groups whose members have different amounts of experience (i.e. interns and trainees learning alongside experienced colleagues), and/or youth and family learners participating in simulations facilitated by professionals?

Establishing group norms and expectations before a simulation can help establish psychological safety. Common norms in simulation include maintaining confidentiality and utilizing the basic assumption that all participants are capable, smart, and want to improve. The establishment of a "fiction contract" can also be helpful; facilitators commit to making the scenario as realistic as possible (with acknowledgment of limitations) and invite learners to maximize the experience by engaging as if the scenario is real. Ideally, participants can decide collectively before the simulation if they wish to establish any other group norms (Rudolph et al., 2014).

Prebriefing before the simulation can help foster psychological safety by clarifying expectations and creating an initial opportunity for learners to ask questions. The length and scope of the prebrief can be adjusted as needed, depending on the learners' needs and the scenario. During the prebrief, facilitators may wish to initiate a discussion of:

- Goals and/or objectives of the simulation
- Group norms
- Roles and expectations of the facilitators and learners
- Logistical expectations
    - Length of the scenario and the debrief
    - Management of other competing duties (for example, will participants' phones be turned off during the simulation and debrief, or do learners and/or facilitators have any other responsibilities for which they need to leave their phones on?)
    - Orientation to modalities used in the scenario (manikins, screen-based technology, etc.)
    - Considerations for working with embedded participants and/or standardized patients, if applicable (Rudolph et al., 2014)

Further, trauma-informed practice and structural and cultural humility can support facilitators in maintaining psychological safety. In the prebrief, for example, facilitators may acknowledge the potential for their inevitable oversights and biases to impact the simulation and invite learners to share feedback to help the facilitators improve. Learners may also be given the option to step out of the simulation and/or debrief if needed (Sagalowsky et al., 2021a).

Debriefing

Debriefing is an essential element of all simulations, as it allows learners to analyze, synthesize, and evaluate their experience, with the goal to improve their performance (Rudolph et al., 2006; Sawyer et al., 2016). The saying "Simulation is just an excuse to debrief" is common within simulation-based education and highlights the necessity of debriefing in the learning process (Sawyer et al., 2016). Debriefing aligns effectively with the child life profession's commitment to reflective practice (Association of Child Life Professionals, 2019). Child life specialists may find overlap between debriefing frameworks and approaches and other forms of reflective practice, such as approaches to clinical supervision.

As with other forms of reflective practice, debriefing incorporates the theory that each individual's actions are driven by unique internal *frames* (sometimes referred to as mental models or frames of reference), which may include "knowledge, assumptions, and feelings" (Rudolph et al., 2006, p. 49). Although the resultant actions are seen in the simulation, the frames are unknown until explored further in the debrief. Facilitators should approach the debrief with curiosity to uncover the learners' frames, as opposed to prior judgment about what those frames are. By asking questions, facilitators can support learners in understanding their frames and how those frames impact their actions. Facilitators can then guide learners to begin developing new frames that may help them consider different actions in the future (Rudolph et al., 2006).

Debriefing commonly occurs after a simulation. However, debriefing may also occur during a simulation, with the scenario paused for debriefing, then restarted. This format allows learners to quickly apply the lessons learned from debriefing, rather than waiting until the next simulation or other opportunities (Sawyer et al., 2016).

Debriefing can be tricky to facilitate while also maintaining psychological safety. Learners may feel vulnerable speaking in a group and/or when discussing aspects of the simulation that they found challenging. Facilitators may wish to share input and critiques to help learners improve but might worry about seeming overly critical or confrontational (Rudolph et al., 2006).

To begin addressing these potential difficulties, facilitators must understand the distinction between debriefing and feedback. Feedback is a one-way conversation (from facilitator to learner) and is facilitator-driven, while debriefing is a two-way conversation between facilitator(s) and learner(s) and is guided by the reflections of the learners (Rudolph et al., 2008; Sawyer et al., 2016). The use of established debriefing frameworks and approaches can support facilitators in sharing critiques and input within a two-way debriefing conversation.

Frameworks organize the process of debriefing for facilitators and learners, providing predictability to both groups. Many debriefing frameworks exist, and facilitators may wish to consider a range of options to find the best fit. A common framework in healthcare simulation is the three-phase model of *reaction*, *analysis*, and *summary* (Sawyer et al., 2016). This framework may be particularly effective when incorporating simulation into child life practice, as it can be used with a wide range of learners (professionals, parents and caregivers, and children and youth), and it is applicable when debriefing both healthcare and non-healthcare scenarios.

Reaction

During the reaction phase, learners are invited to share their initial emotional responses to the simulation. This strategy allows learners to express and/or begin processing any strong feelings before reflecting further on the simulation (Sawyer et al., 2016). Understanding these reactions can help the facilitators calibrate the remainder of the session in response to the learners' feelings and needs. While facilitators structure the subsequent analysis phase to explore the scenario objectives, they should also incorporate some of the topics shared by the learners (Rudolph et al., 2008). When working with children and families in other contexts, child life specialists adjust their approach in real-time based on verbal and non-verbal cues. When debriefing, facilitators should do the same by applying information gleaned from the learners' reactions.

Before shifting to the analysis phase, salient facts of the simulation scenario are clarified (Sawyer et al., 2016). The facilitator(s) may invite a learner to offer this review of key points by briefly summarizing the scenario. Reviewing the relevant facts helps ensure that all learners and facilitators have a shared understanding of the scenario prior to analysis.

Analysis

In the analysis phase, facilitators and learners reflect together on what happened during the simulation. A range of debriefing approaches can be used during this phase. For example, facilitators may choose the *learner self-assessment* approach, in which the plus/delta method is commonly used. Learners are asked to explore what they feel went well (plus) and what actions they want to change in the future (delta) (Sawyer et al., 2016). The plus/delta method supports learners in codifying positive actions to repeat, while also self-identifying areas for improvement. The learner-centered simplicity of plus/delta may make it the preferred debriefing approach for use with children, youth, and families (Mednick et al., 2021). However, a disadvantage of this approach is that it may not uncover learners' frames, thus missing the opportunity for facilitators to help learners understand their frames and create new ones to apply to subsequent scenarios. Furthermore, facilitators may find it challenging to hone in on scenario objectives when using the learner self-assessment approach (Sawyer et al., 2016).

Debriefing with good judgment is another approach that may be used during the analysis phase, instead of or in addition to learner self-assessment. This approach posits that both facilitators' and learners' frames can be valid, and all participants benefit if facilitators are forthcoming about their frames. When learners understand the frame from which a facilitator is guiding a particular discussion point, they can engage in the debrief with less worry about the facilitators' underlying motives or potential assumptions of superiority. As a result, debriefing with good judgment helps flatten hierarchies and foster a psychologically safe environment in which learners can explore their frames (Rudolph et al., 2006).

The direct sharing of facilitators' frames and the goal of exploration rather than imparting information contrasts with other common educational methods. For example, debriefing with good judgment avoids the leading questions frequently employed by the Socratic method. Instead of maintaining an underlying goal of guiding learners to recognize an idea or theme (a motive that may be detected by learners and lead to misunderstandings and/or defensiveness), facilitators pose questions with genuine curiosity and transparency about their purpose. Debriefing with good judgment also avoids the "feedback sandwich" in which a compliment is offered, followed by a critique, and then another compliment. While a "feedback sandwich" may be considered a gentle approach, it can also lack clarity, cause confusion, and convey an unspoken message that areas for improvement should be hidden rather than embraced and discussed (Rudolph et al., 2006).

To share transparent input and the desire to explore learners' frames, facilitators use the speaking style of advocacy-inquiry when debriefing with good judgment. Advocacy-inquiry combines a statement of the facilitator's perspective (advocacy) with a question (inquiry) (Rudolph et al., 2006). The O^3 mnemonic can help facilitators use this speaking style by sharing an Observation, followed by an Opinion, and then an Open-ended question (Sagalowsky et al., 2021b). The words chosen can be adapted to the developmental level of the learner(s).

For example, when debriefing a school-aged child who participated in simulation for preparation before MRI:

- **Observation:** I saw that you were taking deep breaths while laying still during the "practice MRI."
- **Opinion:** I think deep breathing can be a great way to help your body feel calmer and able to stay still.
- **Open-ended question:** What was it like for you to try that deep breathing during the practice MRI?

Or when debriefing a group of adolescent and young adult camp staff preparing to work with children with diabetes:

- **Observation:** After the group identified that the reading on the glucose monitor was very low, I noticed it took several minutes to locate the apple juice.
- **Opinion:** I was concerned that the child's condition could worsen during this time.
- **Open-ended question:** Talk me through the process of locating the apple juice - how did you experience it?

For the advocacy-inquiry speaking style to be effective, facilitators must possess genuine curiosity about the learners' frames. In individual instances in which the facilitator finds that this curiosity is absent, they may consider offering input as *direct feedback.* Facilitators should think about whether, how, and when to use direct feedback based on previously established group norms, learner responses within the debrief, and the need to maintain a psychologically safe environment. Depending on scenario objectives and learner needs, direct feedback may have a role in some simulation-based education (Sawyer et al., 2016).

Experienced facilitators often blend approaches within the analysis phase of debriefing. The PEARLS debriefing script supports both novice and experienced debriefers in selecting and incorporating multiple approaches: learner self-assessment, focused facilitation around specific objectives or other identified issues (using advocacy-inquiry and/or other techniques), and providing information or direct feedback (Bajaj et al., 2018; Eppich & Cheng, 2015). As with other forms of reflective practice, facilitators improve their ease and confidence with the various debriefing approaches (and their ability to toggle between approaches as dictated by learner needs, scenario objectives, and time constraints) through experience and coaching.

Summary

After all scenario objectives (as well as other pressing issues identified by learners) have been addressed, facilitators shift from the analysis phase to the summary phase of debriefing (Eppich & Cheng, 2015). During the summary phase, key learning points are distilled. The summary supports learners in their continued movement through Kolb's cycle by helping them conceptualize lessons learned. Learners can then apply these lessons to their next experience (Rudolph et al., 2008).

Ideally, learners can be invited to drive the summary by each offering a lesson that they will take away and apply to future scenarios. This approach gives learners an additional opportunity to process information for future use while allowing facilitators to informally assess how and if the objectives have been met. Alternately, facilitators can lead the summary by offering a recap of the scenario and/or their perception of the key takeaways. This facilitator-driven approach may be less engaging and meaningful for learners but can be useful when managing time constraints (Eppich & Cheng, 2015).

Additional Debriefing Considerations

Throughout all phases of debriefing, facilitators should monitor for threats to psychological safety and actively mitigate these threats if/when they arise. When working with interprofessional groups of learners, facilitators should pay close attention to rapport management: are all professional identities valued, heard, and respected during the debrief (Auerbach et al., 2018; Loo et al., 2018)? Considering personal identities is vital, too; facilitators must identify and disrupt any microaggressions within the debrief (Sagalowsky et al., 2021a; Vora et al., 2021). Facilitators may find that the aforementioned debriefing approaches (advocacy/inquiry or direct feedback, depending on the circumstances) are useful for addressing microaggressions (Sagalowsky et al., 2021b).

THE FUTURE OF CHILD LIFE IN SIMULATION

Pediatric simulation educators, researchers, technicians, and enthusiasts worldwide are connected via organizations such as IPSS and INSPIRE. Members of these organizations have identified the potential for further innovation in the use of simulation-based education for children, youth, and families as well as the need for research on the impact of both interprofessional simulation and simulation with pediatric patients and their families (Arnold et al., 2018; Grant et al., 2016; Mednick et al., 2021; Palaganas et al., 2016). Child life specialists can help expand the use of simulation in these contexts and apply their research skills to contribute meaningfully to simulation science and the pediatric simulation community.

INSPIRE offers support to both emerging and experienced simulation researchers, including educational opportunities, mentorship, and grant funding. Additionally, both INSPIRE and IPSS include child life specialists in leadership roles within the organizations (International Network for Simulation-based Pediatric Innovation, Research & Education, n.d.; International Pediatric Simulation Society, 2021). This climate of support and inclusivity provides excellent pathways for child life specialists to become involved in simulation and influence the way simulation is used with children, families, and professionals around the world.

The possibilities for further integration of child life and simulation are boundless. Child life specialists can work with simulation centers and programs to create developmentally appropriate, accessible opportunities for children, youth, and families to learn through simulation in healthcare and community settings. The child life profession can create an educational culture in which all child life specialists learn through simulation (both when working toward their initial certification and as part of their continuing professional development) to improve the emotional safety of the populations they serve. As child life specialists envision a future in which emotional safety is assessed, taught, and valued alongside physical safety, they can take a leadership role in incorporating patient-centered psychosocial objectives into simulations for healthcare professionals. Child life specialists can help simulation centers expand their programs to include not only professionals in the hospital, but professionals who work with children, youth, and families elsewhere in the community.

CONCLUSION

By integrating simulation into their practice, child life specialists can provide effective, psychologically safe, developmentally appropriate learning opportunities for children, youth, and families. Child life specialists can also be effective simulation educators and facilitators for professionals who work with these populations. Child life specialists are well-equipped to incorporate simulation into their practice and harness simulation-based education to lead improvements in the psychosocial care of children, youth, and families in healthcare and community settings worldwide.

REFERENCES

Adams, N. E. (2015). Bloom's taxonomy of cognitive learning objectives. *Journal of the Medical Library Association: JMLA, 103*(3), 152–153. doi:10.3163/1536-5050.103.3.010 PMID:26213509

Amar-Dolan, L. G., Horn, M. H., O'Connell, B., Parsons, S. K., Roussin, C. J., Weinstock, P. H., & Graham, R. J. (2020). "This is how hard it is". Family experience of hospital-to-home transition with a tracheostomy. *Annals of the American Thoracic Society, 17*(7), 860–868. doi:10.1513/AnnalsATS.201910-780OC PMID:32267725

Arnold, J. L., McKenzie, F., Miller, J. L., & Mancini, M. E. (2018). The many faces of patient-centered simulation: Implications for researchers. *Simulation in Healthcare: Journal of the Society for Simulation in Healthcare, 13*(3S), S51–S55. doi:10.1097/SIH.0000000000000312

Association of Child Life Professionals. (2019). Child life competencies. *ACLP Official Documents*. https://www.childlife.org/about-aclp/official-documents

Association of Child Life Professionals. (2020). Child life code of ethics. *ACLP Official Documents*. https://www.childlife.org/about-aclp/official-documents

Auerbach, M., Cheng, A., & Rudolph, J. W. (2018). Rapport management: Opening the door for effective debriefing. *Simulation in Healthcare: Journal of the Society for Simulation in Healthcare, 13*(1), 1–2. doi:10.1097/SIH.0000000000000266 PMID:29117095

Auerbach, M., Stone, K. P., & Patterson, M. D. (2016). The role of simulation in improving patient safety. In V. J. Grant & A. Cheng (Eds.), *Comprehensive healthcare simulation: Pediatrics* (pp. 55–65). Springer. doi:10.1007/978-3-319-24187-6_5

Bajaj, K., Meguerdichian, M., Thoma, B., Huang, S., Eppich, W., & Cheng, A. (2018). The PEARLS healthcare debriefing tool. *Academic Medicine, 93*(2), 336. doi:10.1097/ACM.0000000000002035 PMID:29381495

Boyer, T. J., & Mitchell, S. A. (2021). Utilization of embedded simulation personnel in medical simulation. In *StatPearls*. StatPearls Publishing. https://www.ncbi.nlm.nih.gov/books/NBK562294/

Chang, T. P., Gerard, J., & Pusic, M. V. (2016). Screen-based simulation, virtual reality, and haptic simulators. In V. J. Grant & A. Cheng (Eds.), *Comprehensive healthcare simulation: Pediatrics* (pp. 105–114). Springer. doi:10.1007/978-3-319-24187-6_9

Cheng, A., Auerbach, M., Calhoun, A., Mackinnon, R., Chang, T. P., Nadkarni, V., Hunt, E. A., Duval-Arnould, J., Peiris, N., Kessler, D., & INSPIRE Investigators (2018). Building a community of practice for researchers: The International Network for Simulation-Based Pediatric Innovation, Research and Education. *Simulation in Healthcare: Journal of the Society for Simulation in Healthcare, 13*(3S), S28–S34. doi:10.1097/SIH.0000000000000269

Cicero, M. X., & Weiner, D. L. (2016). Simulation for pediatric disaster and multiple casualty incident training. In V. J. Grant & A. Cheng (Eds.), *Comprehensive healthcare simulation: Pediatrics* (pp. 253–264). Springer. doi:10.1007/978-3-319-24187-6_20

Crnjak, E., Kerns, M., Stevens, M., O'Connell, B., & Mednick, L. (2021, Sept. 19). *Child life at end of life: Enhancing psychosocial care through bereavement simulation training* [Poster presentation]. 13th International Pediatric Simulation Symposia and Workshops, IPSSV 2021: A Virtual Experience. https://www.eventscribe.net/2021/IPSSV2021/fsPopup.asp?efp=T05YTlpQQ1oxNTA1Nw&PosterID=427009&rnd=0.944971&mode=posterinfo

Demaria, S. Jr, Bryson, E. O., Mooney, T. J., Silverstein, J. H., Reich, D. L., Bodian, C., & Levine, A. I. (2010). Adding emotional stressors to training in simulated cardiopulmonary arrest enhances participant performance. *Medical Education, 44*(10), 1006–1015. doi:10.1111/j.1365-2923.2010.03775.x PMID:20880370

Diaz, M. C. G., Arnold, J. L., & Robinson, T. (2016). Simulation for patient- and family-centered care. In V. J. Grant & A. Cheng (Eds.), *Comprehensive healthcare simulation: Pediatrics* (pp. 329–340). Springer. doi:10.1007/978-3-319-24187-6_26

Edmondson, A. (1999). Psychological safety and learning behavior in work teams. *Administrative Science Quarterly, 44*(2), 350–383. doi:10.2307/2666999

Eppich, W., & Cheng, A. (2015). Promoting excellence and reflective learning in simulation (PEARLS): Development and rationale for a blended approach to health care simulation debriefing. *Simulation in Healthcare: Journal of the Society for Simulation in Healthcare, 10*(2), 106–115. doi:10.1097/SIH.0000000000000072 PMID:25710312

Gaba, D. M. (2004). The future vision of simulation in health care. *Quality & Safety in Health Care, 13*(Suppl 1), i2–i10. doi:10.1136/qhc.13.suppl_1.i2

Galvez, J., Eisenhower, M., England, W., Wartman, E., Simpao, A., Rehman, M., Lustig, R., & Hribar, M. (2019). An interactive virtual reality tour for adolescents receiving proton radiation therapy: Proof-of-concept study. *JMIR Perioperative Medicine, 2*(1), e11259. doi:10.2196/11259 PMID:33393932

Gordon, J. (2021). Emotional safety in pediatrics. *Emotional Safety Initiative*. https://emotional-safety.org/emotional-safety-in-pediatrics/

Grant, D. J., Grant, V. J., & Cheng, A. (2016). The future of pediatric simulation. In V. J. Grant & A. Cheng (Eds.), *Comprehensive healthcare simulation: Pediatrics* (pp. 401–410). Springer. doi:10.1007/978-3-319-24187-6_31

Harrington, D. W., & Simon, L. V. (2021). Designing a simulation scenario. In *StatPearls*. StatPearls Publishing. https://www.ncbi.nlm.nih.gov/books/NBK547670/

International Network for Simulation-based Pediatric Innovation, Research & Education. (n.d.). *INSPIRE executive board*. Retrieved January 11, 2022, from https://inspiresim.org/what-is-inspire/executive-committee/

International Pediatric Simulation Society. (2021). *The 13th International Pediatric Simulation Symposia and Workshops - IPSSV2021: A virtual experience*. Retrieved January 11, 2022, from https://www.ipssglobal.org/ipssv2021-a-virtual-experience/

Kolb, A. Y., & Kolb, D. A. (2009). The learning way: Meta-cognitive aspects of experiential learning. *Simulation & Gaming*, *40*(3), 297–327. doi:10.1177/1046878108325713

Lateef, F. (2010). Simulation-based learning: Just like the real thing. *Journal of Emergencies, Trauma and Shock*, *3*(4), 348–352. doi:10.4103/0974-2700.70743 PMID:21063557

Loo, M. E., Krishnasamy, C., & Lim, W. S. (2018). Considering face, rights, and goals: A critical review of rapport management in facilitator-guided simulation debriefing approaches. *Simulation in Healthcare: Journal of the Society for Simulation in Healthcare*, *13*(1), 52–60. doi:10.1097/SIH.0000000000000258 PMID:29076968

Maa, T., Heimberg, E., & Reid, J. R. (2016). In situ simulation. In V. J. Grant & A. Cheng (Eds.), *Comprehensive healthcare simulation: Pediatrics* (pp. 153–163). Springer. doi:10.1007/978-3-319-24187-6_12

Mednick, L., O'Connell, B., Graber, K., Roussin, C., & Weinstock, P. (2021). "Ready SIM go": An adapted simulation "service line" for patients and caregivers. *Simulation in Healthcare: Journal of the Society for Simulation in Healthcare*, *16*(2), 120–127. doi:10.1097/SIH.0000000000000448 PMID:32218091

Moslehi, S., Masoumi, G., & Barghi-Shirazi, F. (2022). Benefits of simulation-based education in hospital emergency departments: A systematic review. *Journal of Education and Health Promotion*, *11*, 40. doi:10.4103/jehp.jehp_558_21 PMID:35281376

Nestel, D., & Kneebone, R. (2010). Perspective: Authentic patient perspectives in simulations for procedural and surgical skills. *Academic Medicine*, *85*(5), 889–893. doi:10.1097/ACM.0b013e3181d749ac PMID:20520046

Orgill, B. D., & Nolin, J. (2021). Learning taxonomies in medical simulation. In *StatPearls*. StatPearls Publishing. https://www.ncbi.nlm.nih.gov/books/NBK559109/

Palaganas, J. C., Scott, E., Mancini, M. E., & Stryjewski, G. (2016). Interprofessional education. In V. J. Grant & A. Cheng (Eds.), *Comprehensive healthcare simulation: Pediatrics* (pp. 195–208). Springer. doi:10.1007/978-3-319-24187-6_15

Patterson, S. (2020, Oct. 27). *Pioneering pediatric psychosocial education and the use of simulation based learning* [Conference session]. 12th International Pediatric Simulation Symposia and Workshops, IPSSV 2020: A Virtual Experience. https://www.eventscribe.com/2020/IPSSW2020/fsPopup.asp?Mode=presInfo&PresentationID=783321

Pillai, R. L. I. (2020). We all need a little TLC: An argument for an increased role of child life services in patient care and medical education. *Hospital Pediatrics*, *10*(10), 913–917. doi:10.1542/hpeds.2020-0119 PMID:32887731

Potthoff, L. M., Glotzbecker, M. P., O'Connell, B., O'Neill, N. P., Graber, K. M., Byrne, C. A., Tremmel, J. M., Weinstock, P., & Mednick, L. (2021). SIMDiscovery: A simulation-based preparation program for adolescents undergoing spinal fusion surgery. *Spine Deformity*, *9*(5), 1363–1370. doi:10.100743390-021-00322-6 PMID:33689156

Ramachandra, G., Deutsch, E. S., & Nadkarni, V. M. (2020). A road map for simulation based medical students training in pediatrics: Preparing the next generation of doctors. *Indian Pediatrics*, *57*(10), 950–956. doi:10.100713312-020-2001-9 PMID:33089810

Raphael, B. P., Takvorian-Bené, M., Gallotto, M., Tascione, C., McClelland, J., Rosa, C., Dinan, J., O'Connell, B., & Weinstock, P. (2021). Learning gaps and family experience, nurse-facilitated home parenteral nutrition simulation-based discharge training: Proof-of-concept study. *Nutrition in Clinical Practice: Official Publication of the American Society for Parenteral and Enteral Nutrition*, *36*(2), 489–496. doi:10.1002/ncp.10421 PMID:31589007

Rudder, B. S., Boyd, S. L., Easley, S. A., Nusbaum, J. D., Sherman, A. K., Sommer, D. R., & Schremmer, R. D. (2019). Psychosocial simulation: A novel approach to interprofessional training. *Journal of Interprofessional Education & Practice*, *14*(1), 67–71. doi:10.1016/j.xjep.2018.12.004

Rudolph, J. W., Raemer, D. B., & Simon, R. (2014). Establishing a safe container for learning in simulation: The role of the presimulation briefing. *Simulation in Healthcare: Journal of the Society for Simulation in Healthcare*, *9*(6), 339–349. doi:10.1097/SIH.0000000000000047 PMID:25188485

Rudolph, J. W., Simon, R., Dufresne, R. L., & Raemer, D. B. (2006). There's no such thing as "nonjudgmental" debriefing: A theory and method for debriefing with good judgment. *Simulation in Healthcare: Journal of the Society for Simulation in Healthcare*, *1*(1), 49–55. doi:10.1097/01266021-200600110-00006 PMID:19088574

Rudolph, J. W., Simon, R., Raemer, D. B., & Eppich, W. J. (2008). Debriefing as formative assessment: Closing performance gaps in medical education. *Academic Emergency Medicine: Official Journal of the Society for Academic Emergency Medicine*, *15*(11), 1010–1016. doi:10.1111/j.1553-2712.2008.00248.x PMID:18945231

Sagalowsky, S. T., Agnant, J., Bailey, B., Woodward, H., Duncan, E., Grad, J., & Kessler, D. O. (2021a, Jan. 19). *Addressing inequity and structural competency through simulation: Transformative learning workshop* [Conference session]. International Meeting on Simulation in Healthcare, IMSH Delivers: Simulation - Bringing Learning to Life, Virtual. https://ssh.expoplanner.com/index.cfm?do=expomap.sess&event_id=12&session_id=5278

Sagalowsky, S. T., Kester, K., Woodward, H., Bailey, B., & Catallozzi, M. (2020). Lessons learnt from piloting paediatric patient-focused and family-focused simulation methodology in a clerkship objective structured clinical experience. *BMJ Simulation & Technology Enhanced Learning*, *6*(5), 306–307. doi:10.1136/bmjstel-2019-000532 PMID:35517386

Sagalowsky, S. T., Woodward, H., Evins, J., & Kessler, D. O. (2021b). Responding to microaggressions: Further frameworks from simulation debriefing. *Annals of Emergency Medicine*, *77*(3), 381–382. doi:10.1016/j.annemergmed.2020.10.006 PMID:33618815

Sawyer, T., Fleegler, M. B., & Eppich, W. J. (2016). Essentials of debriefing and feedback. In V. J. Grant & A. Cheng (Eds.), *Comprehensive healthcare simulation: Pediatrics* (pp. 31–42). Springer. doi:10.1007/978-3-319-24187-6_3

Shetty, R., & Nadkarni, V. (2016). Simulation in acute care pediatrics: New paradigms in care. *Journal of Pediatric Critical Care, 3*(3), 35-39. doi:10.21304/2016.0303.00136

Society for Simulation in Healthcare. (n.d.a). *SIM center directory*. Retrieved January 10, 2022, from https://www.SSH.org/Home/SIM-Center-Directory

Society for Simulation in Healthcare. (n.d.b) *V2.0 addendum: Terms related to simulation at a distance*. Healthcare simulation dictionary. https://www.SSH.org/Dictionary

Stunden, C., Stratton, K., Zakani, S., & Jacob, J. (2021). Comparing a virtual reality-based simulation app (VR-MRI) with a standard preparatory manual and child life program for improving success and reducing anxiety during pediatric medical imaging: Randomized clinical trial. *Journal of Medical Internet Research, 23*(9), e22942. doi:10.2196/22942 PMID:34550072

Theilen, U., Fraser, L., Jones, P., Leonard, P., & Simpson, D. (2017). Regular in-situ simulation training of paediatric Medical Emergency Team leads to sustained improvements in hospital response to deteriorating patients, improved outcomes in intensive care and financial savings. *Resuscitation, 115*, 61–67. doi:10.1016/j.resuscitation.2017.03.031 PMID:28359769

Vora, S., Dahlen, B., Adler, M., Kessler, D. O., Jones, V. F., Kimble, S., & Calhoun, A. (2021). Recommendations and guidelines for the use of simulation to address structural racism and implicit bias. *Simulation in Healthcare: Journal of the Society for Simulation in Healthcare, 16*(4), 275–284. doi:10.1097/SIH.0000000000000591 PMID:34398114

Wagner, M., Jaki, C., Löllgen, R. M., Mileder, L., Eibensteiner, F., Ritschl, V., Steinbauer, P., Gottstein, M., Abulebda, K., Calhoun, A., & Gross, I. T. (2021). Readiness for and response to Coronavirus Disease 2019 among pediatric healthcare providers: The role of simulation for pandemics and other disasters. *Pediatric Critical Care Medicine: A Journal of the Society of Critical Care Medicine and the World Federation of Pediatric Intensive and Critical Care Societies, 22*(6), e333–e338. doi:10.1097/PCC.0000000000002649

Woodward, H., & Ching, K. (2020, Oct. 26). *Impact of integrating child life specialists into simulation-based pediatric emergency medicine training* [Conference session]. 12th International Pediatric Simulation Symposia and Workshops, IPSSV 2020: A Virtual Experience. https://www.eventscribe.com/2020/IPSSW2020/fsPopup.asp?efp=Q0JUUERNQkk1Nzk4&PresentationID=782876&rnd=0.5213007&mode=presinfo

Woodward, H., Evins, J., O'Connell, B., & Diezel, K. (2018, May 5). *Simulation in child life practice: The next generation of preparation, education, and interprofessional collaboration* [Conference session]. Association of Child Life Professionals 36th Annual Conference, National Harbor, MD, United States. https://education.childlife.org/products/simulation-in-child-life-practice-the-next-generation-of-preparation-education-and-interprofessional-collaboration#tab-product_tab_overview

Woodward, H., Kessler, D. O., Fenster, D., Jamal, N., Evins, J., & Sagalowsky, S. T. (2017, June 3). *Stirring the pot: Blending medical, interprofessional & patient-centered objectives in simulation* [Conference session]. 9th International Pediatric Simulation Symposia and Workshops, Boston, MA, United States.

Woodward, H., & Patterson, S. (2020, Jan. 18). *Optimal technique to improve child life specialists' skills at cultivating emotional safety for families - A pilot study* [Oral presentation]. ALERT (Advanced Look Exploratory Research Template) presentation for INSPIRE (International Network of Simulation-based Innovation, Research & Education) meeting at 20th Annual International Meeting on Simulation in Healthcare, San Diego, CA, United States.

Yerkes, R. M., & Dodson, J. G. (1908). The relation of strength of stimulus to rapidity of habit-formation. *The Journal of Comparative Neurology and Psychology*, *18*(5), 459–482. doi:10.1002/cne.920180503

KEY TERMS AND DEFINITIONS

Debrief: Guided reflection that supports learners in processing what happened during a simulation and applying lessons to future scenarios.

Distance Simulation: Replicated experience in which participants (learners, facilitators, embedded participants, and/or standardized patients) are in different physical locations. Distance simulation often uses technologies such as video chat platforms and remote controls.

Embedded Participants: Actors trained to portray roles other than patients during simulations.

Fidelity: Realism. Improving the fidelity of a simulation may increase learner engagement.

In Situ: The practice of facilitating simulation in the environment where the learners will use the skills in real life instead of in a replicated environment.

Prebrief: Orientation prior to a simulation to help learners know what to expect.

Psychological Safety: The feeling that interpersonal risk-taking is acceptable and will not lead to negative repercussions.

Simulation: The technique of replicating experiences in a guided learning environment.

Standardized Patients: Actors trained to portray patients during healthcare simulations.

Chapter 3
Organ, Tissue, and Eye Procurement

Alli Reilly
The Living Legacy Foundation of Maryland, USA

ABSTRACT

Organ, tissue, and eye donation is an essential component of healthcare necessary to save and enhance the lives of others. The decision to honor a loved one's designation, or consent to donation on the behalf of an eligible donor, is a choice fraught with a multitude of competing factors which may provide stress among family decision-makers, and the bereavement journey does not end once recovery is completed. Certified Child Life Specialists are expertly equipped with the knowledge, skills, and abilities to effectively and compassionately offer donation opportunities during potentially traumatizing or crisis-laden situations as family services coordinators. As indispensable members of any organ procurement organization, family services coordinators collaborate with clinical recovery coordinators, hospital services individuals, and hospital critical care teams to ensure families are poised to make well-informed decisions, honor their loved one in a uniquely profound and rare way, and provide ongoing bereavement and grief support to families experiencing the loss of a loved one.

SUPPORTING FAMILIES DURING DEATH AND ORGAN, TISSUE, AND EYE DONATION AS A CERTIFIED CHILD LIFE SPECIALIST

Donate Life America (2022) reports that more than 100,000 people are awaiting life-saving transplants throughout the United States. While the transplant waiting list is extensive, fewer than three in every 1,000 people are eligible to provide the gift of life to another through organ donation (Health Resources and Services Administration, 2021), and only 60% of adults are designated or registered organ, tissue, and eye donors. One organ, tissue, and ocular donor, via deceased donation, can save up to eight lives through solid organ transplant, enhance more than 75 lives through the gift of tissue donation, and restore vision to two people (Donate Life America, 2022).

For many families facing end-of-life (EOL) decision-making on behalf of a loved one, organ donation is typically not considered until the family is approached by a representative of an organ procure-

DOI: 10.4018/978-1-6684-5097-0.ch003

ment organization (OPO). There are 57 OPOs throughout the United States, separated by region and population (United Network for Organ Sharing, 2022); each organization is certified by the Centers for Medicare and Medicaid Services. The American Academy of Pediatrics Committee on Hospital Care (2010) "supports the role of OPOs by recommending that all potential donor families be approached in a systematic method by individuals trained in the psychological, social, and medical aspects of organ donation" (p. 823). Methods often include decoupling; a purposeful delay that occurs between the time a family is notified of brain death or the decision is made to compassionately withdraw life-sustaining therapies (WDLST), and when the opportunity for organ donation is presented. Decoupling aims to ensure separation between critical care teams that primarily focus on treating a patient's illness or injury, and an organ procurement organization. This separation occurs in order to effectively and empathically support families through EOL decision making, offering the opportunity for organ, tissue, and eye donation when a patient is eligible (Kao, 2000). Eligible organ donors must be receiving ventilatory support to be considered a viable donation candidate, to ensure potential gifts receive adequate blood circulation and oxygenation; as mentioned previously, the number of people ever in a position to donate their organs is relatively small, fewer than one percent. Tissue and eye donors, however, are considered eligible after the point that an individual's heart stops beating, or cardiac time of death. Following a thorough review of medical records and documentation of the circumstances surrounding the death, eligibility determination for tissue and eye donors is made based on known medical history (i.e., patients diagnosed with cancer with metastases or communicable diseases are often disqualified), active infections at the time of death, and permission from state medical examiners. The amount of possible tissue and ocular donors far exceeds the number of potential organ donors, however exact statistics are not widely available.

OPOs consistently have a number of varying departments within their organizations with unique goals and team configurations. The professionals responsible for providing support and the opportunity for donation to families include, by formal title (Association of Organ Procurement Organizations, 2022):

- Donation and family advocate
- Donor family grief advocate
- Donation liaison
- Family care coordinator
- Family services coordinator
- Family support counselor
- Family support specialist

For this chapter, the role in reference will be referred to as a family services coordinator (FSC), as it is the author's documented title, and an increasing number of FSCs are formally trained as child life professionals. FSC eligibility requirements vary between organizations; however, standard qualifications incorporate knowledge and skills proportional to those of a Certified Child Life Specialist (CCLS) credentialed by the Association of Child Life Professionals (ACLP), along with a minimum of two to five completed years of working with acute or critical care populations, bereavement or palliative care expertise, and master's level education. The preferred background of FSCs includes degrees in psychology, counseling, chaplaincy or pastoral care, social work, and other allied health modalities. Identified interest areas or additional certificates may consist of bereavement and family counseling, clinical assessment skills, and family crisis or trauma-informed support (Association of Organ Procurement Organizations, 2022). Often, degree level is mitigated by additional experience. Additionally, several OPOs cite job requirements and responsibilities of FSCs to include performing thorough electronic medical record review and clinical evaluation of patient referrals to determine patient candidacy. These roles indicate additional eligibility and training requirements in medical terminology competency or skills acquired through experience in nursing education or emergency medical technician training. In a small subset of OPOs, donation professionals responsible for the clinical care and support of consented donors are additionally accountable for in-person psychosocial and family support and are therefore required to have critical care nursing licensure. OPOs have the flexibility to set departmental structures to best support the needs of the families served and activity within the OPO's defined donor service areas.

Scheduled work hours for FSCs are often in 12-hour or 24-hour rotating on-call shifts, with anywhere from 10-15 shifts per month depending on OPO specifications, dedicated simulation or training activities, and departmental support obligations. Due to potentially extensive geographical coverage, travel is often necessary for an FSC to support organ donor activity within the OPO's donor service area, whereas authorization and subsequent family support and updates for families of tissue and ocular donors may be completed from a central office location or remotely.

CCLSs are adequately prepared and skilled to support families of organ, tissue, and ocular donors within OPOs, as defined by each individual organization. Due to extensive credentialing requirements and an array of clinical experiences, CCLSs possess the necessary knowledge, skills, and abilities to comprehensively support families making EOL decisions on behalf of a family member, including offering the opportunity for donation.

SETTING/POPULATION

Because potential organ donors must be receiving mechanical ventilation, initial donation conversations, in-person psychosocial support, and the authorization or consenting process for organ donor families often occurs within hospital intensive care and critical care units or emergency departments. FSCs often travel to many hospitals within their assigned region to collaboratively meet with medical team members and offer the opportunity of donation to qualifying patients' families and decision-makers. Due to the need to travel to many hospitals within an OPO donor service area, FSCs do not frequently have the opportunity to repeatedly work with the same physicians, providers, or critical care nursing team members that they otherwise would be able to form working relationships within a traditional unit-based or service-based child life role.

FSCs who offer opportunities for tissue and eye donation, independent of organ donation (i.e., after a patient's cardiac time of death has been established), may also travel to hospitals and hospice facilities, or utilize telephone communication to reach an individual's legal next of kin to obtain consent, offer grief and bereavement support, and guide families through funerary planning, including any involvement with the medical examiner, as appropriate.

People of all ages and medical histories can be organ, tissue, and eye donors and the need for a life-saving transplant does not discriminate based on demographic factors; however, Donate Life America (2022) indicates that although both donation and transplantation can successfully occur between individuals of different racial or ethnic groups, transplant outcomes are more successful when organs are matched between people of similar ethnic or racial backgrounds. There is currently a disproportionate number of patients—58% of those formally listed and awaiting a life-saving transplant—of African American/Black, Asian/Pacific Islander, Hispanic/Latino, American Indian/Alaska Native, and multiracial descent, indicating that these communities are in greater need of organ and tissue donors (Donate Life America, 2022). Although it is difficult to put into formal practice, some studies indicate that consent or authorization rates for organ, tissue, and eye donation increase when the cultural background of the requester matches that of the family making an EOL decision (Haliko & Arnold, 2002). Several OPOs with significant numbers of minorities within their donor services area seek to recruit and employ professionals with similar backgrounds and bilingual or multilingual skills to more comprehensively support donor families.

The age of donors varies widely; however, adult donors far outweigh the pediatric donor population. The Organ Procurement and Transplantation Network's (2022) data shows that in 2021, there were 13,863 organ donors, with fewer than seven percent of donors in the range of newborn through age 17. FSCs may observe that support provided to pediatric donor patients and their families occurs much less frequently compared to adult donor patients and their families. Nonetheless, donor families benefit from broad-spectrum support throughout the donation process, regardless of the donor's age.

The circumstances of an organ donor's death, including the mechanism of injury, are often traumatic or sudden, rather than due to a chronic illness or diagnosis. In 2021, the most recent year in which data is available, documented causes of death included: asphyxiation (4.9%), blunt injuries (16.5%), drowning (1.1%), drug intoxication (16.2%), gunshot wounds (7.4%), motor vehicle accidents (11.5%), child abuse (0.3%), suicide (8%), and cerebrovascular accident or stroke (24.9%) (Organ Procurement and Transplantation Network, 2022). Due to the nature of such accidents and injuries, families may often be notified of their loved one's hospitalization unexpectedly or when the injury occurs while the decision-maker is not with the patient, causing additional levels of stress. FSCs are pivotal in supporting families through processing a loved one's sudden decline and often demise, helping family members to understand grim prognosis, brain death declaration, and the assessment of a patient's discussed or presumed EOL wishes.

Families of tissue and eye donors, for whom organ donation was not a possibility, may be more prepared for a loved one's death in cases related to chronic illness or cancer, but death by traumatic experiences, as victims of crime, by motor vehicle accidents, and other sudden losses are still prevalent among this population. In scenarios regarding only potential tissue and ocular donation, families often have not been part of decision-making regarding their loved one until the patient's passing and may feel suddenly overwhelmed by the many decisions to be made including funerary planning and estate arrangements. This is exacerbated under circumstances in which there is no warning prior to death and planning needs to commence immediately.

SUPPORT NEEDS OF DONOR FAMILIES

FSCs, including CCLSs and similar professionals, support the needs of all families making EOL decisions on behalf of a loved one regardless of race, socioeconomic status, gender, sexual orientation, religion, immigration status, and ability. While sexual orientation, gender, gender identity, or gender expression does not prevent someone from registering as an organ donor, in regards to tissue and eye donation opportunities, there are often specific, albeit antiquated, situations in which a patient's sexual orientation or gender identity may influence the ability to donate, as mandated by the Food and Drug Administration. Certain social history behaviors may eliminate someone from providing tissue and ocular gifts for safety reasons (Donate Life America, 2022). In addition, all major religions within the United States "support donation as a final act of compassion and generosity" (Donate Life America, 2022). However, some specific denominations may have restrictions in unique ways (i.e., donation for transplantation only, rather than a donation for research or education purposes). FSCs often facilitate chaplaincy support for families making EOL decisions to ensure that faith leaders are involved to provide guidance when uncertainty surrounds a family's donation decision.

In many OPOs, demographics of families will vary by hospital, often reflective of geographic region or location. Because traumatic incidents resulting in death affect all groups of people, it is imperative that CCLSs, and those serving as FSCs, have specific training or experience in health care equity to identify disparities that exist and how such inequalities may impact patients' and their decision makers' healthcare experiences (ACLP, 2020b). According to the ACLP's *Child Life Code of Ethics*, CCLSs "have an obligation to maintain an environment that respects variations in culture, age, gender, race, ethnicity, physical ability, sexual orientation, gender identity/expression, religious affiliation, veteran status, and socioeconomic status" (2020a, p. 1). Boles et al. (2020) supports that "regardless of geographic location or setting, CCLSs employ an individual approach that honors and serves patients and families or all backgrounds, experiences, belief systems and preferences (p. 3).

Eligible patients who become organ donors donate via either a brain death declaration, in which death by neurological criteria is legal and documented after undergoing brain death testing, or when a family makes an often difficult decision to withdraw life-sustaining therapies. Among other reasons, these decisions frequently arise when families reflect on patient wishes, citing the likelihood that the patient expressed a desire not to be maintained on machines, or the family recognizes that a patient's quality of life would be compromised by the medical care needed to remain ventilated and medically supported for a potentially extended period. In both pathways, and as mentioned previously, the cause of the donor's illness or injury is often sudden, due to an accident, drug or alcohol overdose, or a cardiac arrest, among other causes. Shemie et al. (2017) noted "it is recognized that presenting the opportunity for donation to families who are in a stressful, traumatic situation is difficult and must be done with sensitivity to their unique situations, values, and beliefs (p. S17)." The Committee on Non-Heart-Beating Transplantation II (2000) further illustrates that decisions related to donation opportunities are often made within the structure of a crisis; the patient who eventually becomes an organ donor is most often a previously healthy person stricken by a sudden, unanticipated, life-altering event. CCLSs are qualified to provide support rooted in trauma-informed care. Child life certification requires that they possess the knowledge to identify events that may affect families such as loss, traumatic life events, EOL, and grief work (ACLP, 2019). According to Boles et al. (2020), "CCLSs have practiced principles of trauma-informed care long before the term was coined… understanding and facilitating physical and emotional safety, establishing trusting relationships, communicating honestly and accurately, offering choice and control, and using a strengths-based approach to care" (p. 5).

WORK AS A CERTIFIED CHILD LIFE SPECIALIST

Certified Child Life Specialists are adequately prepared and skilled to support families of organ, tissue, and ocular donors in the role of family service coordinators within OPOs. Due to extensive credentialing requirements and an array of clinical experiences, CCLSs possess the necessary knowledge, skills, and abilities to comprehensively support families making EOL decisions on the behalf of a family member, prepare families for donation processes, disclose when a loved one has made a donation decision for themselves, connect families to hospital and community resources, and offer continued follow-up and bereavement or grief support for families whose loved one has died, regardless of donation decision. ACLP's *Position Statement on Child Life Practice in Community Settings* (2018) affirms that child life competencies are easily and often effortlessly applicable to any professional environment, whether primarily pediatric-focused or otherwise, that supports children impacted by crisis or change, as well as their families and their extended support systems. The death or imminent passing of a loved one and subsequent decision-making on the loved one's behalf, including organ, tissue, and ocular donation, in addition to funerary arrangements and estate planning, can affect the entire family unit, often without warning.

A CCLS in the role of an FSC may provide support in a variety of ways, including initiating the donation conversation, developing legacy materials with family involvement, providing bereavement support, offering continuous information regarding the donation processes and associated timelines, proposing or facilitating ceremonies or rituals to honor the donor, and accompanying a donor and their family to the operating room for procurement (Fieten, 2021). Further, FSCs holding the CCLS credential may bear witness to a donor's last moments as a family proxy in certain scenarios, debrief with hospital staff who have cared for a donor and their family members throughout the donation process, offer guidance in confirming funerary plans and accompanying timelines, and provide follow-up grief and bereavement support as needed based on family preference. Ongoing family support after procurement or donation recovery completion may include assisting with memorial planning, organizing annual donor ceremonies of remembrance, and facilitating donor and recipient correspondence or meetings. While the family support role within each OPO may not be entirely standardized, in many organizations, an FSC has the ability and responsibility to support each family in comprehensive ways, with a solid foundation of skills that can be attained by the experience and ongoing work of child life professionals.

While the FSC role is a natural extension of child life work, CCLSs are also increasingly beginning to explore other OPO roles. Additional job positions within an OPO which may be applicable to CCLSs with a career interest in donation may include community engagement and education, liaison work between medical facilities and OPOs, organizational training roles, or executing a working relationship between medical examiner offices, funeral homes, and the OPO team members who directly support donation. As the chapter author has become aware of CCLSs in roles outside of the chapter's focus as an FSC but has no personal or direct experience as a CCLS in such complimentary OPO roles, and documentation of child life professionals in such roles is not prevalent, the responsibilities and job descriptions were not comprehensively evaluated.

Assessment

ACLP's position statement on child life practice in community settings (2018) denotes that the ability to assess the variety of coping reactions or responses in addition to the psychosocial needs of children, families and their immediate supports is an essential goal of child life practice; it is also a pillar of the role of an FSC.

CCLSs regularly identify factors that may impact a family's vulnerability to both stress and trauma and recognize how a particular family may interpret or make meaning of illness or loss (ACLP, 2019). Defined assessment skills and the ability to determine the needs of each family also ensure that when such needs spread beyond the scope of practice, CCLSs make professional referrals and recommendations for additional or complementary services (ACLP, 2018). This is similarly accurate in the role of

FSCs; through either hospital-specific or community-based referrals, recommendations can be offered to families on a case-by-case basis.

Boles et al. (2020) suggests that child life work is founded on the assessment of patient-and-family strengths as well as stressors, exacerbated by treatment factors that threaten family functioning and overall well-being. A similar approach exists for FSCs across many, if not all, OPOs. Specific to organ, tissue, and ocular donation opportunities, Shemie, et al. (2017) assert that:

Families considering donation are in a vulnerable and emotional crisis state during which decision-making can be difficult. As a result, problems with decision-making, attention span, concentrating, and remembering information are common. The attitude, manner, and language used by healthcare professionals involved have been shown to have a significant impact on how families experience and react to the opportunity for donation. (p. S20)

FSCs strive to assess a family's ability to receive and retain information from the critical care team regarding a potential donor's grim prognosis or declaration of death before initiating donation conversations, an additional benefit of decoupling practices. With permission from the medical team, additional time can be offered to families after receiving such updates to ensure that families are prepared and ready to discuss the next steps including donation opportunities, the discontinuation of mechanical support, or extubation. The FSC has the professional responsibility to assess the family's needs, along with the duty to balance the guidelines or policies of the medical institution to support all parties involved. Supplementary to this assessment is the need to continually evaluate the donor family's receptivity to ongoing updates throughout the donation process and respect familial attitudes toward adjustments to the process as it unfolds.

Preparation

As the goal of care transitions from saving a donor's life to supporting the donor management and transplantation process once a family authorizes donation, the OPO's clinical or organ recovery coordinators typically oversee medical care instead of the hospital's critical care team. Because of this transition, it is the responsibility of OPO team members, specifically FSCs, to walk families through the evaluation, allocation, and eventual organ, tissue, and eye recovery process. Regarding preparation by CCLSs, Boles et al. (2020) cite that families cope more effectively with what is understood and expected or anticipated rather than details that may be unpredictable or uncertain. This statement is accurately transferable to organ donation professionals in the FSC role. To minimize the effects of stress, FSCs aim to provide health-literacy appropriate explanations to all family members of a potential donor about the sequence of events and next steps related to donation processes, understandably explaining medical terminology, and allowing the opportunity for families to express their needs and hopes for the experience to support the gift or enhancement of life to another.

It is often the goal of a FSC, in the initial conversation regarding a donation opportunity, to provide a framework and timeline to assist family members in making an informed decision. In the event of a designated and declared donor, an additional goal is targeted to advocate for the needs of each family to ultimately honor the donor's decision or wishes; designated donors have previously documented their intent to donate via their state of residence's motor vehicle or driver's license department, the national donor registry, or an advanced directive. In most states, a designation or donor registration is considered a legally documented decision, similar to an advanced directive or living will. While there are often general steps and timelines associated with donation processes, FSCs rely on interactions with family members, as well as general observations and assessments related to family coping styles, to learn whether these timelines best support the needs of each family. In some cases, FSCs may encourage organ procurement teams to expedite timelines if warranted or encourage the pace to move more deliberately to allow additional time for grieving or for extended family members to visit the hospital to say their final goodbye before organ recovery.

Information provided to families should be clear and concise, presenting each family the opportunity to make an informed decision, including: transparency about hospital and OPO roles or responsibilities, values of donation, patient registry or designation details, a review of donation processes, and any impact on funerary arrangements or additional next steps (Shemie, 2017). Chandler et al. (2017) further state that there is a psychological impact on families when donation opportunities are offered; literature generally supports the expectations that respectful and compassionate care for the deceased and their family; listening for and addressing specific family concerns; and an attitude toward donation that is positive, while not solely procurement-focused; is best for both consent rates and family well-being in coping with loss.

After organ and tissue recovery, families benefit from additional preparation, if applicable, for review by a state's medical examiner or anatomy board, additional medical research organizations, and further funerary planning, including burial options or cremation services. Unless a donor has explicitly documented their wishes in an EOL directive (e.g., advance directive, living will), families often base their decisions and planning on what they feel their loved one would have wanted, and many families verbalize that EOL wishes were never discussed before the donor's injury or hospitalization, leaving family members torn as to how best honor their loved one's legacy. Support is explicitly needed when decision-makers have no previous experience with making EOL arrangements on the behalf of a loved one.

Child life specialists are uniquely poised within a multidisciplinary team to individualize psychological preparation that integrates coping abilities and strengths into the plan of care while supporting families during medical experiences (Grissom et al., 2016). According to the ACLP *Evidence-Based Practice Statement on Preparing Children and Adolescents for Medical Procedures* (Koller, 2008), there are three essential components of preparation: provision of clear and accurate information, encouragement of emotional expression, and the establishment of trust. While the statement reflects the need for effective preparation for children undergoing medical experiences, it also seamlessly translates to the support that FSCs provide to donor families throughout the donation experience. Cleiren and Van Zoelen (2002) specify that it is not only information itself that is critical to family well-being, but rather the relational aspect of sharing information that influences more favorable coping through bereavement.

Developmental Explanations

Certified Child Life Specialists habitually empower families to become active, informed participants in healthcare experiences; merging the domains of practice, CCLSs implement a unique skill set for approaching, involving, and aiding children and their support systems in understanding their or a loved one's care (Boles et al., 2020). The FSC is often in a position to offer or provide support to a parent or caregiver in disclosing information about an adult in the child's life who is critically ill or injured, or who has died. During times of bereavement, CCLSs discuss and validate the need for parents or caregivers to actively continue in their primary parenting role as appropriate (ACLP, 2018), a responsibility that FSCs also employ.

The Beryl Institute (2018) states in reference to CCLSs helping to aid in family understanding:

What is evident in this commitment is that experience is not left to chance. Rather there is evidence-based rigor to this work to provide the best in experience. This is not just expressing empathy and compassion; though important, it goes beyond that. This is expressing a true sense of understanding of the person, the family being cared for, with a clear commitment to helping them have clarity about all that is happening (p. 11).

Family Service Coordinators do not always have the opportunity to provide in-person support to children, grandchildren, or other young minors in a donor's life. However, they are readily available to offer insight and expertise to other caring adults in the young person's network. By helping the adults identify common reactions, potential misconceptions, and address questions that may arise, FSCs support the entire family unit.

Expressive Arts

Opportunities for expressive arts facilitated by a CCLS or FSCs during consented donor management may occur less frequently than expressive arts modalities are used in more traditional child life roles, but the opportunities remain and are prioritized where possible, and often honor the life of the donor to provide a tangible component to the donor's legacy. Boles et al. (2020) propose that:

Healthcare experiences provoke a wide range of psychological and developmental responses in infants, children, adolescents, and their families. To assist children and families in finding the individualized sense of meaning needed to effectively cope with their healthcare encounters, CCLSs expressly offer legacy-building interventions as a way to therapeutically chronicle healthcare...and create lasting memories. (p.37)

CCLSs are skilled in making opportunities for legacies to manifest through self-expression and customized celebration, and it is acknowledged that legacy lasts far beyond death (Boles et al., 2020). Legacy-building projects for organ donor families, including those in which family participation is applicable, are a potentially unique offering compared to what may be typically available in adult critical care settings. CCLSs "fill a compelling void in healthcare – psychosocial support for patients and families as they navigate personal difficulties facing their family throughout hospitalization (or death) of a loved one" (Boles et al., 2020, p. 38). FSCs, similar to CCLSs and unit social work team members, frequently offer opportunities for legacy building and by nature, expressive arts to aid families in celebrating the life of a loved one. Options often include creating ink prints or hand molds, generating musical selections and playlists, offering personalized ceremonies honoring a donor's life as well as the effect that a donor may have on others, creating words and personalized images to honor a donor that may subsequently be used for memorial cards for services, obtaining heartbeat and other audio recordings, and creating other more personalized rituals or keepsake items which may hold enormous value to donor families.

Further, after consented donor management has occurred, and organ, tissue, or eye recovery has been completed, opportunities for families of donors are regularly available through OPO aftercare offerings. Families can participate or opt-out based on their comfort level but are regularly invited to join in a variety of programming designed to allow family members to express their thoughts, feelings, and emotions regarding the donor and their ongoing grief.

Coping

Core child life competencies (ACLP, 2019) illustrate the requirement for CCLSs to demonstrate the ability to support families in coping with stressful events, including those that may be considered traumatic life events, those involving loss or EOL, and grief work. Further, CCLSs must identify factors that may influence a family's vulnerability to stress. To this end, CCLSs implement active listening, empathic responding, self-reflection, and awareness of models of grief; all daily practices which are necessary for FSCs as well. Skills that CCLSs and FSCs employ include empowering and supporting families to self-advocate on behalf of their family members, including donors who cannot do so, demonstrating verbal and non-verbal empathic responses during stressful events, and acting as a team participant in bereavement work on behalf of donor families.

Families who fully engage in accepting death, draw upon support from family, friends, religion, and culture, and further face their grief through bereavement tend to cope better (Dicks, et al., 2017). Additionally, the identification of something positive or meaningful, including the goal of helping others, often helps families to make meaning of an otherwise tragic incident.

Play

Play within the realm of roles and responsibilities of a FSC in an organ procurement setting may not permit a child life professional to fully use a play-based skill set compared to a CCLS in a more traditional setting. Organ donors can be admitted and eventually authorized for donation at almost any hospital, including smaller community hospitals, with either critical or intensive care units and operating room facilities. In hospitals where a CCLS is not employed, FSCs with child life certification support donor families through obtaining visitation permissions for children or grandchildren and providing guided play to understand organ, tissue, and eye donation. In larger facilities, and often academic medical institutions or trauma centers, child life specialists are often available through consulting services to support children or grandchildren of adult patients; thus the opportunity for play-based interventions by an FSC is minimal. In any scenario, it is also imperative that the FSC ensures that defined job requirements are followed in alignment with OPO and hospital policy, and thus play-based support may not be appropriate.

Advocacy

Anthony et al. (2021) report that donation coordinators in their study, team members responsible for facilitating the organ donation process and primarily introducing organ donation to substitute decision-makers or legal next of kin, are primarily responsible for advocating for the needs of families throughout the donation processes. Further, the study suggests that value-positive language, role reframing, and increased education are all applicable and vital strategies to increase organ donation authorization rates, and these practices align closely with advocacy. Generally, FSCs are steadfast advocates for designated donors, those who when given the opportunity and when healthy decide for themselves that should they ever be in a position to do so, they would want to save the life of another. It is the obligation of an FSC to provide families with information and support with the ultimate goal of honoring a designated donor's EOL wish, as a designation or donor registration is considered a legal, binding document of gift.

If the designation is ever challenged by family members, or family decision-makers cite difficulty accepting a loved one's designation, the FSC is in an optimal position to support families in expressing their needs and beliefs surrounding the designation, providing appropriate information to all parties, and aiming to honor the patient's decision. The FSC also advocates for the needs of the family to become supportive of donation processes and potentially acquiesce to first-person authorization stipulations, which are present in all 50 states within the United States.

By communicating effectively with community partners and other professionals, including those within each hospital or critical care setting, the work of an FSC is similar to that of a CCLS in the sense that professionals can share expertise surrounding the psychosocial and developmental needs of the donor families being supported (ACLP, 2018). The Beryl Institute (2018) states in reference to child life professionals that: "A priority that is clear in child life is that the focus is unwavering on the person in front of them versus the system that surrounds them" (p. 14). The same working principles can be said in regards to FSCs working with donor families: while FSCs have the obligation to follow regulatory requirements and hospital or facility policies, due to the liaison-like status between multiple groups, there is an opportunity to fully advocate for families in a variety of ways, and ultimately encourage collaboration among all involved to ensure a donor's gifts are maximized where possible. This advocacy may include assisting with family support for visitation where it was once restricted, discussing permission with local medical examiner entities to ensure legacy opportunities remain possible where appropriate, or ensuring family support and agreement to timeline changes based on predicted transplant recipient needs or due to logistics of recovering surgical teams, including travel.

Family-Centered Care

Patient- and family-centered care is a widely accepted, comprehensive approach to the planning, delivery, and evaluation of healthcare that is founded in mutually beneficial partnerships among healthcare providers, patients, and families. The four pillars of patient- and family-centered care are: dignity and respect, information sharing, participation, and collaboration (Institute for Patient- and Family-Centered Care, n.d.). FSCs strive to support families throughout the organ, tissue, and ocular donation process while addressing each of these core concepts. Goals include ensuring both medical teams and OPOs honor and respect family decisions and choices regarding a loved one's EOL wishes, including the decision to donate organs and tissues; ensuring complete and unbiased information is provided to families with accuracy and empathy; offering opportunities for families to participate in a loved one's care to their level of comfort; and ensuring collaboration between family members, medical teams, and OPO staff, in the delivery of care.

The American Academy of Pediatrics Committee on Hospital Care (2010) asserts:

Organ donation is an integral part of EOL care that provides families with a final decision to make concerning a loved one. Every family should be given the opportunity for organ donation if it is medically appropriate, and it should be the expectation that the family will be approached in a professional, compassionate manner. The decision to donate is one made by the family, not by physicians. (p.826)

This policy statement further suggests that the collaboration between the broader medical community, inclusive of nurses, physicians, clergy, child life specialists, and social workers, in addition to OPO teams, is imperative to supporting donor families (American Academy of Pediatrics Committee on Hospital Care, 2010).

The Beryl Institute's white paper titled *What patient experience can learn from child life professionals* (2018) identifies numerous conclusions illustrating the rationale for CCLSs having a role in a variety of situations that address the human experience of healthcare and supporting the needs of all family members who participate in healthcare encounters. The document reinforces an awareness paramount to the overall patient experience: Teams must address the needs of the people they serve. It can be hypothesized that the role of an FSC within an OPO, with CCLS credentials or similar training and alternate licensure, and in conjunction with the many critical care settings and medical institutions they support, aims to fill a seemingly apparent gap in adult-centered care. As the Beryl Institute (2018) states:

This reveals an opportunity for both an acknowledgment of what child life can bring to bear and what healthcare organizations across the spectrum aspire to achieve in addressing the needs of the patients and families they serve. The questions raised are why are we so caring in pediatric settings only to turn so antiseptic in adult clinical environments? Why do we struggle to engage ideas from child life in adult settings where some cases exist of its benefits and value to all engaged in a care experience? And as many have asked, wouldn't it be nice if we could create a child life-like role elsewhere? (p. 3)

FSCs, with similar attainable goals to those of a CCLS, strive to support all families, defined by a commitment to patient- and family-centeredness. The Beryl Institute (2018) states that a CCLS can be considered a "bridge, a translator and a voice for the patient and family" (p. 10). An FSC can likewise be seen as a liaison between the triad of the OPO and donation processes, the critical care team, and the family, while advocating on behalf of the family's needs first and foremost.

Recommendations from the Committee on Non-Heart-Beating Transplantation II (2000) state that:

Like all care at the end of life, non-heart-beating organ and tissue donation should focus on the patient and the family. As an option for patients and families at the end of life, non-heart-beating donation should:

- follow patient and family wishes as closely as possible
- meet family needs for information, support and follow-up;
- recognize and respect patient and family social, economic and ethnic diversity; and
- follow clear mechanisms for identifying and covering all organ donation costs (p. 21)

Through compassionate and informative interactions with donor families as well as collaboration with medical team members and OPO staff, FSCs are uniquely positioned to promote a culture of patient- and family-centered care regardless of physical location, whether a family declines a donation opportunity or proceeds with donation authorization.

Therapeutic Relationships

Throughout a patient's hospitalization, during the initial donation conversation, and throughout the subsequent steps in the donation process, FSCs support families of organ donors striving to ensure that a family's needs are met, the family is supported and comfortable asking questions or advocating for their loved one, and that comfort exists in the donation decision, regardless of the outcome. While FSCs supporting the families of tissue and ocular donors may have a primary touchpoint directly with the family after a patient's death, and with less time overall compared to the duration of supporting families of organ, tissue, and eye donors, the goals remain similar; ensuring families have an opportunity to cope effectively with their unique circumstances, with an end goal of resilience and peace following the death of a loved one.

The relationship between FSCs and the families they support does not end upon organ recovery, which may differ from the relationship between a CCLS and the patients and families they support, generally only until a patient's discharge. While it is unlikely that a FSC will see donor families in person repetitively after their loved one is a donor, ongoing support and follow-up care is offered to donor families in many, if not all, OPO settings through aftercare events or check-ins, grief and bereavement workshops, and memorial celebrations. In some cases, the facilitation of donor family and recipient family communication and meetings is also a role of the FSC, allowing for further ongoing care and support of the donor family.

The ACLP (2018) affirms "therapeutic relationships established between child life professionals and children, families and their support systems create a safe environment that addresses their vulnerability and fosters positive coping, healing and enhanced resiliency (p.1). Child Life Competencies (ACLP, 2019) additionally emphasize that it is paramount for CCLSs to both initiate and maintain meaningful and therapeutic relationships with children and their families by aligning with components of patient- and family-centered care, effectively communicating with families, identifying values related to sociocultural diversity, and providing resources responsive to the needs of families to promote mastery of the information and experience.

FSCs and CCLSs aim to uphold the components of therapeutic relationships while adhering to professional boundaries and ethical duties.

UNIQUE METHODOLOGIES

While goals and expectations for working with families experiencing trauma and EOL decision making may be similar between FSCs and CCLSs, thus making the FSC role to be a natural fit for a child life professional, there are several regulatory requirements as well as standards of care and job responsibilities that are unique to the FSC.

During the organ procurement process, once a family has verbalized either their support of a patient's designation or has decided to donate on their behalf, FSCs complete OPO specific documentation and authorization forms confirming that a patient's decision-maker or legal next of kin is supportive of donation. Authorizing family members may determine their comfort regarding how donated gifts may be used for transplant, therapy, research, or education; may restrict specific organs or tissues based on family preference or funerary arrangements; and may limit transportation of a decedent for a variety of reasons. It is the responsibility of the FSC to ensure that families understand all information and options available so that both the donor and their family's wishes are respected and honored. Further, FSCs complete a medical and social history on behalf of the donor—the Uniform Donor Risk Assessment Interview—to gather pertinent details regarding the donor's medical and social experiences throughout their lifetime; this ensures the safety of any gifts that may be offered to another. Additionally, FSCs disseminate this information to clinical and administrator-level team members as appropriate as any details can affect the entire donor management phase of a donor case or have the potential to alter a donor's eligibility for donation. These areas and tasks of note are not typically required of CCLSs in traditional child life roles. Many, if not all, OPOs require auditing of consenting processes to verify that all questions are asked appropriately and according to regulatory requirements ensuring the safety of the donor, clinical OPO and hospital team members, and recipients of any donated organs, tissues, or corneas.

EXPANSION OF WORK

The expansion of CCLS-specific work in the realm of the FSC or complimentary OPO support role will continue to grow with time. The author was the first CCLS hired within their organization; just three years later the OPO now employs six full-time FSCs formally trained as child life specialists. As FSC positions are often filled by professionals with social work degrees and counseling licensures, it may be prudent to identify the ways that more diverse educational training and backgrounds within an OPO's family services or support departments may more wholly support organ, tissue, and eye donor families in accessing the best care experience throughout the donation process.

In addition to the identified applicability of a CCLS as an FSC, as the breadth of support CCLSs offer to OPOs expands, additional exploration is needed to evaluate the exact roles, or perhaps hybrid positions, which are a natural extension of child life work in supporting OPO missions, community members, and donor families. Based on the chapter author's anecdotal research, CCLSs hold or would be considered exceptional candidates for a wide variety of roles within OPO settings: community education specialists are tasked with increasing public awareness and donor registration numbers; hospital-to-OPO liaisons may be charged with providing both education and ongoing support to critical care team members who clinically support patients and families in emergency and intensive care settings and may also adopt a goal of increasing appropriate referrals; aftercare and ongoing bereavement support professionals may further provide extensive and ongoing grief counseling and donor-recipient relationships.

CONCLUSION

The Beryl Institute (2018) states:

In very significant ways, the philosophies and values of child life provide a clear blueprint for how to achieve success in experience overall. One question that was continually raised… is why do we not or how come we have been unable to ensure this same level of professional service for those beyond the pediatric setting? That is a question healthcare must ask itself: are all those receiving care deserving of this same level of attention and care?

The child life ideals are not unique for children, though they are focused on them. They are fundamentally the framework for taking care, in the broadest sense, of the patient and family in front of you. They are about supporting all those in the care experience and about ensuring we never lose sight that patient experience is a human business first. (p. 21)

The ACLP (2020a) identifies as one of the main principles in the *Child life code of ethics* that CCLSs demonstrate the competencies of the profession by ongoing efforts to improve professional services provided in varied and diverse settings, and within the community at large.

Dicks et al. (2017) states:

The in-hospital process is rich with opportunities for assisting families as they encounter the first tasks of their bereavement. The potential contribution of social support, togetherness, and inclusion when assisting families to find meaning in their experience and develop healthy bereavement practices should be explored to its fullest. Death also has an impact on work, school, religious, social and geographic communities, and the ripple effect of events at the hospital should receive more attention. (p. 13)

The FSC role in an OPO is a natural extension of child life knowledge, skills, and abilities expanded to a larger group of recipients of services, and not solely focused on children. Goals and strategic initiatives aim to support all families, regardless of background or circumstance, to ensure the donation opportunity is offered to all potentially eligible organ, tissue, and eye donors. Ultimately families are empathically supported regardless of their decision to donate.

As CCLSs continue to explore alternative and non-traditional settings in which their training, education, clinical experiences, and acquired skill-set are necessary and highly regarded, OPO careers should be of consideration, either in the position of an FSC or in an alternative role based upon the CCLS's goals and areas of expertise. All families facing EOL decisions on behalf of their loved one, whether wishes are documented or were never discussed, are deserving of compassionate, professional, informative support to navigate unfamiliar territory and honor their loved one's legacy in a uniquely profound way. Child life specialists, FSCs, and OPO team members alike strive to meet this need for all decedents and their families.

REFERENCES

ACLP. (2018). *Position statement on child life practice in community settings.* https://www.childlife.org/docs/default-source/about-aclp/cbp-on-cl-practice-in-community-settings.pdf

ACLP. (2020a). *Child life code of ethics.* https://www.childlife.org/docs/default-source/aclp-official-documents/child-life-code-of-ethics4232ee9c90156ede9dafff00004f030f.pdf

ACLP. (2020b). *Position statement on diversity, equity and inclusion.* https://www.childlife.org/docs/default-source/aclp-official-documents/statement-on-diversity-equity-and-inclusion

ACLP. (2019). *Child life competencies.* https://www.childlife.org/docs/default-source/aclp-official-documents/child-life-competencies_november-2019-updates

American Academy of Pediatrics Committee on Hospital Care, Section on Surgery, and Section on Critical Care. (2010). Policy statement: Pediatric organ donation and transplantation. *Pediatrics, 125*(4), 822-828. doi:10.1542/peds.2010-0081

Anthony, S. J., Lin, J., Pol, S. J., Wright, L., & Dhanani, S. (2021). Family veto in organ donation: The experiences of Organ and Tissue Donation Coordinators in Ontario. *Canadian Journal of Anaesthesia, 68*(5), 611–621. doi:10.100712630-021-01928-0 PMID:33575991

Association of Organ Procurement Organizations. (2022, March). *Job center*. https://aopo.org/job-center

Beryl Institute. (2018). *What patient experience can learn from child life professionals*. https://www.theberylinstitute.org/store/ViewProduct.aspx?id=11084124

Boles, J., Fraser, C., Bennett, K., Jones, M., Dunbar, J., Woodburn, A., Gill, M. A., Duplechain, A., Munn, E. K., & Hoskins, K. (2020). *The value of Certified Child Life Specialists: Direct and downstream optimization of pediatric patient and family outcomes*. ACLP. https://www.childlife.org/docs/default-source/aclp-official-documents/value-of-a-certified-child-life-specialist_full-report.pdf

Chandler, J. A., Connors, M., Holland, G., & Shemie, S.D. (2017). Effective requesting: A scoping review of the literature on asking families to consent to organ and tissue donation. *Transplantation, 101*(5S-1), S1-S16.

Cleiren, M. P., & Van Zoelen, A. A. (2002). Post-mortem organ donation and grief: A study of consent, refusal, and well-being in bereavement. *Death Studies, 26*(10), 837–849. doi:10.1080/07481180290106607 PMID:12440423

Committee on Non-Heart-Beating Transplantation II, The Scientific and Ethical Basis for Practice and Protocols, Division of Health Care Services, Institute of Medicine. (2000). Non-heart-beating organ transplantation: Practice and protocols. National Academy Press.

Dicks, S. G., Ranse, K., Northam, H., Boer, D. P., & van Haren, F. M. (2017). The development of a narrative describing the bereavement of families of potential organ donors: A systematic review. *Health Psychology Open, 4*(2). Advance online publication. doi:10.1177/2055102917742918 PMID:29379629

Donate Life America. (2022, February 25). *Organ donation statistics*. https://www.donatelife.net/statistics/

Fieten, J. (2021). Specialized resources: Organ donation and transplantation in pediatric care. *ACLP Bulletin, 39*(3), 13–15.

Grissom, S., Boles, J., Bailey, K., Cantrell, K., Kennedy, A., Sykes, A., & Mandrell, B. (2016). Play-based procedural preparation and support intervention for cranial radiation. *Supportive Care in Cancer, 24*(6), 2421–2427. doi:10.100700520-015-3040-y PMID:26634562

Haliko, S., & Arnold, R. (2002, November). *Discussing organ donation with families*. Palliative Care Network of Wisconsin. https://www.mypcnow.org/fast-fact/discussing-organ-donation-with-families/

Health Resources and Services Administration. (2021, September). *Donation after life*. https://www.organdonor.gov/learn/process/donation-after-life

Institute for Patient- and Family-Centered Care. (n.d.). *Core concepts of patient- and family-centered care*. https://www.ipfcc.org/about/pfcc.html

Kao, A. (2000, December). The Physician's Role in Discussing Organ Donation at the End of Life. *AMA Journal of Ethics*. https://journalofethics.ama-assn.org/article/physicians-role-discussing-organ-donation-end-life/2000-12

Koller, D. (2008). *Preparing children and adolescents for medical procedures.* ACLP. https://www.childlife.org/docs/default-source/research-ebp/ebp-statements.pdf

Organ Procurement and Transplantation Network. (2022, March). *National data*. https://optn.transplant.hrsa.gov/data/view-data-reports/national-data/#

Shemie, S. D., Robertson, A., Beitel, J., Chandler, J., Ferre, E., Evans, J., Haun, M., & Torrance, S. (2017). End of life conversations with families of potential donors: Leading practices in offering the opportunity for organ donation. *Transplantation, 101*(5S-1), s17-s26. doi:10.1097/TP.0000000000001696

United Network for Organ Sharing. (2022, March). *Organ procurement organizations*. https://unos.org/transplant/opos-increasing-organ-donation/

KEY TERMS AND DEFINITIONS

Brain Death: Irreversible cessation of brain function, death by neurological criteria, legal death with no brainstem reflexes present.

Decedents: A person who has died.

Designation: An individual's documented decision to donate their organs, tissues, or eyes after death.

EOL: End-of-life.

FSC: Family Services Coordinator.

OPO: Organ Procurement Organization.

Procurement (or Recovery): Consented recovery of a donor's organs, tissues, or eyes following death with the goal of donation for transplantation, research, or education.

WDLST: Withdraw of Life-Sustaining Therapies.

Chapter 4
Palliative Care and Hospice

Danielle Eaves Hernandez
Community Hospice and Palliative Care, USA

Emmalee Tresnan
Community Hospice and Palliative Care, USA

Magellan Taylor-Brickey
The University of Texas Southwestern Medical Center, USA

ABSTRACT

This chapter explores the emerging field of child life specialists' (CLS) role in hospital and community-based palliative and hospice care services. Relying heavily on their knowledge of child development, play, family systems, and grief to support patients and families through the trajectory of one's illness, child life specialists can adapt their skills to provide support in this environment. A CLS cannot change what is happening medically but can promote positive experiences for children involved to mitigate the potential trauma, ideally resulting in more positive psychosocial outcomes. Goals of care for CLSs in these settings can include developmentally appropriate education about a diagnosis, treatment plan, physical changes, prognosis, or end of life; various forms of play and therapeutic interventions for processing and the expression of feelings or emotions; memory-making; legacy building; anticipatory grief support; promoting opportunities to say goodbye; funeral or memorial preparation and advocacy for involvement; and bereavement support.

INTRODUCTION

In 2022, the Childhood Bereavement Estimation Model (CBEM) predicted that 1 in 13 children in the United States would experience the death of a parent or sibling by age 18, equivalent to approximately 5.6 million children (Judi's House/JAG Institute, 2022). This number increased to 1 in 7, or 13.9 million when examining bereaved youth by age 25. Parental and sibling loss is considered an adverse childhood experience (ACE) (Mersky, Janczewski & Topitzes, 2017). Adverse childhood experiences are traumatic events that affect the child's sense of safety and security. ACEs have detrimental effects that last a lifetime (e.g., psychosocial, emotional, physical, cognitive, financial, and educational) (Felitti et

DOI: 10.4018/978-1-6684-5097-0.ch004

al., 1998, Mersky, Janczewski & Topitzes, 2017). Measures examining a child's exposure to adverse experiences and risk for negative outcomes now include loss exposure, including parental and sibling death, as opposed to original studies focusing on forms of abuse and neglect (Finkelhor, 2020, Mersky, Janczewski & Topitzes, 2017).

When considering the causes of death in the 2022 CBEM National Report, life-threatening and life-limiting illnesses such as conditions related to birth, congenital disabilities, cancer, heart disease, and liver disease also leave children and youth at risk for other adverse childhood experiences outside of the death itself. Life-threatening and life-limiting illnesses have the potential for families, and children specifically, to endure prolonged toxic stress, or "extreme, frequent, or extended activation of the stress response that causes distress for the child and may lead to negative psychological and physical health outcomes" (Hornor, 2015).

Toxic stress related to chronic illness can be due to decreases in communication, disruption of daily activities, schedules, and routines, changes in social and familial relationships, emotional distress, the financial impact of illness, role conflicts and strain, and even one's overall health and well-being (Golics, Khurshid, Basra, Salek, and Finlay, 2013; Ell, 1996). In addition, chronic exposure to adverse childhood experiences without adequate support has shown to have the potential for long-term adverse psycho-social outcomes, including depression, anxiety, post-traumatic stress, fear, poorer school performance, lower levels of self-esteem, increased health problems, social-relational problems, and even physical changes to the developing brain (Phillips, 2014; Boullier & Blair, 2018; Eklund, Kreicbergs, Alvariza, and Lovgren, 2020; Bugge, Helseth, and Darbyshire, 2008; Hornor, 2015).

Alternatively, research on adverse childhood experiences showed that those with high positive experiences reported fewer mental and physical health challenges in adulthood. These outcomes lead to increases in resiliency through stable relationships with their caregiver and other caring adults, a sense of purpose, better self-regulation, positive coping skills, and increased social connections among friends and their community (Phillips, 2014; Eklund et al., 2020; Christ & Christ, 2006; Bugge, Helseth, and Darbyshire, 2008; Buchwald, Delmar, and Schantz-Laursen, 2011). The research focused on children's coping with serious illness and death found that families equipped with ample resources and support, such as access to staff with experience in talking to children and support programs, experience increased confidence and more positive psychosocial outcomes for all involved (Barnes, Kroll, Burke, Lee, Jones, and Stein, 2000; Fearnley, 2010; Christ & Christ, 2006; Bugge, Helseth, and Darbyshire, 2008).

Child life specialists in palliative care and hospice have the professional responsibility to advocate for the individualized needs of children coping with a loved one's serious illness or imminent death. Promoting open communication, processing feelings and emotions, developing coping skills, encouraging visitation, memory-making, and legacy building throughout a loved one's illness decreases the potential for long-term adverse effects (Christ & Christ, 2006; Buchwald, Delmar, and Schantz-Laursen, 2011; Barnes et al., 2000).

BACKGROUND

Palliative care and hospice are often used in tandem or interchangeably by providers, patients, and family members. However, palliative care and hospice are two different approaches in medicine focusing on quality of life. Palliative care is a specialty within the medical field focused on symptom management for those facing serious illnesses (Center to Advance Palliative Medicine, 2018, 2022; National Hospice and Palliative Care Organization, 2019). Hospice care provides care for the terminally ill, focused on palliation (comfort) when curative treatment is no longer an option. Hospice care involves medical care, pain management, and emotional/spiritual support. It can be provided inpatient or outpatient and focuses on maintaining quality of life and symptom control. Patients can be admitted to hospice when they have a terminal diagnosis of six months or less.

Palliative Care

A palliative care team consists of professionals that address the physical, mental, emotional, and spiritual needs of children and families facing life-threatening or life-limiting illnesses. This multidisciplinary team works with the medical team focusing on the patient's needs rather than the prognosis. The Center to Advance Palliative Care (2018) notes that over 90% of people who have experienced involvement in palliative care are likely to recommend this service to others. Palliative care has improved a patient's quality of life while reducing symptom burden and hospitalizations, ultimately driving increased patient satisfaction and positive outcomes. More than 1,700 hospitals have palliative care services available for patients and families (Center to Advance Palliative Care, 2018). In addition, palliative care continues to expand into community settings, such as outpatient clinics, skilled nursing, long-term and assisted living facilities, and the home setting.

Hospice

Hospice is a philosophy focused on dying with dignity (NHPCO, 2022; 2022a). Hospice services are available 24 hours a day for patients with a serious illness with a prognosis, or life expectancy, of six months or less and are focused on comfort rather than curative treatment (CMS, 2021). There is a critical difference in hospice care for pediatric and adult patients. While adult patients over the age of 21 follow the guidelines above regarding life expectancy and ceasing curative treatment, pediatric patients up to 21 can receive the benefit of hospice services while also pursuing curative treatment. This law is known as Concurrent Care for Children as part of the Affordable Care Act (ACA) and impacts children who qualify for Medicaid or CHIP, the Children's Health Insurance Program (NHPCO, 2019a). While this advancement in care is beneficial to children with complex, chronic medical conditions, providers still have to ask, "Would you be surprised if this patient died within six months or less should their disease follow its normal course?" (NHPCO, 2022).

Hospice comfort-focused therapies involve a reduction in medical interventions that no longer benefit the patient while increasing focus on pain control, symptom management, and quality of time with those important to the patient (NHPCO, 2022). Once enrolled with hospice, the hospice team assumes responsibility for all aspects of the patient's needs and provides bereavement support following the death of a loved one. A hospice interdisciplinary team typically includes a hospice physician, nurses, aides, social workers, chaplains or other counselors, and trained volunteers who support the patient and family as a loved one nears the end of life or is actively dying. Services are offered at four levels which include: routine, inpatient, continuous, and respite care (CMS, 2021). The Medicare Benefit Policy Manual (2021) defines each level of routine home care as a day on which an individual who has elected to receive hospice care is at home and is not receiving continuous home care. Inpatient care is a day on which an individual who has elected hospice care receives general inpatient care in an inpatient facility for pain control or acute or chronic symptom management that cannot be managed in other settings.

Continuous home care is a day on which an individual who has elected to receive hospice care is not in an inpatient facility (hospital, SNF, or hospice inpatient unit) and receives hospice care consisting predominantly of nursing care, continually at home. Hospice aide or homemaker services or both may also be provided on a continual basis. Continuous home care is only furnished during brief periods of crisis and only as necessary to maintain the terminally ill patient at home. Respite care is a day on which the individual who has elected hospice care receives care in an approved facility on a short-term basis for respite. At certain times, respite may be completed in the home setting. The level of service determines the location of care which could include: a hospital setting, inpatient hospice facility, long-term care, skilled nursing, assisted living facilities, or home.

Some states offer expanded services and programs under the hospice benefit, such as care coordination and case management, expressive therapies, counseling, respite care, and pediatric palliative care services. Therefore, it is necessary to be familiar with national and state guidelines around pediatric hospice care if providing child life services in this setting.

Cultural Considerations

In palliative care and hospice, cultural influences are a core tenet of quality care. As Ferrell (2015) states, "culture shapes how an individual makes meaning out of illness, suffering, and death" (pg. 47). Therefore, increased awareness and education regarding how a patient and family's culture impacts end-of-life decision-making, including family structure, language barriers, and death rituals, are critical components of the child life specialist's professional and ethical responsibility. The Association of Child Life Professionals (ACLP) Position Statement on Diversity, Equity, and Inclusion (n.d.) notes it is the child life specialist's professional responsibility to have an increased awareness of the diverse cultural needs of those served and for child life services to be delivered in a way that achieves and promotes culturally effective healthcare.

Family structure impacts children affected by serious illness and death. Multigenerational households are increasingly common, and varying generations of family members living under one roof can be due to financial hardship, economic crisis, loss of a spouse, and even a family member's health (Keene & Batson, 2010). In addition, families may choose multigenerational living arrangements as part of familial values and traditions. This shift in dynamics can impact roles and responsibilities among family members. For example, grandparents may assume caregiving duties for their grandchildren while parents work to financially support the family (Mustillo, Li, & Wang, 2020).

The potential loss of a loved one is considered a catastrophic experience across cultures, nearly 40% of healthcare providers identify cultural differences as a frequently occurring barrier to adequate palliative care, particularly in pediatrics (Davies et al., 2008; De Trill & Kovalcik, 1997). Cultural norms, religious practices, spiritual beliefs, and healthcare literacy, further complicates the appropriate integration of palliative care. Child life specialists assess cultural beliefs and lived experiences by supporting them on their journey with end-of-life decisions. Child life specialists should not assume that a family only adheres to a particular practice based on race, ethnicity, or religious affiliation. However, providing strengths-based interventions that address families' needs empowers them to make end-of-life choices that align with the family's cultural and spiritual practices (Wiener et al., 2015).

A family's willingness to accept palliative care or hospice services in pediatric and adult settings is challenged when language becomes a barrier. While a parent, spouse, medical power of attorney, or other family members may typically serve as the family spokesperson, one's normative hierarchical family structure is often waived based on the individual who is the most fluent in English leading to a child or adolescent becoming the family spokesperson (Campbell, 2006). Breakdowns in communication can frequently occur, leading to improper diagnosis, inadequate pain management, underutilization of prescription medications, and difficulty in obtaining informed consent between patients and their medical providers (Crom, 1994; Flores & Vega, 1998; Flores et al., 1998, 2000). Thus, when working with families who speak a different language than the providers, it is essential to understand that families can experience additional despair resulting in difficulty acquiring complete information about their person's health status or a physician's recommended interventions (Contro et al., 2002). While using a family member or a colleague can provide convenience for providers, this research emphasizes the need to use trained and credentialed medical interpreters to mediate communication between family and healthcare professionals. Furthermore, it also highlights the importance of intervening when children and teens serve as interpreters child life specialists should advocate for ethically appropriate interpretive services (Field & Behrman, 2003; Randhawa et al., 2003). Using a trained professional for language interpretation helps to identify when word choice results in a culture-related communication barrier.

Recognition of Cultural beliefs plays a role in family choices about sharing what and how healthcare and information about end of life with children. Therefore, the belief system should be assessed throughout care. Early and continued conversations help families process if and how these conversations will happen, in addition to the developmental needs of children and the long-term benefits of involving them in the medical experience, which is imperative to culturally responsive healthcare. Child life specialists promote and advocate for the family's cultural beliefs and practices, recognizing them as tools for coping and resilience (ACLP, 2020).

ADULT PALLIATIVE AND HOSPICE CARE

Parents and caregivers report uncertainty with developmentally appropriate ways of explaining a diagnosis, treatment plan, or physical changes due to illness, incorporating their child into the medical experience, and addressing a potential death (Barnes et al., 2000; Sutter & Reid, 2012; Fearnley, 2010; Taylor, Delevett, Kem, and Miller, 2017). Frequently, communication gaps are due to wanting to protect the child, not adding additional stress or a lack of knowledge regarding a child's understanding based on their developmental level. Often loved ones avoid potential questions about death and dying due to inaccessibility to a provider with this specific skill for support (Barnes et al., 2000; Buchwald, Delmar, and Schantz-Laursen, 2011; Sutter & Reid, 2012). Medical professionals in the adult setting, recognize the need for a member of the interdisciplinary team with the education and training to support children of adult patients.

There are few programs dedicated to supporting children of adult patients. Those that do exist tend to be within palliative care programs and are typically a one-person program or a consultant. These consults often come at end-of-life despite the significant opportunity to partner with families earlier in their medical experience. As adult palliative care teams expand within the medical field, the need for child life specialists continues to increase and awareness for earlier consults becomes evident. While well-meaning adults may avoid difficult conversations out of love and a desire to avoid increasing the stress of a child, many children draw their conclusions based on what is happening due to changes in demeanor, schedules, and routines. Research also shows that children and teens want information regarding a loved one's illness and treatment plan and often exhibit more positive psychosocial outcomes when given updates throughout a medical journey (Christ & Christ, 2006; Fearnley, 2010; McCue, 2014). Providing developmentally appropriate information and explanations allows the child to ask questions guiding how much additional information they would like to know.

Child life specialists, knowledgeable in child development, foster confidence in adults who care for children's immediate and long-term needs by providing education and resources on the importance of including children in a loved one's medical experience and tools to support their children. While there are many aspects of a medical experience, child life specialists can provide education and support on the following (Sutter & Reid, 2012; McCue, 2014; ACLP, 2018):

- How to explain a new or current diagnosis in a developmentally appropriate way
- How to explain a change in the treatment plan, as well as side effects of treatment
- Children's three most common concerns when an adult loved one is seriously ill.
    - *Can I catch it?*
    - *Did I cause it, or Can I fix it?*
    - *Who will do the ____ things while he/she is undergoing treatment?*
- Common physical, behavioral, and emotional changes children and teens can potentially exhibit in response to stress based on their developmental level
- Knowing when to identify risky behaviors that warrant a higher level of care
- An anticipated or unanticipated hospitalization, as well as preparation for visiting the hospital
- Verbal and written scripting for disclosing a poor prognosis, imminent death, or death that has already occurred
- Memory making
- Legacy work
- Education varying forms of grief (i.e., anticipatory, traumatic, complicated, typical) and associated grief responses based on developmental levels
- Acute trauma debriefings
- Acute grief support
- Preparing children for a funeral or memorial service
- Community resources for long-term support.

Before the child life specialist meets with a child, it is imperative to meet with caregivers for an initial assessment. It is essential to identify family desires related to information disclosure, timing, and cultural beliefs. Initial assessment also includes gathering information related to the child's current understanding and the patient's medical status. Often caregivers will ask a child life specialist to take the lead in conversations or assist them in disclosing difficult news to a child. Spreading the conversation over several visits builds trust and rapport while not overwhelming the child with too much information. Regardless of the relationship, illness, or traumatic event, child life specialists model simple, truthful, and developmentally appropriate language and positive coping techniques that continue open communication and support between the adult and child.

At times, children may benefit from one-on-one child life services. Families recognize it is helpful for children to have a trusting adult outside of the family to talk to, process their feelings, and ask questions they may not feel comfortable asking a parent. Children commonly want to protect their parents just as much as parents want to protect their children, so internalization of feelings, worries, concerns, and questions can be a typical response when a loved one is ill.

Child life specialists provide therapeutic interventions to support the child of adult palliative care and hospice patients. Child life specialists support the child and teen, offering appropriate choices, helping control an uncontrollable situation, and assisting in developing a trusting relationship. When meeting with children and teens, it is essential to take the children's development, coping, and relationship with the ill person into account. An initial visit with a child life specialist encourages normalization, deepens rapport, and provides a platform for a child life assessment. Child life specialists engage the child or teen in therapeutic activities and play to determine if the child needs time to feel comfortable talking with the CCLS. Child life specialists assessing support systems determine if a child or teen would benefit from visiting a loved one with other family members of similar ages or a separate visit from others. As outlined in the Association of Child Life Professionals' Standards and Guidelines for Child Life Practice in Community and Non-Traditional Settings, facilitating conversations supported by preparation, expressive arts, and play can help the child return to baseline and debrief before leaving or ending a visit (2020b). Leaving space for a game, coloring, or even a quick dance party are often helpful forms of normalized play. Child life sessions with children of adult patients are intense cognitive and emotional experiences resulting in an inability to focus if returning to school or leads to behavioral and emotional changes in the child. Debriefing after the child life session with the adult caregivers is critical, especially if there are any misconceptions, questions, worries, or needs that the caregivers need to know. It is essential to share the major themes of a session. Hence, the adults involved continue to participate in open communication and supportive measures at home and trust the child life specialist as a provider for future needs. Child life specialists in this setting are encouraged to work with the school system to support the impacted child in all areas of life.

Child life specialists working as part of a multidisciplinary adult palliative care team have opportunities to serve families in inpatient and outpatient settings. This flexibility allows for continuity of care and consistency in a provider for families throughout their medical experience that supports a therapeutic relationship throughout the illness, especially when a patient's illness becomes terminal. Furthermore, when a patient nears death, a child life specialist's role transforms depending on the family's needs. For example, for patients opting for comfort care within the hospital without hospice involvement, the patient continues to be managed by the palliative care team. Therefore, child life will provide services during the patient's death. Depending on the organization, the child life specialist provides acute bereavement support until the family feels services are no longer needed or transitions to a community resource for long-term support (i.e., grief support group, bereavement center, counselor, play therapist). Frequently, these community resources can have wait times for enrollment; therefore, acute grief support provided by the CCLS helps bridge the gap in supportive care and additional changes during the transition.

If a patient enrolls with hospice, three potential outcomes can occur for what hospice care entails:

1. General inpatient contract ("GIP") within the hospital setting
2. Hospice inpatient facility or another form of inpatient facility outside of the hospital
3. Home Hospice

Regardless of which happens, Certified Child Life Specialists work collaboratively to ensure a successful transition and partnership between the child life teams, hospice agency, and hospital system.

A unique difference for hospice child life specialists is the hospice mandate under the Center for Medicare and Medicaid Services (CMS) that stipulates bereavement care for a patient's family members for thirteen months after the death of a loved one (CMS, 2021). As a result, child life specialists working in hospice offer programming in addition to in-home grief support, support groups, family-focused weekend retreats, and summer camps specific for grieving children and teens. Moreover, additional programs are available to families living within the hospice's service area. Thus, child life specialists positively impact each family they serve and their community.

PEDIATRIC PALLIATIVE CARE AND HOSPICE

Child life specialists also provide care for pediatric patients in palliative care and hospice, their siblings, their families, and others in their community. Child life specialists tailor services to each family based on their assessment, focusing on the patient's and family's life, interests, culture, and wishes. Child life specialists have specific skills to support families through these difficult conversations promoting open, honest, and developmentally appropriate conversations with their children regarding diagnosis, treatment plans, prognosis, and end of life.

The preparation and support provided throughout a child's palliative care and hospice experience decreases trauma at end of life, promoting better overall family coping (Eaves, 2010). When afforded the opportunity of hours, days, months, or years, therapeutic interventions can be significantly impactful on the lives of patients and families. In addition, child life specialists are responsible for supporting the patient and their siblings, parents, relatives, and friends by promoting family-centered care practices.

These often include, but are not limited to:

- How to explain a change in the treatment plan, including the involvement of palliative care or hospice care
- Preparing for the transition home
- Common physical, behavioral, and emotional changes children and teens can potentially exhibit in response to stress based on their developmental level and knowing when to identify risky behaviors that warrant a higher level of care.
- Identifying developmentally appropriate interventions to support patients in maintaining control and autonomy through disease progression
- Preparing for an anticipated or unanticipated hospitalization, as well as preparation for visiting the hospital
- Verbal and written scripting for disclosing a poor prognosis, imminent death, or death that has already occurred
- Memory making, including wish trip assistance
- Legacy work
- Assistance in facilitating conversations around wishes at end-of-life
- Education on varying forms of grief (i.e., anticipatory, traumatic, complicated, typical) and associated grief responses based on developmental levels
- Preparing children for a funeral or memorial service, as well as an accompaniment if needed or desired
- Bereavement supports up to 13 months after a loss and community resources for long-term support when needed.

When initially meeting with a family, one of the child life specialist's roles is to help support families in understanding palliative or hospice care. Child life specialists educate the patient and siblings on changes in prognosis and the need for a new service team. This conversation builds rapport with all family members and establishes a healthy, therapeutic relationship between the team and the family and occurs while inpatient, outpatient, or in the patient's home. When families plan to receive services in their home, one must recognize that this is a child's safe place. When transitioning home, transforming a familiar space by rearranging furniture and organizing medical equipment (i.e., hospital bed, oxygen machine, ventilator, pain pump, station with supplies) can be uncomfortable and even scary for the patient and family members. Child life specialists can assist the family in normalizing the environment and experience by decorating the space to make it as comfortable and familiar as possible (Basak, Momaya, Guo, and Rathi, 2019). This simple intervention allows for normalization, mastery, choice and control, and self-expression.

SIBLINGS

The sibling of a medically complex child is sometimes unintentionally forgotten due to a chaotic schedule of appointments and events of the ill child. A more significant proportion of siblings of seriously ill children have been found to fall into at-risk or clinical ranges on measures of behavioral problems, anxiety, and depression, in comparison to normative samples (Alderful, Long, Lown, Marsland, Ostrowski, Hock, & Ewing, 2010). Several studies have found that externalizing problems, such as aggression and delinquency, are more common amongst siblings of children with a life-threatening or life-limiting illness when not acknowledged or supported (Breslau, Weistzman, and Messenger, 2010).

Healthy siblings may have their daily lives compromised in various ways depending on the ill sibling's disease progression, changes in the home environment, concern regarding a sibling's impending death, and the intense medical care and medical professionals coming in and out of the home at all hours (Moyson & Royers, 2012). Unfortunately, these factors often consume the parents' time, energy, focus, and resources, leaving siblings to navigate their own experiences alone or with minimal support. While many of the therapeutic interventions discussed in this section consider the whole family, a child life specialist can provide siblings additional support through one-on-one visits tailored to their needs.

Siblings are entitled to their emotions, reactions, and needs as much as everyone else in the family. Open communication with siblings is imperative for trust and emotional coping, as well as preparing for changes, especially when death is imminent. Child life specialists can empower parents with developmentally appropriate tools to promote the inclusion of siblings in all aspects of this journey while encouraging open communication and choice around the sibling's preferences for inclusion. A child life specialist's professional responsibility is to advocate for the patients and siblings.

THERAPEUTIC INTERVENTIONS

Once a family transitions to outpatient support and the palliative care or hospice child life specialist assumes the primary role in providing psychosocial support. There are several ways to promote developmentally appropriate care for the patient and family, such as play, bibliotherapy, legacy building and memory making, and developmental explanations.

Play

According to the Bill of Rights for Children with Terminal Illness, children "have the right to play, because even though I am dying, I am still a child" (Tristán, 2010). Play is vital to children's learning, processing, coping, and expression. Play supports rapport building, using familiar activities to get to know the child. For example, one can write questions on Jenga blocks that can help the child life specialist, patient, and family get to know one another before beginning difficult conversations. Jenga is a game many children are familiar with and willingly play, but adding the additional component can promote a therapeutic purpose. Play helps children process complex information and stressful situations while developing positive coping strategies. Using play to increase autonomy supports children's choices about materials, engagement, and interactions. Child life specialists and families can engage in therapeutic workbooks like *My Wishes* or *Voicing My Choices* as an interactive way to engage the child in making difficult decisions, such as end-of-life comfort plans or funeral arrangements, in a child-friendly way.

These tools give children the ability to have control and express their desires in uncontrollable situations while also assisting parents and caregivers in incorporating and honoring their child's wishes at end of life. Play encourages the identification, validation, and expression of feelings. It supports coping, increases self-esteem, and promotes connection. Finally, play enhances legacy and memory-making opportunities. The authors discuss this more in the first case study at the end of this chapter.

Bibliotherapy

Bibliotherapy uses books for psychosocial interventions to improve the coping skills of children and youth ages 3–18 (Pola & Nelson, 2014). Child life specialists often use bibliotherapy to facilitate conversations about diagnoses, identify and process feelings, develop positive coping techniques, and begin conversations about grief and loss. When choosing books, child life specialists consider developmental age, family situation, and need. For example, if a child has learned their sibling will die soon, a child life specialist uses the book, *Gentle Willow, to* explain concepts of death and grief in a developmentally appropriate way. Bibliotherapy partnered with therapeutic interventions connected to the story's theme provides opportunities to continue difficult conversations. In *Gentle Willow: A Story for Children About Dying* (*Gentle Willow*), Joyce C. Mills finds ways to remember the willow tree. Child life specialists use the book as a bridge to support a therapeutic intervention on legacy building. Books are beneficial when needing to explain a diagnosis, treatment option, disease progression, death, or when helping a child learn how to identify and cope with varying feelings and emotions (Pola & Nelson, 2014).

Books support transitions to therapeutic interventions by continuing conversations. They provide words and images that validate the experiences of children experiencing a variety of emotions and offer a way for children to express themselves. For example, in the book *How Will They Get That Heart Down Your Throat?: A Child's View of Transplants* by Karen Walton, the child life specialist, suggests decorating a pillowcase or picture frame as a way for the child to feel connected to their mom while she is in the hospital. When facilitating a bedside visit in an intensive care unit with the child, a child life specialist reads *Big Boss Brain: Learning About Traumatic Brain Injuries* by Shannon Maxwell to explain the role of the brain and how traumatic brain injuries impact the body. After reading the book, the child life specialist transitions to preparing the child for what they would see, hear, and experience at the bedside and offers them choices about visiting their sibling. Follow-up activities are offered to support the child's decision while continuing to foster the relationship between the sibling, identify positive coping mechanisms, and express feelings about the significant changes in the sibling.

Legacy Building and Memory Making

Therapeutic interventions focused on legacy building and memory-making are considered core components of the child life specialist's role in palliative and hospice care. Creating a good death experience that frames the end-of-life time period in a way that builds memories, legacy, and honors families' ongoing love and connection, is both possible, doable, and rewarding (Broden, Deatrick, Ulrich, and Curley, 2020). Legacy building and memory-making are two different concepts, though often intertwined. Legacy building is a "process of leaving something behind…one's belongings, one's memories, one's values, and even one's body" (Hunter & Rowles, 2005, p. 328). Memory-making is the intangible aspect of the intervention and promotes positive experiences, building memories during an otherwise stressful and traumatic experience.

Creating keepsakes as part of a patient's legacy allows for tangible items made by the patient, or patient and family, and are cherished after a patient's death. Child life specialists promote a patient's legacy through keepsakes such as handprint and footprint-related artwork, 3D molds, fingerprint jewelry, locks of hair, letter writing, heartbeat recordings and heartbeat strips, voice recordings, videos, and photography. While this is not an all-encompassing list, those facilitating these interventions must be comfortable with the processes and familiarize themselves with techniques, materials, and new ideas to create quality memorabilia.

The average hospice length of stay does not always permit the time or availability of a child life specialist to assist in the completion of keepsakes before a patient's time of death. Although rare, postmortem legacy work may be completed and could occur in a morgue or at a funeral home. Parents found that receiving legacy items was helpful (Brooten et al., 2013; Macnab et al., 2013; Neidig & Dalgas-Pelish, 1991) for those who lost a child, including aspects of hand or footprints, locks of hair, photos of the child, and memory boxes. (Butler, Hall, Willets, and Copnell, 2015).

Memory-making can be a part of legacy-focused interventions but is also a way to celebrate life in ways a patient and family find meaningful. While memory-making may involve elaborate wish trips, it may also include normative everyday events (e.g., reading a book or cooking together, planting a garden), traditions and celebrations (e.g., holidays, graduations, birthdays), and intentional family experiences. The essential aspects are the patient's wishes, the family's wishes, the availability of resources and support, and what is possible, given the patient's medical status and potential time frame.

Developmental Explanations

Providers and parents indicate difficulties finding the correct language and approach to addressing the end of life with a seriously ill child (Wiener, Pao, Kazak, Kupst, Patenaude, and Arceci, 2015). As a result, adults often use euphemisms when talking to children, causing misconceptions about death and dying. Child life specialists in hospice often provide parental education on the importance of honesty when death is nearing through simple, truthful, and developmentally appropriate conversations. Adults are the gatekeepers to information that children receive. Personal experiences, culture, spiritual and religious beliefs, and the influence of others can play a role in how much caregivers choose to share with children. Children and teens facing life-threatening and life-limiting illnesses have a right to the truth

(Tristán, 2010). Ethically, children are entitled to know what is happening to their bodies. When parents embrace these conversations and process them together as a family, children have increased opportunities for processing, clarifying complex information, addressing misconceptions, worries, and concerns, and begin preparing for death. These conversations lead to positive coping throughout end-of-life, as children living with a life-limiting illness who receive open communication about their diagnosis and prognosis experience significantly less anxiety and depression (Last & Van Veldhuizen, 1996).

As end-of-life conversations continue, the child life specialist's primary goal is to encourage opportunities that allow the child a sense of autonomy and control during an unpredictable experience. Most medical training concentrates on treating illness and disease in a curative way. Child life specialists encourage preparation for children and involve them in decision-making about their treatment and care plan determining what the child deems to be a good death (Tristán, 2010). Helpful tools to facilitate these conversations include "*My Wishes" and "Voicing My Choices*," which are child- and adolescent-friendly advanced care planning documents that outline end-of-life wishes addressing physical, mental, emotional, and spiritual needs. These tools assist patients who want to leave their toys or special mementos to family members or friends.

While supporting families as they prepare a child for their death, child life specialists advocate for preparing a patient's siblings. Preparation at the end of life could include the equipment's sights, sounds, smells, medications, and bodily changes the ill child may experience. Working with siblings on a plan of care for when the patient is actively dying provides siblings choice and control regarding how they learn of the death, identify trusted adults and peers for support, and how they choose to say goodbye. Child life specialists provide choices such as whether the sibling wants to be woken up if the death is in the middle of the night or if they want to be home when the patient is actively dying. If the death happens during the day, a child could choose if they want to be picked up from school and by whom, or not told until the end of the day when they arrive home. Children can decide whether to say goodbye to their loved one after they have died and if they want to assist with post-mortem care. It is critical to give siblings the option and control of visiting a loved one and respecting their wishes while also being a support system at the patient's bedside. Although patients may be minimally responsive, the child life specialist can still use language such as "their eyes are closed, but they can still hear" to reinforce communication and continued connection between patients and family members during the final moments.

CONTINUITY IN CHILD LIFE SERVICES

One key aspect to remember when initially meeting with a new pediatric palliative or hospice patient is that they likely have already received some form of support from one or more child life specialists. It is critical to partner with this provider as an added layer of support for the family, just as the palliative care team does with the primary medical team. Through the creation of a partnership, a family receives enhanced and thorough psychosocial support specific to the additional complex needs that arise due to serious illness.

A patient diagnosed with Ewing's Sarcoma has received direct support from the hospital oncology child life specialist for approximately one year, including diagnosis education, procedural preparation and support, emotional coping, and normalization opportunities through frequent hospitalizations for treatment. This patient has two younger brothers. The parents recently learned her cancer has metastasized, and her only option is palliative, non-curative treatment. The family met with palliative care to improve her quality of life and symptom burden. Parents requested that the child life specialist assist them with talking to their daughter about the change in her medical status, including her prognosis, and preparation for upcoming changes to her treatment plan. They also asked for assistance talking to the patient's brothers to discuss the prognosis and navigating conversations with friends. In this situation, the palliative care child life specialist partnered with the hospital's oncology child life specialist. They collaborated to define their roles and responsibilities, leading to continuity of care for the family. In this situation, the hospital oncology child life specialist helped the family explain the disease progression and planned palliative treatment to the patient. The palliative care child life specialist assisted with sibling support and navigating peers.

PROFESSIONAL BOUNDARIES

Professional boundaries are vital to maintaining therapeutic relationships and an important part of self-care. Child life services provided in hospital or outpatient settings have established boundaries for professional and patient-care relationships. Patient's hospital, clinic, playroom, and therapy spaces offer physically defined spaces for work. Healthcare systems provide employee training regarding codes of conduct, setting clear expectations and guidelines for provider and patient relationships. These are in place to protect patients, families, and healthcare professionals. Establishing boundaries assists child life specialists in developing their self-care strategies and identifying interactions that are appropriate to engage in with a family. These rules often include expectations around sharing personal information, continued contact after discharge or death, caring for a family member or friend, protected health information, and even social media (ACLP, n.d). Blurring lines or disregarding a healthcare system's expectations can have significant consequences, including termination. Healthcare professionals in palliative care and hospice are at an increased risk of encountering situations where professional boundaries quickly become blurred, given the intimacy of companioning families through a life-limiting illness or end-of-life. This is especially true when providing home-based services (Sanders, Bullock, and Broussard, 2012; Knatt & Slattery, 2004). Poor professional boundaries can be detrimental to a decline in "personal accomplishment, emotional exhaustion, and desensitization," all factors of burnout (Maslach & Jackson, 1981). Burnout is "a syndrome of emotional exhaustion and cynicism," and healthcare providers are at significant risk for burnout due to the daily work of caring for others (Maslach and Jackson, 1981, p. 99). Professional boundaries establish a therapeutic relationship between the child life specialist, patient, and family and are an important component of self-care.

Time & Patient Load

Child life specialists in palliative care and hospice are working with families in crisis and often fluctuate their hours based on patient and family needs. Child life specialists must assess each circumstance to determine if the situation is a boundary violation. While unintentionally harmful, occasional exceptions can become frequent behaviors (Sanders, Bullock, and Broussard, 2012). To establish boundaries and self-care, child life specialists working with families in crisis must critically evaluate their decisions concerning professional and personal time.

The number of patients on one's census can impact professional boundaries. Although census needs vary, the distance the child life specialist travels, family needs, and the child life specialist's experience and skill impact the number of patients a CCLS can work with per shift. Signs that a census acuity is too high and could lead to burnout include needing to work late or come in early, inability to take a lunch break, completing documentation at home or the next day, and lacking the cognitive ability to process services provided at the end of the workday.

Attachment

In the field of medicine, providers of all kinds supporting those who are chronically ill can develop an attachment to their patients. Attachments form between individuals when one or both provide care in times of need, and attachment-related behaviors can be triggered when one feels threatened, whether perceived or real. While attachment theories focus on the parent-child relationship, attachment is also likely relevant to the clinician-patient and clinician-family relationship (Tan, Zimmerman, and Rodin, 2005). Attachment happens from the patient toward the provider and the provider towards the patient and family. This can be especially true in pediatrics and for children with chronic illness due to providing care during a prolonged time of need and the increased frequency of exposure. Increased attachment from a provider could potentially cause territorial behaviors between service lines, ultimately hurting the patient and family. Viewing services as a partnership rather than a transition of care will allow a family to receive comprehensive and in-depth support while maintaining healthy, therapeutic relationships.

Secondary Trauma

Child life specialists in any environment endure many stressful situations and witness trauma in their day-to-day responsibilities. Engaging in self-care is not only therapeutic but also healing in nature. Unfortunately, while working in palliative care and hospice settings, child life specialists are at an increased risk of psychological issues, secondary trauma, compassion fatigue, and high stress and exhaustion levels due to frequent exposure to cases involving death and trauma (Taylor-Brickey, 2020). In contrast to the common tendency of most individuals, which would be to avoid thinking and talking about death, palliative care, and hospice workers expose themselves repeatedly to the process of dying and death (Samson & Shvartzman, 2018). Direct exposure to traumatic events, such as death, or indirect exposure- hearing about traumatic events from an individual directly affected by it- puts palliative care and hospice child life specialists at the highest risk for burnout among their child life peers and multidisciplinary teams.

Grief

Child life specialists must recognize triggers and be prepared to address emotional distress when working with grieving children and teens. Grief bursts are sudden moments of sadness, sorrow, or other emotional responses that occur in response to a trigger related to the deceased. These triggers occur in the hospital setting and in response to a death anniversary, birthday, a song, or driving by a former patient's neighborhood or funeral home. Palliative care and hospice child life specialists experience triggers due to the environment in which they work. Child life specialists must prioritize self-care to provide the best support for patients and families. Additionally, prioritizing opportunities for support from a trained colleague or community professional (i.e., licensed counselor, psychologist, clergy) is critical to debrief and process the continual exposure to trauma and grief associated with these positions. Regular, continuous support from these mental health professionals can be beneficial for long-term coping and assistance in recognizing when one is embarking on compassion fatigue or burnout.

SELF-CARE

Child life specialists must prioritize upholding professional boundaries and use self-care methods regularly. Self-care is individualized and must be more than a relaxation technique. There must be an in-depth understanding and reflection of oneself to have effective self-care strategies, including professional help. Furthermore, when one is functioning in a one-person program, it is imperative to have a mentor to serve as a clinical supervisor to foster professional growth. It is up to each child life specialist to recognize challenges and advocate for clinical supervision, increased training, or more positions.

As these expanded child life roles continue to grow outside of the pediatric hospital walls, many programs with full-time child life specialists are one-person child life programs. Child life specialists in this setting prove the need for additional positions and find other funding but often work alone. Child life specialists in this role must collaborate with other hospice and palliative care child life specialists for support. While working with individuals on an interdisciplinary team is helpful, the support between other child life specialists in similar roles is beneficial on many levels.

The roles discussed in this chapter involve a significant risk of daily exposure to death and trauma and a strong foundation in child life practice. Child life specialists with experience and training in grief and loss are best prepared to work in palliative care and hospice settings. Having strong professional boundaries and self-care practices helps with longevity in a high-risk position.

CONCLUSION

Outpatient and home-based child life services for pediatric families and children of adult patients provide a continuum of care, so no family is facing serious illness or death alone. All children have a right to their views, understanding, and opinions about the death and dying process and their grief. The Hospice Foundation of America (2008) argues that "it's impossible to protect children from loss. However, adults can teach ways of adapting to loss by including young people in the grieving process." Child life specialists know this to be true, and pediatric families and children of adult patients can benefit from the vast support child life specialists provide to mitigate trauma and prevent unhealthy and severe negative, long-term psychosocial outcomes (AACAP, 2018).

Child life services must be seen as a standard of care in pediatric and adult palliative care and hospice programs. A child life specialist's unique and specific training and educational background in child development, family systems, and coping make child life an ideal fit for guiding and supporting children during the palliative care and hospice experiences. Our professional responsibility is to advocate with the Association of Child Life Professionals for this practice and with NHPCO. While a great deal of work lies ahead, the future is bright for child life specialists to become a permanent and prominent component of pediatric and adult palliative care and hospice care.

CASE STUDIES

Pediatric Hospice Patient

Alexis is a 16-year-old with advanced type 1 Neurofibromatosis. Following the onset of poor balance and difficulty hearing, several inoperable brain tumors were found on her magnetic resonance imaging (MRI). Alexis and her family agreed to enroll in a community-based pediatric hospice program. Upon admission, this family met with a hospice nurse and social worker, which led to a referral for child life services. The child life specialist collaborated with the team about aspects of Alexis' initial admission and important factors of their family dynamics, such as cultural considerations, religious beliefs, disease understanding, and acceptance. The child life specialist contacted Alexis' mom to introduce herself and child life services. During the initial assessment, Alexis's mother openly shared how Alexis's diagnosis has impacted their family dynamics. The child life specialist and Alexis's mother agreed to a home visit to support Alexis and her 14-year-old sister, Emma.

Goals of care established for Alexis and her family included promoting optimal quality of life, pain and symptom management, memory making, and sibling support. Alexis's parents remained open and honest about Alexis's disease progression and prognosis with both of their daughters, which the child life specialist validated and reinforced. The first task that was completed was to desensitize Alexis's new space, as a new hospital bed and medical equipment were going to take over her living room. Emma and the child life specialist turned Alexis's room into a tropical paradise to desensitize the mini-intensive care unit that moved into their home. Over the course of four months, which included Alexis's decline and ultimate death, the child life specialist worked with Alexis to establish her motto and complete her "bucket list." Instead of having a mindset around the increasingly popular motto 'YOLO' (You Only Live Once), Alexis modified this into 'YODO' (You Only Die Once). This motto truly exemplified her philosophy in life. The child life specialist collaborated with a local wish-granting organization to ensure the "bucket list" experiences occurred, such as being able to swim with dolphins, celebrating potentially missed holidays early with her family, and planning all aspects of her celebration of life.

While working with Alexis's sister Emma, it is important to note she was a quiet young lady who had a desire to protect her family. She would only discuss the fear of Alexis dying while outside in the garage. The child life specialist worked with her and her parents to identify coping outlets and support systems. Emma enjoyed playing board games with her sister, and the child life specialist assisted them with creating their own. This not only promoted connection, normalization, and play but promoted a positive memory-making experience during a time of sadness and distress. Additionally, the child life specialist offered Emma several options to create keepsakes that would also promote positive memories and legacy work opportunities. Ultimately, Emma chose to create a canvas of her four family members' handprints and even included their beloved dog's paw prints for their home. Alexis wrote "Ohana'', in reference to the "Lilo and Stitch" movie quote, "Ohana means family and family no one is left behind or forgotten."

The 'YODO' philosophy drove the family's plan of care. Alexis continued to decline, and the child life specialist helped her maintain her ability to communicate through adaptive communication applications to ensure she could speak to her family and vice versa. Alexis texted and typed many of her conversations with her family, friends, and the hospice interdisciplinary team. It was vital for Alexis to be part of the conversations and decisions being made about her medical care and end-of-life choices. Specifically, her parents did not want Alexis to die at home, while Alexis voiced that she wanted to remain home as long as possible. Therefore, once Alexis became unresponsive and was actively dying, she was admitted to the hospice inpatient unit. The child life specialist continued supporting Emma through a comforting presence, developmentally appropriate education about what was happening, opportunities for coping and self-expression, and allowing choices when able for autonomy in an uncontrollable situation.

The child life specialist attended Alexis' celebration of life and reinforced how it honored her final wishes and life. The child life specialist offered bereavement visits for Emma and reinforced grief support for Alexis's family through bereavement resources. Her family expressed sincere appreciation and wanted to share Alexis's story with others. The parents have since participated in two conference panels the child life specialist has moderated. Additionally, her family attended the annual bereavement retreat the hospice organization hosts each year.

**Protective patient information has been changed for HIPAA purposes.*

Adult Palliative Care and Hospice Patient

Ryan was a 35-year-old male with a diagnosis of metastatic colon cancer. He was originally diagnosed four years prior and was hospitalized five times over the past year. Palliative care was consulted for pain management, as his cancer had now spread to his liver and abdomen, and he had biliary stents placed during this admission due to new onset blockage in his bile ducts. When meeting with Ryan and his wife, Caitlin, the palliative care physician and social worker, learned about their three children- Sam (4), Sadie (6), and Sophie (8). They were initially hesitant to accept child life support, as their children were aware of their dad's cancer and felt they "had it under control." A few days later, Caitlin decided she was ready to learn more, and the child life specialist met with her and Ryan at the bedside.

When initially meeting with this family, Ryan was not ready to discuss the reality of his prognosis. At the same time, Caitlin wanted to talk about how to prepare her children for the fact that Ryan may not make it to Christmas. Ryan was open to Caitlin and the child life specialist discussing her concerns further but did not want to be a part of the conversation. Validating how difficult this was for him, Caitlin and the child life specialist stepped into a conference room for an almost two-hour conversation. Sadie and Sophie were aware their dad had cancer, and it was in his colon. They had watched him go through multiple forms of treatment, including surgery, and Caitlin and Ryan had done a beautiful job of being open and honest with their children at each step. Sam had been told his dad was 'sick,' and they used the word 'cancer' with him. They would talk about "daddy getting medicine" and did an excellent job of keeping things at the simplest level for him. Caitlin felt they needed to begin conversations about death but was also fearful of having this conversation "too early" or "too late." She also had a lot of concerns around becoming a single parent and raising three children, as she grew up in a single-parent household and did not want them to grow up with the same "adult responsibilities" she had or with the stigmas that accompany minority children being raised by a single mom. Caitlin and the child life specialist talked a lot about how to prepare children when a parent *could die*, and the children sent her home with written scripting to help her with this conversation. The child life specialist also gave her virtual links to several books she could choose from to help with this conversation as well. Caitlin was well-equipped to talk to her children and support them in preparing for what could come and shared that she would reach out if additional child life support was needed.

Ryan was admitted several times between this initial visit and his final hospitalization. The child life specialist would check in with Ryan and Caitlin each time, and they continued to wait on having this difficult conversation due to feeling it was "too early." They would also talk with the palliative care team about their desire to focus on the quality of life and not spending time in the hospital, yet they struggled to accept that Ryan would benefit from home hospice and continued coming back to the hospital each time he experienced a pain crisis or new physical decline. Ryan's final hospitalization was due to a bloodstream infection that led to sepsis, and he ultimately experienced a cardiac arrest. After multiple rounds of resuscitation, Ryan was intubated and sedated on a ventilator in the intensive care unit (ICU), with support from multiple vasopressors. He was at risk for cardiac arrest again, and Caitlin was faced with a very difficult decision. She changed his code status to a Do Not Attempt Resuscitation (DNAR), meaning if Ryan arrested again, they would not perform CPR, and staff would continue with current therapies of support. She asked about taking him home on hospice, but this was no longer an option. Ryan was too unstable, which also meant inpatient hospice at another facility was no longer an option. After several hours, Caitlin was able to say this was not what Ryan would want, and she wanted to move forward with the decision to withdraw from life-sustaining treatment. She requested to meet with hospice to do a GIP contract, so she would have bereavement support for herself and her children. While this meeting was happening, Ryan's parents brought Sam, Sadie, and Sophie to the hospital. Caitlin asked that the child life specialist help explain what happened to their father and the plan for withdrawing life-sustaining treatment later that evening. Having the opportunity to say goodbye was a must for Caitlin, but Ryan's parents disagreed with this decision. They were very vocal in feeling Sam, Sadie, and Sophie should remember their dad "like he was before" and that seeing him in the ICU would be "traumatizing" for them. The child life specialist was able to help Caitlin by explaining the benefits of having this opportunity and how we would not only prepare them for the visit but also offer them the ability to make an informed choice about visitation. The child life specialist helped Caitlin explain what was happening to her children, and it went something like this: *"Last night, daddy's heart stopped working, but the doctors were able to make it start beating again. Right now, daddy has a machine, called a ventilator, breathing for him because his lungs are unable to breathe on their own. The doctors are doing everything they can to try and help daddy, but his body is so sick from cancer and the blood infection that his body is beginning to shut down. There will come a time very soon when the doctors take the tube out of daddy's mouth, and this will allow his body to breathe on its own. He may breathe on his own for a little while, but there will come a time soon after when his body stops working, and he dies."*

Sam sat in Caitlin's lap and hugged her while Sadie and Sophie had a lot of questions about *why* his body was shutting down. The child life specialist helped them process how cancer had spread throughout Ryan's body, how a blood infection works, and what happens when someone's heart stops beating. Ultimately, they were able to recognize their 'daddy' was dying, and they wanted to see him. Caitlin prepared them for what they would see and hear in the room, how they could talk to their 'daddy,' and he could hear them, but he would not be able to talk back to them. All three children opted to go to the bedside and sat holding Ryan's hand while reflecting on positive memories, things they would miss about their daddy, and verbalizing how much they loved him and would miss him. During this time, Sam, Sadie, and Sophie completed thumbprint hearts for their additional family members as a keepsake, as well as handprint posters for their family. After this, they chose to take a break and joined many extended family members in the ICU waiting area. Ryan's parents said they could not believe how well the kids did and talked about feeling grateful to witness this experience. The bedside nurse also shared in a separate conversation how she was new to the ICU setting and had not experienced a death where kids were involved before. She talked about how appreciative she was to witness this because it changed her views on kids being able to visit at end-of-life.

Caitlin chose to prolong withdrawing life-sustaining treatment for two more days and the child life specialist continued to meet with Sam, Sadie, and Sophie each day as they visited. They read books to help reinforce their understanding of death and their family's belief in Heaven. They created memory boxes and wrote letters/drew pictures that were placed in Ryan's hands during their final time together. Caitlin did move forward with enrolling in GIP hospice, however, due to the relationship the hospital child life team had already established with her children, she was not ready to transition to their child life specialist. The hospital child life specialist facilitated several bereavement visits for acute bereavement support, and this family was ultimately able to transition to the hospice child life specialist for further support at home. Sophie was able to attend a local grief camp that summer, and this entire family signed up to attend a family retreat weekend with the hospice organization later that year.

**Protective patient information has been changed for HIPAA purposes.*

REFERENCES

Alderfer, M. A., Long, K. A., Lown, E. A., Marsland, A. L., Ostrowski, N. L., Hock, J. M., & Ewing, L. J. (2010). Psychosocial adjustment of siblings of children with cancer: A systematic review. *Psycho-Oncology*, *2010*(19), 789–805. doi:10.1002/pon.1638 PMID:19862680

Association of Child Life Professionals. (2018). *Position statement on child life practice for children of adult patients.* Retrieved June 2022, from https://www.childlife.org/docs/default-source/aclp-official-documents/cbp-on-cl-practice-for-children-of-adult-patients_deireviewed.pdf?sfvrsn=4eb5834d_2

Association of Child Life Professionals. (2020). *Child life code of ethics.* Retrieved June 2022, from https://www.childlife.org/docs/default-source/aclp-official-documents/child life code-of-ethics4232ee-9c90156ede9dafff00004f030f.pdf?sfvrsn=5327804d_2

Association of Child Life Professionals. (2020a). *Position statement on clinical supervision and reflective practice.* Retrieved June 2022, from https://www.childlife.org/docs/default-source/aclp-official-documents/clinical-supervision.pdf?sfvrsn=61398c4d_2

Association of Child Life Professionals. (2020b). *Standards and guidelines for child life practice in community and non-traditional settings.* Retrieved June 2022, from https://www.childlife.org/docs/default-source/aclp-official-documents/community-based-standards-and-guidelines_final-approved.pdf?sfvrsn=c7d1864d_2

Association of Child Life Professionals. (n.d.). *Position statement on diversity, equity, and inclusion.* Retrieved June 2022, from https://www.childlife.org/docs/default-source/professional-development/utilizing-ethical-tenets-and-the-child-life-code-of-ethics-to-navigate-social-networking_final.pdf?sfvrsn=d2ec834d_2

Association of Child Life Professionals. (n.d.a). *Utilizing ethical tenets and the child life code of ethics to navigate social networking.* Retrieved June 2022, from https://www.childlife.org/docs/default-source/aclp-official-documents/statement-on-diversity-equity-and-inclusion.pdf?sfvrsn=c4d0864d_2

Barnes, J., Kroll, L., Burke, O., Lee, J., Jones, A., & Stein, A. (2000). Qualitative interview study of communication between parents and children about maternal breast cancer. *BMJ (Clinical Research Ed.)*, *321*(7259), 479–482. doi:10.1136/bmj.321.7259.479 PMID:10948027

Basak, R., Momaya, R., Guo, J., & Rathi, P. (2019). Role of Child Life Specialists in Pediatric Palliative Care. *Journal of Pain and Symptom Management*, *58*(4), 735–737. doi:10.1016/j.jpainsymman.2019.05.022 PMID:31195077

Baverstock, A., & Finlay, F. (2008). What can we learn from the experiences of consultants around the time of a child's death? *Child: Care, Health and Development*, *34*(6), 732–739.

Behrman, R. E., & Field, M. J. (2003). *When Children Die: Improving Palliative and End-of-Life Care for Children and Their Families* (1st ed.). National Academies Press.

Boullier, M., & Blair, M. (2018). Adverse childhood experiences. *Paediatrics & Child Health*, *28*(3), 132–137. doi:10.1016/j.paed.2017.12.008

Breslau, N., Weitzman, M., & Messenger, K. (1998). Psychologic functioning of siblings of disabled children. *Pediatrics*, *67*(3), 344–353. doi:10.1542/peds.67.3.344 PMID:6454107

Broden, E. G., Deatrick, J., Ulrich, C., & Curley, M. A. Q. (2020). Defining a "Good Death" in the Pediatric Intensive Care Unit. *American Journal of Critical Care*, *29*(2), 111–121. doi:10.4037/ajcc2020466 PMID:32114610

Brooten, D., Youngblut, J. M., Seagrave, L., Caicedo, C., Hawthorne, D., Hidalgo, I., & Roche, R. (2013). Parent's perceptions of health care providers actions around child ICU death: What helped, what did not. *The American Journal of Hospice & Palliative Care*, *30*(1), 40–49. doi:10.1177/1049909112444301 PMID:22531149

Buchwald, D., Delmar, C., & Schantz-Laursen, B. (2011). How children handle life when their mother or father is seriously ill and dying. *Scandinavian Journal of Caring Sciences*, *26*(2), 228–235. doi:10.1111/j.1471-6712.2011.00922.x PMID:21950563

Bugge, K. E., Helseth, S., & Darbyshire, P. (2008). Children's Experiences of Participation in a Family Support Program When Their Parent Has Incurable Cancer. *Cancer Nursing*, *31*(6), 426–434. doi:10.1097/01.NCC.0000339250.83571.b0 PMID:18987509

Butler, A., Hall, H., Willets, G., & Copnell, B. (2015). Parents' experiences of healthcare provider actions when their child dies: An integrative review of the literature. *Pediatric Nursing*, *20*(1), 5–20. doi:10.1111/jspn.12097 PMID:25443391

Campbell, A., & Campbell, A. (2006). Spiritual care for sick children of five world faiths. *Paediatric Nursing*, *18*(10), 22–25. doi:10.7748/paed.18.10.22.s18 PMID:17193915

Center for Medicare and Medicaid Services. (2021). *Chapter 9 - Coverage of hospice services under hospital insurance*. Retrieved June 2022, from https://www.cms.gov/Regulations-and-Guidance/Guidance/Manuals/Downloads/bp102c09.pdf

Center to Advance Palliative Care. (2018). *What is palliative care*. Retrieved June 24, 2022, from https://www.capc.org/about/palliative-care/

Center to Advance Palliative Care. (2022). *What is pediatric palliative care*. Retrieved June 25, 2022, from https://getpalliativecare.org/whatis/pediatric/

Christ, G. H., & Christ, A. E. (2006). Current Approaches to Helping Children Cope with a Parent's Terminal Illness. *CA: a Cancer Journal for Clinicians*, *56*(4), 197–212. doi:10.3322/canjclin.56.4.197 PMID:16870996

Contro, N., Larson, J., Scofield, S., Sourkes, B., & Cohen, H. (2002). Family Perspectives on the Quality of Pediatric Palliative Care. *Archives of Pediatrics & Adolescent Medicine*, *156*(1), 14. doi:10.1001/archpedi.156.1.14 PMID:11772185

Crom, D. B. (1994). The experience of South American mothers who have a child being treated for malignancy in the United States. *Journal of Pediatric Oncology Nursing*, *12*, 104–112. PMID:7646829

Davies, B., Sehring, S. A., Partridge, J. C., Cooper, B. A., Hughes, A., Philp, J. C., Amidi-Nouri, A., & Kramer, R. F. (2008). Barriers to Palliative Care for Children: Perceptions of Pediatric Health Care Providers. *Pediatrics*, *121*(2), 282–288. doi:10.1542/peds.2006-3153 PMID:18245419

De Trill, M. D., & Kovalcik, R. (1997). The Child with Cancer. Influence of Culture on Truth-telling and Patient Care. *Annals of the New York Academy of Sciences*, *809*(1), 197–210.

Eaves, D. (2010). Contributions to Pediatric Palliative Care and End-of-Life Support from Child life specialists. *Children's Project on Hospice and Palliative Services*, *20*, 14–15.

Eklund, R., Kreicbergs, U., Alvariza, A., & Lövgren, M. (2020). Children's Views Are Not Taken Into Account in Accordance with Article 12 of the United Nations Convention on the Rights of the Child in the Family Talk Intervention When a Parent Is Cared for in Palliative Care. *Omega*, *85*(1), 126–154. doi:10.1177/0030222820941283 PMID:32659170

Ell, K. (1996). Social networks, social support and coping with serious illness: The family connection. *Social Science & Medicine*, *42*(2), 173–183. doi:10.1016/0277-9536(95)00100-X PMID:8928027

Fearnley, R. (2010). Death of a parent and the children's experience: Don't ignore the elephant in the room. *Journal of Interprofessional Care*, *24*(4), 450–459. doi:10.3109/13561820903274871 PMID:20377397

Felitti, V. J., Anda, R. F., Nordenberg, D., Williamson, D. F., Spitz, A. M., Edwards, V., Koss, M. P., & Marks, J. S. (1998). Relationship of childhood abuse and household dysfunction to many of the leading causes of death in adults: The Adverse Childhood Experiences (ACE) Study. *American Journal of Preventive Medicine*, *14*(4), 245–258. doi:10.1016/S0749-3797(98)00017-8 PMID:9635069

Ferrell, B. R. (2015). *Spiritual, Religious, and Cultural Aspects of Care (HPNA Palliative Nursing Manuals)* (1st ed.). Oxford University Press. doi:10.1093/med/9780190244231.001.0001

Finkelhor, D. (2020). Trends in Adverse Childhood Experiences (ACEs) in the United States. *Child Abuse & Neglect*, *108*, 104641. doi:10.1016/j.chiabu.2020.104641 PMID:32739600

Flores, G., Abreu, M., Olivar, M., & Kastner, B. (1998). Access barriers to health care for Latino children. *Archives of Pediatrics & Adolescent Medicine*, *152*(11), 1119–1125. doi:10.1001/archpedi.152.11.1119 PMID:9811291

Flores, G., Abreu, M., Schwartz, I., & Hill, M. (2000). The importance of language and culture in pediatric care: Case studies from the Latino community. *The Journal of Pediatrics*, *137*(6), 842–848. doi:10.1067/mpd.2000.109150 PMID:11113842

Flores, G., & Vega, L. R. (1998). Barriers to health care access for Latino children: A review. *Family Medicine*, *30*, 196–205. PMID:9532442

Golics, C. J., Basra, M., Salek, & Finlay. (2013). The impact of patients' chronic disease on family quality of life: An experience from 26 specialties. *International Journal of General Medicine*, 787. doi:10.2147/IJGM.S45156 PMID:24092994

Holloway, D., & Wallinga, C. R. (1990). Burnout in child life specialists: The relation of role stress. *Children's Health Care*, *19*(1), 10–18.

Hornor, G. (2015). Childhood trauma exposure and toxic stress: What the PNP needs to know. *Journal of Pediatric Health Care*, *29*(2), 191–198. doi:10.1016/j.pedhc.2014.09.006 PMID:25697767

Hospice Foundation of America. (2008). *Eight Myths about Children and Loss*. Retrieved May 2022, from http://www.agis.com/Document/4477/eight-myths-about-children-and-loss.aspx

Hunter, E. G., & Rowles, G. D. (2005). Leaving a legacy: Toward a typology. *Journal of Aging Studies*, *19*(3), 327–347. doi:10.1016/j.jaging.2004.08.002

Johnstone, M. J., & Kanitsaki, O. (2009). Ethics and Advance Care Planning in a Culturally Diverse Society. *Journal of Transcultural Nursing*, *20*(4), 405–416.

Judi's House/JAG Institute. (2022). *Childhood bereavement estimation model 2022 national report*. Judi's House/JAG Institute. Retrieved June 2022, from https://judishouse.org/research-tools/cbem/cbem-reports/

Judi's House/JAG Institute. (2022b). *CBEM data tables*. Judi's House/JAG Institute. Retrieved June 2022, from https://judishouse.org/research-tools/cbem/cbem-data-tables/

Judi's House/JAG Institute. (2022c). *CBEM by race and ethnicity*. Judi's House/JAG Institute. Retrieved June 2022, from https://judishouse.org/research-tools/cbem/cbem-race-ethnicity/

Keene, J. R., & Batson, C. D. (2010). Under One Roof: A Review of Research on Intergenerational Coresidence and Multigenerational Households in the United States. *Sociology Compass*, *4*(8), 642–657. doi:10.1111/j.1751-9020.2010.00306.x

Knapp, S., & Slattery, J. M. (2004). Professional Boundaries in Nontraditional Settings. *Professional Psychology, Research and Practice*, *35*(5), 553–558.

Last, B. F., & Van Veldhuizen, A. M. H. (1996). Information about diagnosis and prognosis related to anxiety and depression in children with cancer aged 8–16 years. *European Journal of Cancer*, *32A*(2), 290–294. doi:10.1016/0959-8049(95)00576-5 PMID:8664044

Macnab, A. J., Northway, T., Ryall, K., Scott, D., & Straw, G. (2003). Death and bereavement in a paediatric intensive care unit: Parental perceptions of staff support. *Paediatrics & Child Health*, *8*(6), 357–362. doi:10.1093/pch/8.6.357 PMID:20052329

Maslach, C., & Jackson, S. E. (1981). The measurement of experienced burnout. *Journal of Occupational Behaviour*, *2*(2), 99–113. doi:10.1002/job.4030020205

McCue, K. (2014). *How to Help Children Through a Parent's Serious Illness*. St. Martin's Press.

Medicare Benefit Policy Manual. (2021). *Coverage of Hospice Services Under Hospital Insurance*.

Mersky, J. P., Janczewski, C. E., & Topitzes, J. (2017). Rethinking the measurement of adversity: Moving toward second-generation research on adverse childhood experiences. *Child Maltreatment*, *22*(1), 58–68. doi:10.1177/1077559516679513 PMID:27920222

Moyson, T., & Roeyers, H. (2012). The overall quality of my life as a sibling is all right, but of course, it could always be better'. Quality of life of siblings of children with intellectual disability: The siblings' perspectives. *Journal of Intellectual Disability Research*, *56*(1), 87–101. doi:10.1111/j.1365-2788.2011.01393.x PMID:21366753

Mustillo, S., Li, M., & Wang, W. (2020). Parent Work-to-Family Conflict and Child Psychological Well-Being: Moderating Role of Grandparent Coresidence. *Journal of Marriage and Family*, *83*(1), 27–39. doi:10.1111/jomf.12703

National Hospice and Palliative Care Organization. (2019). *Palliative care or hospice? The right service at the right time for seriously ill individuals*. Retrieved June 2022, from https://www.nhpco.org/wp-content/uploads/2019/04/PalliativeCare_VS_Hospice.pdf

National Hospice and Palliative Care Organization (NHPCO). (2019a). *Concurrent Care for Children Requirement*. Retrieved June 2022, from https://www.nhpco.org/palliativecare/pediatrics/pediatric-concurrent-care/concurrent-care-for-children-toolkit/

National Hospice and Palliative Care Organization (NHPCO). (2022). *Comfort care is a common term for end-of-life care*. Retrieved June 2022, from https://www.caringinfo.org/types-of-care/comfort-care/

National Hospice and Palliative Care Organization (NHPCO). (2022b). *Hospice Care: What Is It and What Are the Benefits*. Retrieved June 2022, from https://www.caringinfo.org/types-of-care/hospice-care/

Neidig, J. R., & Dalgas-Pelish, P. (1991). Parental grieving and perceptions regarding health care professionals' interventions. *Issues in Comprehensive Pediatric Nursing*, *14*(3), 179–191. doi:10.3109/01460869109014497 PMID:1841073

Phillips, F. (2014). Adolescents living with a parent with advanced cancer: A review of the literature. *Psycho-Oncology*, *23*(12), 1323–1339. doi:10.1002/pon.3570 PMID:24911540

Pola, A., & Nelson, R. (2014). The impact of bibliotherapy on positive coping in children who have experienced disaster. *Therapeutic Recreation Journal*, *48*(4), 341–344.

Randhawa, G., Owens, A., Fitches, R., & Khan, Z. (2003). Communication in the development of culturally competent palliative care services in the UK: A case study. *International Journal of Palliative Nursing*, *9*(1), 24–31. doi:10.12968/ijpn.2003.9.1.11042 PMID:12560794

Samson, T., & Shvartzman, P. (2018). Secondary Traumatization and Proneness to Disassociation Among Palliative Care Workers: A cross-sectional study. *Journal of Pain and System Management, 56*(2), 245–251. PMID:29729350

Sanders, S., Bullock, K., & Broussard, C. (2012). Exploring Professional Boundaries in End-of-Life Care: Considerations for Hospice Social Workers and Other Members of the Team. *Journal of Social Work in End-of-Life & Palliative Care*, *8*(1), 1, 10–28. doi:10.1080/15524256.2012.650671 PMID:22424382

Sandoval, C. O'Neill, J.; Selwyn, P.; Schietinger, H., editors. (2003). Culture and Care [Electronic version]. A Clinical Guide to Supportive and Palliative Care for HIV/AIDS. http://hab.hrsa.gov/ deliverhivaidscare/files/palliativecare2003.pdf

Searight, H. R., & Gafford, J. (2005). Cultural diversity at the end of life: Issues and guidelines for family physicians. *American Family Physician*, *71*, 515–522.

Sutter, C., & Reid, T. (2012). How Do We Talk to the Children? Child Life Consultation To Support the Children of Seriously Ill Adult Inpatients. *Journal of Palliative Medicine*, *15*(12), 1362–1367. doi:10.1089/jpm.2012.0019 PMID:22978620

Tan, A., Zimmermann, C., & Rodin, G. (2005). Interpersonal processes in palliative care: An attachment perspective on the patient-clinician relationship. *Palliative Medicine*, *19*(2), 143–150. doi:10.1191/0269216305pm994oa PMID:15810754

Taylor, M., Delevett, R., Kem, S. & Miller, M.C. (2017, Spring). Supporting well children in a critically ill adult's world. *Association of Child Life Professionals Bulletin*, 37-41.

Taylor-Brickey, M. (2020). W is for work: From burnout to balance. *Association of Child Life Professionals Bulletin*, (Fall), 20–24.

Thibodeaux, A. G., & Deatrick, J. A. (2007). Cultural Influence on Family Management of Children with Cancer. *Journal of Pediatric Oncology Nursing*, *24*(4), 227–233.

Trill, M. D., & Kovalcik, R. (1997). The Child with Cancer. Influence of Culture on Truth-telling and Patient Care. *Annals of the New York Academy of Sciences, 809*(1 Communication), 197–210.

Tristán, L. Q. (2010). *Rights of a child with a terminal illness*. Poster Palliative Care Center Support Foundation.

Wiener, L., Pao, M., Kazak, A. E., Kupst, M. J., Patenaude, A. F., & Arceci, R. J. (Eds.). (2015). *Pediatric Psycho-Oncology: A Quick Reference on the Psychosocial Dimensions of Cancer Symptom Management*. Oxford University Press.

KEY TERMS AND DEFINITIONS

Burnout: exhaustion of physical or emotional strength or motivation usually as a result of prolonged stress or frustration from overwork or overuse (Merriam-Webster)

Hospice: An organization or facility that provides care for the terminally ill, focused on palliation (comfort) when curative treatment is no longer an option. Hospice care involves medical care, pain management, and emotional/spiritual support. It can be provided inpatient or outpatient and focuses on maintaining the quality of life and symptom control. Patients can be admitted to hospice when they have a terminal diagnosis of six months or less. (My Wishes)

Legacy Building: The process of identifying one's life accomplishments and how one wants to be remembered.

Life-Limiting Illness: An incurable chronic disease or condition that no longer responds to curative treatment.

Life-Threatening: An illness or trauma that is potentially fatal.

Memory Making: The intangible aspect of the intervention and promotes positive experiences, building memories during an otherwise stressful and traumatic experience.

Palliative Care: Palliative care addresses physical, intellectual, emotional, social, and spiritual needs facilitating patient autonomy, access to information, and choice. Palliative care is family-centered, focusing on optimizing the quality of life by anticipating, preventing, and treating suffering.

APPENDIX: RESOURCE RECOMMENDATIONS

Books

Big Boss Brain: Learning About Traumatic Brain Injuries by Shannon Maxwell
Gentle Willow: A Story for Children About Dying by Joyce C. Mills

How Will They Get That Heart Down Your Throat: A Child's View of Transplants by Karen Walton

My Wishes by Aging with Dignity

Voicing My Choices by Aging with Dignity

Foundations

The Songs of Love Foundation
https://www.songsoflove.org/
1-800-960-SONG (7660)

Section 2

Settings

Chapter 5
School

Audra Holst-VanNoord
Lowell Area School District, USA

Jessica Lewin
River Valley School District, USA

Courtney Rosborough
Edmonton Catholic School District, Canada

ABSTRACT

Child life specialists in schools help students, school staff, and families function more cohesively, advocating for the needs of each individual while continuing to prioritize child development. This chapter will outline the student and staff needs that child life specialists are uniquely suited to meet while also giving an overview of interventions, supports, roles, and coping strategies that can be led by a child life specialist within the school setting. Throughout this chapter, one will see how easily a child life specialist can integrate into existing systems or propose a new position within the school environment.

INTRODUCTION

This chapter will examine schools as a nontraditional child life setting and how Certified Child Life Specialists can support students experiencing challenging situations that can negatively impact their optimal development and learning ability. Child life was initially established to meet the needs of children in healthcare. However, the profession's scope of practice and skill set can provide support to children and families in any setting in which children are undergo-

DOI: 10.4018/978-1-6684-5097-0.ch005

ing challenging life events (ACLP, 2018). It is especially important for Certified Child Life Specialists to continue to uphold the competencies of the child profession and understand their scope of practice in any setting in which they may work (ACLP, 2020).

Taking into account that child development milestones change over the school years, this chapter gives an overview of how Certified Child Life Specialists can collaboratively create and use therapeutic interventions in elementary, middle, and high schools. "Child life professionals are uniquely educated and trained to provide children, families, and their support systems opportunities to cope, gain a sense of mastery, engage in self-expression, and promote resiliency" (ACLP, 2018, p.1). Real-life examples will show that Certified Child Life Specialists can support student and staff needs as they take on established roles or by proposing specific child life specialist roles within a school setting.

Suppose a child life role is not available in a school setting. In that case, some Certified Child Life Specialists may take on a school position with another title, such as emotional, behavioral specialist, or coordinator of student support. In contrast, others may repurpose a traditional school role into a child life one. As the ACLP position statement on child life practice in the community (2018, p.1) states, "there is a significant value in including child life professionals in a variety of community-based settings." On average, students spend 180 days or 950 hours at school (Carrington, 2020). Coping skills taught by a child life professional within a school setting can lay a foundation for students to cope with significant challenging events throughout their lives and can be generalized to future healthcare experiences.

Much like in the hospital setting, schools have multidisciplinary teams made up of a variety of professionals. Certified Child Life Specialists integrate into existing student support programs collaborating with other support professionals such as social workers, school counselors, behavior specialists, psychologists, teachers, and administrators on the emotional well-being of children. Using weekly psychosocial rounds or collaborative meetings, schools increase staff communication and awareness of student needs impacting academics and ability to learn. With their collective knowledge, the team focuses on common psychosocial goals, identifies action plans, and maximizes staff involvement.

For schools that have implemented multi-tiered support systems (MTSS), a child life skill set articulating strategies and accommodations for students with various diagnoses can be useful at each level: universal, focused and intensive. School-based child life interventions are grounded in the core child life competencies; however, they may look very different from interventions in the healthcare setting. Child life professionals in a school still focus heavily on the essential goals of child life: building rapport, assessing coping, promoting resilience, minimizing stress, providing therapeutic interventions, and communicating effectively with other professionals (ACLP, 2018). Through proactive support in the classroom, in small groups, and individually, students' psychosocial needs will be met first before attempting academics.

According to Abraham Maslow's hierarchy of needs (1954), students' basic needs must be met before confidence and learning occur. These needs will be more challenging to meet if students are dysregulated, anxious, or stressed. Students' mental health and social-emotional needs have been a challenge for school districts and their administrators for years, with a heavy focus on academics and test scores (Carrington, 2020). In 2021, the Child Mind Institute published a mental health report that states that approximately 35% of children and adolescents have voiced feelings of anxiety, depression, or stress occurring on a regular basis (Child Mind Institute, 2021).

Mental health disorders affect 16.5% of children (about 7.7 million), with almost half of those not receiving necessary treatment from mental health professionals (ACLP, 2020). Unfortunately, American schools employing mental health professionals have an average student-to-counselor ratio of 455 to 1, even though the American School Counselor Association recommends no more than a 250-to-1 ratio (Bray, 2019). While this is the lowest margin for the ratio in over 30 years, improving the numbers alone is only part of the answer. Students need specially trained professionals that can address the vital issues impacting today's children (Lewis et al., 2020).

"Students with positive mental health are resilient and better able to learn, achieve success, and build healthy relationships" in the school environment (Edmonton Catholic Schools [ECS], 2020, p. 24). However, when students experience an overwhelming amount of unaddressed stress, students have challenges meeting social, emotional, and behavioral expectations, affecting school performance (Greene, 2016). Therefore, it is up to the school administration to prioritize and arrange emotionally safe spaces with experienced, educated professionals in order to help students cope with and express their emotions.

The psychosocial duty to positively impact success in the classroom and academic performance usually falls upon school counselors or social workers within the school setting. However, Certified Child Life Specialists are qualified to model and demonstrate expertise in (ACLP, 2018):

- Growth and development issues that occur during the school years
- Developmental assessments that may help with developmentally appropriate learning
- Play and therapeutic interventions at any grade level
- Psychological preparation and preventative support for significant student experiences
- Student and family responses to stress, trauma, or significant student experiences
- Interventions to support coping and resilience in the classroom
- Family systems that may affect behavior in the classroom
- Interpersonal communication with students, families, and school staff
- Grief and loss support for students
- Cultural humility in schools

- Ethics to maximize student wellbeing and minimize stress and trauma
- Collaboration with a variety of disciplines and professionals in a school setting
- Rehabilitation programming for students

School is where children spend most of their day and therefore is an ideal setting for a Certified Child Life Specialist to make a positive impact. Certified Child Life Specialists provide additional specialized support to students and are beneficial members of a collaborative school multidisciplinary team.

BACKGROUND

Within the hospital setting, there has been a growing trend of educational programming and a move toward school reintegration services. Nevertheless, there is still a lack of collaboration between child life departments and school systems. Most child life professionals believe their impact on education services is underutilized (Pershick, 2009). Even though research reflects the benefits of collaboration, the majority of hospital-based Certified Child Life Specialists never communicate with school personnel outside of the hospital due to the lack of time and resources (Pershick, 2009; Heffer & Lowe, 2000). Some child life private practitioners offer support for schools; however, the skill set of a Certified Child Life Specialist can be utilized from within the education system for a more proactive and comprehensive approach.

Nevertheless, child life services are often not fully recognized or understood outside of healthcare settings, resulting in a lack of knowledge on how the child life role could look in the school system. From supporting the family as a whole, educating school staff and peers about a child's illness, to teaching students coping techniques, a Certified Child Life Specialist brings a distinct perspective to a school team on supporting students and creating positive behavior interventions. Due to the COVID-19 pandemic that began in 2020, children have encountered significant life changes to routines, schooling, and healthcare. As a result, they have missed typical milestones and life events while also experiencing a loss of security and safety. In addition, many families have suffered from job loss and economic instability, which is directly linked to unfavorable childhood experiences that can impact social-emotional development, focus in the classroom, and overall health (Centers for Disease Control and Prevention [CDC], 2021). Moreover, the COVID-19 pandemic has also significantly impacted child development regarding academic, emotional, mental, and physical health (Benner & Mistry, 2020). Due to these increased psychosocial needs of students and their families, school systems are overwhelmed.

Navigating school stressors can be difficult for teachers. Greiner, Park, and Goldstein (2022) found that nearly half of teachers reported no formal training about death or family separation, while 93% of teachers say they do not have any bereavement training (Carrington, 2020). A study in Detroit found that over 75% of teachers and school mental health professionals want to learn the best practices to support students impacted by trauma and mental illness (Koschmann et al., 2022). Specifically, teachers need to be prepared to identify and address student mental health in the classroom and be taught strategies or interventions to be more proactive (Deaton et al., 2022).

Using additional mental health staff as an educational enhancer to aid teachers has been shown to improve consultation efforts through established rapport, therefore improving the school system as a whole (Atkins et al., 2010). Certified Child Life Specialists can be integral to student mental health teams to proactively anticipate future stressors, anxieties, or misconceptions before they occur. A Certified Child Life Specialist has expertise in assessing what is developmentally appropriate for children of all ages while also providing interventions and coaching to staff and caregivers.

Schools are seeing a rise in students with chronic illnesses and psychosocial and mental health concerns such as suicide, bullying, and drug use (Weiner et al., 2009; Miron et al., 2019). It is common for students to struggle with a variety of issues, both at school and at home, that can make learning and engagement in the classroom more difficult. Mental health professionals, including school psychologists, social workers, and counselors, are typical members of a multidisciplinary team in most school districts. However, student needs and busy schedules can make it hard to achieve effective collaboration (Berta et al., 2022).

School mental health staff are overwhelmed in almost every state due to large caseload numbers and a lack of accredited professionals, including school counselors, social workers, and child psychologists (Child Mind Institute, 2021). School counselors work to proactively maximize student success through academic strategies, managing emotions, interpersonal skills, and planning for post-secondary options (American School Counselor Association, 2022). However, 1 in 5 students (8 million children) do not have access to a counselor in their school at all (ASCA, 2019). School counselors improve student learning and behavior outcomes; however, lower ratios are necessary for counselors to effectively deliver comprehensive counseling programs to better meet students' academic, career, and social/emotional needs (ASCA, n.d).

School social workers are trained to help students combat mental health and behavior concerns, create positive behavior support plans, aid in academic and classroom management, collaborate with teachers, parents, and administrators, and provide individual and group therapy sessions (School Social Work Association of America, n.d). However, in 2016, 58% of all US public schools did not have access to a social worker (NCES, 2016). Therefore, a lack of licensed mental health professionals leaves a gap in student support services that must be filled.

Certified Child Life Specialists are in a unique position to meet this need and be additional support that collaborates with the multidisciplinary team to disrupt negative trends in anxiety, depression, and isolation through creative interventions, therapeutic play, and coping techniques. "Child life competencies are easily transferable to any professional environment that supports children, families, and their support systems impacted by crisis, challenge or change" (ACLP, 2018, p.1). Through ongoing psychosocial assessments and partnering with school staff, a Certified Child Life Specialist can help students maintain their developmental milestones during challenging situations, ultimately establishing more academically present students.

By using a strength-based, collaborative approach, Certified Child Life Specialists can help students overcome difficulties in the classroom and adapt more effectively to the demands of school stressors when other mental health specialists are unavailable. Applying an evidence-based child life practice within the education system can result in students having fewer behavior problems, higher social self-esteem, and higher rates of adjustment (Heffer & Lowe, 2000). In addition, students can reduce the stress that accompanies the school environment by prioritizing coping strategies learned from Certified Child Life Specialists. This approach "shifts the focus from the prevention of specific problems to a more positive, holistic view of child and youth development" to build resiliency, enhance social-emotional learning, and support student growth (ECS, 2020, p. 24).

CHILD LIFE IN THE SCHOOL

Student Needs

Many challenges that schools face require psychosocial support and the need to promote resilience in combating the negative impacts of trauma and other school stressors. Traditionally, these issues are handled by a school social worker or school counselor, but if a school does not have a mental health professional, it falls on the teachers. "Children who experience trauma struggle with interpersonal relationships, face cognitive deficits (including memory and language development) and overreact to everyday stress" (Pappano, 2014, p.1). Traumatized students have a hypervigilant worldview, making social cues hard to read and minor events triggering. Defiant, disruptive, or aggressive behavior may be a natural stress response, making their ability to cope harder to access than the average student.

Looking at students through a trauma-informed lens, it is clear that these classroom challenges are subject to the increasing prevalence of trauma exposure in children today. More than 68% of children have experienced a traumatic event by the time they are 16, having to constantly function within a survival mode mentality and high levels of toxic stress (Pappano,

2014). The Adverse Childhood Experiences (ACEs) study from 1998 found that more than 50% of children have been exposed to at least one of 10 adversities, such as physical and emotional abuse, neglect, and household dysfunction (Felitti et al.,1998). Although ACEs participants were primarily white and middle class, more diverse studies, like the Philadelphia Urban ACE study of 2015, reached similar conclusions. They also widened the definition of adversity, including witnessing violence, experiencing racism or discrimination, living in an unsafe neighborhood, being bullied, or living in foster care (Cronholm et al., 2015).

Children who have experienced trauma have lower reading proficiencies, decreased GPAs, and higher rates of absences, suspensions, and expulsions. They are more likely to repeat a grade, have behavioral problems, drop out of school, and require special education classes (Bethell et al., 2014). School teachers may not have been given the education and training to de-escalate behaviors and teach coping skills or are spread too thin with other students' needs (Greene, 2016).

Child life specialists are experts in helping children express themselves and supporting the development of coping strategies to build resilience (ACLP, 2016). This is accomplished by creating safe, nurturing environments for children to build their social-emotional intelligence in the home, school, and community (Bethell et al., 2014). Research shows that building resilience can combat the negative effects of trauma that are so prevalent in schools today (Bethell et al., 2016). Child life specialists value therapeutic relationships, communication, and professional collaboration (ACLP, 2001). Child life specialists support their school staff in building non-academic relationships, adjusting student interactions, and creating safe environments filled with regulated voices, discipline alternatives, and flexibility. These proactive teamwork strategies better prepare the school staff to identify and build upon every student's existing strengths and supports (Berta et al., 2022).

Special Education, Chronic Illness, and Medical Conditions

More children with special healthcare needs (chronic illness, developmental disabilities, cognitive impairments, psychiatric disorders) enter the school system and create diversity in the classroom (Weiner et al., 2009). Unfortunately, a school environment sees multiple service gaps for the 20% of children that have a chronic illness in such areas as school re-entry, diagnosis explanation, normalization, socialization, and individual education plans (IEPs), also known as individualized program plans (IPP) (Weiner et al., 2009). Child life specialists can work with members of their school team to help fill the gaps in these areas with traditional child life interventions.

All students who are identified as having special education needs should have an individual education plan/individual program plan (IEP/IPP), depending on the location or school board. Students with IEPs/IPPs receive accommodations and specialized instruction based on their specific disabilities. The IEP/IPP is a student-focused, collaborative plan of action that addresses barriers within the learning environment and communicates student goals and growth while providing a guide for transition planning at the end of the year. It should include the student's interests and learning preferences, assessment data, accommodation ideas, functional impacts, goals, and strategies to meet those goals (Alberta Education, 2006).

With expertise in developmental assessment and therapeutic interventions, child life specialists are a valuable addition to the school's multidisciplinary team collaborating in creating and implementing these strength-based documents. Diagnosis education is integral to this step so that the child, caregivers, and school staff all understand how a diagnosis affects a student's capacity to learn.

Similar to IEPs/IPPs, 504 plans typically provide accommodations for students with mental or physical impairments in the United States. The 504 coordinator can be filled by a variety of school staff, from secretaries to administrators or school counselors. In addition, a child life specialist can be a qualified professional to sit in the position of a 504 coordinator, given their extensive training with various diagnoses typically seen in the hospital setting.

Family-centered care in the school setting advocates for family involvement in supportive and meaningful conversations regarding the child's impairment and assists in identifying proper accommodations that can be made and documented in the child's school profile. Child life specialists working as 504 coordinators collaborate with teachers and staff, similar to how a child life specialist collaborates with the multidisciplinary team in the hospital for patient care plans.

Although other school staff navigate challenging school situations, the expertise in childhood development and diagnoses makes a child life specialist an excellent addition to any school psychosocial support team. With their experience and creative nature, child life specialists can work together with teachers and staff to develop innovative solutions and interventions for student accommodations. It is important for the child life specialist to have organizational skills to file, document, and communicate these accommodations to the student, teachers, administrators, and family members, as well as keep up with yearly reviews and reevaluations for each student.

Family Medical Experiences and Preparation

A more traditional area where child life specialists add value in the school setting is surrounding medical experiences, which in the past were supported by the school counselor or social worker who may not have training in medical play. This includes support for a student who has suffered a medical trauma or is awaiting an upcoming medical treatment. Students may also be supported to understand better the feelings and terminology associated with a loved one going through a medical experience.

Research shows that children living with a chronically ill family member (parent, grandparent, sibling) encounter difficulties in their daily life exhibited in their schooling efforts as well as their mental, physical, and social/emotional well-being (Van der Werf et al., 2019). For example, a student may need to process a medical trauma, prepare for surgery, or understand a new diagnosis, injury, or illness. A child life specialist provides further support to the student, their family, classmates, and staff with developmentally appropriate language, education, and explanation for a student's diagnosis, such as cancer or diabetes.

Developmentally appropriate language and preparation can vary depending on the intended audience. For staff, child life specialists can create scripts for school communication with staff and families. Certified Child Life Specialists may provide whole-class, individual, and group lessons for fellow students. Medical playgroups promote mastery and understanding, including painting, music, making masks, a teddy bear clinic, molding clay, sand tray worlds, drawing, scribble tag, and body outlines.

Creating more traditional child life interventions in a school setting, like school reintegration to transition students from the hospital, fill gaps in services that most hospitals do not have the time or resources to fulfill (Pershick, 2009). From inside the school rather than the hospital, child life specialists provide support for transitions back into the classroom from medical settings and events, such as the hospital, an inpatient mental health stay, or a distressing medical incident. The healthcare knowledge of child life specialists is a huge asset in a school setting, as child life specialists can serve as a liaison between hospitals and schools to coordinate the release of necessary medical information. This ability to collaborate with hospital child life staff and teachers allows child life specialists to provide a smooth transition for students and families.

School Transitions

School child life specialists prepare students and their families for non-medical or medical-adjacent events, such as psychiatric inpatient stays, active shooter drills, visits to a family member in jail, or even a student's visit with probation officers. Usually, a teacher prepares students for school-related transitions. However, a child life specialist can provide additional support using accurate, developmentally appropriate information prior to novel school or life experiences, such as test taking, first days of school, transitioning to a new building, active shooter drills, and more. Preparation for these various school transitions depends on assessing students' developmental and psychosocial needs, a core competency of child life (ACLP, 2016).

In the classroom, preparation may be necessary for a student to successfully move from one activity to the next. Student preparation for transitions may include:

- Role-playing a sequence of events
- Incorporating a classroom daily visual schedule
- Showing a first/then visual (a breakdown of multi-step tasks into concise instructions) prior to moving from a preferred to non-preferred activity (e.g., first clean up, then carpet time)
- Explaining the reason why a situation or change is occurring, such as a substitute teacher or a fire drill
- Going over sensations a student may experience in a new environment, such as a loud music class or feeling warm in a school assembly
- Utilizing verbal warnings or timers
- Making to-do lists or checklists

Separation anxiety and school avoidance are often realities for students who struggle with transitions. Students may fear their caregivers will not come back to pick them up, becoming so emotionally distraught that they vomit at the front doors. Child life specialists provide support to help students of all ages into the school building and advocate for adaptations that keep them in the classroom. Organizing "happy visits" to the school, classroom, and new grade to meet teachers builds positive experiences associated with school. Self-regulation theory suggests that students regulate behavior based on past experiences and information available (Vohs & Baumeister, 2016). This increased competence can be generalized to other similarly stressful situations in or out of the school environment (Gaynard et al.,1998).

Behavior Challenges

One of the most prominent struggles schools face is an increasing number of students with behavioral challenges (Greene, 2016). Some school districts have access to behavior consultants or Board Certified Behavior Analysts (BCBAs) to help staff and students. Unfortunately, half the US counties have no access to BCBAs, while the half with BCBAs do not reflect the recommended 1:15 caseload (Yinglin, Ruther, & Dubuque, 2022). Child life specialists can be additional support in this area for schools.

Dr. Jody Carrington (2020) found that some of the most common diagnoses seen in schools are emotional-regulation-based behavioral diagnosis, such as oppositional defiant disorder (ODD), conduct disorder (CD), and attention-deficit/hyperactivity disorder (ADHD), where applied behavior analysis (ABA) may not be effective. These diagnoses can also mislabel children whose hyperactivity is due to trauma experiences (Carrington, 2020). Observed behavioral challenges can range from crying to full-blown tantrums, with desks being pushed over, chairs being thrown, and people being injured. Child life offers a skill set that complements traditional school roles collaborating with the school counselor or social worker and can also be considered an alternative role to support these students.

Behavior challenges often show themselves when a student is dysregulated, cannot comply with expectations, or engage in school-appropriate behavior. Positive behavior strategies can be embedded within a student's daily routine to increase coping and resilience. Child life specialists work with students of varying ages to develop coping skills, such as:

- Deep breathing techniques
- Positive self-talk
- Meditation
- Mindfulness practices
- Guided imagery
- Movement breaks or sensory courses
- Yoga
- Time in nature

Using play, videos, puppets, drawing, and worksheets provide developmentally appropriate education on coping skills and their effect on the brain and body under stress. A child life specialist collaborating with school counselors or social workers helps students recognize feelings, develop strategies to manage emotions, and understand the impact of their actions on others. In addition, child life specialists teach alternative coping tools and positive behavior replacements, empathy, impulse control, conflict resolution skills, and restorative practices.

When a student needs more individualized strategies to help decrease challenging behaviors, a child life specialist works with school team members to create behavior support plans, behavior contracts or agreements, and use of Check-In/Check-Out (CICO; see Appendix) or Check and Connect interventions. Reward systems, sticker charts, schedules, checklists, or check-ins with supportive adults can assist students in successfully re-engaging with their learning. The student should always be involved in creating the plan to promote autonomy and ownership.

With training provided by the schools, a child life specialist may take the lead or be a consulting member of a team that completes a functional behavior assessment (FBA). These assessments consider a student's background history and analyze data to create a step-by-step, more formalized positive behavior support plan (PBSP). This is a working document that is regularly reviewed and modified to evaluate the effectiveness of interventions and make necessary adaptations. The plan is a visual representation of goals and lists positive behavior supports, lagging skills needing to be taught, and reactive interventions that all staff members and family members can reference. This document creates accountability for the student and an opportunity for building rapport, especially after discipline has occurred. Child life specialists are an additional supportive adult connection that students need to process emotions and promote success in the classroom.

If students' behavior poses a risk to themselves or others, a school child life specialist and other staff may need further training in CPI Nonviolent Crisis Intervention. This training is designed to help professionals provide safe care during crisis behaviors. In addition, child life brings an array of tools that can aid in de-escalation situations, such as distraction, One Voice (Wagers, 2013), and co-regulation. Ideally, how to manage these crisis behaviors are laid out in a crisis management plan that is collaboratively written by school staff. A child life specialist's role is to advocate for non-restrictive holds to be the last resort and facilitate processing for the student post-CPI. After an incident, a child life specialist assists with re-entry into the classroom, provide emotional support and coaching for staff, and offers developmentally appropriate explanations and lessons for other students.

School Crisis

Schools experience a variety of traumas and crises within the community, including natural disasters, shootings, and loss from illness or accidents. Schools must have drills and lockdowns to prepare for bomb, active shooter threats, or fires. School counselors, administration, teachers, and child life specialists work with other mental health professionals to support students and faculty in preparing for such events, processing potential traumatic reactions, and debriefing staff and students post training and events. To stay within their scope of practice, child life specialists make referrals to outside agencies if additional support is required.

Child life specialists may advocate for their role in the school district's crisis team, designing crisis plans and procedures, providing scripts to staff and families, facilitating whole class discussions, and creating opportunities for trauma processing. Other interventions include therapeutic or expressive activities helping students and staff cope with potential grief or loss and reduce anxiety. According to the Child Life Code of Ethics (2020), child life specialists make referrals or work with other mental health team members to refer families to outside resources should a student need further assistance. Having a child life specialist who is knowledgeable in developmentally appropriate explanations of crises, effective communication of next steps, leading and organizing school crisis responses, and creating safe, therapeutic, healing environments would be an asset to the school system working with or in place of mental health counselors.

Death and Bereavement

Statistics from the National Center for School Crisis and Bereavement (NCSCB) and the Coalition to Support Grieving Students (2020) show that nine in 10 children will experience the death of a family member or close friend. More specifically, one in 20 students will lose one or both parents by the time they graduate high school (Schonfeld, 2015). Additionally, nearly 70% of teachers are aware of at least one student who has experienced the loss of an immediate family member or close friend in the past year (American Federation of Teachers [AFT] and New York Life Foundation, 2012). However, only 7% of teachers have bereavement training (Carrington, 2020).

School staff is often provided with little or no training, resulting in a lack of confidence in navigating student challenges that accompany death and bereavement (McManus & Paul, 2019). As a result, classroom teachers observe students experiencing difficulty concentrating, decreased engagement, chronic absenteeism, lower quality work, and fewer completed assignments (AFT and New York Life Foundation, 2012). Usually, these situations are handled by school counselors or social workers, but having a child life specialist with specific crisis and bereavement experiences can relieve other school staff and provide much-needed, specialized support for students and families.

Child life specialists organize bereavement interventions such as a response plan after a death, providing space for processing, therapeutic activities, and scripting for staff and families. Additionally, school child life specialists provide developmentally appropriate explanations of death with whole classes, small groups, and individual activities to help children cope, such as:

- Active listening
- Expressive art
- Memory or worry boxes
- Reading books about death and coping
- Restorative circles with opportunities to share
- Journaling

By the age of 18, five million children will have experienced death in their family (Burns et al., 2020). A child life specialist is one of many psychosocial staff that can provide one-to-one support for these children and their families by communicating family wishes to staff/students and educating teachers and administration on how to discuss grief using developmentally appropriate considerations. They can also serve as a point person for families to connect them to outside resources, such as nonprofits that specialize in crisis, grief, or counseling.

Mental Health and Suicide

Multiple protective and risk factors affect students' mental health, but most can fit into one of three categories: individual attributes, social circumstances, or environmental factors (ECS, 2020). According to the Child Life Competences, child life services are prioritized by a child's susceptibility to stress and trauma (ACLP, 2016). Child life also recognizes the diversity of individual strengths and needs, acknowledging a student's support systems and community links (ACLP, 2001). Therefore using an ecological lens to examine student's mental health, child life specialists view the child within their multiple ecosystems not just as their behaviors or suicidal ideation (Bronfenbrenner, 1981).

Child life specialists do not complete suicide assessments in the healthcare setting. However, it is common for staff without mental health backgrounds or training to complete the suicide assessment in a school setting. Child life specialists collaborating with school counselors or social workers provide support for mental health issues or suicidal ideation accessing additional training available to increase their confidence and competency by providing suicide assessments, support for self-injury, and resources for students and families.

School support staff, including child life specialists, should use an evidence-based tool to conduct suicide assessments and create safety plans. Child life specialists collaboratively work with their school district to create suicide protocols for district-wide consistency and safety. Suppose a hospital evaluation or inpatient stay is recommended. In that case, a release form should be signed so the child life specialists can communicate with hospital staff, advocate for child life and teacher support in the hospital and provide insight to hospital social workers working with the student.

Child life specialists provide safe, therapeutic, and healing environments (ACLP, 2001). By explaining the impact of environmental designs on human behavior, child life specialists are within their scope of practice to coordinate a student's school re-entry after an inpatient stay. Safety plans and coping plans should be created in communication with hospital and school staff. The child life specialist works with families, connecting them with outside counseling services. Since child life professionals' scope of practice encompasses life events that can influence typical growth and development, they aim to minimize the risk of long-term effects for friends of students who have died by suicide and potentially decrease the risk for students that are self-harming (ACLP, 2018).

Diversity, Equity, and Inclusion (DEI)

According to Principle three of the Child Life Code of Ethics (2020), "Certified Child Life Specialists have an obligation to maintain an environment that respects variations in culture, age, gender, race, ethnicity, physical ability, sexual orientation, gender identity/expression, religious affiliation, and socioeconomic status (ACLP, 2020, p.1). Therefore, child life specialists provide emotional support and coping techniques for students within the LGBTQIA+ community, working towards creating safe spaces for them in school settings.

Some schools may form a Genders and Sexualities Alliance (GSA) to create a safe space for students who identify as LGBTQIA+ and their straight or cisgender peers who may be allies to the community. A GSA in a school has been shown to increase school attendance, heighten students' perceptions of belonging within their school, and achieve greater support for those within the LGBTQIA+ community from teachers, staff, and administration (Ioverno et al., 2016). This safe space allows students to feel supported by their peers, socialize with those similar to them as well as those who are allied with their LGBTQIA+ peers and advocate for positive change within the school and community. Support for sexual minority students can be seen in staff interceding when made aware of negative or homophobic comments, thus creating a safer environment overall (Ioverno et al., 2016). Child life specialists may serve as an advisor for this group.

To support individual students, child life specialists work with students and families to create gender support plans and gender communication plans while equipping staff to support the social-emotional needs of students. With the student's permission, Certified Child Life Specialists provide education to staff and administration regarding a student's pronouns, how to handle conversations with a student's family if the family is unaware of their child's gender identity, or common terms and phrases used in the LGBTQIA+ community and how to use those terms appropriately. Additionally, the child life specialist provides coaching and training for staff on how best to support LGBTQIA+ students through appropriate language and scripting.

Child life specialists work toward ensuring that policies and procedures in a school district are culturally responsive, promoting equity, safety, and inclusion not only for gender-diverse students but also for students of diverse races, religions, socioeconomic statuses, languages, disabilities, and ethnicities. As part of trauma-informed discipline, the Certified Child Life Specialist work alongside other psychosocial support staff to educate students who have used racial or homophobic slurs at school on relevant topics such as respect and tolerance, positively impacting learning and the learning environment. Child life specialists present on diversity, equity, and inclusion for staff and students with the goal of creating a sense of belonging for all students and educating students individually and in groups about empathy and tolerance.

Restorative Practices

Restorative practices are an evidence-based approach many schools use to promote inclusion grounded in trauma-informed care. This approach proactively builds relationships and a sense of community to prevent and address conflict and wrongdoing (Schott Foundation for Public Education, 2014). Child life specialists aim to establish and maintain a therapeutic and healing environment, allowing an opportunity to teach students skills and improve future behavior in a safe space (ACLP, 2001). After appropriate training, Certified Child Life Specialists may take on a role of facilitating, advocating for, and growing restorative practices in the school. Through restorative conferences, proactive and reactive circles, children are allowed to have a voice and time to process, along with learning how to build healthy relationships and conflict resolution and communication skills. This intervention aligns with the child life skill to provide input about facility design to promote orientation, comfort, healing, culturally inclusive materials, security, and normalization while also seeking professional development based on the population served (ACLP, 2001).

Students Experiencing Homelessness

Under the federal McKinney-Vento Act (1987), every local educational agency is required to designate a liaison for homeless children and youth. This role assists students and families who may be experiencing homelessness. The McKinney-Vento liaison position is usually filled by administrators, counselors, or clerical staff. However, it should not be filled by school resource officers or other law enforcement personnel (California Department of Education, 2019). Child life specialists have served in this position district-wide.

The term "homelessness" has traditionally been associated with living on the street been associated with living on the streets or in a shelter. However, students experiencing homelessness may be undergoing a variety of circumstances (National Center for Homeless Education [NCHE], n.d.), such as:

- Living in a hotel due to a house fire with no home insurance
- Living with their grandparents as a last option before needing to go to a shelter
- Experiencing an economic hardship
- Being removed from their home and staying with a relative or friend with no primary caregiver present (this is referred to as an unaccompanied youth)

The McKinney-Vento liaison's job is to identify these families, ensure they have transportation to school, provide support during a traumatic time, and connect families to resources to help rebuild what was lost.

Child life specialists are familiar with traumatic situations, given their experience in the hospital. For example, it is common to encounter families experiencing an unexpected loss or fatal prognosis, teenagers recovering from attempted suicides, or children receiving care for an injury due to abuse. Although primarily an administrative position, child life specialists functioning as the McKinney-Vento liaison gain insights into students' lives, deepening understanding of students' lived experiences and increasing psychosocial support that prioritizes inclusion for all students.

Staff Needs

Staff Coaching and Wellness

Coaching and staff support have become a crucial need in schools as the many challenges mentioned above have put new demands on teachers, all confounded by the stress of the COVID-19 pandemic. Teachers and school staff show the highest burnout rates in years (Chesak et al., 2019). A recent survey by the National Education Association (2022) reveals that 55% of its members are looking to retire or leave the profession early. Training in Mental Health First Aid is helpful for staff to increase knowledge and ability to address the mental health needs of a school community and their own mental health.

Historically, even though teachers are at the front line in supporting our students' psychosocial needs, they have not been equipped with the tools needed to provide psychosocial support. Although 95% of educators report a high level of concern for student's mental health, 85% state they need more training, specifically in mental health and mental health disorders (Moon et al., 2017).

Similar to supporting nurses in a hospital, child life specialists support teachers in a school, coaching them on strategies that encourage positive behaviors, functioning as extra support in the classroom, and validating staff feelings. Skilled in positive coping strategies, child life specialists promote staff self-care and wellness while also helping a child advocate for their needs to be met in more appropriate ways (ACLP 2018). Child life specialists present professional development, have one-on-one conversations with staff, facilitate self-care groups for staff, and provide emotional support and guidance after a crisis or death in the school system.

Classroom Environments

Traditionally, child life specialists build rapport with the child, the family, and the medical team. Similarly, school child life specialists must build rapport to collaborate with school staff effectively. This rapport enables classroom environments to empower further collaboration between teachers, students, and all school personnel. Child life specialists using a trauma-informed environmental checklist direct conversations with teachers regarding their students' psychosocial and developmental needs. This collaboration creates learning environments where students feel safe, heard, and cared for. Universal classroom strategies can be implemented to improve the classroom environment, positively impacting student behaviors and learning. Mindfulness activities like music and grounding, neuroscience-based movement and brain breaks, or visual daily schedules decrease stressful transitions and increase student coping. Child life recommendations create safe, therapeutic, and healing environments for students based on the assessment of development, life experience, and culture of the teacher and students.

SOLUTIONS AND RECOMMENDATIONS

Child Life Interventions

Trauma-Informed Care

The development of trauma-sensitive practices within the school system is at the core of the child life specialist work in any setting (Pappano, 2014). This involves shifting the mindset from asking, "What is wrong with them?" to "What happened to them?" (Perry & Winfrey, 2021). Child life specialists offering professional development provide school staff with knowledge about trauma-informed approaches to support all students in the school system, not just students with a history of trauma. Certified Child Life Specialists educate staff on the impact of trauma on a student's brain, body, ability to learn, and behavior in the school environment (Cole et al., 2013). Within a trauma-informed framework, the inclusion of diversity, equity, and inclusion is vital to all facets of the school system.

With increased behavioral challenges, schools are rethinking the traditional school discipline approach (Greene, 2016). This has historically consisted of exclusionary practices, such as out-of-school suspension and expulsion. However, failing to teach replacement behaviors, these methods contribute to students falling further behind, dropping out, and experiencing other negative outcomes.

Due to the harmful effects of these exclusionary practices, new discipline techniques are needed to keep students in school, using discipline as an opportunity to educate and build new skills. An example of this is an intentional in-school suspension program that incorporates reflection and processing, social-emotional learning, and practicing coping techniques. Keeping students in school keeps them closer to supportive adults, like child life specialists, who have time, training, and skills to create safe spaces where students learn self-regulation tools to prevent future occurrences and keep students in school rather than falling behind academically.

No child likes to be disciplined. However, natural consequences and restorative discipline are essential for helping children develop a foundation for self-discipline (Nieman & Shea, 2004). Child life specialists provide preparation for students before and after discipline happens. They facilitate processing and recovery tactics to help students return to baseline before returning to the classroom. By practicing healthy coping strategies as a replacement behavior, accountability and problem-solving will occur more easily.

Child life specialists use regulation or reflection sheets, which help students process emotions before a challenging behavior, identify how another person was feeling, and understand the difference between expected and unexpected school behaviors. By using these sheets, the Certified Child Life Specialist helps students cultivate understanding and empathy while preparing the student before or after a disciplinary meeting.

Providing validation and a listening ear encourages students to be more receptive to the necessary discipline of negative behaviors. Coaching school staff and administrators to implement "connection before correction" promotes discipline within a supportive relationship, resulting in less repeated negative behaviors (Carrington, 2020).

Social-Emotional Learning

The Collaborative for Academic, Social, and Emotional Learning (CASEL) breaks down social-emotional learning (SEL) into five competencies: "self-awareness, self-management, social awareness, responsible decision making, and relationships skills" (CASEL, n.d.). When students master these competencies, they can empathize with others, achieve cultural competence, problem-solve, utilize coping techniques when stressed, and better understand their own thoughts and feelings (CASEL, n.d.).

The overall goal of SEL is to help students understand and manage their emotions, make good decisions, practice empathy, and cultivate healthy relationships. There are many benefits to having social-emotional learning in schools, including increased academic scores and positive social behaviors, more time on task, and a more empathetic school climate due to feelings of attachment and connectedness at school (PATHS Program LLC, n.d.). Ultimately, the goal is for students to succeed not only in school but also in their future careers and community endeavors.

Child life specialists bring competencies in play and child development that aid in social-emotional learning, whether through the creation of a curriculum or implementing a pre-made, evidenced-based curriculum. To implement a SEL curriculum effectively, education should start with the adults in the building to create a universal language. Child life specialists can facilitate this training for school staff to promote whole-school participation and accountability.

Conversations with teaching staff direct lesson themes to help build up SEL skills in a classroom. SEL can be utilized individually with students, in group sessions, or by teaching whole-class lessons. With younger students, whole-class activities may look like reading a book on a psychosocial or social-emotional topic and then doing a hands-on or gross motor activity. Using as many multimodal strategies as possible to encompass different learning styles is important. These activities can help with classroom management and create a sensory-safe environment for all students.

In middle school, students are presented with whole-class subjects revolving around healthy friendships, bullying, social media, boundaries, and coping with stress. Often this responsibility falls to teachers when there is little or no psychosocial support. Child life specialists are uniquely equipped with a background in processing, developmentally appropriate language, preparation, and helping children talk about difficult experiences, can fill the gap in schools by providing support in the classroom, programming for students, and education for staff.

Coping Skills

A student should be taught coping strategies while they are regulated to strengthen neurological pathways, making it easier to access skills when dysregulated. The child life specialist functions as an additional safe, regulated adult in the classroom to serve as a role model, prompting the student through calming techniques, and leaving the teacher available to continue teaching the class.

The therapeutic relationships that child life specialists build with students are key in these emotionally charged situations. Evidence shows that when students are emotionally unavailable, their academic learning abilities become inaccessible (Carrington, 2020). It is only from a safe attachment that a child can be taught to regulate their emotions and problem-solving.

School Coping Spaces

Sensory spaces create an environment for students of all abilities to self-regulate, rebalance, and meet their sensory needs (Biel et al., 2009). Students experience fluctuations in their regulation throughout the school day due to a variety of stressors: environmental, social, emotional, and physical. Child life specialists can assess students' responses to these stressors and recognize feelings of frustration, anxiety, and anger as stemming from student dysregulation.

Students may not have access to strategies to recover, which is why they need to be pre-taught techniques when they are regulated. Ultimately, school staff want students to be capable of regulating at their desks. However, a child life specialist may first need to teach a student how to regulate in a sensory room, hallway, or at the back of the classroom.

Regulation bins for each classroom can be created by a school child life specialist in collaboration with an occupational therapist. Each bin may look different to assist with classroom coping based on student needs. These bins may include:

- Wiggle cushions
- Weighted lap lizards
- Fidget blankets
- Kinetic sand
- Sand timers

Because information processing may be slower during times of stress, regulation bins will help a student independently overcome stressors in their own workspaces. Regulation bins can be used in the classroom as a whole or within specific calm-down spaces.

Calm-down corners are a type of trauma-informed intervention that a child life specialist enhances in a school setting. They are considered safe spaces within the school walls that can be found anywhere, from a classroom corner to a hallway cubby or even the school office. In the hospital, child life specialists typically carry a distraction kit; in the school setting, this kit is transformed into a calm-down space.

In a calm-down space, visual and written prompts are used to teach students skills and how to use tools appropriately and independently. Coping tools might include:

- Sensory balls
- Fidgets
- Pinwheels
- Bubbles
- Coloring books
- Journals

- 5-4-3-2-1 mindfulness technique
- Progressive muscle relaxation
- Yoga poses
- Guided imagery

An agitated student will use these calm-down corners to cope with emotions by decompressing in a bean bag chair, drawing, squeezing a stress ball, or practicing deep breaths.

Students who experience more extreme challenges with focus, high emotional stress, or overwhelm due to environmental stimuli may need an intentionally created space to return to an optimal state of readiness to learn. A sensory room contains dynamic seating, feelings visuals, timers, bubble tubes, and fiber-optic lighting to aid in de-escalation. These rooms are not to be considered as restrictive or time-out spaces, but are supervised, safe areas for staff and students. Since a child life specialist is not always available in the moment of escalation, they can provide training for support staff on how to use the space appropriately with students.

Child Life Integration

Caregiver Involvement

Caregivers may sometimes be reluctant to work with school staff due to previous difficult experiences they had with the education system. Child life specialists build therapeutic relationships, grow trust, and help re-establish the school as a safe place for families and staff to collaborate.

"Certified Child life specialists empower children and families to become informed and active participants in their experiences" (ACLP, 2020, p.14). Through active communication between caregivers and staff about students' academics and coping, family-centered care is implemented to keep information uniform, help caregivers cope, and provide guidance on the best practices to support the student in the process. This is especially important in situations of truancy, chronic absenteeism, and discipline issues but is also critical for children in vulnerable families, such as refugees, immigrants, or minorities.

Group Work

The Association of Child Life Professionals (2018) states in their position statement for child life practice in community settings that child life specialists are qualified and trained to minimize stress and anxiety by facilitating interactions within a group setting for children experiencing similar traumatic or life events. This can include mediating amongst a peer group to promote self-advocacy and strengthen communication skills or facilitating a group that focuses its efforts on supporting children who may have lost a loved one and need a space to remember or grieve. Within a group setting, children can build resilience and leave with an understanding that they are not alone in their thoughts, feelings, or grief.

Anti-Bullying and Friendship Groups

Middle and high school are a pivotal time in developing peer relationships and impacting students' well-being. Words and actions of peers can be highly influential during this time. Child life specialists can facilitate and mediate difficult conversations between peers to resolve misunderstandings and address hurtful actions or words.

Bullying often occurs on social media and digital platforms. Many students are experiencing heightened anxiety due to the inability to know when the bullying may take place. As social media allows full access, anytime and anywhere, it is unclear when the hurtful words or actions may occur (Singh et al., 2018), which can lead to heightened stress, anxiety, and depressive symptoms (Martínez-Monteagudo et al., 2020). However, a more empathetic student body emerges when students understand each other. Child life specialists support students, those that are bullied and those that are the bully. Using restorative practices that promote empathy and expressive arts to encourage identification, validation, and sharing of feelings, child life specialists teach coping skills regulating students' emotional reactions when bullied but also in hopes of decreasing bullying.

Grief Group

With their expertise in grief and loss and promoting resilience, a child life specialist provides a safe space for students experiencing loss (ACLP, 2018). Mr. Rogers says, "When we can talk about our feelings, they become less overwhelming, less upsetting, and less scary. The people we trust with that important talk can help us know that we are not alone" (Rogers, n.d.). Child life specialists can lead or work in collaboration with a school counselor or social worker to run bereavement groups that focus on remembering students' loved ones who passed away. In addition, they normalize the grief process by introducing students to others who are facing the same or similar loss.

Social Skills Groups

Supporting a child's healthy relationships is one way a child life specialist promotes resilience through therapeutic interventions (ACLP, 2018). Facilitating social skills groups is one way this can be done, and working in collaboration with other professionals is helpful in creating a well-rounded group. For example, child life specialists collaborate with the school's social worker to run groups around themes of recess or LEGO® to gain buy-in from students to participate and engage in social skills groups.

LEGO® Club uses LEGO®-themed building activities to focus on following directions, paying attention, active listening, working in a group, regulation, and body awareness. Recess Club focuses more on asking peers to play appropriate games for recess time, naming feelings, and problem-solving.

Expressive play groups are used to work with students experiencing divorce in their family or struggling with big worries. These groups may use puppets, drawings, sand play, clay, storytelling, and music to help students express their big emotions, build coping strategies, enhance self-esteem, and regain positive thoughts through play.

Peer-to-Peer

Through the START Project created by Grand Valley State University in Michigan, children in Michigan often participate in the Peer-to-Peer program, which can be led by a child life specialist, teacher, or social worker with the appropriate training. This program pairs an upperclassman with a student with special needs. Social relationships with peers have been shown to increase the quality of life. In regards to those with disabilities, peer relationships can elevate self-esteem, provide confidence and support when socializing with others, and allow the student with the disability to stay in the inclusive classroom environment rather than transition out of class to be with peers with similar disabilities (Biggs & Carter, 2016).

During this experience, upperclassmen form connections with students whose educational experiences may be different from their own. Child life specialists may serve as the Peer-to-Peer coordinator and provide opportunities for mentoring for upperclassmen to better understand their peers by educating them on different disabilities using modalities like articles and videos. A child life specialist's knowledge of development supports opportunities to brainstorm and problem-solve when challenges arise between peers.

Individual Sessions

Expressive Arts

A child life specialist aids in processing emotion, traumatic event, experience, or thought by utilizing expressive arts to help a student cope. "Expressive art therapies, including visual art therapy, have the potential to help adolescents manage developmental tasks and attain the skills necessary to be resilient in times of stress" (Lindsey et al., 2018, p. 2).

Students are provided choices regarding their creative outlet to foster autonomy over their creative expression. Every student processes differently; some may find benefit in verbal processing, while others may experience the most breakthroughs by using their hands through writing, drawing, or coloring. In the same way, that child life specialists provide patients with appropriate choices for normalization or therapeutic play in the hospital setting, a school child life specialist may provide students with choices for how they process their feelings (writing, music, art, or verbally), thus impacting and increasing a student's emotional intelligence (Drigas & Papoutsi, 2018). Normalizing that there is more than one way to process emotions and teaching students how to move through emotions in a healthy way cultivates a positive school culture.

Therapeutic Play

Therapeutic play usually involves broad-based play activities with a targeted goal. Whether working alone or collaborating with psychosocial team members, child life specialists use therapeutic play to support students dealing with challenges that may impact their ability to learn.

The child life value of play states that "play facilitates healing, coping, mastery, self-expression, creativity, achievement, and learning, and is vital to a child's optimal growth and development" (ACLP, 2001, p.1). Play also allows a student to explore or rehearse how a social situation may transpire or process emotions in a way that is not appropriate in real-life contexts, like using a punching bag to release aggression rather than punching a peer. As a result, students regain their former level of functioning in the classroom, enhance self-esteem to initiate tasks, adjust to life challenges, and develop individual coping strategies for upcoming changes (ECS, 2020).

When a student is stressed, staff may see changes in their play behaviors due to the perceived lack of safety or unpredictability of a challenging situation. Pretend play, unstructured therapeutic play, or free play prevents or reduces anxiety and distress by allowing students to identify and express their emotions and gain control of their environment (ACLP, 2020). A child life specialist does not always need to lead the play, but rather supervise, track what they see, or purposely modify the play to reinforce effective emotional regulation or peer interactions.

Child-led play during centers, small groups, or even pull-outs allows for the student to gain mastery, confidence, and connection. As students play out their emotions and feelings at a distance with toys, they become better at expressing their feelings in everyday exchanges with peers and staff. Child life specialists build therapeutic rapport through play. They provide a safe environment for students to express feelings through appropriate aggressive play, which could be construed as inappropriate in other contexts (e.g., bursting balloons, pounding clay, throwing scrunched-up paper).

Creating play opportunities aids in literacy skills, facilitates relationship building, develops cause-and-effect thinking, practices problem-solving, allows for processing stressful situations, and helps students learn social skills (Drewes & Schaefer, 2015). A child life specialist can use observations of a student's play to assess interactions with their environment, critical developmental factors, self-control, and emotional regulation. They can then help facilitate developmentally appropriate learning through play for students that require academic accommodations.

Documentation

Child life specialists communicate effectively with other professionals by documenting observations and assessments. They should create notes after sessions with a student and share them with the appropriate stakeholders. Each note should include a brief, objective update of a student's progress and any beneficial strategies that aid in the student's coping. Discussions with the school team or family should be documented to note items to revisit.

At the end of the year, child life specialists complete transition summaries to provide a snapshot of student information for the new grade teacher or new school if a student is moving. Key strategies that the student depends on for success in the classroom should be listed within this document. It is important to collect data indicating how many students a child life specialist sees, specific student needs, and what interventions were implemented to illustrate the position's impact on school leadership.

CHILD LIFE SCHOOL PROPOSAL

When a child life role is not established in a school district, a proposal is often necessary to illustrate the rationale behind creating a full-time child life position in the school setting. The proposal highlights the numerous benefits a child life specialist would afford to school staff, students, and families. The proposal should be concise while presenting the full scope of the child life role, making sure to use language and research pertinent to the specific school setting.

Child life specialists eager to enter the school setting will likely have to educate school administrators on the benefits of child life and the differences between a child life specialist and other, more familiar school mental health roles, such as a school counselor or social worker. They may find success in targeting schools with open positions related to student mental health, asking them to consider meeting these needs with the role of a child life specialist.

Data and research increasingly prove the effectiveness of child life in school settings and have been beneficial in securing child life school positions.

CONCLUSION

Greater collaboration between schools, families, and health care must be established from an ecological framework (Bronfenbrenner, 1981). As students move through different developmental ages, they interact with multiple systems that influence how they cope. A student's behavior is not simply impacted by what is happening in the school. Child life values that students communicate their needs through words, play, and behavior. Child life specialists, therefore, observe, listen and facilitate communication with those who may be misunderstood or need support to be heard (ACLP, 2001).

Child life specialists work alongside professionals from multiple systems in a student's world as school staff members. Child life specialists work closely with the family and school personnel at the microsystem. As different institutions interact, a child life specialist can navigate communication between healthcare professionals, the school, and caregivers. Although a student may not have direct contact with their exosystem, a child life specialist can consider specific exosystem impacts when supporting a student in the classroom. Finally, as a profession, child life has knowledge, training, and skills related to the mesosystems that impact student behaviors, such as sociocultural diversity. "Regardless of the setting, child life specialists have a responsibility to provide clinical, ethical and sociocultural-sensitive care that aligns with the ACLP Standards of Clinical Practice and supports its commitment to upholding diversity, equity and inclusion" (ACLP, 2020, p.1).

Students who have experienced trauma or have disabilities are often prioritized in the school for needing additional support. However, many neurotypical, well-adjusted students with good attendance and involved parental figures are often overlooked. These students may also have emotional, physical, or mental needs that are not supported due to the lack of mental health professionals: grief in losing a pet, an unexpected visit to the hospital, or school immunizations. By providing more education and coaching to teachers and caregivers, child life specialists employed in a school system can further bridge the communication between home and school. Students will thrive when caregivers understand and prioritize the interactions between their students' diagnoses, mental health struggles, and academic learning.

Schools will continue to need more psychosocial support to combat the issues created by crises such as the COVID-19 pandemic. Employing child life specialists enhances a school's ability to build students' resilience by filling a gap in service. Future areas to address will include the expansion of culturally responsive and trauma-informed school systems to address issues of identity and demographics, increasing tolerance and leading to a more empathetic student body. Research needs to be done on the efficacy of child life specialists in school systems and the effects on SEL, mental health, trauma, and resilience. Data collection and research are needed to show the impact of child life on decreasing disciplinary actions, increasing mental health and coping, and increasing test scores in the school environment. As diversity, equity, and inclusion continue to be a priority for schools, child life specialists are a complementary profession to expand multidisciplinary teams educating staff to move this work forward.

As the profession grows and enters the community, schools are a natural setting for employing child life specialists. Child life services in all school settings are a proactive way to increase students' ability to cope in multiple environments. As a leader of change, the child life profession will transform organizational thinking surrounding the impact of school suicide risk teams, community health centers, and outside resources on school campuses.

Throughout this chapter, it is evident that schools have been issued a challenge with the significant unmet psychosocial needs of their students. School mental health professionals are usually underrepresented, and community organizations have extremely long wait lists. For the most part, the quantity of students that need mental health support is unmatched by school resources. This must be improved by increasing resources and staff support.

The foundations for child life in the school and healthcare settings are much the same: increased coping, empowering others to manage stress, helping others to talk about difficult topics through play, developmentally appropriate preparation, therapeutic activities, and more. As the child life role expands into new areas, interventions are adapted to meet the school environment's specific needs while staying within the child life scope of practice. Making appropriate referrals and respecting other professionals in the multidisciplinary team allows a child life specialist in a school to use flexibility and creativity to support students appropriately.

There is an overwhelming need for additional psychosocial services in the school setting, and child life specialists effectively fill this need. The school is an incredibly exciting environment where the expertise of a child life specialist, as part of a dynamic psychosocial team, can add value to the lives of students and their families.

REFERENCES

Alberta Education. (2006). *Individualized program planning*. https://education.alberta.ca/media/384992/indidivualized-program-planning-2006.pdf

American Federation of Teachers and New York Life Foundation. (2012). *Grief in the classroom*. https://www.newyorklife.com/assets/foundation/docs/pdfs/NYL-AFT-Bereavement-Survey.pdf

American School Counselor Association. (2019). *School Counselors Matter*. https://www.schoolcounselor.org/getmedia/b079d17d-6265-4166-a120-3b1f56077649/School-Counselors-Matter.pdf

American School Counselor Association. (2022). *School Counselor Roles and Ratios*. https://www.schoolcounselor.org/About-School-Counseling/School-Counselor-Roles-Ratios

American School Counselor Association. (n.d.). *Empirical Research Studies Supporting the Value of School Counseling*. https://www.schoolcounselor.org/getmedia/7d00dcff-40a6-4316-ab6c-8f3ffd7941c2/Effectiveness.pdf

Association of Child Life Professionals. (2001). *Mission, values, vision, and operating principles*. https://www.childlife.org/docs/default-source/the-child-life-profession/mission-vision-values.pdf

Association of Child Life Professionals. (2016). *Child Life Competencies*. https://www.childlife.org/docs/default-source/the-child-life-profession/childlifecompetenciesjune2016.pdf?sfvrsn=2

Association of Child Life Professionals. (2018). *Association of Child Life Professionals position statement on child life practice in community settings*. https://www.childlife.org/docs/default-source/about-aclp/cbp-on-cl-practice-in-community-settings.pdf

Association of Child Life Professionals. (2020). *The value of Certified Child Life Specialists: Direct and downstream optimization of pediatric patient and family outcomes*. https://www.childlife.org/docs/default-source/the-child-life-profession/value-of-cclss-full-report.pdf

Association of Child Life Professionals. (2020). *Child Life Code of Ethics.* https://www.childlife.org/docs/default-source/certification/child-life-code-of-ethics.pdf?sfvrsn=2

Atkins, M. S., Hoagwood, K. E., Kutash, K., & Seidman, E. (2010). Toward the integration of education and mental health in schools. *Administration and Policy in Mental Health, 37*(1-2), 40–47. doi:10.100710488-010-0299-7 PMID:20309623

Benner, A. D., & Mistry, R. S. (2020). Child development during the COVID-19 pandemic through a life course theory lens. *Child Development Perspectives, 14*(4), 236–243. doi:10.1111/cdep.12387 PMID:33230400

Berta, S., Blonsky, H., & Wogan, J. (2022). *Developing your school's student support teams: A practical guide for K-12 leaders, student services personnel, and mental health staff.* CRC Press. doi:10.4324/9781003240266

Bethell, C., Combojav, N., Solloway, M., & Wissow, L. (2016). Adverse childhood experiences, resilience and mindfulness-based approaches: Common denominator issues for children with emotional, mental, or behavioral problems. *Child and Adolescent Psychiatric Clinics of North America, 25*(2), 139–156. doi:10.1016/j.chc.2015.12.001 PMID:26980120

Bethell, C., Newacheck, P., Hawes, E., & Halfton, N. (2014). Adverse childhood experiences: Assessing the impact on health and school engagement and the mitigating role of resilience. *Health Affairs, 33*(12), 2106–2115. Advance online publication. doi:10.1377/hlthaff.2014.0914 PMID:25489028

Biel, L., Peske, N., & Grandin, T. (2009). *Raising a sensory smart child: The definitive handbook for helping your child with sensory processing issues.* Penguin Books.

Biggs, E. E., & Carter, E. W. (2016). Supporting the social lives of students with intellectual disability. In *Handbook of research-based practices for educating students with intellectual disability* (pp. 243–262). Routledge.

Bray, B. (2019). *One school counselor per 455 students: Nationwide average improves.* Counseling Today. https://ct.counseling.org/2019/05/one-school-counselor-per-455-students-nationwide-average-improves/

Bronfenbrenner, U. (1981). *The Ecology of Human Development.* Harvard University Press. doi:10.2307/j.ctv26071r6

Brown, A. (2008). *The school setting. Child Life Beyond the Hospital.* Child Life Council, Inc.

Burns, M., Griese, B., King, S., & Talmi, A. (2020). Childhood bereavement: Understanding prevalence and related adversity in the United States. *The American Journal of Orthopsychiatry, 90*(4), 391–405. doi:10.1037/ort0000442 PMID:31999137

California Department of Education. (2019). *Designating Liaisons for Students Experiencing Homelessness.* https://www.cde.ca.gov/sp/hs/cy/documents/designatingliaisons.docx

Carrington, J. (2020). *Kids these days: A game plan for (re)connecting with those we teach, lead & love.* IMPress Books.

Centers for Disease Control and Prevention. (2021). *COVID-19 parental resources kit.* https://www.cdc.gov/mentalhealth/stress-coping/parental-resources/index.html

Chesak, S. S., Khalsa, T. K., Bhagra, A., Jenkins, S. M., Bauer, B. A., & Sood, A. (2019). Stress Management and Resiliency Training for public school teachers and staff: A novel intervention to enhance resilience and positively impact student interactions. *Complementary Therapies in Clinical Practice, 37*, 32–38. doi:10.1016/j.ctcp.2019.08.001 PMID:31445365

Child Mind Institute. (2021). *The impact of the COVID-19 pandemic on children's mental health: What we know so far.* https://childmind.org/wp-content/uploads/2021/10/CMHR-2021-FINAL.pdf

Cole, S. F., Eisner, A., Gregory, M., & Ristuccia, J. (2013). *Creating and advocating for trauma-sensitive schools.* Massachusetts Advocates for Children.

Collaborative for Academic, Social, and Emotional Learning. (n.d.). *What is the CASEL framework?* https://casel.org/fundamentals-of-sel/what-is-the-casel-framework/

Cronholm, P. F., Forke, C. M., Wade, R., Bair-Merritt, M. H., Davis, M., Harkins-Schwarz, M., Pachter, L. M., & Fein, J. A. (2015). Adverse Childhood Experiences: Expanding the Concept of Adversity. *American Journal of Preventive Medicine, 49*(3), 354–361. doi:10.1016/j.amepre.2015.02.001 PMID:26296440

Deaton, J. D., Ohrt, J. H., Linich, K., Wymer, B., Toomey, M., Leris, O., Guest, J. D., & Newton, T. (2022). Teachers' experiences with K-12 students' mental health. *Psychology in the Schools, 59*(50), 932–949. doi:10.1002/pits.22658

Drewes, A. A., & Schaefer, C. E. (2015). *School-Based Play Therapy* (2nd ed.). John Wiley & Sons Inc.

Drigas, A. S., & Papoutsi, C. (2018). A new layered model on emotional intelligence. *Behavioral Sciences (Basel, Switzerland)*, *8*(5), 45. doi:10.3390/bs8050045 PMID:29724021

Edmonton Catholic Schools. (2020). *Mental Health Strategic Plan*. https://sbecsdstor.blob.core.windows.net/docs/9115d70a-5ccc-4a1f-8273-a4176310f7a1_ECSMENTALHEALTHBROCH1920.pdf

Felitti, V. J., Anda, R. F., Nordenberg, D., Williamson, D. F., Spitz, A. M., Edwards, V., Koss, M. P., & Marks, J. S. (1998). Relationship of childhood abuse and household dysfunction to many of the leading causes of death in adults. The Adverse Childhood Experiences (ACE) Study. *American Journal of Preventive Medicine*, *14*(4), 245–258. doi:10.1016/S0749-3797(98)00017-8 PMID:9635069

Gaynard, L., Wolfer, J., Goldberger, J., Thompson, R., Redburn, L., & Laidley, L. (1998). *Psychosocial care of children in hospitals: A clinical practice manual from the ACCH child life research project*. Child Life Council, Inc.

Greene, R. W. (2016). *Lost and found: Helping Behaviorally Challenging Students (and, While You're At It, All the Others)*. Jossey-Bass.

Greiner, C. M., Park, J., & Goldstein, S. E. (2022). Teacher trainees' experience with and beliefs about responding to students' challenging life events. *Teaching and Teacher Education*, *111*, 103603. doi:10.1016/j.tate.2021.103603

Heffer, R. W., & Lowe, P. A. (2000). A review of school reintegration programs for children with cancer. *Journal of School Psychology*, *38*(5), 447–467. doi:10.1016/S0022-4405(00)00046-7

Ioverno, S., Belser, A. B., Baiocco, R., Grossman, A. H., & Russell, S. T. (2016). The protective role of gay–straight alliances for lesbian, gay, bisexual, and questioning students: A prospective analysis. *Psychology of Sexual Orientation and Gender Diversity*, *3*(4), 397–406. doi:10.1037gd0000193 PMID:28042585

Koschmann, E., Jacob, R., Robinson, J., Foster Friendman, M., Foster, A., Rodriguez-Quintana, N., Vichich, J., Smith, M., & Rajaram, H. (2022). Mental health needs in a large urban school district: Findings from a web-based survey. *Health Services Research*, *57*(4), 830–841. Advance online publication. doi:10.1111/1475-6773.13924 PMID:35243624

Lewis, T., Jones, K. D., Militello, M., & Meisenhelder, R. (2020). A Clear and Consistent Focus on Students: Principals' Perceptions of the Role of School Counselors. *Journal of School Leadership*, *32*(1), 3–26. doi:10.1177/1052684620972067

Lindsey, L., Robertson, P., & Lindsey, B. (2018). Expressive arts and mindfulness: Aiding adolescents in understanding and managing their stress. *Journal of Creativity in Mental Health*, *13*(3), 288–297. doi:10.1080/15401383.2018.1427167

Martínez-Monteagudo, M. C., Delgado, B., Díaz-Herrero, Á., & García-Fernández, J. M. (2020). Relationship between suicidal thinking, anxiety, depression and stress in university students who are victims of cyberbullying. *Psychiatry Research*, *286*, 112856. doi:10.1016/j.psychres.2020.112856 PMID:32062285

Maslow, A. H. (1954). *Motivation and Personality* (1st ed.). Harper.

McManus, E., & Paul, S. (2019). Addressing the bereavement needs of children in school: An evaluation of bereavement training for school communities. *Improving Schools*, *22*(1), 72–85. doi:10.1177/1365480219825540

Miron, O., Yu, K., Wilf-Miron, R., & Kohane, I. S. (2019). Suicide rates among adolescents and young adults in the United States 2000-2017. *Journal of the American Medical Association*, *321*(23), 2362. Advance online publication. doi:10.1001/jama.2019.5054 PMID:31211337

Moon, J., Williford, A., & Mendenhall, A. (2017). Educators' perceptions of youth mental health: Implications for training and the promotion of mental health services in schools. *Children and Youth Services Review*, *73*, 384-391. doi:10.1016/j.childyouth.2017.01.006

National Center for Education Statistics. (2016). *Number and percentage of public schools by presence of counselors, psychologists and social workers on staff and selected school characteristics*. https://nces.ed.gov/surveys/ntps/tables/ntps1516_027_s1n_04.asp

National Center for Homeless Education. (n.d.). *The McKinney-Vento definition of homeless*. https://nche.ed.gov/mckinney-vento-definition/

National Center for School Crisis and Bereavement and the Coalition to Support Grieving Students. (2020). *Supporting grieving students in schools*. https://grievingstudents.org/wp-content/uploads/2020/06/TTM-Combined-May-31-2020.pptx

National Education Association. (2022). *Poll results: Stress and burnout pose threat of educator shortages.* https://www.nea.org/sites/default/files/2022-02/NEA%20Member%20COVID-19%20Survey%20Summary.pdf

Nieman, P., & Shea, S. (2004). Effective discipline for children. *Paediatrics & Child Health*, *9*(1), 37–41. doi:10.1093/pch/9.1.37 PMID:19654979

Pappano, L. (2014). "Trauma-sensitive" schools: A new framework for reaching troubled students. *Harvard Education Letter, 30*(3), 1–5.

PATHS Program LLC. (n.d.). *PATHS® curriculum research: Research-based with proven outcomes.* https://pathsprogram.com/paths-research

Perry, B. D., & Winfrey, O. (2021). *What happened to you? Conversations on trauma, resilience, and healing.* Melcher Media Inc.

Pershick, S. (2009). *Child Life Specialists' Perspective on Collaboration with Schools.* Ryerson University.

Rogers, F. (n.d.). *He helped us with our feelings.* https://www.misterrogers.org/articles/he-helped-us-with-our-feelings/

Schonfeld, D. (2015). *Grieving children: An essential role for schools.* https://www.etr.org/blog/my-take-grievingchildren/

School Social Work Association of America. (n.d.). *Role of School Social Worker.* https://www.sswaa.org/school-social-work

Schott Foundation for Public Education. (2014). *Restorative practices: Fostering healthy relationships and promoting positive discipline in schools.* https://schottfoundation.org/sites/default/files/restorative-practices-guide.pdf

Singh, P. P., Kumar, V., & Sadeeq, M. (2018). Cyber bullying as an outcome of social media usage: A literature review. *Indian Journal of Public Health, 9*(12).

Van der Werf, H. M., Luttik, M. L. A., Francke, A. L., Roodbol, P. F., & Paans, W. (2019). Students growing up with a chronically ill family member; a survey on experienced consequences, background characteristics, and risk factors. *BMC Public Health, 19*(1), 1–8. doi:10.118612889-019-7834-6 PMID:31703664

Vohs, K. D., & Baumeister, R. F. (2016). *Handbook of self-regulation: Research, theory and applications* (3rd ed.). The Guilford Press.

Wagers, D. (2013). Speaking up for children undergoing procedures: The ONE VOICE approach. *Pediatric Nursing, 39*(5), 257. https://onevoice4kids.com/ PMID:24308094

Weiner, P. L., Hoffman, M., & Rosen, C. (2009). Child life and education issues: The child with a chronic illness or special healthcare needs. In R. H. Thompson (Ed.), *The Handbook of Child Life: A Guide for Pediatric Psychosocial Care* (pp. 310–326). Charles C Thomas.

Yinglin, M. E., Ruther, M. H., & Dubuque, E. M. (2022). Trends in geographic access to Board Certified Behavior Analysts among children with autism spectrum disorder, 2018-2021. *Journal of Autism and Developmental Disorders*. Advance online publication. doi:10.100710803-021-05402-0 PMID:34985719

ADDITIONAL READING

Alber, D. (2015). *A little scribble spot: A story about colorful emotions*. Diane Alber Art LLC.

Carrington, J. (2020). *Kids these days: A game plan for (re)connecting with those we teach, lead & love*. IMPress Books.

Faber, A., & Mazlish, E. (2012). *How to talk so kids will listen and listen so kids will talk*. Scribner Book Company.

Forbes, H. T. (2012). *Help for Billy: A beyond consequences approach to helping challenging children in the classroom*. Beyond Consequences Institute LLC.

Greene, R. W. (2021). *Lost and found: Unlocking collaboration and compassion to help our most vulnerable, misunderstood students (and all the rest)* (2nd ed.). Jossey-Bass.

Hewson, K., Hewson, L., & Parson, J. (2015). *Envisioning a collaborative response model: Beliefs, structures, and processes to transform how we respond to the needs of students*. Jigsaw Learning.

Maynard, N. & Weinstein, B. (2019). *Hacking school discipline: 9 ways to create a culture of empathy & responsibility using restorative justice*. Times 10 Publications.

Perry, B. D., & Winfrey, O. (2021). *What happened to you? Conversations on trauma, resilience, and healing*. Melcher Media Inc.

Siegel, D. J., & Bryson, T. P. (2012). *The whole-brain child: 12 revolutionary strategies to nurture your child's developing mind*. Bantam.

KEY TERMS AND DEFINITIONS

504 Plan: Plans used in schools to remove barriers and give equal access to students with disabilities. 504 plans provide modifications or accommodations to enhance learning and add support so all students can participate in public education or any schools that receive public funding.

Behavior Challenges: In a school setting, a student's behavior is considered challenging when it is unsafe for themselves or others, or if it is significantly impacting their ability to learn and join in on everyday routines. For example: aggression, tantrums, impulsivity, elopement, screaming, swearing, refusal to follow instructions, repetitive movements.

Environmental Checklists: When implementing universal strategies in a classroom, staff must identify internal environmental conditions that may impact a student's academic performance. Simple steps can be completed to transform a space to be more inclusive for all types of learners.

Functional Behavior Assessment (FBA): A process used to identify and understand challenging behaviors, while also coming up with possible solutions and more appropriate, alternative behavior. Once a challenging behavior is defined, observations and data is collected. After developing a hypothesis of why the behavior is occurring, staff can create and implement strategies to increase positive behavior. A positive behavior support plan is then created to identify scripts, skills to be taught and individual interventions for the student.

Genders and Sexualities Alliance (GSA): Student-led group to provide those who identify with LGBTQIA+ community as well as their allies a safe space to educate, advocate, and support one another.

Individual Program Plan (IPP): Is a student-focused, collaborative action plan that addresses barriers within the learning environment, communicates student goals and growth, while also providing a guide for transition planning at the end of the year. Can also be known as an Individual Education Plan (IEP), Special Education Plan (SEP), Student Support Plan (SSP), Individual Support Plan (ISP), depending on the location or district. This plan identifies goals for students with disabilities (intellectual, physical, medical, learning, hearing, visual, communication, behavioral or emotional) and disorders, which may include General Anxiety Disorder (GAD), Depression, Oppositional Defiant Disorder (ODD), Conduct Disorder (CD), Autism Spectrum Disorder (ASD), Fetal Alcohol Syndrome (FASD), Tourette's, fine and gross motor delays.

Multi-Tiered System of Support (MTSS): A proactive, school-wide approach that is committed to ensuring equitable education for all students by utilizing universal (whole class), focused (small group), and intensive (individual) strategies. This system provides a framework for instruction, assessment and support so that staff can work collaboratively with students, families, and community partners. It is inclusive of all students, but is not considered special education. It is student focused and responds to all their unique strengths and needs to increase student success. Integrating this approach into a school environment, staff can address student's academic, behavioral, and social-emotional health needs preventatively.

Non-Violent Crisis Intervention: Interventions that help keep staff and students safe during crises such as assaultive, disruptive, or out-of-control persons. Training focuses on prevention, de-escalation, personal safety, and physical intervention.

Positive Behavior Support Plan: A plan created after completing a Functional Behavior Assessment (FBA). It is a working document that is continually evaluated and redesigned if strategies are not working or next steps need to be made. This proactive plan focuses on the function of behavior by looking at changing the environment the behavior occurs, the lagging skills leading to the behavior, and how the behavior is reinforced. This plan aims to decrease challenging behaviors and increase appropriate, functional behaviors instead.

Restorative Practice: An approach that focuses on strengthening the community, building healthy relationships, and conflict prevention and resolution. It is a social science that aims to improve relationships and repair any harm that has been done. All parties are included and treated with dignity to create a positive and equitable school culture.

Sensory Spaces: An intentionally created area in a school that supports students' need to self-regulate by stimulating or calming their senses. This therapeutic space may contain a variety of multi-sensory resources and stimuli that help reduce stress or fulfill a need for sensory input in an appropriate way. Once a student is calm, they can re-engage with learning.

Social-Emotional Learning (SEL): Is the process of developing the self-awareness, self-control, and interpersonal skills that are vital for school, work, and life success. SEL helps kids identify their feelings, understand and communicate with others, build strong relationships, and make good, empathetic decisions. Students are better able to cope with everyday challenges and benefit academically, professionally, and socially.

Strength-Based Approach: Has multiple definitions based on which profession it comes from. Social work focuses on relationship building and creating community networks for a client. Teaching, it is about being self-reflective in their practice and understanding how they impact their students. As a child life specialist in a school, this approach is more about focusing on the strengths of others (students, staff, families). Instead of identifying deficits, this practice is holistic and multi-disciplinary to work with an individual to promote their success and wellness.

Trauma-Informed: An approach that realizes the prevalence of trauma, recognizes how trauma impacts individuals and their development, responds to trauma and resists re-traumatization. Trauma-informed care focuses on including safety, choice, trustworthiness, collaboration, and empowerment.

APPENDIX

Figure 1. Check-In/Check-Out (CICO) template

STUDENT NAME

Check In-Check Out

0 = no effort

1 = effort for half the class

2 = full effort all class

	1st Hour	2nd Hour	Study Hall	3rd Hour	4th Hour	5th Hour	6th Hour
Be Alert (be present and awake in class)	0 1 2	0 1 2	0 1 2	0 1 2	0 1 2	0 1 2	0 1 2
Be Social (when appropriate talk to your peers and engage in open discussions in class)	0 1 2	0 1 2	0 1 2	0 1 2	0 1 2	0 1 2	0 1 2
Be Respectful (acknowledge teacher when spoken to)	0 1 2	0 1 2	0 1 2	0 1 2	0 1 2	0 1 2	0 1 2
Be on Task (complete work in class and use time wisely)	0 1 2	0 1 2	0 1 2	0 1 2	0 1 2	0 1 2	0 1 2
Teacher Initials							

Chapter 6
Prison

Genevieve Lowry
https://orcid.org/0000-0002-9639-5830
Bank Street College of Education, USA

ABSTRACT

This chapter focuses on the role of the child life specialist working with families affected by incarceration. Children and families are at increased risk due to trauma exacerbated by arrests, incarceration, and re-entry. This chapter will focus on the ways a child life specialist working in jails, prisons, detention centers, and in communities with schools, non-profits, and faith-based organizations can provide developmentally appropriate explanations, preparation, play, expressive arts, and coping, facilitating opportunities that foster relationships and understanding while promoting resilience.

INTRODUCTION

The author of this chapter provided specific programming for incarcerated caregivers. The ideas for the role of a child life specialist outlined in this chapter originated from discussions with parents and caregivers experiencing and being affected by incarceration, as well as the author's experience and knowledge as a Certified Child Life Specialist in both traditional and community settings. This chapter describes how a child life specialist would benefit those affected by incarceration and the staff working within a corrections facility. The role of the child life specialist, as described in this chapter, could also be incorporated into schools, nonprofits, and faith-based organizations working to support those affected by incarceration or at risk for incarceration or re-entry post-incarceration.

Throughout this chapter, the author defines those affected by incarceration as individuals who have been incarcerated, children of those who are incarcerated, and families, including foster families that care for the children of incarcerated individuals. Although the chapter focuses on caregivers and parents in jails and prisons, the author recognizes that child life services and many of the interventions described would also benefit at-risk youth, justice-involved youth, and those committed to juvenile detention centers.

DOI: 10.4018/978-1-6684-5097-0.ch006

BACKGROUND

Statistics, Settings, and Disparities

According to Sawyer and Wagner of The Prison Policy Initiative (2022), the American criminal justice system holds almost 2 million people in 1,566 state prisons, 102 federal prisons, 1,510 juvenile correctional facilities, 2,850 local jails, 186 immigration detention facilities, and 82 Indian Country jails, as well as in military prisons, civil commitment centers, state psychiatric hospitals, and prisons in the U.S. territories. The same report articulated that of those incarcerated, nearly half of state prisoners (47%) and more than half of federal prisoners (57%) reported having at least one minor child. Among minor children of parents in state prison, 1% were younger than 1, about 18% were ages 1 to 4, and 48% were 10 or older. The average age of a minor child among parents in federal prison was 10 years old. An estimated 13% of minor children of federal prisoners were age 4 or younger, and 20% were aged 15 to 17.

Before working within jails or prisons and community agencies, one must first understand the types of settings, statistics, and disparities that affect and contribute to the stress of those affected by incarceration. Most justice-involved persons are incarcerated in either jail, state or federal prison, or juvenile detention centers. Jail is a locally operated, short-term facility where justice-involved persons typically await trial and sentencing for up to 364 days and those sentenced to less than a year. Prison is a state or federally operated, long-term facility. Prisons are for incarcerated individuals sentenced to 365 days or longer. Federal prisons prohibit parole, so the amount of time served is significantly higher than the average time served in state prison (Crime Museum, n.d). In addition, those under the age of 18 reside in juvenile detention centers unless tried and convicted as an adult.

A child life specialist must understand the racial disparities affecting Black, Indigenous, and People of Color (BIPOC) experiencing incarceration or justice-involved persons or youth. According to The Sentencing Project (2021), Black Americans are imprisoned at five times the rate of White Americans. In addition, those that identify as Latinx have 1.3 times the incarceration rate of Whites, making it clear that the "outcome of mass incarceration today has not occurred by happenstance but has been designed through policies created by a dominant White culture that insists on suppression of others" (p.4). The toll is steep for families affected by incarceration, as it disrupts relationships through lost connections. Communities suffer from losing parents whose absence leaves families in tatters through lost jobs, income, homes, and hope. Many families will experience financial stress as the added burden of lost revenue, legal and court fees, and phone calls and commissary costs can leave families struggling to make ends meet (Annie E. Casey Foundation, 2016).

A demographic analysis commissioned by the Association of Child Life Professionals (2018) states that the typical Certified Child Life Specialist is a 34-year-old White female (Lookabaugh & Ballard, 2018). Although a profession of predominantly White women, any child life specialist, regardless of race, would benefit from education and training on how the justice and correctional systems perpetuate and promote racism and anti-Blackness that have led to the increased incarceration of BIPOC. Principle 3 of the Child Life Code of Ethics states:

Certified Child Life Specialists have an obligation to maintain an environment that respects variations in culture, age, gender, race, ethnicity, physical ability, sexual orientation, gender identity/expression, religious affiliation, veteran status, and socioeconomic status (Official Documents of the Child Life Council, 2020).

The ACLP Position Statement on Diversity Equity and Inclusion (2020) envisions Child Life Specialists building a "culturally effective, inclusive, and equitable profession that aligns with and supports our patients, workforce, and the communities that we serve" for CCLS to "create safer spaces that foster mutual understanding, respect, and growth" (ACLP Official Documents, 2020). This requires education, training, and reflection on practice that examines the work to root out bias and privilege while identifying areas for growth and learning.

Due to the increased criminalization of poverty, Child Life Specialists should acquire anti-racist training to deepen their understanding of how mass incarceration has affected primarily black and brown communities as a first step toward examining and identifying one's bias. In addition, Child Life Specialists working with those affected by incarceration should develop reflective practices that support examining clinical work, boundary issues, and areas of bias and racism. Without understanding the lived experiences of others and one's position and privilege, or lack thereof, Child Life Specialists cannot effectively amplify the voices of those families they serve and could cause further harm to the families they are trying to support. Therefore, it is the obligation, and ethical responsibility of any child life specialist working with families affected by incarceration, especially those who identify as White, to obtain additional education and training focused on racial consciousness and cultural humility that examines positionality, privilege, and implicit bias.

RATIONALE FOR ROLE OF THE CHILD LIFE SPECIALIST

Child Life Specialists' innovative approach to care and resourcefulness makes them a good fit for working in settings that require structure and strict guidelines to function and maintain safety. For example, a child life specialist in healthcare settings follows the rules and regulations to protect and safeguard children and families coming to medical centers for treatment. Infection control, visitation policies, and confidentiality are regulations that dictate how a child life specialist practices. The Child Life Competencies explicitly state that Certified Child Life Specialists must have "the ability to implement child life services within the structure and culture of the work environment" (ACLP Official Documents, 2020). Within the prison system, rules and regulations are in place to safeguard incarcerated individuals, employees, and visitors. Working within the confines of these structures, a child life specialist respects the need for those regulations and finds ways to provide child life interventions within those structures. The role of the child life specialist is to provide opportunities for expression, education, and coping with the existing safety nets. According to the Child Life Code of Ethics (2020), "Certified Child Life Specialists demonstrate the competencies of the child life profession by continuous efforts to improve professional services and practices provided in the diverse settings in which they work and in the community at large." Child Life Specialists should advocate for examining systems and policies that limit the possibility of relationships and connections. The child life specialist in these settings suggests evidenced-based practices that support programs or changes grounded in research and theory. The child life specialist works with prison staff to develop safe ways to meet the needs of families visiting or communicating with an incarcerated loved one while also considering the safety of those who live and work in prison.

Certified Child Life Specialists are integral to the social and emotional well-being of families affected by changes due to separation, trauma, grief, and loss. Child Life Specialists support coping responses, minimize stress and coping, prepare children and families for life experiences, promote independence and self-esteem, and communicate and advocate for children and families as multidisciplinary team members (ACLP, Official Documents, 2020).

NEEDS ASSESSMENT

Parental incarceration is an adverse childhood experience affecting long-term health, education, and quality of life outcomes (Felitti et al. 1998). Children affected by incarceration experience upheaval in family systems due to short and long-term separations, changes in financial stability, and food insecurity.

Incarceration of a loved one puts children at increased risk for issues associated with social-emotional development and attachment, school readiness, and educational achievement. Dichter et al., (2020) cite a number of studies that indicate incarceration of a loved one significantly impacts executive functioning and cognitive skills including children as young as three may exhibit aggressive behaviors. Additionally, economic challenges due to incarceration may lead to food insecurity, residential and housing instability, and homelessness. Family relationships can be strained and often experience disruptions and dissolution of the family due to incarceration. Children and teens are exposed to and experience trauma responses as witnesses to arrests, physical searches (stop and frisk), environmental searches (home or car), and trauma associated with visiting a loved one in jail or prison. According to a document from the International Association of Chiefs of Police on Safeguarding Children of Arrested Parents, parental arrest or incarceration can harm a child's physical, mental, social, and emotional well-being (2014). Minimizing trauma experienced by children at the time of parental arrest and then throughout incarceration leads to lessening this risk (International Association of Chiefs of Police, August 2014, as cited in Report of the Attorney General's National Task Force on Children Exposed to Violence, 2012). The stigma associated with incarceration makes children not want to discuss or share experiences. Stigma isolates them from opportunities that could help them develop coping tools and access information and education about the incarceration of their loved ones, as well as isolates them from outlets for expression. The stigma becomes a wedge that keeps children from asking adults for help in their schools, churches, and sports teams, decreasing their likelihood of receiving social support (Luther, 2015). Children affected by incarceration are also at risk for mental health and developmental issues. According to The Annie E. Casey Foundation (2016), the trauma of being separated from a parent and lacking sympathy or support from others can increase children's mental health issues, such as depression and anxiety, and hamper their educational achievement.

Hairston (1991) suggests that maintaining family relationships throughout incarceration leads to decreased recidivism and improved mental health and family reunification after release. A child life specialist could also work with schools and community organizations, providing information, training, and support that addresses stress and trauma for children with an incarcerated loved one while decreasing stigma and increasing a sense of wellness and resilience. The role of the child life specialist as part of the prison system or as a contracted professional or consultant could enhance the lives of incarcerated individuals and their families, leading to stronger relationships and potentially decreasing the risk of recidivism (Hairston,1991).

Including a Certified Child Life Specialist as part of a jail/prison team, community, and nonprofit agency may improve children's and families' wellness. A child life specialist using child-centered play assesses children's emotional states and misconceptions to determine the child's and family's needs. Providing interventions through play, art, and movement, the child life specialist offers non-threatening ways for children to tell their stories, strengthen relationships, support developmental milestones, and promote coping skills. A child life specialist working with justice-involved families can support existing programs and staff and create and develop programs that foster resilience. Including a child life specialist as part of school personnel or community programming can decrease stigma by increasing the understanding of the needs of children affected by incarceration. Because the role is not diagnostic, a child life specialist is uniquely qualified to work with populations that often experience distrust of a system. A child life specialist will provide a non-judgmental opportunity, grounded in play, that only seeks to deepen understanding of the experience, situations, and emotional responses and to learn which tools will better manage them. The Association of Child Life Professionals developed a set of competencies highlighting how a child life specialist uses child development, ecological models, and strengths-based approaches to support children and families in crisis. This chapter will focus on the following child life competencies that support Child Life Specialists working with those affected by incarceration: (ACLP Official Documents, 2020)

- The ability to assess the developmental and psychosocial needs of infants, children, youth, and families
- The ability to initiate and maintain meaningful and therapeutic relationships with infants, children, youth, and families
- The ability to provide opportunities for play for infants, children, youth, and families
- The ability to support infants, children, youth, and families in coping with stressful events
- The ability to provide teaching specific to the population served, including psychological preparation for potentially stressful experiences, with infants, children, youth, and families.
- The ability to function as a member of the service team

DEVELOPMENTAL FRAMEWORKS

Throughout the chapter, child life practice, program development, and interventions are influenced by and grounded in developmental theories such as Erikson's social-emotional theory, stating that trust is foundational to the development of attached relationships (1950). Child Life Specialists, informed by Vygotsky's Zone of Proximal Development, scaffold children's understanding of previous traumatic experiences by building a bridge supporting new information while using and reaffirming existing skills and knowledge (Bedrova & Leong, 2007). Child Life Specialists, grounded in the Developmental Interaction Approach, support development through inquiry and engagement with hands-on learning opportunities that reflect children's lived experiences and relationships (Franklin, 2000). Versed in child development, CCLSs have the tools necessary to understand children's reactions and responses to the incarceration of a loved one across development. Understanding how familial, cultural, and societal factors affect the growth and development of individuals provide Child Life Specialists with a framework for understanding how these factors and systems are interrelated, interact with each other, and impact development (Christiansen, 2016). Using Bronfenbrenner's Ecological Systems theory, the child life specialist considers relationships between the incarcerated loved one and child, the developmental age of the child, proximity to jail or prison, and attitude and support of the custodial caregiver. The model offers the child life specialist a deeper understanding of factors that conflict or contribute to supportive relationships of those affected by a loved one's incarceration. Both development and ecological theories provide the child life specialist with information used to develop tools and strategies that foster relationships. Child life practice grounded in child development and children's lived experiences, interests, and connections equip the CCLS to identify family strengths rather than negative characteristics, viewing the family as resourceful and resilient even when faced with adverse conditions (Stoerkel, 2020).

Fostering Resilience

According to Mullane-Morgan (2018), parental incarceration itself is a symptom of existing trauma and a direct cause of trauma. Parental incarceration is a strong predictor of childhood trauma due to the overlapping racial, social, and structural disadvantages experienced by most children of incarcerated parents. The skills of the child life specialist outlined in the Child Life Competencies can be viewed as mitigators of trauma. According to the American Psychological Association (2022), resilience is the development of coping strategies that promote flexibility and adaptation to life's circumstances, mental and emotional fortitude to adjust to internal and external factors, and supportive relationships and community resources. A child life specialist provides distraction for anxiety-producing events, validating feelings, acknowledging experiences, and supporting the natural roles of the family, increasing a child's ability to cope with adverse experiences and fostering resilience in children and families. Focusing on ecological systems and developmental factors, the CCLS can teach and evaluate methods to enhance resilience (Southwick et al., 2014). Society wants to believe that justice-involved people are "bad parents," so the separation and breakdown of families and communities are justified. However, "many families impacted by incarceration are not broken or torn apart but are refigured and reimagined. The level of love and strength is evident in the way they can remain a family despite the criminal justice system's best efforts to distance them" (Hollins, 2022, p.31). Incorporating family strengths is integral to delivering developmentally appropriate information and choosing coping strategies that decrease stress for those affected by incarceration. Child Life Specialists facilitate supportive adult-child relationships, build a sense of efficacy and control, and encourage self-regulatory skills like deep breathing, meditation, and music that foster resilience (Center on the Developing Child, n.d). A child life specialist seeks out sources of faith, hope, and cultural traditions that support resilience by using information shared by the family as foundations for psychological preparation, coping, expressive arts, and play (Center for the Developing Child, n.d).

Hobfoll et al. (2007) identified the five essential needs of children during and after mass disasters and violence: safety, efficacy, regulation, hope, and connection. These frameworks can also foster resilience in those affected by incarceration. Incarceration is an assault on the family and community, as its devastating effects can be felt emotionally, psychologically, financially, and physically (Annie E. Casey Foundation, 2016). A child life specialist can develop activities and events that support and encourage sharing cultural and faith-based traditions with their children. Tapping into these experiences supports a positive foundation that fosters love, respect, and family identity and decreases feelings of shame as families come together in a shared vision of hope and resilience. Tools such as play, expressive arts, and developmental explanations support a child's sense of efficacy. Children and teens are prepared for and learn about the prison environment, master regulating emotions for upcoming visits through mindfulness, and continue relationships with loved ones through letters, games, and activities shared despite distance and time. The child life specialist supports children and families through new and stressful environments and circumstances by scaffolding existing information and skills, both newly learned and existing information, that develops skills that foster the protective factors that promote resilience.

Issues of Separation

It is widely understood that secure attachments with a primary caregiver are imperative for developing healthy relationships. Attachment is an emotional bond between infant and primary caregivers that result in a sense of security or trust in those that care for them, the environment, and ultimately oneself (Keller, 2018). Relationships grounded in trust, routine, and consistency support the parent and child in developing strong attachments and a sense of safety and security. Incarceration poses challenges to the formation and continuation of attached relationships, and in this regard, incarceration is comparable to other prolonged absences (Turney, 2019). Institutional policies, frequent disruptions in contact and interaction with caregivers, and the effects of separation on supportive and continued relationships affect the social-emotional development of children and their relationships with their caregivers (Dargis & Mitchell-Somaza, 2021). Other factors, such as children placed in kinship or foster care, distance, and visiting costs, will determine the ability to maintain or foster relationships. These relationships are often on a spectrum that ranges from loving, committed relationships to contentious or non-existent relationships, adding a whole other layer of possibility or difficulty to fostering meaningful connections with children. Navigation of parent-child relationships is a significant stressor for families affected by incarceration (Dargis & Mitchel-Somaza, 2021). A specific skill set and experience in settings where separation is a factor equips the child life specialist to assess and provide interventions that support families facing separation due to incarceration.

Long-term reductions in parental involvement are often caused by location of the jail or prison, finances, and transportation. Therefore, when justice involved people are unable to engage with their children this potentially leads to children growing accustomed to and suffering from separation (Turney, 2019). Depending on the child's developmental age when separation occurs, the number of prolonged separations and the strength of the relationship at the time of separation can affect how the child copes, the continuation of the relationship, and social-emotional and school outcomes (Dargis & Michel-Somoza, 2021). When the family cannot visit their child in the hospital, Child Life Specialists seek strategies that support communication and connection between the patient and family. Infants and young children have extreme reactions to separations when faced with new and potentially threatening environments. During hospital admission, Child Life Specialists will assess families using the Stress Potential Assessment addressing criteria regarding children's reactions to the previous separation, such as drop off at preschool or when a parent leaves the room for a shower or coffee break (Hollen et al., 2018). Understanding the impact of separation from a loved one, Child Life Specialists working with those affected by incarceration use similar assessment questions to support young children and families. Child Life Specialists address strategies to ease the separation at the time of arrest, after in-person or online visits and phone calls, and during reunification and re-entry. The child life specialist working with children and families to develop strategies that support the continuation of relationships will seek ways to decrease separation stress through normalization, preparation, and coping. Collaborating with prison staff, a child life specialist identifies stress points for children and families and decreases separation anxiety by supporting parents in meeting their children's social, emotional, and behavioral needs. For example, a child life specialist can maintain parent-child relationships beyond visits and phone calls by collaborating with nonprofit organizations that allow parents to make digital recordings of themselves reading a child's favorite story, singing a lullaby, or sharing a family tradition.

During the author's experience facilitating a parent discussion group, parents expressed resistance to encouraging their children to call or visit them in jail. Parents shared that they felt awkward talking on the phone. They stated they felt unsure of how to engage with their young child or teen in meaningful conversation and experienced increased stress when the child could not touch or hug the parent due to most jails having a no-touch visitation policy. Due to the distress of saying goodbye, caregivers in the group shared that they chose not to communicate or limited their calls and letters to only the caregiving adult. The discussion group provided the child life specialist and participants who had found ways to stay connected to their children to share strategies grounded in strengths and developmental theory. The discussion group offered a safe space to consider their path and experiment with ideas to support and connect with their children.

Developing and supporting children's existing routines is one way to ease separation by promoting children's sense of predictability. Knowing what to expect next helps children feel safe in new or threatening environments. However, routines are complicated when a loved one is incarcerated. Visitation, phone calls, and letters are monitored, often requiring money and may entail several security requirements (Dargis & Mitchell-Somaza, 2021). The author worked with the participants on routines they could implement during visits and phone calls, potentially decreasing separation stress for children and youth. The CCLS working with the incarcerated caregivers encouraged hello and goodbye practices, worked with them to establish patterns for conversation such as who asks a question first and rituals for ending the call, and developed a set of recurring questions to alleviate the pressure often experienced during visits and phone calls. A child life specialist can model games such as peek-a-boo that reinforce validation and acknowledgment of children's fears and anxiety about missing a loved one (Gaynard et al.,1998).

For older children and teens, separation from a parent due to incarceration can have lasting effects on a child's sense of self and identity. To maintain the lines of communication with loved ones in meaningful ways, a child life specialist draws from experiences with hospitalized families to promote supportive relationships. For example, working with the incarcerated caregiver to write letters, mail drawings, or develop stories together using mail, phone, or other modes of communication approved by the prison. Finding ways to support communication with a loved one from prison or jail requires an investment on the part of an incarcerated caregiver and the cooperation of those caring for the children of incarcerated caregivers. All involved will need to encourage and facilitate connection even when children may have strong emotional responses and reactions, such as refusing to respond to a caregiver's communication. Child Life Specialists can support family connections and attachment through creativity and innovation, working with families to accept what each can give while developing strategies that foster communication and routines through letter writing, phone calls, and visits when appropriate.

Opportunities for Play

A child life specialist uses play to engage children and families in non-threatening ways to examine events or topics that could be stressful. A child life specialist working with children affected by incarceration uses play and expressive arts to create safe spaces for children to learn about, understand, and process the experience and the emotional toll. Play provides a supportive modality for children and youth to tell their stories, gain control, and rewrite the trauma (Gordon & Paisley, 2018). Play offers a safe way to engage with big feelings while also modeling for caregivers tools to navigate children's and teens' emotional responses and reactions to a loved one's incarceration. Child-led open-ended play allows children the space to begin to process big feelings and emotional responses and an opportunity to mitigate misconceptions, correct misinformation, and decrease anxiety and stress through physical outlets. Play offers children affected by incarceration a sense of control and mastery. The child life specialist uses open-ended materials and empathic responses that encourage children to lead the play. Children can recreate events using dolls, little people, and small police and rescue vehicles, encouraging voice and agency as they determine different outcomes or practice regulatory skills.

For younger children, play also offers an outlet to express feelings, physically releasing tension and stress felt in the body. For example, working in waiting areas before visits, a child life specialist provides children with toys or games, coloring, books, and stories as they wait, fostering positive relationships with jail and prison staff, providing open-ended play opportunities, and decreasing the anxiety of both child and caregiver. These interactions could support feeling cared for and attended to while potentially easing transitions and diffusing emotions. The child life specialist may also work within an organization as part of a multidisciplinary team developing support or playgroups that amplify the voices of children and youth, supporting efficacy and control in their own lives.

A child life specialist encourages exploration in non-threatening ways that promote conversation and questions. Providing materials for inquiry exploration and discovery supports children's recreation of experiences and imagining different outcomes leading to an understanding of the environment, activities, and relationships in adult spaces (Franklin, 2000; Cohen et al., 2016). A CCLS facilitating the play provides a safe space, materials, and empathic responses that validate children's feelings and experiences. Child Life Specialists trained in therapeutic play techniques create safe spaces for children to re-enact experiences and create alternative outcomes as they process those experiences leading to better-developed, more sustained, and more productive play (Cohen et al., 2016). By demonstrating, rehearsing and practicing with small dolls, police cars, cardboard boxes, and other materials to re-enact arrests, prison, or visitation, children have the opportunity to gain mastery and control of a situation where they have little to none. Providing play opportunities can disrupt potentially harmful outcomes as the child builds "meanings through representation and organizes these into coherent sequences into the form of stories" (Franklin, 2000, p. 50). These "stories" offer the child life specialist a way into the child's mind that helps them assess what types of intervention or support a child may need to cope with a loved one's incarceration. In this way, the play also provides opportunities to state and reiterate that a loved one's incarceration is not the child's fault.

Certified Child Life Specialists often use movement, art, and games to engage with children and families in the hospital. For older children and teens, play with the CCLS might involve board or card games used to develop rapport and normalize spaces or as the medium that allows the youth to feel comfortable, relaxed, and share something about themselves. Although materials brought into the jail or prison are often limited, a CCLS working in these settings can strive to create a fun environment that supports diverse learners, fostering discussion, reflection, and the ability to join in what feels most comfortable for each child or teen.

Regardless of age, physical play offers a way to engage the body. Many children experience stress in the body—nervous energy, tantrums, and stomachaches are examples of how children and youth manifest stress and trauma. Providing outlets for energy through physical play helps children expend energy and release anxiety and stress to cope with upcoming changes, adverse experiences, or emotional outbursts due to the increased stressors associated with a loved one's incarceration.

Play can happen anywhere—waiting areas before visits with loved ones; community and faith-based agencies and organizations; schools, and homes. Temporary play spaces can be created using movable furniture and mats that delineate space or portable items brought into spaces and removed when the child life specialist leaves.

Play is also a way for parents to connect with children in meaningful and fun ways, support attachment and relationships, and promote developmental milestones. For example, prison nursery programs for those who gave birth while incarcerated promote attachment and bonding between caregivers and infants while supporting incarcerated parents' rehabilitation (Goshin & Byrne, 2009). A CCLS could provide new parents and infants with a child-friendly and stimulating environment that supports the infant's development and the self-confidence of a new parent. In addition, Child Life Specialists, with an additional certification in infant massage, could provide instruction that supports parent-child interactions, potentially improving outcomes for bonding, infant development, and parent and child mental health (Porter et al., 2015).

Some prisons offer play spaces and programs for incarcerated parents to engage with children in non-threatening, normalizing ways. A child life specialist could enhance and expand these programs by developing and working with existing staff to develop parenting classes, parenting support groups, and educational workshops to provide resources, information, and opportunities to discuss topics relevant to the family's circumstances. A child life specialist experienced in supervising play spaces in healthcare settings, maintaining materials and supplies, orienting and training volunteers, and observing parent-child interactions fosters strong relationships using strengths-based approaches. In settings where there is not an existing play space or daycare, a child life specialist can work toward finding funding resources and materials to develop programs that strengthen the connections between incarcerated caregivers and their families while facilitating ties to their communities through education and support. (Kazura & Toth, 2004).

Preparation and Developmental Explanations

Engaging with caregivers who are incarcerated, a child life specialist supports caregivers in developing developmentally appropriate language that explains incarceration, arrest, addiction, court, visitations, sentencing, and re-entry, while supporting relationships and the core concepts of family-centered care. Including discussions of developmental approaches to understanding right and wrong provides a framework for the participants to begin to shape language that feels comfortable to them as experts of their children. To respect caregivers' wishes and roles, Child Life Specialists include caregivers in decision-making. For example, discussing language choices, what and how much information they would like to share, and collaborating with parents to honor the family's experiences and choices improves relationships with children, family, and staff (Institute for Patient and Family-Centered Care, n.d). By providing caregivers with a developmental overview of stages and theories, a child life specialist and the caregivers can work together to develop developmentally appropriate explanations that align with a caregiver's parenting style.

Children need developmentally appropriate language to understand the terminology associated with the correctional system. Developing language that supports children's understanding will help children share concerns, fears, and misconceptions, leading to children being able to process and develop coping skills to mitigate and navigate anxiety brought on by the incarceration of a loved one. Information that is kept from children, leaving them unaware of their caregiver's circumstances, can make it more difficult for them to feel secure and trust those around them (Glesner, 2012). When children do not have adequate information and are in unfamiliar settings or stressful situations they often fill in the blanks with fears, misconceptions, and untruths. Children may become scared, confused, and upset when a parent is arrested and placed in jail or prison. They may blame themselves, others, or systems involved in the imprisonment of a loved one. The adults in their lives, under immense pressure themselves, are often unsure of what to tell children, how to tell their children, or even if to tell children what is happening and how it may affect them. When children and families receive accurate information, they can better understand and cope with some of the stress they may experience when a loved one is incarcerated (New Jersey Department of Corrections et al., 2007).

A child life specialist can work to decrease parents' apprehension by discussing the importance of honesty. In this author's experience, the participants in the parenting discussion group chose not to tell children they were incarcerated and instead created elaborate stories such as a job that is far away, that they are attending college in another state, or hospitalization and illness. Participants shared that the false story felt like a better choice than the truth of incarceration. A child life specialist addresses this by asking parents about their worries and fears about telling the child the truth. Caregivers may become concerned that children are not old enough to understand, will fear for the loved one's safety, or be ashamed of the loved one. A child life specialist provides opportunities for conversations about honesty, creating dialogue regarding children's reactions and responses to a loved one's incarceration. Whether working with a group or individually, using non-threatening activities such as MadLibs™—filling in nouns, adjectives, and adverbs—without knowing the full context of the story provides the foundation for a discussion about honesty without increasing anxiety, guilt, or shame. Reflecting on how the MadLibs™ becomes a story even when facts are missing makes it clear that when children do not have all the information, they will just fill in the blanks based on whatever information they know or think they know. Activities where caregivers discuss the importance of honesty and developmentally appropriate explanations provide a non-judgmental way to connect what they have or have not shared with children and behavioral, academic, and relational responses to the parent's incarceration. Providing opportunities to reflect on children's expression of feelings, behavior, and how to respond by naming, validating, and acknowledging the behavior as an expression of their children's feelings leads to a deepening understanding of the connection between the trust built through the provision of developmentally appropriate explanations and connections to their children's behavior and the caregiver's response to it.

The child life specialist must respect the children's and families' values and not judge their decisions or push them to do something they are not ready to do. Instead, the child life specialist must provide a safe space for incarcerated caregivers to share their rationale and choices (Institute for Patient and Family-Centered Care, n.d). Giving parents the space to assess their own needs and reason to hide information allows them to examine their fears and determine a path forward that aligns with their comfort level and parenting style. For those who are justice-involved, there is incredible shame and guilt associated with being incarcerated (Dargas & Mitchel-Somoza, 2021). Encouraging them to share their story with their children and supporting them with tools and developmentally appropriate language choices offers caregivers a different way to envision their relationship. One that is developmentally appropriate but, more importantly, is grounded in honesty and trust.

Child Life Specialists work with children and teens to break down adult concepts and information using analogies, familiar experiences, and chunking information into manageable amounts for children to understand. A Certified Child Life Specialist provides "teaching, specific to the population served, including psychological preparation for potentially stressful experiences, with infants, children, youth, and families" (Association of Child Life Professionals, Official Documents, 2020). Working with caregivers, a child life specialist provides developmentally appropriate language that allows children to begin to understand and process potentially stressful experiences. Child Life Specialists identify basic terminology, processes, and expected care plans for the population (Association of Child Life Professionals, n.d). Children who feel knowledgeable or prepared for stressful events may experience a reduction in their distress and promote successful coping in the future (Boles, 2018). For example, children in early childhood may respond to the description of incarceration as a "time out" since that is a familiar language for many young children. Therefore, it is essential to scaffold unknown or new information with what is known and familiar using developmentally appropriate language (Boles, 2018). Using "time out" for incarceration with young children, Child Life Specialists scaffold unknown or new information with known information, supporting children's learning and understanding of complex topics or concepts.

Visiting a loved one in jail or prison is a particular stress point for children and families affected by incarceration, both emotionally and practically. In addition, prison staff frequently view visits as problematic (Dixey & Woodhull, 2012). A child life specialist working within the prison or jail system may provide psychological preparation to decrease anxiety about visiting a loved one in jail or prison. Although a lack of contact with their child may have negative consequences for the prisoner, bringing their children into the prison environment may not feel appropriate and limit any positive effects (De Claire & Dixon, 2015). In addition, caregivers' concerns for their children's experience visiting a loved one may prevent those incarcerated from encouraging their children's visits. Therefore, psychological preparation and developmental explanations at critical stress points, from arrest to re-entry, can decrease stress and trauma. Similar to the work of a traditional CCLS working in pre-operative preparation programs in hospitals, families affected by incarceration would be provided with developmentally appropriate language and tools to talk about and prepare for upcoming changes in their lives, including preparation and coping tools focused on visiting an incarcerated loved one.

Using play as the foundation for preparation, a child life specialist might engage children and families in waiting areas, schools, homes, or community spaces, providing step-by-step information regarding a visit. Preparation aims to decrease stress and anxiety and increase control and predictability of potentially overwhelming life experiences. Providing families with developmentally appropriate information will increase children and families' emotional adjustment (Goldberger et al., 2018). The setting and types of visits will determine the materials and type of preparation. For example, in "no-touch" settings where families are separated by thick plexiglass and talk using handheld phones, a child life specialist supports developmental explanations with hands-on materials encouraging children to manipulate and practice coping strategies to better proceed through the experience (Goldberger et al., 2018). Child Life Specialists prepare children for each step, including security screenings, pat-downs, and potentially long waits. The CCLS who familiarizes with the rules regarding touching and hugging, dress codes, and what can and cannot be brought to a visit will decrease family stress, leading to smoother processes. Rehearsing events, using dolls and small toys, or role-playing helps children to develop coping strategies to decrease fear and anxiety. Through the provision of developmental explanations and sensory experiences, psychological preparation could, have potentially positive effects on interactions between families and the jail and prison staff, making transitions to visits smoother when children and families know what to expect and what is expected of them (Gaynard et al.,1998). Prepared families enter spaces feeling less anxious and ready to engage, fostering positive interactions where families spend time talking with each other rather than trying to relax following a stressful event.

Preparation needs to be considered at all critical points of incarceration. Preparing families for visits is one stress point; another may be re-entry and returning home. Re-entry can be stressful for families as they navigate changes in relationships, probation rules, and possibly post-traumatic stress (De Veaux, 2013). The child life specialist working with incarcerated individuals before their release prepares them for how relationships with children may have changed. In addition, the CCLS supports the understanding of reactions and responses of children to their loved one's return and develops strategies for building and fostering positive relationships and potential explanations about their experience. For example, the author's experience has been that participants of the parenting discussion group felt both excited and anxious about a return home and needed a space to discuss fears, explore strategies for re-engagement with family, and have conversations about positive discipline and overindulgence. A child life specialist, working both leading up to re-entry and after, can provide a space for the caregivers to establish new routines, participate in current ones, and provide tools for the caregiver to learn how to navigate and support their children's reactions.

Expressive Arts

Expressive arts— music, movement, poetry, photography, drawing, painting, and many others—provide humans with an outlet that is beyond words. Maxine Greene (1995) states that the arts "may now and then move us into spaces where we can envision other ways of being and ponder what it might signify to realize them" (p. 135). For children using art to express their experiences and emotions, often it is the process that gives value and acceptance to those feelings. The arts provide opportunities to deepen one's self-understanding while sharing that with others. Those who have experienced trauma often find it difficult to express their feelings in words. Young children may shut down or tantrum, and older children and teens will act out or misbehave, punished for the behavior, which may be the body's way of coping with stress (Morgan-Mullane, 2018). Emotional labor, as defined by Hochschild (2003), is the "work a person does to induce or suppress feelings to sustain an outward countenance that produces the proper state of mind in others" (p. 7). Those affected by incarceration use energy to manage their genuine emotions to please others and make them comfortable (Hollins, 2022). As Hochschild refers to it, this energy or labor requires daily effort. It is energy that could be better used to develop relationships, and developmental milestones, learn in school and support oneself and family.

A child life specialist provides opportunities to express, vocalize, share, and cope with those feelings, creating space for understanding, curiosity, imagination, aspiration, and hope. A CCLS uses the arts to support children and families' expressions and understanding of themselves. The child life specialist does not use the arts to diagnose but creates a safe space to engage and explore. Using modalities such as poetry, music, or visual arts allows the participants to express themselves in ways that decrease anxiety while exploring safe methods of emotional expression while doing something enjoyable (Rollins, 2018). Although the child life specialist is limited by materials brought into the jail, poetry, music, and movement are accessible when thought about creatively. These art experiences can tap into emotions in ways that offer safe structures to share, discuss, and process ideas that can be expanded upon, are new, or unfamiliar.

The arts provide opportunities for choice and control as children or adults determine what color, song, or words to replicate experiences and emotions. There is no wrong way to engage in the arts, as the child life specialist creates opportunities for expressing one's feelings of grief, loss, anger, or joy. A child life specialist's facilitation of an individual session with a child, teen, or caregiver, or with a group or family may use expressive art activities to provide a platform for participants to dip into their creative parts. One example of this is writing poetry. Whether they are working together or individually to identify words that describe themselves or their child(ren), what it means to be a parent, or looking to the future, writing poetry can help to foster hope and develop resilience.

Other examples are mask-making, examining emotions—those we hide (inside a mask) and those we share with the world (outside the mask). Another example is throwing wet paper towels at a target of things that make one angry, facilitating safe ways to express and release anger. Through these and other art-making activities, the child life specialist offers opportunities for expressing, exploring, and discovering feelings. In addition, art provides the vehicle for assessment and intervention by creating an outlet and space to share that is non-judgmental, safe, and controlled. As a result, a Certified Child Life Specialist can assess how children and families cope while using art to identify strengths, connect with supportive relationships, and foster coping tools.

A child life specialist uses bibliotherapy to support children, youth, and teens to understand their own experiences. Books offer an opportunity to see oneself represented in the character of a story while decreasing stigma as readers envision themselves in someone else's experience (Bishop,1990). Books are also a way for caregivers to support children while incarcerated. In addition, they provide outlets for understanding emotions through the identification of characters and stories. Finally, books offer a way for adults to provide support and motivation (Clutter, 2018). For example, *My Daddy Is In Jail* by Janet M. Bender provides simple drawings, language and activities to enhance discussion with young children. *From the Desk of Zoe Washington* by Janea Marks is the story of a young girl who wants to know more about her dad who is incarcerated and addresses issues of family, hope and justice for the middle grade reader. Although not specific to incarceration, the author was asked by a father in the discussion group for suggestions of books he could share with his spouse about grief and loss to read for his children who had lost a beloved grandparent. Although he could not be physically present, he was finding ways to continue his role as a father and support his wife and family from jail. With support from the child life specialist, this father used books to offer his children a roadmap and provided examples of coping, hope, and healing through characters that demonstrate resilience (Walker et al., 2020).

Community or School Liaison

A child life specialist working within the corrections system could also support incarcerated caregivers by helping to establish appropriate efforts to continue connections with their children and identify ways to build and foster relationships from prison. By connecting with nonprofit organizations and schools, a child life specialist can function as a liaison with outside agencies, supporting the participation of the incarcerated caregiver in their children's lives. Schools may also help address the needs of families by ensuring that all parents can participate in school activities, such as parent-teacher conferences (Turney, 2019). Having an advocate for families at the jail or prison who works with schools and community organizations potentially increases the success of caregivers continuing to be active participants in their children's lives. Assumptions are often made about parents who are incarcerated. A child life specialist as liaison to communities and schools provide education and awareness about incarceration, decreasing stigma and potentially increasing funding sources and grants for programming.

PARENTING DISCUSSION GROUPS WITHIN JAIL AND PRISONS

The following is based on a parenting discussion group facilitated by a CCLS in a jail. However, it can be used as a template for other caregiver discussion groups and groups for children, youth, and teens.

A Certified Child Life Specialist often provides opportunities for informal and formal discussions between caregivers, parents, and guardians in healthcare settings. It is an opportunity for caregivers to share their experience of having an ill child and to develop relationships with others who also relate to common challenges. Most importantly, it is a space where caregivers can support each other with ideas, strategies, and techniques for caring for a hospitalized child. Similarly, studies suggest several benefits of parenting education for incarcerated parents "including improving family stability, strengthening family bonds, and teaching positive parenting practices which strengthen parent-child relationships and improve child outcomes" (Kamptner et al. p.64, as cited in Sandifer, 2008). According to Luther (2015), criminality and incarceration do not negate the positive impact of some incarcerated or formerly incarcerated caregivers. Therefore, caregivers need opportunities for quality parenting education during incarceration that guide how to support children from behind bars and help prepare families for navigating the parent-child relationship leading up to and during re-entry post-incarceration.

Although the setting is different in many ways, the goals of the parenting discussion group at the jail are the same as those established and facilitated by a child life specialist in the hospital setting. A CCLS as a facilitator of parenting discussion groups using skills in psychological preparation and coping, as well as knowledge of development, offer incarcerated caregivers the tools to figure out how they can encourage, support, and advocate for their children. According to Luther (2015), incarcerated caregivers need guidance on parenting from prison or jail. Discussion groups provide a space to focus on parenting from within prison, during re-entry, and throughout re-engagement with children and families after release. Parenting roles within groups ranged from those involved in their children's lives to participants with children who are grown adults, those with children who have limited or no contact with them, and those with younger siblings, grandchildren, or other children who are vital to them in their lives. A caregiver discussion group provides a safe space to foster and strengthen existing bonds and grieve lost opportunities while exploring possible reconnection and reconciliation. According to Dargis and Mitchell-Somoza (2021), more work must be done to aid parents and caregivers in making decisions regarding parental involvement. Child Life Specialists offer a neutral position to discuss the needs of the child, family, and incarcerated individuals seeking to balance the benefits of contact and how that is achieved.

Participants in a caregivers' discussion group would be encouraged to share their experiences of being an incarcerated caregiver, thus supporting others' learning and understanding of the effects of incarceration and potentially supporting each other toward connected relationships with their children. Often it is the caregivers who have chosen to be honest with children who have the most significant impact on others. The child life specialist amplifies these voices rather than speaking as an expert. The parenting discussion group challenges them to find innovative ways to stay connected to loved ones, foster relationships, and continue to parent from jail or prison. Creating a safe space to discuss parenting skills provided opportunities for participants to reflect on how they parent and were parented. A child life specialist using experience and knowledge of children and child development includes parenting skills as an integral component of discussions. These discussions can foster resilience in caregivers and children by improving "parental mental health, strengthen family bonds, and deter parents' re-offending" (Kamptner, 2017, p.64).

Establishing overarching goals for a parenting discussion group provides a safe structure in which participants understand the nature of the group, the opportunities for the participants to learn about themselves and their children, and strategies for supporting their children and themselves as parents. The goals also provide a framework that guides the child life specialist's role in working with incarcerated caregivers. With a focus on developmentally appropriate language and psychological preparation, a child life specialist can provide caregivers with strategies to engage with their children from within an institution as well as learning tools that support the management and complicated dynamics that may be a result of incarceration (Dargis & Mitchell- Somoza, 2021). The caregiver discussion group provides a space to talk about frustrations while encouraging the sharing of strategies and experiences of others so that they understand they are not alone. By asking open-ended questions, the child life specialist encourages discussion and sharing of potential ideas for engagement and connection among the group participants. As a result, the participants provide lived experiences and knowledge of what is potentially possible, working together to formulate strategies and tools that foster and build relationships with their families.

As a parenting discussion group facilitator, the author established routine and structure in each session, developing trust so participants could better explore the topics and share personal experiences. Not all the participants have happy childhood memories. The facilitator allowed participants to pass or to share whatever came up for them, using the moment to demonstrate ways to acknowledge those experiences, validate their feelings, and refrain from judgment. Each session began with activities that offered an alternative way to enter conversations chosen by the participants. These activities decreased feelings of vulnerability and created an entry point for engagement by using humor, music, and movement to build trust, lighten the mood, and foster relationships among the facilitator and participants (Pierce et al., 2015). The author organized each session around a discussion topic, with the flexibility for participants to discuss what is important to them, promoting a sense of control. It was essential to this author that participants felt ideas were not sprung on them but generated by them.

CONCLUSION

Challenges

This chapter outlines and describes ways a child life specialist might engage with jail and prison populations to support and foster relationships with their children. However, there are challenges to the role that Child Life Specialists should consider before deciding if working with those affected by incarceration is the right fit. Correctional facilities are governed by strict rules, regulations, safety measures, and routines. They are simultaneously routine-driven and unpredictable. A child life specialist wanting to pursue a role within a jail or prison must develop a comfort level with the prevalence of guns, rules that feel restrictive and is invasive for those visiting loved ones, and the possibility of witnessing violence. Child Life Specialists working in jails and prisons should also consider their own safety. Identifying triggers, coping tools and supportive staff may increase physical and improve emotional safety. Governments that preside over local and federal correctional facilities can move slowly regarding change. A CCLS who wants to or does work in correctional facilities will need patience and perseverance to justify changes, as well as the ability to provide research and supporting literature to support any new ideas or changes. Funding sources are also challenging, and few positions are designated for the psychosocial needs of children and families within correctional facilities. Writing proposals and grants and seeking funding to support positions or programmatic ideas will be challenging for any Certified Child Life Specialist working with this population. Collaboration in care is key to implementing program ideas successfully and supports children and families in any setting. CCLS are accustomed to working with interdisciplinary teams with similar goals of psychosocial care. Collaborations in correctional facilities will likely be with social workers, correctional officers, and local sheriffs who govern agencies. Child Life Specialists must be aware of the difference in goals and outcomes for some professionals, it is safety first. Child Life Specialists must learn to work within those parameters while staying within their scope of practice.

Areas of Growth

The idea of a child life specialist working in a jail or prison is already new. However, a child life specialist could function as a consultant to correctional facilities, local law enforcement, or government agencies, creating book lists for children, adolescents, and adults. They could create resources such as tip sheets, lists of websites, and organizations offering caregivers easily accessible and cost-effective materials vetted and organized by the CCLS. A child life specialist could participate in creating and distributing available brochures developed by state and local government agencies. A child life specialist would provide a developmental perspective on topics such as what to expect when visiting a loved one, how to talk to children about jail and prison, and the types of questions children and teens may have about incarceration to introduce or reinforce information. As a consultant or contract worker, a child life specialist could participate in the creation of play spaces and daycares, family events, and support groups for those affected by incarceration. A child life specialist working with various agencies developing normalizing experiences supports caregivers' involvement in celebrations and recognizes children's milestones and transitions, promoting family routines that may closely connect to what would be experienced by families in the home, school, and community. For example, CCLS can work with organizations to facilitate events such as parent-child dances, gift exchanges, and cards for birthdays and holidays. Child Life Specialists can support parents' participation in parent-teacher conferences, provide audio or video tools to read bedtime stories, or build routine and structure through regular letter writing, emails, or phone calls. Collaborating with psychosocial teams within juvenile detention settings, Child Life Specialists develop programs and groups to foster regulation skills that teach and encourage mindfulness, meditation, and deep breathing. Certified Child Life Specialists supporting the development and education of justice-involved and at-risk youth or those re-entering the community or transitioning to adult prisons can offer opportunities to participate in art experiences creating space for expression, development of interests, and prosocial behaviors. Using the same skills to work with children and families affected by incarceration, a Certified Child Life Specialist can provide preparation when teens arrive, establish rules and routines, and prepare them for re-entry. Providing developmental explanations, play, coping, and expressive arts support relationships and resilience and provide hope to those who may struggle to see a future beyond their current existence.

REFERENCES

Association of Child Life Professionals. (2022). *ACLP Official Documents* Retrieved from https://education.childlife.org/aclp

American Psychological Association. (2022). *Resilience*. http://www.apa.org/topics/resilience

Annie E. Casey Foundation. (2016). *A Shared Sentence: the devastating toll of parental incarceration on kids, families, and communities*. The Annie E. Casey Foundation.

Bender, J. M. (2019). *My Daddy Is In Jail*. Youth Light Inc.

Bodrova, E., & Leong, D. (2007). *Tools of the Mind: The Vygotskian approach to early childhood education*. Pearson/Merrill Prentice Hall.

Boles, J. (2018). Preparing children for healthcare encounters. In J. Rollins, R. Bolig, & C. Mahan (Eds.), *Meeting Children's Psychosocial Needs Across The Health-Care Continuum* (2nd ed.). PRO-ED.

Bishop, R. S. (1990). Mirrors, Windows, and Sliding Glass Doors. *Perspectives: Choosing and Using Books for Classroom, 6*(3), 1-2 https://scenicregional.org/wp-content/uploads/2017/08/Mirrors-Windows-and-Sliding-Glass-Doors.pdf

Center on the Developing Child Harvard University. (n.d.). *Resilience* Retrieved March 15, 2022, from https://devhcdc.wpengine.com/science/key-concepts/resilience/

Clutter, L. B. (2018). Spiritual *Needs in Children's Health Care Settings.* In R. Thompson (Ed.), *The Handbook of Child Life* (2nd ed., pp. 349–410). Charles C Thomas.

Cohen, D. H., Stern, V., Balaban, N., & Gropper, N. (2016). Recording children's behavior in dramatic play. In *Observing and recording the behavior of young children* (6th ed., pp. 66–90). Teachers College Press.

Crime Museum. (n.d.). *Types of Prisons.* Retrieved February 17, 2022, https://www.crimemuseum.org/crime-library/famous-prisons-incarceration/types-of-prisons/

Dargis, M., & Mitchell-Somoza, A. (2021). Challenges Associated with Parenting While Incarcerated: A Review. *International Journal of Environmental Research and Public Health, 18*(9927), 1–16. doi:10.3390/ijerph18189927 PMID:34574849

De Claire, K., & Dixon, L. (2015). The Effects of Prison Visits From Family Members on Prisoners' Well-Being, Prison Rule Breaking, and Recidivism: A Review of Research Since 1991. *Trauma, Violence & Abuse, 18*(2), 1–15. PMID:26330175

De Veaux, M. (2013). The Trauma of the Incarceration Experience. *Harvard Civil Rights-Civil Liberties Law Review, 48*, 257–277.

Dichter, H., Ruprecht, K., & Tomlin, A. (2020). Exploring Early Care and Education Policy for Young Children of Incarcerated Parents. *Zero to Three, 40*(4), 51–58. https://hdl.handle.net/1805/28132

Dixey, R., & Woodall, J. (2012). The significance of "the visit" in an English category B prison: Views from prisoners, prisoners' families, and prison staff. *Community Work & Family, 15*(1), 29–47. doi:10.1080/13668803.2011.580125

Erikson, E. (1950). *Childhood and Society.* W.W. Norton & Company.

Felliti, V. J., & … . (1998). Relationship of childhood abuse and household dysfunction to many of the leading causes of death in adults. The Adverse Childhood Experiences (ACE) Study. *American Journal of Preventive Medicine, 14*(4), 245–258. doi:10.1016/S0749-3797(98)00017-8 PMID:9635069

Franklin, M. B. (2000). The Meanings of Play in the Developmental-Interaction Tradition. In N. Nager & E. K. Shapiro (Eds.), *Revisiting a progressive pedagogy: The developmental interaction approach* (pp. 47–71). SUNY Press.

Gaynard, L., Wolfer, J., Goldberger, J., Thompson, R., Redburn, L., & Laidley, L. (1998). *Psychosocial Care of Children in Hospitals: A clinical practice manual from the ACCH Child Life Research Project.* Child Life Council.

Glesner, T. (2012). Addressing the Needs of Children of Incarcerated Parents. A Publication of the University of Vermont, James M. *Jeffords Center*, *2*(2), 2–4.

Greene, M. (1995). Chapter 11: Texts and Margins. In Releasing the Imagination: Essays on Education, the Arts, and Social Change. (3rd ed., 134–151). John Wiley & Sons

Goldberger, J., Lumbering Mohl, A., & Thompson, R. (2018). Psychological Preparation and Coping. In R. Thompson (Ed.), *The Handbook of Child Life* (2nd ed., pp. 268–312). Charles C Thomas.

Gordon, J., & Paisley, P. (2018). Trauma-Focused Medical Play. In L. Rubin (Ed.), Handbook of Medical Play Therapy and Child Life (pp. 154-172). Routledge.

Goshin, L. S., & Byrne, M. W. (2009). Converging Streams of Opportunity for Prison Nursery Programs in the United States. *Journal of Offender Rehabilitation*, *48*(4), 271–295. doi:10.1080/10509670902848972 PMID:19865610

Hairston, C. F. (1991). Family Ties During Imprisonment: Important to Whom and for What? *Journal of Sociology and Social Welfare*, *87*, 87–104.

Hobfoll, S. E., Watson, P., Bell, C. C., Bryant, R. A., Brymer, M. J., Friedman, M. J., Friedman, M., Gersons, B. P., De Jong, J. T., Layne, C. M., Maguen, S., Neria, Y., Norwood, A. E., Pynoos, R. S., Reissman, D., Ruzek, J. I., Shalev, A. Y., Solomon, Z., Steinberg, A. M., & Ursano, R. J. (2007). Five Essential Elements of Immediate and Mid–Term Mass Trauma Intervention: Empirical Evidence. *Psychiatry*, *70*(4), 283–315. doi:10.1521/psyc.2007.70.4.283 PMID:18181708

Hochschild, A. R. (2003). *The Managed Heart: Commercialization of Human Feeling*. University of California Press. doi:10.1525/9780520930414

Hollen, E., Clark, E., LeBlanc, C., & Skinner, L. (2018). Assessment and Documentation in Child Life. In R. Thompson (Ed.), *The Handbook of Child Life* (2nd ed., pp. 195–229). Charles C Thomas.

Hollins, W. Q. (2022). *Supporting Children of Incarcerated Parents in Schools Foregrounding Youth Voices to Improve Education Support*. Routledge.

Institute for Patient and Family-Centered Care. (n.d.). Retrieved on April 5, 2022, from https://www.ipfcc.org/about/pfcc

International Association of Chiefs of Police. (2014). *Safeguarding Children of Arrested Parents*. The Bureau of Justice Assistance, U.S. Department of Justice.

Kamptner, L. N. (2017). Evaluating the Efficacy of an Attachment-Informed Psychotherapeutic Program for Incarcerated Parents. *Journal of Prison Education and Reentry*, *4*(2), 62–81. doi:10.15845/jper.v4i2.1058

Kazura, K., & Toth, K. (2004). Playrooms in Prison: Helping Offenders Connect with Their Children. *Corrections Today*, *66*(7), 128–130, 132.

Keller, H. (2018). Universality claim of attachment theory: Children's socioemotional development across cultures. *Proceedings of the National Academy of Sciences of the United States of America, 115*(45), 11414–11419. doi:10.1073/pnas.1720325115 PMID:30397121

Lookabaugh, S., & Ballard, S. (2018). The Scope and Future Direction of Child Life. *Journal of Child and Family Studies, 27*(5), 1721–1731. doi:10.100710826-018-1031-6

Luther, K. (2015). Examining Social Support Among Adult Children of Incarcerated Parents. *Family Relations, 64*(4), 505–518. doi:10.1111/fare.12134

Marks, J. (2020). *From The Desk of Zoe Washington*. Katherine Tegan Books.

Morgan-Mullane, A. (2018). Trauma-Focused Cognitive Behavioral Therapy with Children of Incarcerated Parents. *Clinical Social Work, 46*(3), 200–109. doi:10.100710615-017-0642-5 PMID:30100639

Nellis, A. (2021). *The Color of Justice: Racial and Ethnic Disparities in State Prisons*. The Sentencing Project.

New Jersey Department of Corrections, Divisions of Programs and Community Services, Office of Transitional Services. (2007). *"What About Me?" When a Parent Goes to Prison: A guide to discussing incarceration with your children*. Author.

Pearce, E., Launay, J., & Dunbar, R. I. M. (2015). The ice-breaker effect: Singing mediates fast social bonding. *Royal Society Open Science, 2*(10), 150221. Advance online publication. doi:10.1098/rsos.150221 PMID:26587241

Porter, L. S., Porter, B., McCoy, V., Bango-Sanchez, V., Kissel, B., Williams, M., & Nunnewar, S. (2015). Massage–Parenting Enhancement Program on Recovering Substance-Abusing Mothers' Parenting Stress, Self-Esteem, Depression, Maternal Attachment, and Mother-Infant Interaction. *Asian Nursing Research, 9*(4), 318–327. doi:10.1016/j.anr.2015.09.002 PMID:26724241

Rollins, J. A. (2018). The Arts in Children's Healthcare Settings. In J. Rollins, R. Bolig, & C. Mahan (Eds.), *Meeting Children's Psychosocial Needs: Across the Health-Care Continuum* (2nd ed., pp. 119–165). PRO-ED.

Sawyer, W., & Wagner, P. (2022). *The Prison Policy Initiative*. Retrieved on February 17, 2022 day, from https://www.prisonpolicy.org/reports/pie2022.html

Southwick, S. M., Bonanno, G. A., Masten, A. S., Panter-Brick, C., & Yehuda, R. (2014). Resilience definitions, theory, and challenges: interdisciplinary perspectives. *European Journal of Psychotraumatology, 5*. doi:10.3402/ejpt.v5.25338

Stoerkel, M., & Sc, E. (2020). What is a strength-based approach? *On Positive Psychology*. Retrieved on March 23, 2022, from https://positivepsychology.com/strengths-based-interventions/

Turney, K. (2019). Understanding the Needs of Children with Incarcerated Parents: What Educators Should Know. *American Educator, 43*(2), 22–28.

Walker, S. L., Connery, C., Blackson, G. N., Divine, T. F., Walker, T. D., Williams, B., Finke, J. A., & Bartel, K. (2020). Developing Resilience in Youth with Incarcerated Parents: A Bibliotherapeutic Blueprint with Tween and Young Adult Literature Chapter Books. *Journal of Correctional Education, 71*(2), 37–56. https://www.jstor.org/stable/27042207

Yogman, M., Garner, A., Hutchinson, J., Hirsh-Pasek, K., & Michnick Golinkoff, R. (2018). The Power of Play: A Pediatric Role in Enhancing Development in Young Children. *Pediatrics*, *142*(3), e20182058. doi:10.1542/peds.2018-2058 PMID:30126932

KEY TERMS AND DEFINITIONS

Commissary: A "store" that incarcerated individuals can purchase with money made in prison or provided by family to purchase additional items not available from the jail or prison.

Jail: Jail is a locally operated, short-term facility where justice-involved persons typically await trial and sentencing for up to 364 days and those sentenced to less than a year.

No-Touch Visits: Families are typically separated by a thick plexiglass wall during visits. Visitors communicate using handheld phones attached to the wall.

Prison: Prison is a state or federally operated, long-term facility. Prisons are for incarcerated individuals sentenced to 365 days or longer.

Re-Entry: A term used to define the period following the release of a previously incarcerated person from jail or prison.

Recidivism: When a previously incarcerated individual reoffends.

APPENDIX

Specific Needs of Women Who Experience Incarceration and Addiction

Briana McDonald; *Blue Monarch, USA*

Research shows that white females held the largest population (42%) of incarceration for conviction of drug offenses, while African American followed at (32%) and Hispanic (37%) (Carson & Anderson, 2016). While the percentage of incarcerated women increases, so does the percentage of incarcerated mothers. The incarceration of mothers is especially problematic as most are the primary caregivers of their families, requiring mothers to place children in temporary care settings with family members or foster care. According to The National Survey of Substance Abuse Treatment Services (N-SSATS), a total of 15,961 substance abuse treatment facilities were reported in 2019 (*Quick statistics. National Survey of Substance Abuse Treatment Services,* 2019). Of these treatment facilities, 12,970 offered additional education and counseling services for the family (*Quick statistics. National Survey of Substance Abuse Treatment Services,* 2019). While many residential drug rehabilitation programs do not allow children to reside with their mothers while in treatment, there has been a shift towards developing programs where women can get the treatment they need while still caring for their children. It is in this type of setting that the role of the child life specialist will be discussed.

Role of Child Life Services

Certified Child Life Specialists (CCLS) play a unique role in the transitional process as children adjust to various changes during their mother's recovery from addiction. The role of the CCLS in a residential facility is to design and implement pediatric programs, therapies, and activities to help children cope and adjust to various changes throughout the recovery experience. With an in-depth knowledge of child development, therapeutic age-appropriate interventions, coping techniques, and child supportive services, Child Life Specialists play an integral role helping children recover from past stress and traumatic events of their parent's addiction. The effects of a substance use disorder (SUD) not only affect the individual, but the entire family, including children (Lander, Howsare, and Byrne, 2013). The goal of the child life specialist in the residential facility is to provide educational assistance, psychosocial services, developmentally appropriate coping techniques, and minimize levels of stress and anxiety for children. This can be done by providing experiences that allow for expression of feelings and provide opportunities for play to promote a sense of understanding and mastery during their caregiver's recovery experiences. A CCLS also helps to reduce the negative impact of stressful and life-changing events that can affect the child's development, health, and emotional well-being. By implementing child life services within a residential facility, Child Life Specialists can help children develop strong family relationships, long term coping skills, and promote a sense of resilience.

Transitional Support and Preparation

Adjusting to any new environment, especially a long term residential facility, can be particularly stressful on any child and family member. Children can be uncomfortable and confused when transitioning into new environments. Children process information from the world around them much differently than adults. They have distinct needs for managing the effects of stress and trauma. Without the assistance of a professional who understands their unique perspective, children of all ages may experience emotions such as fear, shame, confusion and loneliness. These thoughts, feelings, and emotions can potentially inhibit their natural development and have lasting negative effects on their wellbeing. When mothers focus on their recovery journey, it is not uncommon for their children to feel neglected while also adjusting to a new environment of the residential facility. Parents do not always know the right way to help manage their child's residential experience, much less know how to support them when transitioning into new and maybe uncomfortable surroundings. Child life services are integral to understanding what a child may need to successfully transition into a residential facility. Child Life Specialists can also help children gain a better understanding of their new environment while correcting any common misconceptions. Some common questions and misunderstandings children may have while coping and adjusting to a residential facility include (but are not limited to):

What is this place?
Why are we here?
How long are we going to be here?
Did I do something to bring us here?
My mother says she is "sick", but she doesn't look sick?
When will my mother get better?
How long will it take for my mother to heal?
Will I get sick like my mother?

It is important to consider each question and concern with care. Child Life Specialists can help guide these conversations with children by providing developmentally appropriate language to support concerns, gain a better understanding of their mother's previous addiction, and correct any misconception.

Reunification

Oftentimes mothers recovering from addiction do not have custody of their children when entering rehabilitation. For example, one child may be in guardianship of a family member, while another child may be in foster care or state's custody. Another child may even be adopted. It is not uncommon for children and their siblings to be separated due to their family's history of addiction. However, if a mother regains custody of her child while in recovery, the objective of the CCLS is to help provide supportive services during the mother and child's reunification process. This can be done by creating an individualized pre-entry framework through developmentally appropriate conversations, education, teaching, and preparation with the child and mother. Poor transitions from one environment into another can negatively influence behavioral outcomes and meaningful participation in everyday life experiences. Incorporating an initial assessment from a child life specialist upon arrival into a residential facility can help mitigate those risks for children; especially with the reunification process. In effort to reduce negative impacts of reunification on children, CCLSs must be able to determine whether the child is at risk for experiencing any negative psychological sequelae. Given that the quality and intensity of a child's reaction to reunification can be influenced by many variables, Child Life Specialists must consider the most significant variables when conducting assessments. Some examples of these variables include (but are not limited to); temperament, behavior, age, gender, development, any parental anxiety or distress, parental presence and involvement, previous living conditions, relationship with previous caregiver, post traumatic trauma or stress, and their ability to cope.

A CCLS's role is to sustain a supportive and motivating environment for all children to achieve optimal reunification with their families during their recovery experience. This can be done by developing trusting relationships that foster a sense of safety, security, and normalcy. It is important to recognize and demonstrate that reunification for all children is top priority. A child life specialist can help demonstrate this by meeting the psychosocial, physical, mental, and emotional needs of children transitioning into their new home environment at the rehabilitation facility. Child Life Specialists play a unique role in the reunification and integration process by conducting reassessments; to provide tailored resources in educational assistance, psychosocial services, and developmentally appropriate coping techniques during recovery from family addiction designed for individual children and family members. The goal is to increase the success of reunification through the provision of support that can assist a family long after they have graduated from the residential rehab facility and integrated back into society.

Since rehabilitation can be offered in lieu of time served, it is not uncommon for incarcerated women to receive furlough and enter a residential drug abuse program (RDAP). RDAP is a voluntary, 500-hour, nine- to twelve-month program of individual and group therapy for federal prisoners with substance abuse problems. Due to the voluntary nature of the program, if a prisoner withdraws from residential drug abuse program or is discharged before completion, they are immediately transferred back to their last prison. This can be problematic, especially if the mother has been reunified with her children at any point of time during the RDAP. Child life services play an integral part in understanding the child's emotional and social needs if they are removed from their mother again for reincarceration. Child Life Specialists hold a very important role helping RDAP administrators and mothers understand the mental and emotional needs, not only of the child but also components of any other child community peers within the residential program. The CCLS can act as a bridge between these groups. Child Life Specialists contribute to the residential program through their in-depth knowledge of the program and the developmental needs of the child (Laser-Maira & Nicotera, 2011). The presence of an external support person, such as a child life specialist, is fundamental to resilient outcomes (Laser-Maira & Nicotera, 2011). While administrators and other staff members can help children reduce levels of stress in certain environments, Child Life Specialists help them to persevere in other healthy and positive ways.

These life-altering events can leave parents with questions such as:
"How will I tell my child I am going back to jail?"
"Who will receive care of my child?"
"Will they be safe?"
"Will my child be okay without me?
"I don't want my child thinking they are at fault for me going back to jail."

It is important to consider each question with care and help facilitate and support each child while guiding challenging conversations. This can be done by providing an individualized plan for each child.

Fostering Resilience

According to Rutter (1987), resilience is defined as the ability to deal with life's challenges in a positive and productive manner. For example, this might be the ability to bounce back from stress, adversity, failure, challenges, or even trauma. Resilience is what helps children navigate through stressful situations. Since children of addicted parents are often faced with more challenges and adversity than children of sober parents, it is important they learn effective coping skills to help deal with challenging situations. Proper support from trusted adults and Child Life Specialists within the residential facility can help establish long-term coping skills to use in stressful situations and assist in building resilience. Resilient children are more likely to take healthy risks. They are curious, brave, trusting of their instincts, work towards their goals in life and solve problems independently (Hurley, 2018).

Child life services help children build resilience and confront challenging situations by teaching them how to solve problems independently through effective coping skills. Child Life Specialists can help children learn how to cope effectively with stress and feel better prepared to overcome life's challenges. Some positive ways a child life specialist can help develop positive coping skills include (Building Resilience in Children, n.d.):

Learning what has helped the child deal with previous stressful situations.
Modeling positive coping strategies.
Helping children focus on individual strengths to build competence.
Creating a safe environment for them to share their innermost thoughts, feelings, and emotions.

Child Life Specialists can help assess psychosocial needs, promote resilience, minimize stress, and ultimately help mothers and their children cope with new or stressful situations throughout the residential program.

CONCLUSION

Certified Child Life Specialists understand how toxic stress and traumatic events affect a child's normal activity level, lifestyle, education, self-esteem, and social relationships (Yeo & Sawyer, 2005). Each reunification experience will be different for each child; with the guidance of a child life specialist, children can successfully reunify with their mother and family members.

REFERENCES

Building Resilience in Children. (n.d.). Retrieved from https://www.healthychildren.org/English/healthy-living/emotional-wellness/Building-Resilience/Pages/Building-Resilience-in-Children.aspx

Carson, E. Ann, and Anderson, Elizabeth, "Prisoners in 2015" (Washington, DC: US Dept of Justice Bureau of Justice Statistics, Dec. 2016), NCJ250229, p. 14 (state) and p. 15 (federal).

Hurley, K. (2018, September 26). How to Build Resilience in Children: Strategies to Strengthen Your Kids. Retrieved from https://www.psycom.net/build-resilience-children

Importance of early childhood development. (n.d.). Retrieved from https://www.child-encyclopedia.com/importance-early-childhood-development

Lander, L., Howsare, J., & Byrne, M. (2013). The impact of substance use disorders on families and children: From theory to practice. *Social Work in Public Health, 28*(3-4), 194–205. doi:10.1080/19371918.2013.759005 PubMed

Laser-Maira, J. A., & Nicotera, N. (2011). *Working with adolescents: a guide for practitioners*. Guilford Press.

Rutter, M. (1987). Psychosocial Resilience and Protective Mechanisms. *The American Journal of Orthopsychiatry, 57*(3), 316–331. doi:10.1111/j.1939-0025.1987.tb03541.x PubMed

Quick statistics. National Survey of Substance Abuse Treatment Services. SAMHSA.gov. (2019). Retrieved April 12, 2022, from https://www.samhsa.gov/data/quick-statistics-results?qs_type=nssats&state=United+States&year=2019

Yeo, M., & Sawyer, S. (2005). Chronic illness and disability. In R. Viner (Ed.), *ABC of Adolescence* (pp. 16–18). Blackwell.

Chapter 7
Law Enforcement

Jessica Foster
Charles County Sheriff's Office, USA

Amelia Ryan
Police Athletic League of KCMO, USA

ABSTRACT

Child life specialists working with law enforcement are valuable in providing direct support and timely intervention in the community. This chapter discusses the implementation of a child life specialist in the role of a victim services provider including practical applications of interventions and opportunities for further consideration. With additional training on law enforcement basics and criminal justice processes, child life specialists have the expertise necessary to bridge the gap between law enforcement and victims of crime. This chapter also introduces the positive impact of employing Certified Child Life Specialists in the police athletic league setting. It illustrates the importance of the role of child life working in the urban community setting with youth and police officers to help normalize the environment, encourage positive coping techniques, and support and advocate for youth and families' psychosocial needs.

INTRODUCTION

Law enforcement officers serve to ensure safety in the community through preventing and investigating crimes, community policing, and countless other obligations. The presence of law enforcement in the community enables officers to build rapport and establish the agency as a trusted source of support. Similar to law enforcement officers, child life specialists are uniquely trained to support the community through knowledge of trauma-informed care, development, and family systems. Child life specialists have used their competencies and integrated into law enforcement settings for years. The following chapter will describe two different roles Certified Child Life Specialists (CCLS) have taken on within law enforcement to support the officers and the community they serve. The first as a victim services provider and the second as a CCLS in a Police Athletic League.

DOI: 10.4018/978-1-6684-5097-0.ch007

CHILD LIFE AS A VICTIM SERVICES PROVIDER

Most often, when an individual encounters the police it is due to involvement in a crime as either a suspect or a victim. A crime may involve a traffic violation that leads to a car accident where a victim sustains injuries that involve hospitalization and rehabilitation. A crime may occur as an armed robbery, a domestic or sexual assault, a burglary, reckless endangerment, rape, or murder. While law defines crimes based on various classifications, a crime, regardless of the severity, can affect a victim's well-being in several ways. Crime has the potential to impact physical, psychological, social, spiritual, and financial aspects of a victim's life. To assist victims of crime, a victim services provider serves as an additional resource to expand community support. A Certified Child Life Specialist in the role of a victim services provider has the ability to evaluate a victim's needs, create and implement a plan of care to address those needs, and guide a victim to additional resources and support as appropriate.

History

In the late 1960's, a report authored by the President's Commission on Law Enforcement and Administration of Justice brought national attention to the study of crime. More significantly, the report highlighted the fact that studies neglected to address the victims of crime. The recognition of crime victims spurred conversations that subsequently revealed several challenges within the criminal justice system. Though little was known about the significance of the role of crime victims at the time, further surveys that stemmed from the President's Commission report indicated that victims were underreporting crime. Research showed that success rates of prosecutions were low as a direct result of victims and witnesses not cooperating in the criminal justice process. Underreporting and the lack of cooperation was due to the lack of support for victims of crime. With national attention on the needs of crime victims, the United States experienced a shift in the early 1970's when the Department of Justice prioritized research on the needs of crime victims and funding for victim-witness programs. As a result, the role of the victim services provider was established in the criminal justice system.

Until the early 2000's, victim services programs within police departments were uncommon (Parker, 2001). The growth of crime victim support beyond the investigation was slow to gain momentum. In support of expansion, the Austin Police Department shared several benefits of direct victim services support based on their experience. Advocates found that victim services support provided a substantial tool to improve relationships with the community, increase conviction rates to hold offenders accountable, and serve as a natural gateway for victims of crime to seek and receive necessary mental health support (Parker, 2001). Law enforcement officers in departments across the country wear several hats, often due to a lack of resources. Realistically, the role of counselor or victim advocate should not be the responsibility of an officer, but rather a victim services provider who works in collaboration with law enforcement to serve the community (Anonymous, personal communication, March 17, 2022).

The Role of Victim Services

The role of a victim services provider is to make certain that victims of crime have the necessary support after a traumatic event, during an investigation, or after an arrest of a suspect. Victim services providers work to ensure victims of crime are aware of their rights as a victim established by law, to provide support for victims and/or family members or friends that are present at the scene of a crime, and to refer victims of crime to appropriate resources and support services. This requires victim services providers to work directly with police officers, as well as local and regional support providers. In building working relationships, an efficient program allows police officers to use victim services providers as a resource when additional support is necessary to avoid impeding on an investigation or crime scene preservation. As an officer shared,

having a victim services coordinator present alleviates the pressure we face in supporting victims of crime during criminal investigations, so that we can place our utmost focus on the investigation. On less critical scenes where there is not an immediate need for victim services presence, victim services has provided officers with electronic and print resources that we can utilize as necessary allowing us to offer victims support in that moment (Anonymous, personal communication, March 8, 2022).

The value in quality victim services support benefits the work of police officers and support providers who collectively work to serve their surrounding communities. A commander of the criminal investigations division of a law enforcement agency that has a victim services program stated,

Victim services has become crucial to the law enforcement mission over the past several decades. As the nature of crime continues to evolve, so must law enforcement response to the needs of victims who are affected by these crimes. The victim services function allows for officers and detectives to concentrate vigorously on the investigation at hand, while the victim services representative can tend to the needs of the victim. This could be in the short term, to assist with the victim's emotional and physical needs with a personal touch or provide resources for immediate shelter, food, clothing, and health care for the victim. It can also be with the long-term needs, such as providing information and contacts for advocacy organizations, counseling services, or welfare agencies. Victim services can also be crucial in helping victims understand the legal process, and can assist the victim in navigating the steps involved in criminal justice proceedings that are often complicated and emotional (J. Pratta, personal communication, March 11, 2022).

The Office for Victims of Crime, which is a component of the Office of Justice Programs of the United States Department of Justice, wrote a handbook about the law enforcement response to victims of crime. The handbook discusses the critical role of a victim services provider and states that the initial interaction that law enforcement has with victims of crime and the manner of the response "is critical in determining how victims cope, first with the immediate crisis and, later, with their recovery from the crime" (as cited in Parker, 2001, p. 1). Police departments across the country are continually expanding their support for victims of crime. Given the extensive processes involved in the criminal justice system, a prosecutor's office handles less than 25% of major crimes (Parker, 2001). Therefore, more than 75% of victims of crime do not have access to victim services support unless a program is available within the police department (Parker, 2001). A victim services provider within law enforcement enables an immediate response that benefits police officers and the community.

Who do Victim Service Providers Serve?

Victim services providers within law enforcement encounter the community whenever and wherever a crime has occurred. Crime has no boundaries. Though a victim services provider can support a victim of any crime, a victim services provider most often works with individuals who have been victims of the following types of crimes:

- Homicide
- Suicide
- Rape
- Assaults
- Reckless endangerment
- Human trafficking
- Threats and/or harassment
- Accidental injury
- Fatal motor vehicle collisions

While certain factors can mitigate crime, crime has the potential to happen everywhere and the potential to happen to anyone. Therefore, victim services providers work with individuals of all ages, genders, religions, races, and ethnicities. Victim services providers work with individuals with all levels of physical and cognitive ability, as well as individuals of all levels of socioeconomic status. Cultural humility is important in establishing positive, trusting relationships with a diverse community. Differences exist in cultures that include communication styles, values, and family definitions (Johnson as cited in Rollins et al., 2005), which can be factors that impact a victim's response to a crime. Without an awareness and knowledge of an individual's culture or needs, such a response has the potential for misinterpretation. For instance, certain cultural groups speak in a loud volume, which can be perceived as anger when that is not the intent. Some cultural groups may perceive touch as comfort, whereas others perceive touch as taboo or an invasion of personal space (Johnson as cited in Rollins et al., 2005). Effort to gain cultural humility of the community where a victim services program operates is necessary in delivering appropriate support.

In addition, the type of victimization and the demographic of a victim are also important factors in determining need. The needs of crime victims can fluctuate over time as victims process the psychological or physical effects of the crime they experienced. Crime has the potential to present a stressful situation that is often traumatic for individuals involved. Prolonged or repeated stressors increase the risk of adverse development or health effects. For children, effects may not be evident until adolescence or adulthood (Franke, 2014). For children and adults, adverse effects can be evident in coping, mental health, or physical illnesses. The goal of victim services programs is to provide the necessary support that promotes wellness, healthy development, and resilience.

Education

For many years, volunteers who had a desire to support law enforcement and their community filled the role of a victim advocate. However, as the field of victim services has evolved, there has been a progression towards advanced degree and professional certification requirements. Professional certification requires victim assistance providers to have field experience in a victim support role, applicable educational training, and continuing education in the field of victim services (Roper Victim Assistance Academy of Maryland [RVAAM], 2019). While there is still variation in requirements necessary for the role of a victim services provider across regions, the cohesive movement towards advanced education and field experience promote continued growth in the field. A Certified Child Life Specialist (CCLS) has the education and field experience well suited for the victim services role within a law enforcement agency. A commander within the criminal investigations division of a law enforcement agency shared his thoughts based on direct experience working with a victim services provider with a child life background.

Today's law enforcement agencies must transition from handling victim/witness services in a business-like manner, such as sending letters or surveys to victims, to having more personal interactions with victims and witnesses. It is essential that law enforcement hire victim services personnel who have backgrounds in fields such as counseling, psychology, child life, or family service related fields. With these backgrounds, they are qualified to provide on-scene support to persons involved in tragic incidents. These personal interactions are comforting for the victims and benefit law enforcement because it establishes a trusting relationship. Victims and witnesses who feel as though law enforcement is truly there to help and cares about them as individuals will be more willing to provide information and cooperate during an investigation, which in turn helps to hold an offender accountable (A. Celia, personal communication, March 11, 2022).

Child life specialists who work in a traditional hospital environment provide support for patients and their families during traumatic, stressful, or challenging situations that often involve heightened emotions and responses. Their expertise allows for the implementation of preventive and supportive interventions (Association of Child Life Professionals [ACLP], 2018). In the community, a victim of crime may also experience traumatic, stressful, or challenging situations that involve heightened emotions and responses. As the Association of Child Life Professionals outlines in their Standards and Guidelines for Child Life Practice in Community Based and Non-Traditional Settings, transitioning to work with victims of crime in the community is achievable with training and continuing education that is specific to law enforcement and the criminal justice field in order to deliver competent care (ACLP, 2018). While the foundational education and training is transferable, the processes and language used in law enforcement and victim services is immensely different from the medical field and traditional child life programs. Thus, additional training and continuing education is necessary.

Intervention

Effective victim support programs operate on a model that addresses psychological, practical, and information needs (Huang, 2018). When a crime occurs, timely intervention is critical. Intervention involves ensuring that a victim has appropriate information about the law enforcement response to the crime that has occurred and the investigative process, information about their involvement in criminal justice proceedings as a victim of a crime, and information about their rights as a victim of a crime as defined by law. Intervention also ensures that an individual is able to address practical needs that affect daily living including safe shelter, prescription medications, legal expenses, and advocacy, as well as making necessary notification to an employer or a child's school. The third category, psychological needs, is often not necessary to address in the immediacy of victimization (Huang, 2018). As Maslow's hierarchy of needs describes, the most basic needs, physiological and safety needs, must be met prior to addressing psychological needs (McLeod, 2007). Once an individual's basic needs are satisfied, such as shelter, food, and security, then an individual can begin to address their psychological needs including counseling or therapy. While there are several factors that influence a victim's needs, a person-centered approach or family-centered approach, depending on the situation, should be taken into consideration in order to provide individualized support for a victim of crime. A victim services provider is able to deliver the individualized attention to meet these needs while allowing law enforcement officers to focus on a criminal investigation.

One officer described the scene of a death investigation where the presence of a victim services provider was not only valuable, but critical in allowing the officers on scene to conduct their investigation. The victim's mother was present on scene and refused to leave her child's side. She was in shock, emotional, and unable to process information. The officers on scene diverted their attention to support the victim's mother, which hindered the investigative process and impacted the timeline of crime scene preservation and evidence collection. A victim services provider arrived on scene with the purpose of providing support for the victim's mother. The victim services provider conducted a brief, informal assessment to determine the mother's immediate needs, provided emotional support in an effort to build rapport and a therapeutic relationship, and assisted in providing information in an effort to prepare the victim's mother for the processes involved in her situation. Through collaboration, the victim services provider and officers on scene worked to ensure that the victim's mother had a safe and sufficient plan to address her immediate needs. Due to building rapport on scene, the victim services provider established a connection with the victim's mother that permitted her to gain a sense of trust and comfort that allowed continual support throughout the investigation to address more long-term needs. According to the investigating officer, "having a victim services provider on scene who was capable and had the skills necessary to provide support for the victim's mother during such a traumatic situation was instrumental in allowing us to complete our investigation thoroughly and effectively" (Anonymous, personal communication, March 11, 2022).

Child life specialists have a unique perspective of children and families that provide a valuable opportunity in the community environment. As standards of clinical practice outlined in the Association of Child Life Professional's Position Statement on Child Life Practice in Community Settings states, child life specialists work to promote and advocate for normalization in a child's environment, assess psychosocial needs, and minimize stress and anxiety (ACLP, 2018). All of which are aspects that serve to improve family functioning as a whole. These standards of clinical practice are evident in the work of victim services providers in law enforcement.

Practical Application

The nature of crime means that an emergency has occurred and an immediate response is necessary. Similar to a trauma response in a hospital emergency department, child life specialists have the expertise to respond in the community. The following section will provide insight into the role of a victim services provider in law enforcement and will examine how a child life specialist can provide services in collaboration with police officers and the community. Program goals of any child life specialist include using available information about a case to create a care plan that is appropriate for those who are involved and subsequently adapting the care plan as needed (ACLP, 2018). When a crime occurs and an officer determines that the support of a victim services provider is necessary, several steps occur to ensure a victim has appropriate support.

Step 1: Obtain basic information about the individuals involved in the incident and the known details of the incident (Note: Initial information is provided through a phone call, as a victim services provider is not automatically dispatched to a scene)
Step 2: Gather applicable materials or resource information that may be used at the scene of the incident (Note: As a victim services provider, it is important to have materials and resources that are accessible, easy to transport, and readily available when needed)
Step 3: Once on scene, review any updates with the investigating officer and discuss an initial care plan (Note: The term care plan is not common in law enforcement. It is important to have an awareness of the language of the profession and adapt language to what is appropriate for the environment. To an officer, plan of action is the common phrase for care plan)
Step 4: Approach the victim(s) to introduce services and conduct an assessment

Step four described above is vital, as it provides an opportunity to build rapport with the victim(s). It is an opportunity to hear the victim's perspective, determine their immediate needs, and adjust the care plan accordingly. Building therapeutic relationships with individuals in the community assists to address vulnerability, promote healthy coping, and foster resiliency (ACLP, 2018). Child life specialists working in a victim services role within law enforcement are also valuable in bridging the gap in understanding child development, human development, and psychology. Generally, police officers do not have education on such subjects beyond what may have been received at the high school level or delivered during training sessions that are presented through their local agency. Expertise in such subjects provides a significant opportunity for police officers to gain awareness and adapt support in an effort to deliver developmentally appropriate and competent service within the community.

Functions of Play

Child life services include opportunities for play (ACLP, 2018). Play is how children learn about the world around them, how children process information, and how children cope. Play is also how children express their concerns (Thompson & Stanford, 1981). While there are several classifications and purposes for play, The Association for Play Therapy, Inc. identifies play as a tool for communication, a method for self-expression, and an aide in alleviating psychosocial injury (Bolig as cited in Rollins et al., 2005), three components that are critical and included in a victim services care plan for engagement during an investigation. Play is a universal language regardless of location or environment, and can be a valuable tool for victim services providers working with children and families in the community. A crime often presents an unfamiliar situation, an opportunity to play can provide a sense of normalization and comfort.

Few resources are needed for play. A child life specialist in the role of a victim services provider is able to use minimal materials to foster a play opportunity during engagement with children and families. While this play experience may seem to lack purpose to those who are unfamiliar, a child life specialist is able to lead guided play or allow an opportunity for child-directed play with given materials that present valuable information for an investigation or creation of a plan of care. Through observing play, a child life specialist is able to help identify emotions, spark conversation, and assist children in being a valuable part of the investigative process. All through an activity that is a normal element of a child's life – play.

Psychological Preparation

Victim services providers usually encounter community members for a brief period of time. Though interactions are limited, psychological preparation is a valuable tool to use when working with victims of crime who have experienced stressful situations. The processes involved in investigations and criminal justice proceedings vary greatly depending on the crime. There is also variation in processes among regions or agencies. A lack of information including knowing what to expect can create additional stress, worry, or concern. The role of victim services is to provide accurate explanations and present information in a manner that is appropriate for an individual's level of understanding (Thompson & Stanford, 1981). A lack of information can also create misconceptions or cultivate fears. Appropriate preparation provided by a child life specialist in a victim services role serves to alleviate stress and eliminate fears. Child life specialists receive education in psychology including human development, bereavement, hospitalization and illness, and family relationships. Child life specialists are trained to break down complicated, unfamiliar information into developmentally appropriate language. Using this knowledge, child life specialists can create materials that are developmentally appropriate to educate and support children and families in the community.

Law enforcement officers work with the community during some of the most challenging moments of their lives. Conversations about crimes, especially major or violent crimes, can be difficult for adults and children. Child life specialists who work in a victim services role can implement resource materials that provide developmentally appropriate preparation and education. For instance, consider a fatal accident. A child is hit by a car and dies on scene as a result of injuries sustained in the accident. The accident occurs during daytime hours when other children and adults are present. Therefore, multiple adults and children in the neighborhood witness the accident and the aftermath of the accident. Police officers and emergency medical personnel arrive on scene and, once it is determined that the child has died, their focus becomes crime scene preservation and evidence collection, a process that can last several hours. Officers request that a victim services provider respond to the scene for additional support. A brief assessment with neighbors reveals that several adults are uncomfortable talking with their children about the accident and are unaware of how to explain the accident to their children. The adults in the neighborhood also experience a range of emotions that require opportunities for processing. Common questions include –

- What do I say to my child when they ask questions about the accident?
- How do I explain to my children that the child has died?
- How do I prepare my children to return to school where they may hear other children talk about the accident or ask questions?

The victim services provider is able to work with adults in the neighborhood to provide examples of appropriate language, as well as lists of appropriate resource materials and local support services. This role allows the agency to provide family-centered care for all who are involved. In addition, child life specialists in the role of victim services provider can create resource materials to assist adults in the community. Specific to the situation described above, a developmentally appropriate book to assist adults in talking with children about death is a valuable tool. Such a book can include general information on grief, for instance, developmental responses to grief and how to support children through their grief. The book can be distributed in an effort to promote appropriate conversation and support as the adults and children in the neighborhood continue to process their own experiences. Victim services support in this type of situation alleviate stress and fear that adults face in providing support for their children, promote education, and provide an opportunity to address misconceptions about death.

Assessment

With limited time available to interact with victims of crime, victim services providers often use informal techniques to conduct assessments. Similar to a hospital-based program, an informal assessment involves a multidimensional estimation of a victim's vulnerability and their ability to cope effectively (Gaynard et al., 1990). Variables used in developing an estimation of vulnerability and ability to cope include chronological and developmental age, prior experiences with law enforcement and the criminal justice system, coping skills, financial resources, circumstances of the crime, misconceptions, and current knowledge of the situation (Gaynard et al., 1990). Child life specialists are invaluable in providing opportunities for coping. The ability to process information while under stress has been widely researched for years. The concept described by Gaynard and colleagues (1990) depicts a cyclical pattern that indicates that stress levels and interpretation of a threat rise when little information is available, which in turn lead to high levels of emotional distress. In continuing the cycle, high levels of emotional distress inhibit cognitive processing (Gaynard et al., 1990). This cycle is applicable across environments including children and adults in the community who are victims of crime.

While oftentimes a victim services provider works with adults in the community, helping the parents or caregivers helps the children. By assisting a caregiver with managing stressors and creating a healthy environment, victim services programs help to mitigate adverse responses in children (Franke, 2014). Using a family-centered care lens, a child life specialist is trained to assess the family unit as a whole and as individuals and uses the assessments to provide appropriate services. Child life specialists are trained providers skilled at coaching parents and caregivers in an effort to involve the family unit as a whole in the processes involved. For a victim services provider, this is highly valuable in increasing involvement in the investigative process, which in turn improves the experience and outcome of the criminal justice processes.

Trauma-Informed Care

Victims of crime often experience situations that are not only stressful, but also traumatic and life altering. Part of the investigative process involves interviews with victims and witnesses. When deemed necessary, an interview may occur in an interview room at a local police station. Typically, interview rooms are consistent with what is depicted on a television show. The room has bare, white walls with a table, chairs, and recording equipment of some form. An environment that can feel threatening and uninviting. A child life specialist is trained to have an awareness of non-verbal messages transmitted through an environment (Thompson & Stanford, 1981). Minor alterations to the environment can decrease the risk of re-traumatization. For instance, the creation of a care and comfort interview room provides a less threatening atmosphere based on trauma-informed care. In particular, a care and comfort interview room is valuable for a special victims unit that works with victims of sexual assault or domestic violence. This type of interview room allows a victim to feel comfortable in a safe space, which subsequently can improve the interview process (Cienfuegos, 2019). A care and comfort interview room includes soft furniture rather than wooden or plastic furniture. It includes neutral colors and white noise machines

(Cienfuegos, 2019). Though a minor change, such an awareness provides significant improvements that benefit police officers and victims of crime, especially victims who are processing trauma. Child life specialists have the awareness to advocate for trauma-informed environmental changes that can change the outcome.

Death Notifications

Part of the law enforcement role in investigations is providing death notifications to next of kin. A victim services provider is a part of the team that can deliver a death notification alongside law enforcement. The focus of law enforcement in the process is to deliver facts and answer questions with known information about a case at the time. The presence of a victim services provider alleviates the burden on law enforcement of ensuring that next of kin have appropriate emotional support, as well as psychological preparation of what to expect in the process of an investigation and how to proceed. As discussed previously in the chapter, a culturally sensitive response is also key. Certain cultures have specific beliefs pertaining to rituals or appropriate emotional expressions when dealing with death (Pearson as cited in Allen et al., 2009). Applying the principle of cultural humility to the delivery of a death notification is a task for victim services providers to assist law enforcement in promoting positive relationships with the community. The presence of a victim services provider at the scene of a death notification also serves as a gateway to ensure that family members have appropriate information about grief and bereavement, including available grief support services.

Child life specialists have education on death, dying, and bereavement, as well as specialized training in providing bereavement support. Appropriate grief support begins at the time of notification. A child life specialist is trained to deliver competent support at the time of notification that is developmentally appropriate, sensitive to an individual's needs, and permits an emotionally-supportive conversation. A child life specialist is trained to initiate therapeutic expression that serves as a gateway to long-term grief support. When a victim services provider is unable to be present at a death notification, a child life specialist in the role of a victim services provider can provide education for police officers that teaches such competent support.

Advocacy and Family-Centered Care

Victim services providers advocate for victims and witnesses of crime. A law enforcement officer is tasked with investigating a crime, identifying a suspect, making an arrest, and subsequently participating in the criminal justice processes to hold an offender accountable. While an officer interacts with a victim for investigative purposes, an officer's focus is on the crime. That is where collaboration with a victim services provider is key. A victim services provider with a background in child life is able to advocate for the victim(s) and witness(es) by considering their perspective based on education and experience.

Look at the following scenario. A death occurs in a home where children are present. Patrol officers and emergency medical personnel arrive at the home and determine that the victim has died due to injuries sustained by suicide. Due to the nature of the incident, detectives are called to the scene to investigate. With appropriate consent, the children are transported to the police station for an interview. Once the interview is finished, the children leave with a family member without their primary caregiver. As the investigation continues, the children participate in subsequent interviews. Immediate family now has care and custody of the children due to the circumstances of the investigation.

The implementation of a victim services program can transform that experience for the children and family members involved. With the presence of a victim services provider with a child life background, the children and their family receive developmentally appropriate support throughout the entire process. As an advocate for the children and their family, who are victims of a crime, the children have an opportunity for child-directed play while at the police station. Despite their recent traumatic experience, the children engage in play as a manner of coping and self expression. Play provides a sense of normalcy in their world, which is impacted dramatically by the loss of a family member in a traumatic manner. Through observations of child-directed play, a victim services provider can assess what the children are thinking and how the children are feeling. This information helps guide a plan of care.

Considering family-centered care, a plan of care involves developmentally appropriate education for the children and their family. The victim services provider uses individualized resource materials to provide psychological preparation for the processes that the children and family will experience during their interactions with law enforcement and the criminal justice system. The resource materials offer accurate information and suggestions for appropriate language to address misconceptions, answer questions, and alleviate fears. This interaction allows the victim services provider to build rapport and establish a trusted source for the children and family members involved. Continuing the investigation, the victim services provider is present during interviews. Their presence offers a somewhat familiar face, which promotes a safe space that enhances the interview process. Education also involves information for family members on grief and bereavement for children. In this scenario, the children are now in the care and custody of family members that are not their primary caregivers. It is essential that those family members understand how to assist the children in processing their grief, what appropriate grief responses look like, and how to determine when additional bereavement support is necessary. The victim services provider is able to deliver this information during timely intervention.

FUTURE CONSIDERATIONS

The potential for the growth of victim services programs within law enforcement is tremendous, especially for providers with a child life background. Considering education and professional experience, victim services providers have the potential to collaborate with law enforcement in detention centers, funeral home directors in funeral homes, forensic investigators, medical examiners, and other first responders including firefighters and emergency medical personnel. Expansion to detention centers would benefit detention center personnel, inmates, and their families, and add value to programs focused on family-centered support. Possible considerations include the implementation of a family visitation program led by victim services providers with a background in child life in collaboration with detention facility personnel. A family visitation program would offer developmentally appropriate preparation and education on what to expect during a visit with a family member at a detention center, as well as family support during visitation to enhance the opportunity for a positive experience. Proper preparation for a visit will allow family members to maximize time spent with loved ones instead of utilizing visitation time to explain processes or address misconceptions. Preparation can include developmentally appropriate resource books or videos created by a child life specialist that are secure and only accessible with appropriate permissions, as to respect an individual's privacy. A family visitation program would also include guided family activities that are appropriate for the environment. Guided activities foster opportunities for family engagement, creativity, self-expression, and normalization in an environment that is often restrictive and intimidating, especially for children during visitation.

Partnerships with funeral homes provide value in offering similar support. Victim services providers with a background in child life have the knowledge and skills to collaborate with funeral home directors to offer opportunities for legacy building with families that have lost a loved one to violent crime. Legacy building can include handprint or thumbprint activities, as an example. The concept would allow family members to engage in memory making activities that would not be available otherwise due to circumstances of the crime. In turn, family members have a tangible means to hold onto memories of their loved one. Investigations of violent crimes often include extensive, arduous processes that are unavoidable. For instance, a victim of a homicide will be transported to a medical examiner for a more detailed investigation of the crime. A process that can take weeks or months. This presents a waiting period where families are unable to proceed with funeral arrangements, a ceremony that often provides a sense of closure and is vital in the course of processing grief. While these processes are unavoidable, psychological preparation can aid to avoid a negative experience in light of a traumatic situation.

The expansion of victim services in collaboration with first responders or local emergency medical personnel affords tremendous potential for providers with a child life background. Having a home base within a local law enforcement agency permits timely and direct intervention with the community. Other considerations for expansion can include –

- Psychological preparation and procedural support for forensic examinations at a local medical center for children and adults who are victims of sexual assault or rape
- Education for first responders including police officers, firefighters, and emergency medical technicians on human development and developmental disorders, as well as suggestions for ways to appropriately provide services for individuals with various disorders
- Collaboration with school resource officers and students to provide education on victimization and available resources
- Implementation of support programs for children and family members impacted by the loss of a loved one due to violent crime, including grief support groups or summer camps

Victim services programs are a vital component of law enforcement. The expertise of a child life specialist in the role of a victim services provider adds tremendous value to support for an agency. Infusion of this type of service into law enforcement enhances confidence and trust between officers and the community that they serve (anonymous, personal communication, March 24, 2022). Working alongside police officers, a victim services provider ensures agency personnel are able to place their utmost attention on an investigation while ensuring victims of crime have the individualized attention necessary to support their well-being and resiliency. The process begins with establishing a community connection through outreach. Given the nature of crime, the implementation of appropriate support and intervention is likely in the immediacy of or following an event. Therefore, increasing awareness of victim services support and providing community education is fundamental in promoting preparedness. The inclusion of child life interventions supports opportunities for assessment, psychological preparation, education, procedural support, and play, all of which a child life specialist is trained to do. The passion, education, and professional experience that a child life specialist brings to the table in a law enforcement environment is transformative in the victim services role.

In addition to child life specialists serving as victim services support specialists within law enforcement, child life specialists have also served within specific programs hosted by law enforcement. One such example is the Police Athletic League In Kansas City, MO.

CHILD LIFE SERVICES IN A POLICE ATHLETIC LEAGUE

The Police Athletic League (PAL) of Kansas City, Missouri (KCMO) is a nonprofit organization staffed by two sergeants, four officers and two Certified Child Life Specialists(CCLS). PAL is a national program currently operating in approximately 300 police departments across the country. The KCMO PAL center is located in the East Patrol Division of the Kansas City Police department. It is located in a zip code with one of the highest violent crime rates in Kansas City (Kansas City Police Department, 2020). The center is a multi-level building with an indoor basketball court, weight room, kitchen area, computer lab, boxing space, a newly renovated wellness and resilience room for child life specialists' programming, and a 500-meter track with green space for outdoor activities. PAL serves area youth, ages 8-18, weekdays between 3:00 and 8:00 p.m. Activities offered include boxing, soccer, pickleball, volleyball, expressive art, running, baseball, weightlifting and basketball. The PAL youth have the opportunity to develop positive, trusting relationships with police officers in their neighborhood in a safe, non-threatening environment. Police officers, in turn, develop and strengthen understanding, trust, empathy and advocacy skills for urban youth through consistent, positive non-enforcement interactions.

According to the "Young Child Risk Calculator" from the National Center for Children in Poverty, there are 34,218,709 children under age 9 in the United States. Forty percent (40%) of them live in low-income families. Many of these children experience additional risk factors: households without English speakers, large families, low parental education, residential mobility, single-parent, teen mother and non-employed parent. (National Center for Children in Poverty, n.d.). The definition of economic hardship resulting in "low income" is a family whose income is less than 200% of the poverty guidelines determined by the Department of Health and Human services. The 2022 national poverty guidelines for all states excluding Hawaii and Alaska for a family household of three is $23,030 per year. (Department of Health and Human Services, n.d.) PAL serves between 50-75 urban youth daily, roughly 65% Hispanic, 30% African American and 5% Caucasian. PAL offers various daily activities and a meal for each participant. PAL youth come from diverse home backgrounds including single-parent, two parent, multi-generational, English as a second language, bilingual, first-generation immigrant, refugee, and foster care homes. Many PAL youth have parents and caregivers who work multiple jobs and/or face intermittent unemployment. PAL youth experience daily risk factors, e.g. exposure to trauma, economic vulnerability, limited access to healthcare and resources, undocumented caregivers, unsafe neighborhoods and incarcerated family members. PAL provides youth with opportunities to socialize, exercise, and engage in community activities that otherwise may not be readily available due to limited finances, resources and transportation.

The child life specialists at KCMO PAL coordinate the Wellness and Resiliency program. At-risk PAL youth need a safe, trauma-informed environment to relax and process their experiences and build resiliency. The PAL child life specialists adhere to the Association of Child Life Professionals Values Statements. Their commitment to relationships built on trust, respect and professional competence contribute to the development of confidence, resilience, and problem-solving skills that enable individuals and families to deal effectively with challenges to development, health and well-being (Association of

Child Life Professionals, n.d.). Child life specialists incorporate mindfulness techniques, yoga, expressive arts, preparation, coping skills, various therapeutic play modalities and self-regulation skills into working with youth in the PAL environment.

In order to develop and establish a collaborative approach to working with youth, PAL child life specialists offer educational inservices to the KCPD captain, sergeants and officers working at the center. The training focuses on child development, the stress response system, evidence-based research including the Adverse Childhood Experiences (ACEs) study and the importance of trauma-informed care with an emphasis on building resilience. Child life specialists incorporate a strengths-based model to reinforce natural attributes and highlight the importance of providing a consistent, positive adult presence in the lives of youth experiencing high risk factors. In referencing Academic Pediatrics:

"Resilience research and discoveries of neuroplasticity and epigenetics help explain the wide variation in the effect of ACEs and trauma, highlighting the capacity to heal, build resilience, and buffer effects through nurturing relationships and environments and self-care." (Bethell et al., 2017, S37)

One of the initial goals of the child life specialists when assessing youth needs at PAL was to advocate for a designated space for child life programming. Child life specialists observed youth making statements like, "I can feel my heart beating in my stomach and I don't like it" while exhibiting uncomfortable non-verbal body language, i.e., covering ears with hands related to the noise level in the gymnasium and enclosed kitchen dining area. The child life specialists recognized the need for a specific space to be used in a similar fashion to the playroom in a hospital setting. The PAL sergeants and board of directors approved this request, permitting the renovation of an extra locker room and bathroom to be constructed into a child life space. The child life specialists envision a multitude of therapeutic interventions, activities and special events taking place in this area. In the interim period, the child life specialists use the computer lab and outdoor space to accommodate the requests of youth sensitive to the overstimulating nature of the gymnasium or populated dining area.

Child life specialists at PAL provide daily interventions to assess the ongoing psychosocial needs of youth. The majority of youth who attend programming walk directly to PAL from school or get dropped off after school by a parent, sibling or family member. Upon arriving, PAL youth sign in and have free time to play in the gym or talk with staff. Child life specialists help normalize the PAL environment, offer active and reflective listening, and engage with youth through play to best assess and meet youth needs. Child life specialists remain visible and present, eager to model adaptive coping techniques when youth show signs of dysregulation, i.e. fast-paced sporadic breathing, increased heart rate, verbal outbursts, etc.

Certified Child Life Specialists incorporate the Circle of Courage resiliency model into work with PAL youth and staff. This model highlights children's universal needs of belonging, mastery, independence and generosity. (Starr Commonwealth, 2019) Child life creates an environment of belonging through accepting, listening and encouraging youth of various ages and backgrounds to feel seen, heard and safe in the PAL environment. Child life encourages youth to verbalize thoughts, feelings and insight regarding the PAL environment, i.e., interests, dislikes, special events, activities offered. Child life specialists strive to provide individualized and group interventions that allow youth the opportunity to learn, grow, fail and succeed in mastering various skills. Child life specialists routinely assess the unique and varying needs for youth independence, confidence and mastery through implementing child-driven play and offering developmentally appropriate activities.

PAL youth need opportunities for social emotional growth through consistent healthy relationships with peers and adults outside of their home and school setting. PAL offers older teenage participants the opportunity to mentor and model positive behavior to younger participants through their involvement on the Youth Advisory Board (YAB). Child life specialists at PAL developed YAB to cultivate the four main protective factors of resilient children: supportive adult-child relationships, a sense of self-efficacy and perceived control, adaptive skills and self-regulatory capacities and sources of faith, hope and cultural traditions (Starr Commonwealth, 2019, 4). Through involvement in monthly meetings and ongoing youth-initiated activities, the PAL Youth Advisory Board fosters independence, generosity, self-efficacy skills and a sense of mastery through goal setting and advocating for the needs of area youth and community.

Child life specialists help prepare PAL youth for various school-related experiences including transitions to a new school, testing, try-outs for extracurricular activities and engaging in healthy ongoing peer interaction. Child life specialists observe, listen and develop "care plans for individuals or groups based on assessment of the child's development, temperament, coping style, culture, spirituality, potential stressors, family needs, and social supports." (Association of Child Life Professionals, 2020) Child life trained professionals empower youth by teaching body and emotional awareness and labeling, rehearsal of coping techniques, and self-regulation skills.

When the Wellness and Resiliency program began at the KCMO PAL in 2020, the COVID-19 pandemic led the majority of area schools to shut down in–person school. In a stressful, confusing and overwhelming time, PAL became one of the few places where local youth could feel empowered to have some independence, control, choices and the opportunity to socialize in- person with peers. PAL child life specialists encouraged youth to label, express and process emotions and feelings related to the losses and adjustments the pandemic created. PAL child life specialists provided materials for healthcare play giving youth opportunities to work through fears, misconceptions and experiences while gaining a sense of mastery over an ongoing universal situation. Child life specialists helped create a safe, consistent space for youth to paint, write, act, run, play, laugh, cry and move through their experiences.

The overall nature and goals of the PAL environment create a meaningful opportunity for the addition of child life specialists. Meeting urban youth in a play-driven environment creates the opportunity for caring adults to develop trusting relationships on the youth's level. The American Academy of Pediatrics states that, "Play is crucial to a child's social, emotional and cognitive development and is even more critical during adversity or stress points in a child's life." (Romito et al., 2021, p. 3) Child life specialists spontaneously jump into a game of basketball, Uno or volleyball, and quickly develop rapport with youth while assessing personality, stress potential, coping style, etc. Play naturally allows the brain and body to expand its capacity for joy, creating resilience and fostering hope. Child life specialists give voice and choice to PAL youth when possible, allowing them to build confidence and gain a sense of mastery in their lives. Child life professionals, regardless of setting, help weave an emotional and psychological safety net for youth and families. Including Certified Child Life Specialists in standard care protocols cultivates positive development and, most importantly, resilience. (Boles et al., 2020)

The Police Athletic League offers athletic programs that allow youth to release physical energy through organized play. Child life specialists offer mindfulness activities, yoga and stretching following activities such as martial arts and boxing to help youth gain a sense of body awareness and control. Incorporating breathing techniques and sensorimotor exercises strengthen youth's ability to focus the mind and body on the present and gain a sense of mastery and control over self. Mindfulness has been shown to activate the brain regions involved in emotional regulation and lead to changes in the regions related to body awareness and fear. (Van Der Kolk, 2014, p.211)

Child life specialists utilize outdoor green space to give PAL youth opportunities to engage in both cooperative and unstructured free play. Due to traffic, high crime rates and homelessness in the neighboring areas, the majority of PAL youth do not have access to play freely in parks, woods, or green spaces. Child life specialists promote outdoor therapeutic play and expressive art activities, using simple low-budget items such as magnifying glasses, bubbles, paint, yarn, water, and sidewalk chalk. When the weather permits, PAL youth routinely ask child life specialists to have one-on-one time while walking the track to talk or debrief about school events, friendships, or family concerns. Bessel Van Der Kolk states, "Feeling listened to and understood changes our physiology; being able to articulate a complex feeling, and having our feelings recognized, lights up our limbic brain and creates an "aha moment." (Van Der Kolk, 2014, p.234) Child life specialists are trained to work through typical and creative means to utilize these moments to support the continued growth and healthy development of PAL youth.

PAL child life specialists continue to build on and enrich the diverse programming available to area youth. Child life will continue to employ a family-centered approach to interventions. In building on the strengths and success of the Youth Advisory Board (YAB), child life specialists hope to create a Family Advisory Board where parents, caregivers and older siblings will feel empowered to give voice to their needs, hopes and dreams in a supportive environment. Using the newly renovated child life space at PAL will provide opportunities to build volunteer programs such as community art initiatives, animal-assisted interventions, and continued collaboration with area organizations.

Child life specialists in community, non-traditional settings such as PAL can harness the power to change and impact entire communities. Child life specialists possess a professional background that is highly adaptable to a variety of urban settings working with children, youth and families. The Substance Abuse and Mental Health Services Administration (SAMHSA) suggests community resilience must be a factor in community safety; community trust, including law enforcement and the judicial system; opportunities for all; peer and family support; and embracing historical gender, and cultural diversity. (Ortiz, 2019, 475-476) The incorporation of child life practice into the Police Athletic League environment is promising and leads the profession to discover new applications for the advocacy and skillset of a child life specialist.

REFERENCES

Allen, K. E., Bell, J., Brown, C. D., Cross, J., Davitt, K., Desai, P. P., Fenn, L. D., Gaynard, L. L., Goldberger, J., Hicks, M., Hoffman, M., Hollon, E. C., Jessee, P. O., Johnson, B. H., Klinzing, D. G., Klinzing, D. R., McCue, K., McLeod, S. M., Mohl, A. L., . . . Wojtasik, S. (2009). The handbook of child life: A guide for pediatric psychosocial care. Academic Press.

Association of Child Life Professionals. (2020a). *Child Life Code of Ethics*. https://www.childlife.org/docs/default-source/aclp-official-documents/child-life-code-of-ethics4232ee9c90156ede9dafff00004f030f.pdf?sfvrsn=5327804d_2

Association of Child Life Professionals. (2020b). *Standards of Clinical Practice*. https://www.childlife.org/docs/default-source/aclp-official-documents/4-standards-of-clinical-practice.pdf?sfvrsn=893e8c4d_4

Association of Child Life Professionals. (n.d.). *Mission, Values, Vision, and Operating Principles.* https://www.childlife.org/docs/default-source/the-child-life-profession/mission-vision-values.pdf?sfvrsn=61b804d_2

Association of Child Life Professionals. (2018). *Standards and guidelines for child life practice in community based & non-traditional settings.* https://www.childlife.org/docs/ default-source/aclp-official-documents/community-based-standards-and-guidelines_final-approved.pdf?sfvrsn=c7d1864d_2

Bethell, C. D., Solloway, M. R., Guinosso, S., Hassink, S., Srivastav, A., Ford, D., & Simpson, L. A. (2017). Prioritizing Possibilities for Child and Family Health: An Agenda to Address Adverse Childhood Experiences and Foster the Social and Emotional Roots of Well-being in Pediatrics. *Academic Pediatrics, 17*(7, 7S), S36–S50. doi:10.1016/j.acap.2017.06.002 PMID:28865659

Boles, J., Fraser, C., Bennett, K., Jones, M., Dunbar, J., Woodburn, A., Gill, M. A., Duplechain, A., Munn, E. K., & Hoskins, K. (2020, January). *The Value of Certified Child Life Specialists: Direct and Downstream Optimization of Pediatric Patient and Family Outcomes.* https://www.childlife.org/the-child-life-profession/value-proposition-statement#:~:text=The%20goal%20behind%20the%20Child,youth%2C%20families%2C%20and%20organizations

Cienfuegos, S. J. (2019, November 18). APD unveils soft interview rooms to ensure trauma-informed approach. *Hilltop Views.* https://www.hilltopviewsonline.com/20750/news/apd-unveils-soft-interview-rooms-to-ensure-trauma-informed-approach/

Franke, H. A. (2014). Toxic stress: Effects, prevention, and treatment. *Children (Basel, Switzerland), 1*(3), 390–402. doi:10.3390/children1030390 PMID:27417486

Gaynard, L., Wolfer, J., Goldberger, J., Thompson, R., Redburn, L., & Laidley, L. (1998). *Psychosocial care of children in hospitals: A clinical practice manual from the acch child life research project.* Child Life Council.

Huang, L. (2018). Unmet needs and service satisfaction of victim support for the direct and indirect victims of serious violence: Results from a cross-sectional survey in Taiwan. *PLoS One, 13*(2), 1–16. doi:10.1371/journal.pone.0192905 PMID:29466463

McLeod, S. (2007). Maslow's hierarchy of needs. *Simply Psychology.* https://www.simply psychology.org/maslow.html

Ortiz, R. (2019, September-October). Building Resilience Against the Sequelae of Adverse Childhood Experiences: Rise Up, Change Your Life, and Reform Health Care. *American Journal of Lifestyle Medicine, 13*(5), 470–479. doi:10.1177/1559827619839997 PMID:31523212

Parker, S. G. (2001). *Establishing victim services within a law enforcement agency: The Austin experience.* Office for Victims of Crime. https://www.ncjrs.gov/ovc_archives/bulletins/evs_3_2001/welcome.html

Rollins, J. A., Bolig, R., & Mahan, C. C. (2005). *Meeting children's psychosocial needs across the health-care continuum.* Pro-ed.

Romito, B., Jewell, J., Jackson, M. (2021, January). AAP committee on hospital care, & association of child life professionals. Child Life Services. *American Academy of Pediatrics, 147*(1).

Roper Victim Assistance Academy of Maryland. (2019, September). *Certification*. https://www.rvaam.us/certification.html

Starr Commonwealth. (2019). *Children of Trauma and Resilience Guidebook*. www.starr.org

Thompson, R. H., & Stanford, G. (1981). *Child life in hospitals: Theory and practice*. Charles C. Thomas.

Van der Kolk, B. (2014). *The body keeps the score: Mind, brain and body in the transformation of trauma*. Penguin UK.

ADDITIONAL READING

Charles, C. Thomas. Association of Child Life Professionals. (2018). *Position statement on child life practice in community settings*. https://www.childlife.org/docs/ default-source/aclp-official-documents/cbp-on-cl-practice-in-community-settings_deireviewed. pdf?sfvrsn =62b5834d_2

KEY TERMS AND DEFINITIONS

Crime Victim: An individual who has directly or indirectly had a crime committed against him or her.

Investigation: The process that a law enforcement officer uses to assess and solve a crime.

Psychological Preparation: Providing developmentally appropriate information on a given topic using various modalities.

Victim Services Provider: A professional who works to ensure that victims of crime have appropriate resources, information, and support.

Chapter 8
Child Advocacy Center

Victoria Isaacson
Yale New Haven Children's Hospital, USA

Samantha Ainsworth
Yale New Haven Children's Hospital, USA

ABSTRACT

The nature of a visit to a child advocacy center (CAC) following an allegation of child abuse has the potential to be challenging for children and their non-offending caregiver for a variety of reasons. Within a CAC, Certified Child Life Specialists are able to call upon their unique skill set to support children throughout the many elements of a forensic evaluation process. In an effort to reduce anxiety, enhance coping, and provide developmentally appropriate play and education opportunities for children in this setting, child life specialists serve as integral members of the multidisciplinary team (MDT). In their active role, child life specialists are able to collaborate with community MDT members to creatively and effectively support children throughout the forensic evaluation process. The need for child life involvement in CACs and during the investigative forensic evaluation process is highly valuable when reflecting on the benefit and overall experience for children and their families.

INTRODUCTION

Child abuse and neglect occur in every social class. According to the Centers for Disease Control and Prevention (2022), 1 in 7 children has experienced child abuse or neglect in the past year. More than four million reports are made each year to child protection agencies in the United States when there is concern for a child's safety and well-being (Childhelp, n.d.). After a report is made, if it is accepted, an investigation follows. Not all investigated reports are substantiated: the 2020 Maltreatment Report indicates the victimization rate is just under nine victims per 1,000 children in the U.S. population (U.S. Department of Health & Human Services, Children's Bureau, 2022, p. 20). The investigative process that follows a report of child abuse has great potential to be traumatic for a child and their caregivers. The involvement of Certified Child Life Specialists (CCLS) can drastically reduce the negative impact of the investigation of children. Certified Child Life Specialists possess knowledge and clinical skills

DOI: 10.4018/978-1-6684-5097-0.ch008

that enhance the child's ability to engage during the investigative process. They also support the critical roles of the non-offending caregiver, forensic interviewers, medical providers, and other multidisciplinary team members.

COMMUNITY RESPONSE TO CHILD ABUSE ALLEGATIONS

Although each state's definition of child abuse may vary, federal legislation informs these definitions. The U.S. Department of Health & Human Services, Children's Bureau (2022) summarizes the federal Child Abuse Prevention and Treatment Act to describe child abuse as "any recent act or failure to act on the part of a parent or caretaker, which results in death, serious physical or emotional harm, sexual abuse or exploitation," or sex trafficking of a child (p. 17). Child sexual abuse is defined as sexual activity with a child by an adult, adolescent or older child (Prevent Child Abuse America, n.d.). About 90 percent of child victims know their abuser, but not all perpetrators are in a caretaking role. There are times the perpetrator is also a minor who may be older and more powerful than the victim (Finkelhor, 2012). Additionally, sexual abuse can involve both contact and non-contact incidents. Exposure to pornography and communication in a sexual manner online is also considered child abuse.

A report of suspected child abuse to a child protection agency triggers a response from a multidisciplinary team of professionals. Experts across many disciplines, including but not limited to child protection, law enforcement, medicine, forensic interviewing, victim advocacy, mental health, and child life, are likely involved in the multidisciplinary team response. These professionals are responsible for investigating the abuse allegation and offering services to the child victim and their non-offending caregivers. Ideally, a child advocacy center (CAC) manages the multidisciplinary team response to ensure that high-quality, comprehensive care is delivered in child-friendly environments (National Children's Alliance, n.d.). In the absence of a coordinated effort from a CAC, children may be interviewed by the multidisciplinary team, who may not have the training to gather information from a child in a developmentally appropriate way. In the child advocacy center model, children participate in an evaluation process that includes a forensic interview with a specially trained professional and a non-urgent forensic medical evaluation from a child abuse pediatrician or other specially trained practitioners. Forensic interviews are recorded and observed in real-time by other multidisciplinary team members involved in a child's case to prevent the need to interview a child multiple times. After the forensic evaluation is completed, information is shared among the multidisciplinary team to effectively care for and support the child and caregivers throughout this process.

Many child advocacy centers work to become accredited through the National Children's Alliance (NCA) by exhibiting service excellence across 10 different standards of practice (National Children's Alliance, n.d.). While accredited CACs are compelled to demonstrate how they oversee the multidisciplinary team and ensure that each standard of practice is upheld, the specific organizational structure and the nature of providing services for each child advocacy center varies across rural, suburban, and urban communities (Westphaln et al., 2021). Differences among CACs exist regarding the number of agencies that are located at each CAC, how many services are offered on-site, and whether services are delivered by CAC staff members or by partner agency staff (Herbert et al., 2018). Despite these differences across CACs, a universal goal is to foster cross-agency work.

COMPONENTS OF A FORENSIC EVALUATION IN A CHILD ADVOCACY CENTER

Even with differences across CACs, the general components of a forensic evaluation include a forensic interview, forensic medical evaluation, screening for pregnancy and sexually transmitted infections, and referrals for advocacy, mental health, and ongoing support services. The duration of a child's and caregivers' visits to a CAC varies. An appointment may range anywhere from one to three hours, depending on the services provided.

Forensic Interview

A forensic interview is structured in a way that asks a child open-ended questions to gather a narrative explanation of events a child may have experienced or witnessed. Professionals who are trained in child development, the dynamics of child abuse, and forensic interviewing protocols conduct these interviews. Interviewers tailor questions to match a child's developmental ability. There are times when anatomical drawings are used during interviews, and these drawings become evidence in the investigation. Forensic interviews are typically audio and video recorded and/or observed in real-time by law enforcement, child protective services, and other multidisciplinary team members. One benefit to the multidisciplinary team presence during a forensic interview is the opportunity for professionals to give feedback to the interviewer and provide additional questions to ask the child. It is important to note that caregivers are typically not allowed in the interview room, nor are they permitted to observe the interview. This means children must be able to separate from caregivers in order to engage in the forensic interview.

Forensic Medical Evaluation

Irrespective of how much time has passed since the suspected abuse occurred, children may have worries or concerns about their bodies. Part of the forensic evaluation is a medical evaluation that may include a non-invasive, yet comprehensive physical exam conducted by a trained medical provider. Unlike rape kits completed in the emergency department, the forensic examination is not urgent and has much in common with a typical well-child physical examination. Even though about 95% of the time, significant findings related to the suspected abuse are not detected, these examinations play a vital role in offering reassurance, education, and medical support or interventions to a child (Heger et al., 2002). Along with traditional medical equipment, the forensic medical exam also includes the use of a colposcope device or similar video or recording equipment for external anogenital examination. These devices have the capability to capture photos but do not touch the child. They illuminate and magnify the anogenital area from a distance. This assists the medical provider, allowing them to identify and record any medical findings accurately. A crucial element of the forensic medical examination is that it is offered as a choice. Restraints are not used, and the child has the ability to end the exam at any point.

Pregnancy & Sexually Transmitted Infection Screening

Not all children who are victims of suspected abuse require pregnancy and sexually transmitted infection (STI) screening. However, this level of testing may be useful even if the child is asymptomatic, as some sexually transmitted infections may not present symptoms. The decision to offer pregnancy and STI screening is made on an individual basis following a conversation with the medical provider. Testing can be done through the collection of urine specimens, oral or anogenital swabs, and/or blood samples. If either a pregnancy or STI screening test is positive, the child is offered appropriate medical care and follow-up services.

Advocacy, Mental Health, and Ongoing Support Services

As members of the multidisciplinary team, advocates fulfill an important role for the child and caregivers during the forensic evaluation process. Advocates meet with the non-offending caregiver during the investigative process to offer services such as emotional support, assistance in securing resources, help to navigate the victim compensation application, and facilitating information sharing between caregivers and the multidisciplinary team. Once connected, caregivers may be continuously supported by advocates through court proceedings. Child advocacy centers also work in partnership with agencies to connect children to specialized mental health services to support their healing process. There is often close collaboration among mental health practitioners and the multidisciplinary team.

The Multidisciplinary Team Collaboration

Active engagement from the multidisciplinary team is the common denominator in supporting children and caregivers during the forensic evaluation process. Ideally, the multidisciplinary team becomes involved with a child and caregivers at the onset of the investigation, following the initial report of abuse. Law enforcement professionals focus on whether a crime has been committed, whereas child protective services workers determine the safety of the child while under their guardian's supervision. Forensic interviewers conduct interviews with children, and medical providers offer medical services as needed. Certified Child Life Specialists help children cope during the forensic evaluation process. Advocates and mental health clinicians work to offer ongoing support services to both the child and caregivers. Meanwhile, state attorneys help guide the criminal investigation and prosecute alleged perpetrators. Although each professional has their designated area of expertise throughout this process, collaboration across disciplines is critical in providing comprehensive care to children and caregivers that best supports the healing process.

RATIONALE FOR CHILD LIFE SERVICES IN A CHILD ADVOCACY CENTER

The Child Life Value Proposition Statement highlights how Certified Child Life Specialists design interventions by combining the knowledge of children and caregivers within a developmental framework with the ability to craft an individualized approach that centers on trauma-informed care (Boles et al., 2020). The Association of Child Life Professionals (ACLP) Position Statement on Child Life Practice in Community Settings further validates using child life services to support children, families, and their support systems amid challenging life events, both in hospital settings and within the community. Specific education and training "equip child life professionals with an understanding of the unique perspective of children, families and their support systems and an ability to advocate their needs to others" (Association of Child Life Professionals [ACLP], 2021). Child advocacy centers are listed as one of many potential community-based settings where the child life skill set is both needed and applicable. The National Children's Alliance also recognizes Certified Child Life Specialists as among the professionals who could deliver services within the context of a CAC. In 2017, the NCA published an updated edition of *Standards for Accredited Members* that acknowledges the need to support children and caregivers in navigating unfamiliar legal and community systems, coping with fears and anxiety experienced by the child, and a better understanding of the process through ongoing education, information, and support. These statements reinforce the value of child life involvement during the forensic evaluation process in a CAC environment.

SCOPE OF PRACTICE

Rapport Building and Play

Play is often recognized as the universal language among children. Play is a powerful tool that allows children to communicate, explore, and learn without bounds (Jessee & Gaynard, 2018). Certified Child Life Specialists hold the ability to incorporate play as a means of reducing children's anxiety and misconceptions while increasing overall coping in stressful situations (Burns-Nader & Hernandez-Reif, 2016). In child advocacy centers, child life specialists are closely involved with children and caregivers experiencing stressful situations. Developing rapport quickly and using play is paramount when working with alleged child abuse victims. Child life specialists apply the power of play in a child-friendly setting with an intentional purpose that carries throughout the child's forensic evaluation. During appointments, while information is obtained from the child's caregivers, the CCLS has an opportunity to establish rapport with the child through play and normalizing conversation. This child-directed interaction foreshadows how the child will engage with other professionals during the forensic evaluation. Additionally, this protected time allows the CCLS to assess the child's ability to cope with various elements of the process. Similar to play experiences in the hospital setting, it is important to match the child's affect in terms of their coping, development, and comfort level. While some children do not have difficulty engaging or initiating play, others require more of an adjustment period or, when appropriate, may prefer to spend time in the playroom alone.

In order to maintain objectivity in the investigation of suspected child abuse, Certified Child Life Specialists intentionally offer child-directed play to avoid leading the child in any way. Landreth (2012) emphasizes the importance of incorporating child-directed play to help professionals quickly establish rapport and trust with children. Affording a child the flexibility to determine how play takes place, what materials to use, and whom to involve in the play activities is a simple way to empower the child throughout the forensic evaluation process. These child-directed interactions deliberately foreshadow how the child will engage with the multidisciplinary team and provide the child with freedom of choice and control. Child life specialists are able to facilitate conversation through play that mimics the conversation style they will experience during the forensic evaluation process. Cued invitations that encourage a detailed narrative (e.g., "Tell me all about that") or option posing questions (e.g., "Do you like coloring, painting, or something else?") are intricately woven throughout the play experience with the child. This type of purposeful dialogue allows the child to hear specific words and phrases while engaging in a non-threatening play experience. Through active participation and observation in this play, CCLSs gather valuable insight into the child's overall development, language ability, level of understanding of the visit, and how they may cope throughout the forensic evaluation process.

Orientation and Education

Children may be anxious, fearful, or unsure of new, potentially stressful experiences due to a lack of control and familiarity (Lerwick, 2016). The elements of preparation and education provided by a CCLS have been proven to directly reduce these feelings in children navigating stressful experiences (Brewer et al., 2006). Within the context of a CAC, child life specialists orient children to the setting and offer developmentally appropriate education related to the anticipated sequence of events of the forensic evaluation. Children receive specific information related to the forensic interview process, the medical examination, and, when appropriate, testing for sexually transmitted infections (STIs) and pregnancy. This education is presented to a child prior to the start of their participation in a forensic evaluation. As a result, child life specialists are mindful to facilitate neutral and open-ended dialogue that mirrors the interaction a child will have with a forensic interviewer and medical provider. Due to the sensitive nature of appointments, child life specialists carefully craft their approach to orienting and educating a child while providing information that meets the child's specific needs. While this type of intervention from a child life specialist is typically considered preparation, CCLSs in CACs more often refer to this element as the orientation process. This language is chosen in an effort to mitigate concerns about the possibility that the CCLS will coach or lead a child during an active investigation. On the contrary, there is no such preparation for the child about what to say; rather, there is an orientation for the child about what to expect. Once rapport has been established, the child is oriented to the CAC to aid further understanding of the sequence of events and details related to the visit. Ideally, child life specialists show the child each of the rooms they will visit during the appointment. The process of educating children mimics the actual flow of the child's visit, introducing experiences in chronological order.

When equipped with accurate and age-appropriate information, children are better able to cope with and adjust to difficult or new situations (Jaaniste et al., 2007). Therefore, having child life specialists in a CAC provide children with accurate details in an experiential manner increases overall coping and engagement in the forensic evaluation process while offering the child accurate information to reduce anxiety and misconceptions. Consider the benefits of bringing a child to the forensic interview room. With this element, the child can physically see the room before the start of their interview. Additionally, they are able to sit in the exact chair they will be in for the interview, further orienting them for the experience to come. During this time, child life specialists are able to inquire about the child's understanding of the visit by asking an open invitation question to the child (e.g., "Tell me what you know about your visit today"). Regardless of the child's response, child life specialists are intentionally informing the child the purpose of the visit is to ensure they are safe and healthy. From there, a CCLS can correct misconceptions and offer developmentally appropriate information related to the sequence of events. Due to the sensitive nature of the visit and the involvement of law enforcement, child life specialists carefully engage with the child and avoid asking leading questions in an effort not to elicit details about the abuse scenario. Certified Child Life Specialists explain key elements of the forensic interview, such as interacting with the interviewer and the style of questioning that is used. Certified Child Life Specialists also identify and discuss the items inside the interview room, such as the note-taking paper and the audiovisual equipment.

With an in-depth knowledge of child development, child life specialists need to tailor the orientation process to meet the unique needs of each child. A common element of the forensic interview focuses on the function and use of the audio and visual equipment. Forensic interviews are typically audio and video recorded and observed in real-time by law enforcement, child protective services, and the multidisciplinary team. Video cameras are often used to record forensic interviews, as these interviews later become documented evidence. Due to age-appropriate egocentrism, the idea that video cameras allow observers to watch and listen from another room can be abstract and challenging for young children to comprehend. Therefore, upon further assessment, it is left to the discretion of the CCLS to determine how and when it is appropriate to identify this element for children. Video cameras are discussed in a non-threatening way and identified as a tool that allows the necessary multidisciplinary team members to watch and listen to the interview from an observation room. Children are often reassured that using video cameras limits them from repeatedly answering questions related to the investigation. Children actively participate in the orientation process when they gain a visual understanding of how the cameras operate. Certified Child Life Specialists use experiential teaching methods by allowing the child to both view and demonstrate the functions of the cameras.

The forensic medical exam may be a challenging experience for a child. With that in mind, offering the medical exam as a choice is a valuable piece of the process. Certified Child Life Specialists use their skill set and expertise to provide detailed preparation for the medical exam to reduce anxiety, offer appropriate choices, address misconceptions, and increase overall coping. To further enhance the experiential element of preparation, children accompany the CCLS to the exam room to learn about the medical provider and the elements that make up the medical exam. Children are provided sequential information regarding medical equipment, in the order of most to least familiar. The forensic medical exam is comparable to a typical well-child exam, with a few exceptions. This comparison affords the child a sense of competence as they learn about a new experience. It is communicated to older children that the forensic medical exam is not equivalent to a gynecological pelvic exam. The child life specialist may invite the child to demonstrate knowledge of familiar medical equipment, such as a stethoscope, while also providing information about tools that may be new to them, such as a colposcope. When necessary, children may require screening for pregnancy and sexually transmitted infections. Child life specialists are able to offer preparation and developmentally appropriate education related to this type of testing. Providing an opportunity for active participation and manipulation of the tools creates a full sensory preparation experience for the child. While the fundamental components of the orientation for a forensic evaluation generally remain consistent, Certified Child Life Specialists adjust and personalize the orientation experience based on the child's age, developmental level, interest in learning, and overall affect.

Procedural Support

Past research exemplifies how child abuse evaluations are anxiety-producing events for children and their caregivers. Many children have fears about the evaluation, specifically their forensic medical exam (Marks, Lamb & Tzioumi, 2009). The medical exam allows trained medical professionals to provide the child reassurance, access to medical care, and any necessary health education following suspected abuse. Generally, the forensic medical exam is comparable to a well-child physical exam. However, due to the nature of the visit, it may still be a threatening, emotional, or anxiety-provoking experience for the child. In an effort to offer the child the utmost level of control, the medical exam is always presented as a choice. At times, decisions on whether the child will have a medical exam are discussed between the child, caregiver, and medical provider.

Certified Child Life Specialists in a CAC offer procedural support services to every child for the forensic medical exam and STI screening. Depending on the child's age, coping style, developmental level, and personal preference, varying methods of alternative focus are implemented. Common regulating techniques such as diversional conversation, handheld fidget items, and deep breathing are applied during the exam, and blood draws for STI screening when appropriate. Additionally, procedural support from a child life specialist allows the medical provider to focus on completing the exam, as well as supporting the non-offending caregiver who may be present in the room. Another valuable role of a CCLS during the medical exam is acting as an advocate for the child. During the exam, the child life specialist will intently observe the child's facial expressions, nonverbal behaviors, and a potential shift in affect. The child life specialist's observation of the child's cues can lead to advocating for a break and reinforcing the child's selected choices during assessed stress points of the medical exam.

Assessment and Advocacy

Similar to the role of child life in healthcare settings, child life specialists are likely to spend a great deal of time working directly with children during visits to a child advocacy center. Certified Child Life Specialists use the time spent with children as an opportunity to assess the child across myriad variables. Comparable to how typical child life assessments are conducted, child life specialists rely on knowledge of child development, coping styles, temperament, and the potential impact of stressful experiences to gain insight into a child's perspective (Hollon et al., 2018). Within a CAC, there is a unique approach to how a CCLS develops informal assessments seeking specific information, using a supportive but neutral method. During play and preparation experiences, child life specialists collect information through direct behavioral observation and pose open-ended questions. Assessment data gleaned from a child using child-directed communication techniques helps child life specialists adjust services to promote a child's positive coping and engagement throughout the forensic evaluation process. Child life specialists' detailed observations are essential for members of the multidisciplinary team to support their work with the child.

Children arrive at forensic evaluations with various degrees of understanding about the reason for a visit. Non-offending caregivers may feel anxious to provide information, leading to some children entering appointments with very little knowledge about what will occur. Alternatively, some children are provided details about the evaluation by caregivers or the multidisciplinary team before arrival and may have expectations about what to anticipate. Child life specialists can first ask the child a general open invitation question, exploring their understanding of the reason for the visit. A child's response to these prompts (e.g., "Tell me what you know about today's visit") can demonstrate their knowledge and ability to comprehend open-ended inquiries. From there, child life specialists can clarify misconceptions about the visit and provide appropriate education based on a child's answer. Certified Child Life Specialists are also trained to identify a child's level of anxiety and capacity to cope during stressful situations. Similar to healthcare encounters, both verbal and behavioral cues can signal a child's emotional state during a forensic evaluation. How readily a child is able to separate from caregivers and interact with a CCLS might also indicate how the child will engage with the multidisciplinary team during the process. A noticeable shift in a child's affect may occur as information about the visit is received. Once these changes are observed, child life specialists help children acknowledge which aspects of the visit might be stressful and create a plan to implement appropriate coping strategies (Goldberger et al., 2018).

In contrast to visits in other clinical settings, children tend to have more control over their level of engagement throughout a forensic evaluation in a CAC. While it is the goal and hope that every child who comes to a CAC completes a forensic interview, receives a medical exam if necessary, or connects with mental health services, some children simply are not ready to participate. Gaining insight into a child's willingness to engage in the forensic evaluation helps child life specialists anticipate how the child will respond throughout the process. During interactions with a child, Certified Child Life Specialists can determine how receptive a child is to meeting with the multidisciplinary team. A child's engagement in dialogue, whether it is normalizing conversation or a more focused exchange about aspects of the evaluation, supports a child life specialist's assessment of a child's readiness. Increased anxiety about disclosing abuse to professionals could be one explanation for a lack of cooperation. Schaeffer et al. (2011) also conclude that some children delay disclosure due to threats made by perpetrators, real or assumed relationships with perpetrators, or fears about what would happen if they told someone of the abuse. These same concerns may present barriers to a child's participation during various components of a forensic evaluation. Conversely, some children approach the evaluation eager to share their story and spontaneously disclose. This information sharing might take place at any point during a visit but most commonly occurs during play interactions. Spontaneous disclosure from a child to a child life specialist might be a positive predictor of the child's readiness. However, discrepancies about the details of the abuse might incidentally occur as a child discloses to more individuals, which then presents a challenge for law enforcement. Therefore, it is critical for a child life specialist to avoid gathering additional information after a child discloses outside the forensic interview. Following a spontaneous disclosure, child life specialists should thank the child for sharing the information and provide reassurance that the CAC is a safe place to discuss those types of experiences. If the forensic interview has not yet been completed, child life specialists should also remind the child of the importance of disclosing to the forensic interviewer during the interview. Given the uncertainty of how a child may present for a visit, importance of a child life specialist's assessment of the child's readiness to disclose and engage in the process is invaluable.

Establishing a developmental assessment of a child is important. Cognitive developmental theories help predict how children think based on age, but individual differences exist among children in the same age group (Turner, 2018). Likewise, Saywitz & Camparo (1998) found that age-related differences in a child's memory, suggestibility, language and reasoning skills will influence how a child engages in a forensic interview. Therefore, Certified Child Life Specialists seek to gain as much information as possible about the child's developmental abilities. Given the open-ended format of the forensic interview, a child's ability to formulate responses relies heavily on their capacity to interpret the questions and apply cognitive skills to communicate with the forensic interviewer. A child's vocabulary, particularly the words used for body parts, is valuable information for child life specialists to learn. Children may label body parts with words that differ from anatomical terms. Forensic interviewers are intentional when using a child's specific words to avoid confusion. Comprehension of basic concepts like counting and time units is extremely relevant. During an interview, a child is asked to recall details such as when, where, or how many times abuse occurred. Forensic interviewers may also ask the child to describe an episode of abuse in sequential order of beginning, middle, and end. Through play and preparation experiences, child life specialists are uniquely positioned to gather an assessment and share findings with other professionals interacting with the child.

Certified Child Life Specialists communicate their assessment of the child with the multidisciplinary team. This communication allows the multidisciplinary team to understand better the child's overall coping, level of engagement, and demeanor. Child life specialists assume an advocacy role, relaying relevant information about the child's unique needs. Child life specialists share information with the multidisciplinary team about the preferred name and pronouns a child uses in an effort to encourage others to address the child during any interactions respectfully. Recommendations made by child life specialists regarding a child's developmental level help prepare forensic interviewers and medical providers to use vocabulary and sentence structures that will be understood by the child. When child life specialists share observations about a child's readiness and levels of anxiety, the multidisciplinary team is better equipped to anticipate which components of a visit might induce stress and approach these junctures more delicately. A collective awareness about the child's choices regarding elements of the forensic evaluation process not only sets reasonable expectations for the multidisciplinary team about the child but also increases the child's sense of control. Ultimately, involvement of child life through interventions of assessment and advocacy fosters increased positive interactions among the child and members of the multidisciplinary team throughout the forensic evaluation process.

Children with Diverse Needs

Understanding that the forensic evaluation process can be challenging for children for a variety of reasons, it is important to recognize the potential impact this process may have on children with varying needs and abilities. It is valuable to consider the positive influence the inclusion of a Certified Child Life Specialist within a CAC may have on children using the facility. Adaptation of care provided to children is a critical component of a CCLS's role but is especially important when working with children of diverse needs throughout the forensic evaluation process. Participation in a forensic evaluation process requires that a child be able to engage verbally. This is particularly true for the element of the forensic interview, as this interview is legal evidence for the investigation. Child life specialists in CACs often support children with differing cognitive abilities or language barriers. When appropriate, a child's specific communication tools may be used to support both the child's engagement and the child life specialist's ability to assess the child and meet their needs properly. Children who are diagnosed with developmental delays, cognitive disabilities, or autism require a more comprehensive assessment of their abilities. Forensic interviewers and medical providers may need to shift their approach to engage with a child of varying abilities appropriately. Certified Child Life Specialists deliver assessment information to these professionals to prepare them to interact with the child and advocate for meeting the child's individual needs.

In addition to serving children who are alleged victims of abuse, CACs may also support children who are witnesses to the abuse of a loved one or witnesses to a murder. Supporting child witnesses may present a different level of challenges for providers and the child and caregivers due to the sensitive nature leading to a visit. Likewise, children from immigrant families may also need a higher level of emotional support during the forensic evaluation process. These individuals face a variety of barriers, including but not limited to language and cultural needs, immigration status, and involvement with the legal and child protection systems. While CACs typically serve children and their caregivers, they may also provide support to developmentally delayed adults when appropriate. These adults may require assistance from child life specialists to understand and sign consent papers. Child life specialists may also provide interventions to individuals with developmental delays or variations similar to those provided to typically developing children. Within the bounds of what is acceptable from a legal standpoint, CCLSs are able to use creative techniques and thorough assessment skills to afford individuals who have experienced or witnessed abuse every opportunity to participate in the process.

Documentation

Certified Child Life Specialists document the care provided to demonstrate their work in a comprehensive way that is then accessed by other professionals as needed (Hollon et al., 2018). The mechanics of documentation can vary across clinical settings, yet the core elements remain consistent. In a CAC, verbal information sharing transpires regularly among the multidisciplinary team. In addition to this highly valued communication, accurate and timely, written documentation of child life interactions in the child's protected record is not only a critical component of care but is also supportive of the investigative proceedings of child abuse.

Due to the sensitive nature of a CAC referral, there are special considerations for child life specialists completing written documentation. Child life specialists can be subpoenaed to testify should the investigation lead to a trial. Typically, years pass before the case is tried in court. Documentation containing concrete details about interactions with a child will enhance a CCLS's ability to recall the account later. Child life specialists should note their impressions of a child, including how a child appears to be coping. It is particularly important to record in detail what the child verbalizes about their understanding of the reason for a visit. Child life documentation should outline the child life interventions offered and provided. When there is direct child life involvement, observations on how the child responded to various components of the evaluation process should also be noted. Any disclosure a child shares related to an abuse allegation should be clear in the child's confidential record, using the child's specific language and phrasing. Ultimately, reliable and accurate written documentation is beneficial to child life specialists in their function as active members of the multidisciplinary team.

Community Involvement

While direct care remains to be the central focus of the child life specialist's role, it is just as important to build relationships with community partners and have a visible presence within the community. Multidisciplinary teams hold routine meetings where professionals review the status of child abuse cases. Child life specialists contribute to case discussions by offering knowledge and insight based on their assessments and interactions with children during the forensic evaluation process. Child life specialists also have the opportunity to gather pertinent information for incoming child abuse referrals during the multidisciplinary team meetings. Attending these meetings regularly offers CCLSs the opportunity to establish relationships with the multidisciplinary team, increasing the likelihood of collaboration in future situations. As members of the multidisciplinary team, child life specialists provide education about child life involvement to the multidisciplinary team who are new to working with the child abuse population, to professionals from other CACs who are unfamiliar with the benefits of child life services, and to emerging professionals from a variety of disciplines.

There is also the potential for child life specialists and multidisciplinary team members to partner and create shared resources and tools that will positively influence the child and caregiver's experience. A visit to a CAC can be overwhelming, and some children and caregivers may not fully process what will take place. Certified Child Life Specialists understand how to develop tangible educational resources to support an individual's understanding of a stressful experience. Both caregivers and children benefit from materials and audiovisual media that are readily accessible and provide education about the forensic evaluation process. Informational handouts might include simple and clear descriptions of the process, pictures of the CAC child-friendly environment and its staff, and tips on preparing a child for a visit. A virtual tour can introduce a child and caregivers to the CAC setting while explaining each visit aspect. Children might also benefit from materials such as coloring pages or coloring books that include pictures of the CAC for a child to fill in, along with brief descriptions of what takes place. While child life specialists possess the skills to develop these valuable products, their distribution depends on the multidisciplinary team making contact with children and caregivers after an initial report is made.

High-quality relationships with community partners allow child life specialists to establish connections in the larger community. These connections can, in turn, lead to increased child life involvement and expansion of child abuse awareness and prevention initiatives aimed at providing education to children and at-risk youth, caregivers, and professionals who serve as mandated reporters. In the United States, 37 states have adopted Erin's Law (Erin's Law, n.d.). This legislation requires all public schools to implement a prevention-oriented child abuse program for kindergarten through 12th-grade students. In some cases, victim advocate agencies are charged with this task and deploy the services of a community educator. These individuals work to connect with local school systems, establish clear communication of prevention education program content and goals, and teach the curriculum either in person or virtually. However, there is great potential for CCLSs to join these local agencies to amplify their efforts in order to reach as many youths in the community as possible. Regardless of specific settings, these collaborative endeavors hone in on topics such as body safety, personal boundaries, responses to abuse, internet safety, healthy relationships, and exploitation prevention strategies. Certified Child Life Specialists are well-suited to adjust specific language included in child abuse prevention curriculums and implement effective teaching methods that best meet the developmental needs of various age groups.

It is also possible for child life specialists to play a greater role in community outreach. For example, April is Child Abuse Prevention Month, and many CACs plan events throughout the month to raise public awareness about child abuse. These efforts may take the form of organized community presentations, fundraising events, or social media campaigns. Typically, local and state officials participate, as do local businesses, non-profit organizations, and student groups. Having experience in working with diverse groups of individuals, combined with an understanding of how to communicate information to a broad audience, makes child life specialists an important part of community outreach strategic planning.

POTENTIAL BARRIERS

As previously noted, the National Children's Alliance (2017) recognizes the value in initiating child life services in a child advocacy center. Aside from other challenges child life specialists encounter in a work setting, funding and the acceptance of child life's role by the multidisciplinary team are two of the more significant obstacles to establishing child life services with suspected victims of abuse. Depending on fiduciary relationships, it can be challenging for a CAC to create a child life specialist's position using the agency's budget. One possible solution is to request grant money from the Crime Victims Fund. In 1984, the Victims of Crime Act (VOCA) was enacted, thus establishing the Crime Victims Fund and a means for the federal government to subsidize state and local programs that support victims of crime (U. S. Department of Justice, Office for Victims of Crime, n.d.). Deposits are sourced from the collection of fines, forfeited appearance bonds, and special assessments from individuals and corporations convicted of federal crimes. Money is distributed to state-level victim service offices, which then release grant opportunities to non-profit and public organizations that provide direct services to victims of crime. The VOCA grant is just one potential source of funding. Child advocacy centers may also solicit funds from other grants or private donors to employ Certified Child Life Specialists to work with child victims of abuse. Once a position is established, some of the multidisciplinary team may not be familiar with the role of child life or recognize the benefits of having a Certified Child Life Specialist on the team. Therefore, it is important to clearly delineate the role and responsibility of a child life specialist, highlighting the unique lens child life specialists possess to focus on the specific needs of a child during a visit to the CAC.

FUTURE DIRECTIONS

The case for child life in CACs has the potential to extend beyond the services outlined thus far. Future directions include more outreach in the community, which could mean joining community partners to train mandated reporters who work in local agencies, schools, and healthcare institutions. Planned collaboration between mental health clinicians and child life specialists could lead to a handoff of care that supports the development of trusting relationships and facilitates a child's positive coping during future therapy sessions. Similar to how victim advocates provide services to caregivers beyond visits at a CAC, child life specialists could also support children later in the investigative process. State's attorney professionals could consult a Certified Child Life Specialist when preparing children for court appearances. The use of developmentally appropriate language and teaching methods from a CCLS has the potential to educate a child about court proceedings effectively, thus enhancing a child's understanding and ability to engage with state's attorneys during the final phase of the criminal investigation. Further, there is also the potential for child life specialists to explore becoming forensic interviewers. The foundational knowledge of child development and expertise in working with children of varied abilities combined with additional training about forensic interviewing protocols, the dynamics of child abuse, and trauma-informed care would make child life specialists successful candidates to transition into forensic interviewer roles. In general, the role of a child life specialist in CACs is not yet widely known. Therefore, more research is needed to demonstrate the efficacy of clinical interventions in this type of setting. These findings can then be used to help expand the reach of child life services in CACs and obtain funding to secure stable positions.

CONCLUSION

With almost 1000 child advocacy centers in the country, there is a great opportunity for Certified Child Life Specialists to join multidisciplinary team professionals in their efforts to provide quality care and support to children who are victims of abuse. Although not yet widely adopted, child life specialists' value and importance in a CAC during a child's forensic evaluation process is patently evident. CAC visits may be stressful and potentially anxiety-provoking for children and caregivers for a myriad of reasons. With the understanding that child life specialists aim to reduce anxiety, increase coping, and support children through potentially stressful situations, the value of their involvement in the forensic evaluation process is clear. Certified Child Life Specialists have the unique ability to support children throughout this process by facilitating the power of play, offering developmentally appropriate education, providing supportive interventions, and advocating for specific needs. Incorporating child life services in the child advocacy center guarantees a dedicated professional who is solely committed to helping children navigate the forensic evaluation process.

REFERENCES

Association of Child Life Professionals. (2021). *Position statement on child life practice in community settings*. ACLP Official Documents. https://www.childlife.org/docs/default-source/aclp-official-documents/cbp-on-cl-practice-

Boles, J., Fraser, C., Bennett, K., Jones, M., Dunbar, J., Woodburn, A., Gill, M. A., Duplechain, A., Munn, E. K., & Hoskins, K. (2020). *The value of Certified Child Life Specialists: Direct and downstream optimization of pediatric patient and family outcomes*. Association of Child Life Professionals. https://www.childlife.org/docs/default-source/aclp-official-documents/value-of-a-certified-child-life-specialist_full-report.pdf

Brewer, S., Gleditsch, S. L., Syblik, D., Tietjens, M. E., & Vacik, H. W. (2006). Pediatric anxiety: Child life intervention in day surgery. *Journal of Pediatric Nursing*, *21*(1), 13–22. https://doi.org/10.1016/j.pedn.2005.06.004

Burns-Nader, S., & Hernandez-Reif, M. (2016). Facilitating play for hospitalized children through child life services. *Children's Health Care*, *45*(1), 1–21. https://doi.org/10.1080/02739615.2014.948161

Centers for Disease Control and Prevention, National Center for Injury Prevention and Control, Division of Violence Prevention. (2022). *Preventing child abuse and neglect.* https://www.cdc.gov/violenceprevention/pdf/can/CAN-factsheet_2022.pdf

Childhelp. (n.d.). *Child abuse statistics*. https://www.childhelp.org/child-abuse-statistics/

Erin's Law. (n.d.). *What is Erin's Law?* https://www.erinslaw.org/erins-law/

Finkelhor, D. (2012). Characteristics of crimes against juveniles. Durham, NH: Crimes Against Children Research Center.

Goldberger, J., Thompson, R. H., & Mohl, A. L. (2018). Psychological preparation and coping. In R. H. Thompson (Ed.), *The handbook of child life: A guide for pediatric psychosocial care* (2nd ed., pp. 268–316). Charles C. Thomas Pub. Ltd.

Heger, A., Ticson, L., Velasquez, O., & Bernier, R. (2002). Children referred for possible sexual abuse: Medical findings in 2384 children. *Child Abuse & Neglect*, *26*(6-7), 645–659.

Herbert, J. L., Walsh, W., & Bromfield, L. (2018). A national survey of characteristics of child advocacy centers in the United States: Do the flagship models match those in broader practice? *Child Abuse & Neglect*, *76*, 583–595. https://doi.org/10.1016/j.chiabu.2017.09.030

Hollon, E., Clark, E., LeBlanc, C., & Skinner, L. (2018). Assessment and documentation in child life. In R. H. Thompson (Ed.), *The handbook of child life: A guide for pediatric psychosocial care* (2nd ed., pp. 195–229). Charles C. Thomas Pub. Ltd.

Jaaniste, T., Hayes, B., & von Baeyer, C. L. (2007). Providing children with information about forthcoming medical procedures: A review and synthesis. *Clinical Psychology: Science and Practice*, *14*(2), 124–143.

Jessee, P. O., & Gaynard, L. (2018). Paradigms of play. In R. H. Thompson (Ed.), *The handbook of child life: A guide for pediatric psychosocial care* (2nd ed., pp. 230–267). Charles C. Thomas Pub. Ltd.

Landreth, G. L. (2012). *Play therapy: The art of the relationship* (3rd ed.). Routledge.

Lerwick, J. L. (2016). Minimizing pediatric healthcare-induced anxiety and trauma. *World Journal of Clinical Pediatrics*, *5*(2), 143–150. https://doi.org/10.5409/wjcp.v5.i2.143

Marks, S., Lamb, R., & Tzioumi, D. (2009). Do no more harm: The psychological stress of the medical examination for alleged child sexual abuse. *Journal of Paediatrics and Child Health*, *45*(3), 125–132. https://doi.org/10.1111/j.1440-1754.2008.01443.x

National Children's Alliance. (2017). *Standards for accredited members*. https://nationalchildrensalliance.org/wp-content/uploads/2015/06/NCA-Standards-for-Accredited-Members-2017.pdf

National Children's Alliance. (n.d.). *How the CAC model works & NCA's national standards of* accreditation. https://nationalchildrensalliance.org

Prevent Child Abuse America. (n.d.). *Child sexual abuse prevention*. https://preventchildabuse.org/waht-we-do/child-sexual-abuse-prevention/

Saywitz, K., & Camparo, L. (1998). Interviewing child witnesses: A developmental perspective. *Child Abuse & Neglect*, *22*(8), 825–843. https://psycnet.apa.org/doi/10.1016/S0145-2134(98)00054-4

Schaeffer, P., Leventhal, J. M., & Asnes, A. G. (2011). Children's disclosures of sexual abuse: Learning from direct inquiry. *Child Abuse & Neglect*, *35*, 343–352. https://dx.doi.org/10.1016/j.chiabu.2011.01.014

Turner, J. C. (2018). Theoretical foundations of child life practice. In R. H. Thompson (Ed.), *The handbook of child life: A guide for pediatric psychosocial care* (2nd ed., pp. 34–54). Charles C. Thomas Pub. Ltd.

U. S. Department of Health and Human Services. Children's Bureau. (2022). *Child maltreatment* 2020. https://www.acf.hhs.gov/sites/default/files/documents/cb/cm2020.pdf

U. S. Department of Justice, Office for Victims of Crime. (n.d.). *Crime victims fund*. https://ovc.ojp.gov/about/crime-victims-fund

Westphaln, K. K., Regoeczi, W., Masotya, M., Vazquez-Westphaln, B., Lounsbury, K., McDavid, L., Lee, H. N., Johnson, J., & Ronis, S. (2021). Outcomes and outputs affiliated with children's advocacy centers in the United States: A scoping review. *Child Abuse & Neglect*, *111*, 104828. https://doi.org/10.1016/j.chiabu.2020.104828

KEY TERMS AND DEFINITIONS

Colposcope: Specialized medical equipment used to examine and document the anogenital areas of the body if necessary.

Forensic Interview: A neutral discussion that takes place between a child and a trained forensic interviewer to elicit details about an event the child experienced or witnessed.

Forensic Medical Exam: A non-urgent physical evaluation that takes place as part of a child abuse investigation to assess overall health and potential injury.

Non-Offending Caregiver: An adult who is responsible for the care and supervision of a child victim of abuse. This individual is also not the alleged perpetrator under investigation and may accompany a child to the evaluation.

Sexually Transmitted Infection: A disease that spreads from person to person through sexual contact.

Chapter 9
Disaster Relief

Lindsey Murphy
Missouri State University, USA

ABSTRACT

Child life specialists have been supporting children and families in disaster relief settings for years. It is imperative to understand the needs of children affected by disasters and continue to integrate child life services to best support the psychological and emotional outcomes of children and families. This chapter will define disasters and the disaster management cycle, overview key factors in assessing children's needs related to disasters, identify how child life services are utilized during each phase of disaster relief, and identify future opportunities for child life services in disaster relief.

INTRODUCTION

Approximately 400 natural disasters and 35 armed conflicts occur worldwide each year. In 2021, nearly 10,500 people lost their lives due to disastrous events such as the Haiti earthquake and flooding in India (AON, 2021). Active shooter incidents are on the rise; in 2000 the United States Federal Bureau of Investigation (FBI) reported 3 incidents, by 2020 that number increased to 40 (*Active Shooter Incidents 20-Year Review, 2000-2019*, 2021). About 73 million children live in the United States in 2022, approximately 13.9% of those children have been exposed to a disaster and a fourth of those will experience multiple disasters during childhood (Becker-Blease et al., 2010; United States Census Bureau, 2022).

With increasing numbers like this, it is imperative to understand the impact these disastrous events have on children. Certified Child Life Specialists can support resilience by implementing effective interventions to the most vulnerable populations. This chapter will define disasters and the disaster management cycle, overview key factors in assessing children's needs related to disasters, identify how child life services are used during each phase of disaster relief, and identify future opportunities for child life services in disaster relief.

DOI: 10.4018/978-1-6684-5097-0.ch009

DEFINING DISASTERS

Disasters can be broadly or narrowly defined. In general, disasters are natural or human-made events that cause sweeping damage, hardship, and/or loss of life across one or more strata of society (Bonanno et al., 2010; R. W. Perry, 2018). The Federal Emergency Management Agency (FEMA) defines disaster as:

An event that results in large numbers of deaths and injuries; causes extensive damage or destruction of facilities that provide and sustain human needs; produces an overwhelming demand on state and local response resources and mechanisms; causes a severe long-term effect on general economic activity; and severely affects state, local, and private sector capabilities to begin and sustain response activities. (Emergency Management in the United States, n.d.)

There is not one universal categorization of disasters, however, consistency does exist in that they tend to be organized into 2-3 categories: 1) natural disasters 2) human-made disasters, and 3) a third variation that includes disasters such as technological, infrastructure, or public health disasters. Natural disasters include events such as: flooding, hurricanes, tornadoes, earthquakes, and wildfires. Human-made disasters include events such as: incidence of mass violence, school shootings, terrorism, and human conflicts. Examples often put into the third category include: pandemics, building or bridge collapses, transportation crashes, nuclear reactor incidents, and gas explosions.

The key differentiation between an emergency and a disaster is in the size of the event and the resources needed to support and manage the event. Disasters are larger scale, sweeping across a community, and require response and recovery services that are greater than what local entities can provide. Whereas, emergencies are typically smaller in size and resources needed are usually matched locally. Disaster declarations largely decide the resources requested to support the community impacted by the disaster. Declarations are first declared at the local level; once those resources and local capabilities are expected to be exceeded or are exceeded, the state is requested to respond. This repeats at the state and federal level as needed. For example, when a tornado occurs, the local emergency responders, hospitals, and other local community resources are the first on the scene providing support and help to rescue survivors. As those resources are overwhelmed, additional support from nearby communities is requested. From there the disaster response circle broadens to include state resources and support; if needed federal and international resources are requested. Due to this structure, it is imperative that child life services collaborate with disaster management organizations, managers, and officials on all levels: local, state, federal, and international to maximize their reach and effectiveness and decrease their response time.

RESPONDING TO DISASTERS - THE DISASTER MANAGEMENT CYCLE

Disaster management requires that a variety of disciplines, practitioners, academics, professionals, volunteers, governmental agencies, non-governmental agencies, and international organizations coordinate efforts to respond to and reduce, avoid, or mitigate the potential losses that occur when disasters strike. For this collaborative work, the disaster management cycle focuses on four phases: mitigation (or prevention), preparedness, response, and recovery (*Emergency Management in the United States*, n.d.). Figure 1 is the Disaster Management Cycle used to organize efforts to support communities during disasters.

Figure 1. The Disaster Management Cycle

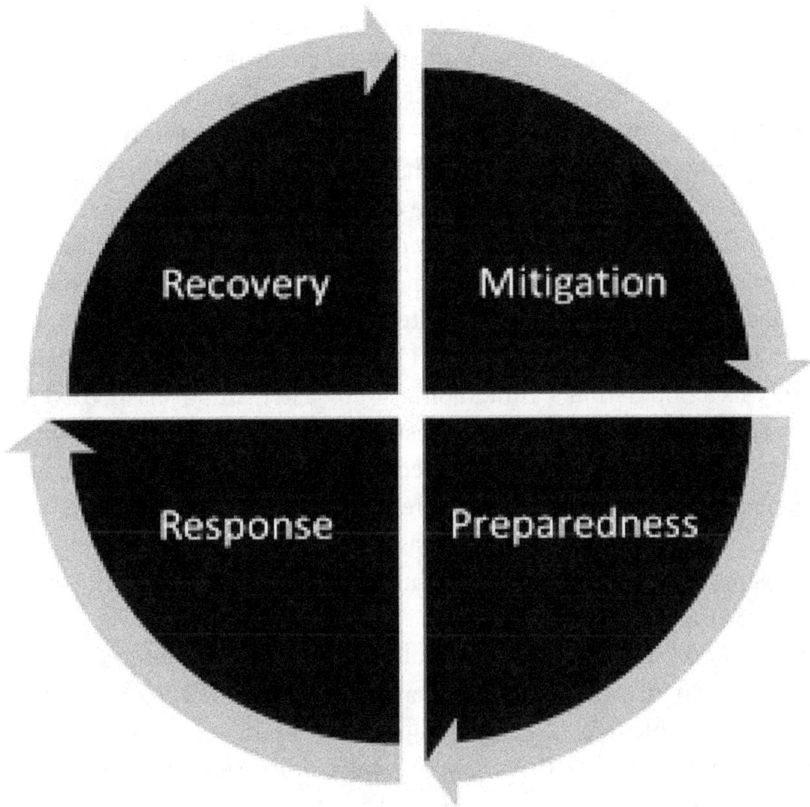

- **Mitigation (or prevention):** focuses on the prevention and analysis of risk and reducing the likelihood of disasters happening or them impacting the community.
- **Preparedness:** focuses on efforts such as helping communities get ready by creating, testing, and rehearsing disaster policies and procedures. This phase will often include training volunteers to mobilize effectively during a disaster response. For disasters that provide early warning (e.g., hurricanes and tsunamis) this is a critical period.
- **Response:** this phase includes the disaster itself and the immediate response to save lives and prevent further damage. The previously created disaster action plans get put into motion and often media coverage and resources are at their height.
- **Recovery:** the focus of this phase is to return the community to its pre-disaster state or better. Rebuilding and creating sustainable economic activity are important work during this phase. This phase sometimes takes several years or decades.

Communities are always in a phase of the disaster management cycle and importantly, some communities that are more disaster prone can find themselves in multiple phases at one time and in certain phases for a longer period than others.

VULNERABILITY TO DISASTERS

Global trends such as population increases, deforestation, unplanned urbanization, and over-farming/degradation of soil are all factors that have made the natural environment more susceptible to the impact of natural hazards (Olsson & Barbosa, 2019). Wisner, Blaikie, Cannon, and Davis (2004) assert that "disaster occurs where hazards meet vulnerability." Vulnerability is not only determined by the natural environment but by a population's social environment as well. A social stratum that puts a group of people at an economic disadvantage will often force them to inhabit natural environments that are more susceptible to natural hazards. For example, a poorer population is more likely to settle in a flood plain or on the slope of a volcano, land that is deemed undesirable by more privileged populations. In addition, overcrowding and overuse of the land ultimately erodes the soil, making inhabitants even more susceptible to flooding, avalanches, mudslides, etc. (Wisner et al., 2004). Political and economic factors also contribute largely to a population's vulnerability to disaster. Impoverished communities are more likely to use subpar and shoddy materials for construction of homes and construct public buildings with little or no safety standards. They have less access to the resources and information that can and would mitigate the impact of a disaster, and they are less likely to have the social protection that more privileged communities would have in the event of substantial loss. It is alarmingly evident that not only are poorer populations more vulnerable to natural hazards, but they are innately and consequently less equipped to withstand them.

Children have been found to be incredibly resilient in the path of disasters and trauma. In fact, children are believed to be more resilient than adults (Masten & Narayan, 2012; Norris et al., 2002). However, children are also more vulnerable to chaos and disruptions from disasters and more likely to be severely impaired than adults (Bonanno et al., 2010; *National Commission on Children and Disasters. 2010 Report to the President and Congress*, 2010; Quinn et al., 2016). It is important to understand the differences between vulnerability and resilience. Vulnerability is the capability of being physically or emotionally wounded. Resiliency is the capability to recover from or adjust easily to misfortune or change. Children are vulnerable in the sense that they are very much dependent on others for basic needs (safety, food, connection, etc.). However, children are resilient in the sense that they are still rapidly developing, forming neural connections, and making sense of their world. This means their brain demonstrates more plasticity, flexibility, and ability to recover. Their systems adapt and repair easier than adults. If their basic needs are provided for and there is a break in stress a child can learn adaptive coping skills and rise out of stressful situations positively.

Despite children's resiliency, children are vulnerable to disasters. Identifying those vulnerabilities is crucial to limit their lasting effect and encourage resiliency. With an increase in frequency of disasters over the last several decades, it is important to assess the effect of disasters on the mental and behavioral health of children and families (Halpern & Vermeulen, 2017). By identifying the impact these disasters have, child life specialists working in disaster relief and mental health can most efficiently and effectively respond to children's needs. The goal is to limit the damage from these disasters through effective interventions that are delivered to the most vulnerable children, ultimately supporting their resiliency.

IMPACT OF DISASTERS ON CHILDREN AND FAMILIES

Normative Reactions

All children impacted by a disaster will have some typical reactions to the event. It is when these reactions are prolonged or cause disruption in everyday living that they become more worrisome. Normative reactions are closely tied to overall development and should be viewed as normal and healthy. Common normative reactions of children include hyperactivity, increases in crying, clinginess, attention seeking behaviors, trouble sleeping or eating, short-term developmental regression (e.g., talking, crawling, potty-training), and changes in behaviors such as withdrawal or increased aggression. The role of the child life specialist is to recognize normative reactions as typical developmental reactions and keep them from becoming long term effects on development or more serious psychological concerns (e.g., depression, anxiety, post-traumatic stress disorder).

There is a heavy focus on the psychological impact disasters have on individuals. Most often studied are the internalizing reactions and psychological outcomes of post-traumatic stress disorder (PTSD) and symptoms (PTS), depression, and anxiety (Pfefferbaum et al., 2014). While the most often cited externalizing reactions include grief, suicide ideations, substance abuse, behavior problems, and cognitive effects. Taking a closer look at these internalized and externalized reactions to disasters will assist child life specialists in understanding the mental health effects of disasters on children and families.

Post-traumatic Stress Disorder or Symptoms, Depression, and Anxiety

Disasters cause a myriad of psychological responses from survivors. Post-traumatic stress disorder, depression, and anxiety are the most researched outcomes measured in children. Post-traumatic stress disorder is generally estimated to occur in less than 30% of the affected population of children, noting elevated symptoms in the more acute phases of disaster relief (hours to months post-disaster) that continue to decline over the first year (Bonanno et al., 2010; Chen & Wu, 2006; La Greca et al., 1996). Moderate post-traumatic symptoms are estimated to occur in about 50% of youth during the acute phase post-disaster (La Greca & Silverman, 2009). Blaze & Shwalb (2009) identified the top three predictors of PTS following Hurricane Katrina in children were storm exposure, relocation time, and loss of resources. For many children, their homes and communities are places of stability and provide a safe, stable environment that enables growth and development. When families are relocated post-disaster a once familiar, safe, and stable environment is disrupted and often lost. In a study looking at Hurricane Floyd survivors, children's homes that were flooded were three times more likely to have post traumatic symptoms than those whose homes were untouched (Russoniello et al., 2002).

Reviews of depression rates among children post-disaster are varied, ranging from 7.5-44.8% (Pfefferbaum, Jacobs, Houston, et al., 2015). Depression and anxiety are even more prevalent in disasters that have a significant death-loss rate and in individuals with pre-existing depression and anxiety symptoms (Bonanno et al., 2010).

Grief

Grief is the universal response to the loss of someone or something to which an attachment has been formed. Disaster inevitably brings great amounts of loss (both death and non-death) and grief to its survivors. Most individuals will experience typical grief reactions (e.g., intense sadness, dysphoria, intrusive preoccupation with loved one, transient cognitive disorganizations, health problems, impaired role functioning) that gradually diminish in intensity over time, creating a new normal. However, 10-15% of individuals will experience more severe, enduring grief responses such as "traumatic grief" or "complicated grief" (Bonanno et al., 2007). Traumatic grief is the intrusion of trauma symptoms into the bereavement process (Cohen et al., 2006). Complicated grief is the persistence of acute grief or the development of complications in the context of the grief process (Dyregrov et al., 2015). These are sometimes also referred to as "prolonged grief" or "Prolonged Grief Disorder (PGD)." Halpern and Vermeulen (2017) discuss several factors related to disasters that complicate the grief survivors experience:

- Traumatic memories of the disaster (or death) and/or physical injuries themselves
- Multiple deaths and/or losses at once
- Recognizing that others may be dealing with more extensive losses, causing them to downplay their need to mourn
- Unresolved issues with the deceased and/or urgent decision making that must happen due to the sudden and unexpected nature of disasters
- If a disaster is human made, dealing with anger, blame, and a desire for justice
- If the survivor received and ignored a warning that could have been life-saving, that survivor may experience self-blame, guilt and shame; if the deceased ignored a warning, the survivor may experience anger towards the victim that then becomes guilt ridden
- Media attention may force survivors to constantly face reminders of their loss and/or force them publicly mourn
- Post-disaster conditions (e.g., inability to recover remains, damage to place of worship) may interfere with funeral and mourning rituals

Understanding the complicated grief of disaster survivors is important to further assess suicide ideations and substance abuse that may arise.

Suicide Ideation & Substance Abuse

Suicide ideations and substance abuse are most prominent in those that had pre-existing ideations or abused substances prior to the disaster impact (Bonanno et al., 2010). Interestingly, there is speculation that there may be increased substance use among adolescent survivors of disasters, likely associated with disaster exposure (Chemtob et al., 2010; Chen & Wu, 2006; Hoven et al., 2005).

Cognitive Effects

Cognitive deficits have often been linked to traumatic life events, such as disasters. Without proper interventions, these deficits can lead to long-lasting issues and affect many developmental outcomes. Amid experiencing a traumatic event (e.g., a disaster) the brain becomes aroused, and it becomes difficult to process information. It is when this arousal state does not return to baseline that cognitive impairments pose further threats to development. The sense of safety must be reestablished and affirmed to relieve the brain of this arousal state. Scrimin et al. (2009) found that children who had been exposed to the Beslan school hostage crisis had significant difficulties in attention, memory, and visual-spatial performance.

Research demonstrates the cognitive effects of disasters and trauma lead to a decline in school functioning and increases in alcohol use, routine disruptions, attention, and memory deficits (Pfefferbaum, Jacobs, Houston, et al., 2015).

Despite the devastation disasters bring, many of those enduring a disaster will not suffer serious psychological harm. In fact, disasters produce multiple patterns of outcomes, including post-traumatic growth. Surprisingly to some, psychological distress and post-traumatic growth can co-exist. The right amounts of stress (not overwhelming or debilitating) can spur healthy growth and development.

Post-Traumatic Growth

Disasters often encourage growth as people are pushed to adapt and learn new things about themselves and their world. Post-traumatic growth (PTG) is positive change that is experienced as a result of major loss or trauma (Cryder et al., 2006). Pfefferbaum et al. (2015) identify three types of PTG including: psychological (e.g., changes in self and values), interpersonal (e.g., changes in relationships), and functional gains (e.g., strategies for coping) that arise after a disaster (Tedeschi & Calhoun, 1996). In a study evaluating PTG in children after a major hurricane in North Carolina, results indicated that beliefs about competency are related to post-traumatic growth. Further, a supportive social environment and ruminative thinking were associated with positive competency beliefs (Cryder et al., 2006). Disasters often activate survival mechanisms that rally one's coping abilities and push adjustment in the face of distress; it is this very process that allows post-traumatic growth and stress to co-exist (Pfefferbaum, Jacobs, Houston, et al., 2015).

FACTORS THAT INFLUENCE THE EFFECT OF DISASTERS ON CHILDREN & FAMILIES

Exposure

There is a dose-response relationship between disaster exposure and negative effects on individuals (Pfefferbaum, Jacobs, Griffin, et al., 2015). It is important to note that proximity to an event does not equate to exposure, but rather specific aspects of exposure that determine risk. Aspects of exposure that assist in creating adverse outcomes include perception of threat; subjective reactions of others; extent of disruption, destruction, injury and death; child-specific disaster experiences such as being injured, witnessing the disaster or its physical effects, and loss and/or death of loved ones (Furr et al., 2010). Disaster exposure is one of the most influential factors for children's post-disaster psychological outcomes (La Greca & Silverman, 2009).

Personal Factors

Development

Children's development inevitably influences the effect the disaster has on them. Their emerging cognition underpins children's abilities to understand and process traumatic events. It also influences the specific way in which children react and adapt to traumatic situations. In addition to cognitive changes rapidly developing throughout childhood, children's emotions, self-regulation, social connections, belief systems, and many other functions are also contributing to their coping, understanding, and reactions to disasters. Further, it is important to recognize that disasters can also influence the process of normative development. Typical developmental tasks become challenged in the face of insecurity, uncertainty, and unfamiliarity, when children's worlds are disrupted. Infants may experience the disaster through the attachment and emotional bonds of their caregiver. Toddlers, developing a sense of autonomy and control, may experience the disaster through separation anxiety and decreased routines. For preschoolers once potty-trained, this may mean a reintroduction to bed wetting behaviors. Preschoolers also exhibit egocentric cognition and socioemotional processes, along with magical thinking, leading them to assume guilt for events in which they could not have caused (e.g., the disaster itself, the loss of a pet or home). School-agers, just beginning to logically think, may exhibit issues with attention and focus leading to a decline in academic performance due to hypervigilance. They also increase in their ability to perspective take and therefore may also be dealing with the effects of the disaster on others. Adolescents typically gaining a better sense of identity and with the ability to think abstractly, may experience the disaster as a disruption in their identity (e.g. the way they defined themselves, their neighborhoods, their families) and increased concern for the long-term implications of the disaster (e.g., financial costs to their family and communities) (Pfefferbaum et al., 2014).

Likewise, there are critical periods in development when certain systems are more vulnerable to disruption and more adaptive in other ways. Children under three years old have increased neural connections and plasticity; nearly 90% of brain growth takes place during these early years (Szalavitz & Perry, 2010). When introduced to small doses of stress, this may cause positive growth and development. However, when overwhelming amounts of stress are presented (and often continue) the brain becomes exacerbated. The increases in synaptic pruning and strengthening of learned survival behaviors may actually become maladaptive (Masten & Narayan, 2012; Szalavitz & Perry, 2010).

Quinn et al., 2016, evaluated identified stressors in children and adolescents after superstorm Sandy hit New Jersey in 2012, killing 117 people (one of the deadliest in the U.S.). Preschoolers were found to exhibit an increased fear of storms and concern for others. Further, disaster themes in the preschoolers' play were seen up to one year after the event. Knowing that preschoolers heavily rely on routine and are heavily reliant on familiar, trusted caregivers, it makes sense that their stressors would include that of other loved ones. Stressors for school-age children included being fearful of weather reports, rain, and anticipatory flooding. Anxiety was a common effect on children who were school-age and can manifest itself in physiological ways such as headaches and stomachaches (Ball et al., 2014). Adolescents reported the most significant stressors and disruptions to their lives. Adolescents indicated increased feelings of depression, anhedonia (inability to experience pleasure from activities), and anxiety (Quinn et al., 2016).

Gender

Gender can also play a role in the presentation of the effects of disasters on children. In a study conducted with children and adolescents one year after a super-cyclone in India, girls reported more startle reactions, depressive symptoms, and feelings of guilt. Males reported more avoidance coping techniques (trying not to think about the event), disruptions in academic performance, and feelings of isolation, worry, anhedonia, and an overall lack of concentration (Kar & Bastia, 2006). Quinn et al. (2016) similarly found that girls overall reported being upset, afraid, or sad more often than boys who demonstrated more psychosomatic symptoms (aches and pains). Research has also drawn attention to the sex differences in interpretation of exposure among males and females and normative differences in internalization and externalization of behaviors for males and females (Masten & Narayan, 2012). This makes it difficult to isolate the role of gender when seeking to understand the effects of disasters on children, it is likely that a myriad of factors contribute to observed gender differences.

Pre-Event History

Children have a limited number of life experiences to contextualize disasters; they lack fully developed concepts of time and perspective. They are more likely to catastrophize an event and develop more intense feelings of helplessness. Their ability to understand a disaster as a one-time versus perpetual event influences their reactions. Therefore, it is important to evaluate the context and experiences children have related to disasters. If children are mentally and emotionally stable pre-event they are likely to be in a better place to activate adaptive coping skills. If children are already mentally and emotionally unstable, they will likely become overwhelmed more easily by a disastrous event.

Family Factors

Families are the central circle that provide context safety. Children's reactions are heavily influenced not only by a family's demographics, but also their caregiver's reactions to the disaster, the quality of their relationship to that caregiver, the interactions between the two that take place, and their caregiving style.

Demographics

Demographics such as income, caregiver education attainment, minority status, and occupation have been found to contribute to children's disaster reactions. In a grounded theory study utilizing head of household survivors with school-age children affected by Hurricane Katrina participants described a pile-up of negative life events (e.g., social isolation, limited opportunities, financial insecurity, witness to early death and/or violence, teen pregnancy), Katrina just being one of them. The described pattern of negative life events emerged as both a risk factor (accumulated stress reactions) and a resilience factor (disaster support brought resources that weren't accessible prior) (Hawkins, 2009). Literature does assert that lower socioeconomic status is associated with overall increases in unfavorable outcomes (Pfefferbaum, Jacobs, Houston, et al., 2015). It is also important to recognize that disaster-prone areas tend to house people with lower incomes, less sturdy housing, and less resources overall (Halpern & Vermeulen, 2017).

Caregiver Reactions, Interactions, and Style

Caregiver reactions to stressful events are strong predictors of child adjustment. Social cognitive theory and social referencing affirm this basic developmental nature for children to take cues from their trusted caretakers and respond based on learned behaviors (Santiesteban et al., 2012). Essentially caregivers serve as not only a strong genetic basis for children's coping, but also as the children's first role-models for coping. High caregiver stress is a strong predictor of children's post-disaster maladjustment (Houston et al., 2016; Pfefferbaum, Jacobs, Houston, et al., 2015). McDermott & Cobham (2012) surveyed 145 families of children ages 8-12 years evaluated association between family functioning in the post-disaster environment and child mental health symptoms. The disaster exposed group demonstrated double the family dysfunction and had more internalizing affects (e.g., anxiety and depression). Recognizing the coping resources caregivers have and supporting their coping is one of the most influential factors to decreasing the negative effects of disasters on children (Pfefferbaum, Jacobs, Houston, et al., 2015; Quinn et al., 2016). Positive caregiver-child relationships also have a positive effect on children's psychological outcomes. Children who have caregivers who generally seem unavailable to support their children experience great stress symptoms. Whereas, children whose caregivers participate in cognitive reframing, are supportive, and encourage and accept emotional expression tend to experience less distressing symptoms post-disaster (Costa et al., 2009). Finally, it is important not to overlook the influence of culture on caregiving styles; the same caregiving style can be both adaptive and maladaptive in various cultures (Pfefferbaum, Jacobs, Houston, et al., 2015).

Social Factors

Media Coverage and Effects

Disasters inevitably require media attention to distribute important information, help publicize resources, etc. However, the media has a critical responsibility in influencing the spread and effect on children's coping and recovery in the wake of disasters. Adults must be aware and monitor the exposure children receive of disasters through media outlets. For children already exposed to the disaster, additional media exposure often results in re-traumatization as young children are not able to differentiate a replay from real-time and thus may experience the same traumatic event each time they view it through media (Bhushan & Sathya Kumar, 2009). High levels of media coverage and exposure have been associated with increased adverse disaster effects on children (Pfefferbaum, Jacobs, Griffin, et al., 2015).

Social Support

Social support comes in many forms (e.g, parents, mentors, teachers, friends, communities) and has been associated with better adjustment and psychological outcomes post-disaster (Pfefferbaum, Jacobs, Houston, et al., 2015). Unfortunately, there is often an inverse relationship between available social support and disaster exposure (Banks & Weems, 2014). Therefore, support services must be aimed at increasing opportunities. When survivors become overwhelmed it is easy to lose hope when few social supports are available; it is imperative that disaster relief provides social support on the scene as quickly as possible. Likewise, it is also helpful in the healing process for survivors to assist others in their own community – helping survivors recognize their strengths can encourage them and provide hope (Halpern & Vermeulen, 2017).

Disaster Characteristics

Individual's reactions to disasters depend on a myriad of factors as discussed above, in addition specific characteristics of the disaster can also help assess the degree of impact on children. These characteristics that greatly impact effects on the individual and community include: the cause, size, expectedness, and timing of the disaster g (Halpern & Vermeulen, 2017).

Cause: Natural or Human-Made

A single disaster can both be human-made and natural. While the cause of a disaster is not always clear, research has identified that emotional reactions to disasters do differ based on cause. People tend to emotionally recover from natural disasters easier than human made disasters. Natural disasters often are unpreventable and therefore people experience less personal responsibility or blaming of others. Survivors of natural disasters' most prominent emotional reaction is helplessness due to a perceived lack of control over the situation (Halpern & Vermeulen, 2017). Human-made disasters tend to be perceived as preventable and therefore cause survivors feelings of anger, revenge, and guilt. This can also be exacerbated by the perception of intentionality (from a pure accident in operations like a train wreck to an intentional mass destruction like an active school shooting). Children are much more vulnerable to human-made disasters due to their inherent dependence on adults to provide a safe and nurturing environment. When an adult or even another child causes harm, this alters their worldview and sense of safety on a much deeper developmental level.

Size: Scope, Intensity, and Duration

Scope is the extent to which the disaster has caused harm across a community, this directly relates to when and how much help and resources are available. If a disaster is large in scope, it impacts the access to those immediate local resources that might have also been impacted (first responders, electric/water, and hospitals). It may also impact the availability and access to school settings which often provide a sense of normalcy, routine, and respite for families affected. Intensity often refers to the human costs of the disaster, the injuries and deaths. Disasters with high intensity leave survivors often dealing with a multitude of losses and grief at the same time. Finally, the duration to which the disaster affects a community affects individuals' reactions. Duration can be the tangible time the disaster was actively happening or the length of time the impacts of the disaster are felt (Halpern & Vermeulen, 2017). If duration is long, families experience exhaustion which inevitably causes challenges for their mental and physical availability to help and support their children well.

Expectedness: Warning or Sudden

The emotional and psychological reactions from survivors of disasters is also closely tied to whether the event was expected or not expected. Expected events cause less intense emotional reactions as they afford people the opportunity to take action to protect, decrease harm, or even sometimes avoid a disaster's impact (Halpern & Vermeulen, 2017). Simply put they offer some sense of control over an impending situation. Some disasters give significant warning (e.g., hurricanes), while others, minutes to hours (e.g., tornadoes). The warning gives people not only time to physically react, but also to psychologically prepare. It is important to note that what people do during this warning phase significantly impacts the emotional reaction afterwards. Those children who put on their helmets and shoes and sit in a basement during a tornado warning will likely be able to recognize how those actions provided some level of safety to them. Those that get stuck in denial and don't take action tend to feel guilt or shame. Unexpected disasters (e.g., earthquakes and shootings) tend to cause people to feel overwhelmed, helpless, and have increased vulnerability. Survivors tend to feel less guilt due to the nature of the event being unexpected, but are more susceptible to the feelings of insecurity and unpredictability they experienced both physically and psychologically.

Timing

When a disaster occurs (e.g., day/night, winter/summer) can have a significant impact on the emotional reactions of survivors. If a disaster occurs in the middle of the night when children are sleeping, they are much more likely to experience trouble physically getting to a safe place as recovery operations are difficult in the dark, separation from caregivers and disorientation are more intense (Halpern & Vermeulen, 2017). Children are also much more likely to suffer more significant issues sleeping since the disaster struck during this time of subconsciousness. If a disaster happens during the day, families may be separated due to school and jobs, whereas, at night families tend to be more proximal in terms of location to each other. Timing may also refer to season or weather-related conditions. Did a disaster occur in the middle of the winter, when freezing temperatures make it hard to survive without shelter, or did it occur in the middle of summer, where it's easier to survive outside, but water access is essential? Timing may also refer to events happening - did it happen during traffic hour and first responder and parents/ children connecting was delayed? Did this happen right before an adolescent's first prom? The timing of a disaster is personalized to each family and child and therefore the emotional reactions are as well.

Understanding the many factors that influence the effect a disaster will have on children and families is essential. Child life specialists and other professionals must assess each of these factors in order to best identify the needs, support, and services that will be most effective with children and families. Nearly everyone that experiences a disaster will demonstrate normative or non-normative stress response symptoms post-disaster, these must be supported to minimize the long-lasting and even more detrimental psychological effects.

INTERVENTIONS

Five Essential Needs of Children Affected by Disasters

Hobfoll et al. (2007) combined evidence-based and clinical expertise from around the world of the most effective treatment for those exposed to disasters. Through this process, consensus was reached on the five-empirically supported intervention principles that should guide and inform intervention efforts in the early (immediate hours) and mid-term (several months after) stages of disaster relief. These evidence-informed principles include promoting a sense of safety, promoting a sense of calm (through regulating the body's nervous system), promoting a sense of self-efficacy and community efficacy, promoting connection, and instilling hope. It is essential that child life specialists and other disaster relief professionals focus on meeting these needs of children in the aftermath of disasters.

Sense of Safety

It is the very nature of disasters that create a threat to individuals and a community's sense of safety. Things that once were indestructible, are now destroyed. In human-made disasters, trust that was assumed in human nature, has now been severed. Promoting a sense of safety becomes of utmost importance to those affected by the disaster. Children and caregivers are at increased risk due to the nature of child development and family life to rely on this sense of trust, protection, and safety (Pynoos et al., 2005). When individuals' safety is at threat (e.g., during disaster or crisis) the survival mechanism and neurobiological response is to fight, flight, freeze, or faint. It is this natural response that allows humans to survive, however, it is when the nervous system is unable to sense increased safety after a threat that the responses become troublesome (Hobfoll et al., 2007; B. Perry & Szalavitz, 2008). It is essential that both physical and psychological safety be resumed. Even when the disaster event itself has passed, many survivors' destroyed worldviews prevent them from reaching psychological safety which can later cause further psychological disorders. Psychological safety is much harder to restore, but necessary. Some tangible efforts to instill safety might include helping to find loved ones, encouraging routines, and providing clear, consistent communication that minimizes rumors from spreading. It is also important that re-exposure to the trauma is limited (media usage, excessive conversation, etc.), especially to children who are cognitively less capable of distinguishing a replay from reality (consecutive traumas). Limiting media and monitoring conversations around children can help to instill a sense of safety by decreasing the threat or experience of consecutive traumas through re-exposure.

Regulation

Although, Hobfoll et al. (2007) identified the need to promote a sense of calm, child life specialists typically use regulation as it is grounded in developmental theory. As the autonomic nervous system responds to the threat with increases in adaptive hormones, this response also encourages hypervigilance and adaptive increases in anxiety to anticipate further threat or danger to one's well-being. Further, heightened emotionality and distress symptoms are typical in the first weeks following a disaster (Hobfoll et al., 2007). It is important that this state of being does decline in the aftermath of the actual disaster or trauma. Promoting self-regulation to survivors is essential in eliminating continued states of heightened anxiety, which have been shown to increase likelihood of agitation, depression, and somatic problems (Shalev & Freedman, 2005). A few techniques to encourage a sense of connection in survivors includes: therapeutic grounding (gentle reminders of threat no longer being present), breathing training (deep breathing to avoid hyperventilation and to counter anxious emotionality), yoga (mindfulness practices and muscle relaxation exercises), guided imagery, psychoeducation (e.g., education on post-disaster management, coping, typical reactions) and structured training for problem-focused coping strategies (breaking the problems into manageable pieces, increasing a sense of control and productive progress). Finally, integrating interventions that involve activities that are typically positive in nature (e.g., play, music, exercise) can assist communities in regulating (Hobfoll et al., 2007).

Self- and Community Efficacy

By nature, disasters bring a sense of helplessness and loss of control. Things individuals once felt were secure and confident in their ability to keep secure, are now destroyed. Survivors must regain their sense of self-efficacy post-disaster. Self-efficacy is the belief that an individual's actions are likely to generate positive outcomes (Bandura, 1997). Likewise, the community also experiences this lack of control and helpfulness. Collective efficacy is the sense that one belongs to a group that is likely to experience positive outcomes. It is maybe even more important for individuals to learn their ability to cope with traumatic events that can be helpful, not just a general sense of self-efficacy (Benight & Harper, 2002;

Hobfoll et al., 2007). It is often once self and community efficacy is restored that both begin recovering through mitigation of future threats (e.g., building stronger buildings, preparing emergency kits, installing hurricane graded windows). One way child life specialists help children to restore efficacy is by allowing the child to be the expert and authority, promoting child led play and encouraging the child to direct the adult's play, and empowering children by providing appropriate choices. For some, it may also be helpful to engage children in strength-based approaches, seeking out how their strengths could be an asset to the community and helping the child to remember times pre-disaster when those strengths were helpful to others.

Connection

Social support and connectedness are extremely important in the aftermath of trauma, stress, and disasters. Not only can it provide a sense of tangible support for information related to recovery (e.g., shelter and resource availability), but it also provides a support system for others who are likely experiencing similar things. Extensive worldwide research indicates that social support is linked to better emotional well-being and recovery following mass-trauma (Altindag et al., 2005; Hobfoll et al., 2007; Norris et al., 2005). Fostering these healthy connections is important to enhance individual outcomes post-disaster. In disasters that require evacuation and relocation, known social support systems are likely inaccessible. Special focus must be placed to help survivors maintain and foster social support structures in their new environments. Among family members, individuals' level of exposure and coping strategies may differ, helping family structures to identify these differences and recognize strengths within the family is important to support family connectedness. Finally, it is essential to recognize that not all forms of social support increase feelings of connectedness (e.g., those that minimize individual's perceptions of problems, those that don't validate emotional reactions), and interventions aimed at promoting connectedness must do so skillfully to foster a sense of community, not rivalry (Hobfoll et al., 2007).

Hope

Individuals and communities enduring disasters often experience a "shattered worldview" and catastrophizing which both lead to a sense of hopelessness. Many times, survivors are faced with devastating financial losses that once provided a sense of safety and opportunity. Inevitably, hope is lost among this devastation. Interventions must focus on helping survivors' step by step through the processes of accessing resources and putting their lives back together. This is often accomplished through Multi-Agency Resource Centers (MARCS) or Family Assistance Centers (FACS) set-up by the American Red Cross and/or FEMA, depending on the disaster declaration. Child life specialists should support children and families in identifying hope. This can be done by helping children to recognize the people making a difference in their community and the progress that has been made. It is essential to continue to validate the child's own experience and current feelings, while also providing opportunities to instill hope.

Certified Child Life Specialists are educated, trained and competent professionals equipped to serve children and families affected by disasters (Association of Child Life Professionals, 2022). One evidence-informed intervention that supports these five essential needs that Certified Child Life Specialists should provide immediately is Psychological First Aid.

Psychological First Aid (PFA)

Psychological First Aid (PFA) is a set of practical early interventions and principles administered by clinicians and non-clinicians to address emotional distress following a stressful or traumatic event (e.g., disaster). The goal of PFA is to stabilize psychological and behavioral functioning, facilitate psychological and behavioral adaptation, and promote access to further care if needed. The major elements of psychological first aid include: establishing contact, addressing basic needs, protecting from further harm, listening and gathering information related to mental health needs and psychosocial concerns, providing reassurance and education, responding to distress and psychological symptoms, assisting with coping and problem solving, and connecting the individual with support systems and formal services if needed (North & Pfefferbaum, 2013). PFA is short term, focuses on symptom reduction, promotes healing (not exploring previous wounds), focuses on interrelated practical, physical, and emotional needs, and deals in the here and now (Halpern & Vermeulen, 2017). Much of the theoretical basis for PFA comes from Abraham Maslow's theory of human motivation (1943) or hierarchy of needs. Maslow (1943) described a series of hierarchical needs that must be met, in order: 1) physiological needs (e.g., food, water, shelter) 2) safety needs (e.g., helping survivors avoid subsequent danger and establish emotional and psychological safety) 3) belongingness and love (listening, encouraging survivors to reconnect with positive social supports), 4) esteem needs (prestige and feelings of accomplishment – not actually addressed with PFA), 5) self-actualization (achieving one's full potential - not actually addressed with PFA) (Halpern & Vermeulen, 2017; Thomas, 2005).

It is important to recognize that all children affected by disasters can benefit from child life services. In the disaster mental health field, a three-tier system is most often utilized to determine the most appropriate mental health interventions for survivors. In general, it includes psychosocial support to the broad population, specialized interventions for those with severe, persistent distress and impairment, and specialized treatment for high-risk children that need more attentive psychiatric care (Ursano, 2007). The first tier is aimed for those individuals with low to moderate levels of exposure (universal populations) to prevent the onset of psychological, behavioral, and functional problems. Tier 1 interventions (general) are psychosocial in nature and focus on strengthening coping skills, encouraging typical development, normalization, and positive adjustment. Child life specialists provide children in this tier with a safe space to engage in open-ended child directed play. They are present with children and encouraging social connections and validating feelings experienced. Tier two is aimed for those individuals with moderate to severe levels of exposure (selected populations) to decrease psychological distress, promote normal development, and adaptive post disaster adjustment. Tier two interventions are for those with elevated risk for negative psychological outcomes (e.g., PTSD, depression). Tier two interventions for child life specialists would look like engaging with a child one on one, promoting, rehearsing, and practicing coping skills, while also assessing the need for more specialized mental health services. Finally, tier three interventions (highly specialized) are aimed for those with severe and persistent distress (indicated populations) beyond typical reactions post-disaster. Individuals needing these interventions likely meet criteria for one or more psychological disorders and would need to be referred to treatment from a licensed mental health professional.

Given the effect disasters have on children and families and the evidence for interventions available it is reasonable to explore the specific role a Certified Child Life Specialist serves in the delivery of effective psychosocial services during each emotional phase of a disaster.

EMOTIONAL PHASES OF A DISASTER & CHILD LIFE INTERVENTIONS

Evaluating the emotional phases of a disaster will help in describing the child life services that would be most effective in each phase. There are four main phases of a community's emotional response to a disaster, these include the heroic, honeymoon, disillusionment, and reconstruction phases (DeWolfe, 2000). Figure 2 depicts the emotional phases of a disaster.

Figure 2. The Emotional Phases of a Disaster

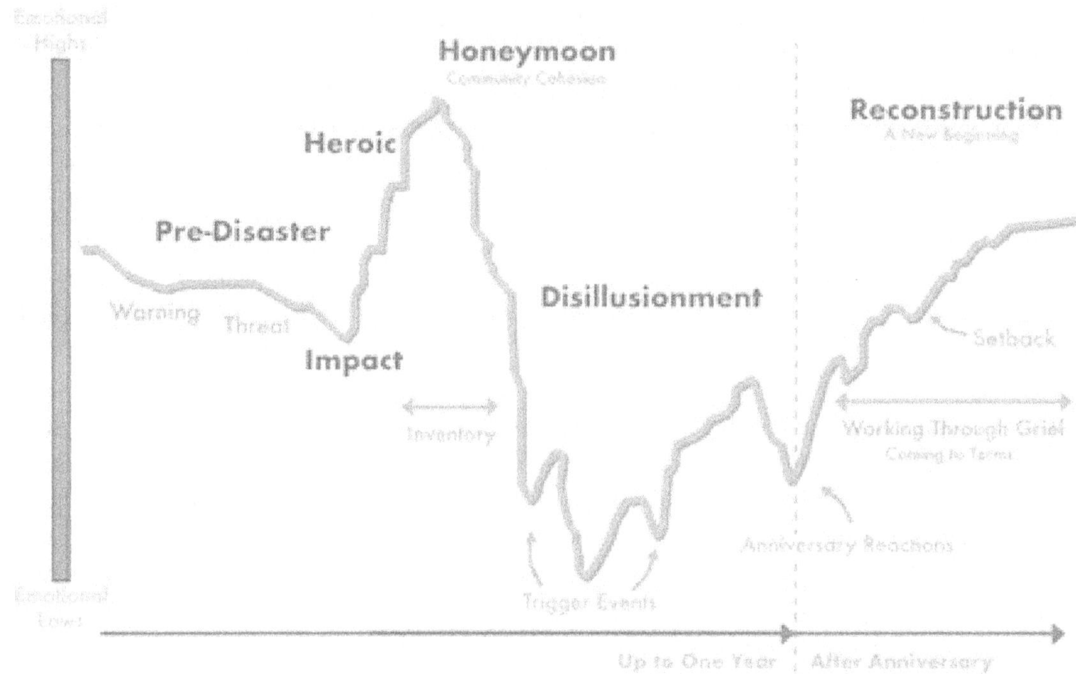

Heroic Phase

The heroic phase (approximately the first 72 hours) is in the immediate aftermath of a disaster's impact. Individuals often feel shocked but are energized and helping others in the community initiating rescue efforts and providing emotional support. It is also during this phase that physical first aid and medical care may be necessary. Healthcare encounters, procedures, and injuries can be traumatic for children any day, in the aftermath of a disaster it is likely that coping responses and resources may be overwhelmed (e.g., caregivers unavailable, routine disrupted, safety and security threats). Immunizations, sutures, splinting, and non-invasive physical exams are likely to be extremely difficult for children in this chaotic and unfamiliar setting.

It is during this phase that child life specialists most acutely would function much like they do in the hospital setting within emergency departments providing developmentally appropriate education and procedural support, coping skills support, and family support (Krebel et al., 1996). Children could greatly benefit from child life services interventions and support while undergoing medical care in the makeshift alternative settings and hospitals after a disaster. For example, following Hurricane Dorian, CCLSs deployed to the Bahamas with Child Life Disaster Relief. Medical clinics had been established to provide physical exams and immunizations for children displaced from their homes. CCLSs worked alongside doctors and nurses to provide preparation and coping support for children and families during these medical encounters.

In addition to medical care support, child life specialists in this phase would also be able to provide psychological first aid and potentially minimize further exposure to the disaster itself. Strategies for providing psychological first aid have been outlined earlier and the desire for trained professionals to complete this work has also been recognized (*National Commission on Children and Disasters. 2010 Report to the President and Congress*, 2010). Establishing rapport, being present, and providing initial emotional support within times of heightened emotional distress has been shown to increase children's responses to later support (Vernberg & Vogel, 1993). Child life specialists support this need as they provide psychological first aid to children and families undergoing stressful events daily in the healthcare setting and are therefore well versed in carrying these steps out in community settings. Efforts to eliminate further exposure to the disaster would mirror efforts child life specialists make to minimize trauma in the healthcare setting (e.g., limiting visual and sensory exposure to grotesque images of the disaster and rescue efforts).

Honeymoon Phase

The honeymoon phase (approximately a week-month post-disaster impact) is when many outside resources begin pouring in. There is typically an overall sense of optimism and security as help and supplies are abundant (DeWolfe, 2000; Halpern & Vermeulen, 2017).

Child life specialists in this phase provide developmentally appropriate, safe, therapeutic spaces for children to engage in child-directed play. Their vast knowledge of play as a healing modality would benefit the services currently being offered in spaces such as a MARC (Multi-Agency Resource Center), FAC (Family Assistance Centers), and/or shelters. Children in this phase benefit from some sense of normalcy and routine. When children are living in shelters, providing therapeutically minded play spaces can assist in this process. Children may follow a routine such as this: wake, dress, breakfast with family, play space, lunch with family, play space, dinner with family, bedtime. Children in this phase also benefit from open-ended child-directed play opportunities to begin processing their experiences in a supported environment. Child life specialists are trained to be present with children in this way and support children by providing appropriate materials and creative outlets for this process to take place. Appropriate materials might include cars and emergency response vehicles, boats, art supplies, unspecified dolls and people (e.g., no Elmo's or Dora's that already have personalities and their own stories), blocks, boxes, puzzles, etc. Child life specialists recognize the importance of the children's process in play and aim to be a supportive presence engaged with children in this process (not directing or leading). For example, CCLSs working with children after Hurricane Dorian assessed the fear that was expressed by children and families living in a shelter when the wind would blow. CCLSs invited children and families outside to play with bubbles on a windy day. As children held bubble wands up in the air, the wind would lift bubbles into the air. Children and families began to laugh as they ran and caught the bubbles, rebuilding associations with wind in their brains. Similarly, CCLSs assessed the connection children had to the natural elements of sand and water after living on an island. As the shelter was not near the beach, CCLSs brought buckets of sand and water to the shelter for play. Some children engaged in sensory play with the sand and water, while others played out their hurricane experience by burying cars and houses in the sand and then washing them clean with water.

Normative developmental tasks and the needs of children under stress (e.g., safety, control, mastery, socialization, validation) guide the philosophy of these play centers. Yule (2006) did specialized work with children following the 2005 tsunamis and provided insight into the fact that non-governmental organizations providing opportunities for play need training to address fears, intrusive memories, and poor concentration with children. These volunteers are likely to lack competence in assessing a child to delineate progressive, therapeutic play that is a useful part of recovery from a disaster versus signs of deeper, more serious issues that need more directed psychological follow-up by licensed psychological professionals.

Finally, child life specialists provide much needed psychosocial support, psychological first aid, and psychoeducation to children and families during this phase as well. Child life specialists are specifically trained to provide developmentally appropriate psychosocial care to help children and families effectively cope with traumatic situations and should be used during this phase of disaster relief. Often caregivers have questions regarding how to talk to the children about the disaster, deaths, or other losses experienced. Child life specialists are specifically trained and equipped to engage in these educational and supportive conversations with caregivers to promote coping within the entire family.

Disillusionment Phase

The disillusionment phase (approximately a month to two-years post-disaster) is experienced when relief agencies and outside support start to withdraw. Individuals in the community feel exhaustion and sometimes resentment for the perception that relief agencies did not fulfill their promises (DeWolfe, 2000; Halpern & Vermeulen, 2017).

During this phase, child life specialists can support children and families through continued supportive presence and psychosocial interventions in more formalized settings (e.g., grief support centers, inpatient hospitalizations, schools, camps). It is also imperative in this stage that formal referrals to mental health professionals would be necessary, child life specialists having spent time with the children in the immediate phases post-disaster would be in an optimal position to assess potential longer-term risks and make referrals to appropriate professionals in the community. In inpatient hospital settings, children more severely injured might be undergoing surgeries to reconstruct physical damage endured during the disaster. Further, those with permanent physical changes and losses would benefit from a child life specialist helping them to adapt to this new way of life. These therapeutic interventions are commonly used by child life specialists who work with children undergoing new diagnosis and trauma (e.g., PICU, hematology/oncology, rehabilitation units). Finally, psychoeducation of caregivers would also be an important role of the child life specialist during this phase. Caregivers often find themselves more emotionally and physically available during this stage and may have increased questions about behavioral responses and ways to help their children. Child life specialists are well versed in communicating supportively and effectively with caregivers regarding their children's needs.

Reconstruction Phase

Finally, the reconstruction phase is when survivors and the community resume responsibility of reestablishing functionality. Individuals have increased enthusiasm as members of the community create a new normal and bring hope to their futures (DeWolfe, 2000; Halpern & Vermeulen, 2017).

Efforts of mitigation and preparation take place during this phase and children benefit from engaging in this process (UNICEF, 2007). Child life specialists assist children in preparations for disasters using their developmentally appropriate knowledge and experience working with children. One such program that is a good model and avenue for child life specialists to support this phase is the "Pillowcase Project" (American Red Cross, 2022). The pillowcase project, funded by The Walt Disney Company and administered through the American Red Cross, teaches children coping skills to use during emergencies and offers tips and tools to help them prepare for future emergencies. Another aspect of this phase is anniversaries and other triggering events. Child life specialists can work with communities, families, and children to prepare for, memorialize, and plan appropriate and supportive events and activities to commemorate and be sensitive to children and adults' experiences.

EXPANDING THE ROLE OF CHILD LIFE IN DISASTER SETTINGS

Child life specialists have been working in disaster relief settings for years through organizations such as Child Life Disaster Relief. They have supported children experiencing natural disasters (e.g., the hurricanes off the Gulf of Mexico and in the Bahamas, wildfires in California, and tornadoes in Missouri), as well as human made disasters (e.g., the 2017 Las Vegas Harvest Music Festival shooting and the 2016 Pulse Nightclub shooting in FL) (Child Life Disaster Relief, 2022). However, there is ample opportunity to continue to grow child life services in this setting.

Child Life Disaster Relief (CLDR) is a nonprofit with a vision to develop a coordinated and global network to ensure that children in disasters and crises have the tools and support needed to promote positive coping and resilience. Child Life Disaster Relief's mission is to empower and support children and families in crises by integrating child life professionals' services into impacted communities through individualized direct services, community outreach, education, and research (Child Life Disaster Relief, 2022). Child Life Disaster Relief continues to participate and integrate as members of disaster management planning and response teams in their communities. Child life volunteers are active advocates, leaders, and members within their communities and regions related to policy and procedures when it comes to planning for and supporting children and families during disasters.

Child life specialists should continue to build partnerships with local emergency response teams for quick, immediate disaster response support to children and families. They should integrate and advocate for their roles on community crisis response teams and continue to build relationships with emergency responders and organizations day in and day out. Through the establishment of these relationships with key groups, child life specialists will be best positioned, trusted, and relied upon to respond to disasters in their communities.

Finally, child life specialists should continue to seek funded positions within the disaster relief field. Through the consistent support and presence of a child life specialist, children and families will best receive the benefits of child life services, leading to increased resilience and coping in the face of disasters.

REFERENCES

Active Shooter Incidents 20-Year Review, 2000-2019. (2021). [File]. U.S. Department of Justice Federal Bureau of Investigation. https://www.fbi.gov/file-repository/active-shooter-incidents-20-year-review-2000-2019-060121.pdf/view

Altindag, A., Ozen, S., & Sir, A. (2005). One-year follow-up study of post-traumatic stress disorder among earthquake survivors in Turkey. *Comprehensive Psychiatry*, *46*(5), 328–333. doi:10.1016/j.comppsych.2005.01.005 PMID:16122532

American Red Cross. (2022). *The Pillowcase Project*. https://www.redcross.org/get-help/how-to-prepare-for-emergencies/teaching-kids-about-emergency-preparedness/pillowcase-project.html

AON. (2021). *2021 Weather, Climate, and Catastrophe Insight*. AON. https://www.aon.com/getmedia/1b516e4d-c5fa-4086-9393-5e6afb0eeded/20220125-2021-weather-climate-catastrophe-insight.pdf.aspx

Association of Child Life Professionals. (2022). *ACLP Official Documents*. https://www.childlife.org/the-child-life-profession/official-documents

Ball, J., Bindler, R., & Cowen, K. (2014). *Child Health Nursing: Partnering with Children and Families*. Pearson.

Bandura, A. (1997). *Self-efficacy: The exercise of control*. Academic Press.

Banks, D. M., & Weems, C. F. (2014). Family and peer social support and their links to psychological distress among hurricane-exposed minority youth. *The American Journal of Orthopsychiatry*, *84*(4), 341 352. doi:10.1037/ort0000006 PMID:24999520

Becker-Blease, K. A., Turner, H. A., & Finkelhor, D. (2010). Disasters, victimization, and children's mental health. *Child Development*, *81*(4), 1040–1052. doi:10.1111/j.1467-8624.2010.01453.x PMID:20636681

Benight, C. C., & Harper, M. L. (2002). Coping self-efficacy perceptions as a mediator between acute stress response and long-term distress following natural disasters. *Journal of Traumatic Stress*, *15*(3), 177–186. doi:10.1023/A:1015295025950 PMID:12092909

Bhushan, B., & Sathya Kumar, J. (2009). Emotional Distress and Post-traumatic Stress in Children: The Impact of Direct Versus Indirect Exposure. *Journal of Loss and Trauma*, *14*(1), 35–45. doi:10.1080/15325020802537047

Blaze, J. T., & Shwalb, D. W. (2009). Resource loss and relocation: A follow-up study of adolescents two years after Hurricane Katrina. *Psychological Trauma: Theory, Research, Practice, and Policy*, *1*(4), 312–322. doi:10.1037/a0017834

Bonanno, G. A., Brewin, C. R., Kaniasty, K., & Greca, A. M. L. (2010). Weighing the Costs of Disaster: Consequences, Risks, and Resilience in Individuals, Families, and Communities. *Psychological Science in the Public Interest*, *11*(1), 1–49. doi:10.1177/1529100610387086 PMID:26168411

Bonanno, G. A., Neria, Y., Mancini, A., Coifman, K. G., Litz, B., & Insel, B. (2007). Is there more to complicated grief than depression and post-traumatic stress disorder? A test of incremental validity. *Journal of Abnormal Psychology, 116*(2), 342–351. doi:10.1037/0021-843X.116.2.342 PMID:17516766

Chemtob, C. M., Nomura, Y., Rajendran, K., Yehuda, R., Schwartz, D., & Abramovitz, R. (2010). Impact of maternal post-traumatic stress disorder and depression following exposure to the September 11 attacks on preschool children's behavior. *Child Development, 81*(4), 1129–1141. doi:10.1111/j.1467-8624.2010.01458.x PMID:20636686

Chen, S.-H., & Wu, Y.-C. (2006). Changes of PTSD Symptoms and School Reconstruction: A Two-year Prospective Study of Children and Adolescents after the Taiwan 921 Earthquake. *Natural Hazards, 37*(1–2), 225–244. doi:10.100711069-005-4671-y

Child Life Disaster Relief. (2022). *About us.* Child Life Disaster Relief. https://cldisasterrelief.org/about-us/

Cohen, J. A., Mannarino, A. P., & Deblinger, E. (2006). *Treating trauma and traumatic grief in children and adolescents.* The Guilford Press.

Costa, N. M., Weems, C. F., & Pina, A. A. (2009). Hurricane Katrina and youth anxiety: The role of perceived attachment beliefs and parenting behaviors. *Journal of Anxiety Disorders, 23*(7), 935–941. doi:10.1016/j.janxdis.2009.06.002 PMID:19577899

Cryder, C. H., Kilmer, R. P., Tedeschi, R. G., & Calhoun, L. G. (2006). An exploratory study of post-traumatic growth in children following a natural disaster. *The American Journal of Orthopsychiatry, 76*(1), 65–69. doi:10.1037/0002-9432.76.1.65 PMID:16569128

DeWolfe, D. (2000). *Training manual for mental health and human services workers in major disasters* (2nd ed.). U.S. Department of Health and Human Services.

Dyregrov, A., Salloum, A., Kristensen, P., & Dyregrov, K. (2015). Grief and Traumatic Grief in Children in the Context of Mass Trauma. *Current Psychiatry Reports, 17*(6), 48. Advance online publication. doi:10.100711920-015-0577-x PMID:25940038

Emergency Management in the United States. (n.d.). Federal Emergency Management Agency. Retrieved March 10, 2022, from https://training.fema.gov/emiweb/downloads/is111_unit%204.pdf

Furr, J. M., Comer, J. S., Edmunds, J. M., & Kendall, P. C. (2010). Disasters and youth: A meta-analytic examination of post-traumatic stress. *Journal of Consulting and Clinical Psychology, 78*(6), 765–780. doi:10.1037/a0021482 PMID:21114340

Halpern, J., & Vermeulen, K. (2017). *Disaster mental health intervention: Core principles and practices.* Routledge. doi:10.4324/9781315623825

Hawkins, R. (2009). Same as It Ever Was, Only Worse: Negative Life Events and Poverty Among New Orleans Katrina Survivors. *Families in Society, 90*(4), 375–381. doi:10.1606/1044-3894.3922

Hobfoll, S. E., Watson, P., Bell, C. C., Bryant, R. A., Brymer, M. J., Friedman, M. J., Friedman, M., Gersons, B. P., De Jong, J. T., Layne, C. M., Maguen, S., Neria, Y., Norwood, A. E., Pynoos, R. S., Reissman, D., Ruzek, J. I., Shalev, A. Y., Solomon, Z., Steinberg, A. M., & Ursano, R. J. (2007). Five essential elements of immediate and mid–term mass trauma intervention: Empirical evidence. *Psychiatry*, *70*(4), 283–315. doi:10.1521/psyc.2007.70.4.283 PMID:18181708

Houston, J. B., First, J., Spialek, M. L., Sorenson, M. E., & Koch, M. (2016). Public Disaster Communication and Child and Family Disaster Mental Health: A Review of Theoretical Frameworks and Empirical Evidence. *Current Psychiatry Reports*, *18*(6), 54. Advance online publication. doi:10.100711920-016-0690-5 PMID:27086315

Hoven, C. W., Duarte, C. S., Lucas, C. P., Wu, P., Mandell, D. J., Goodwin, R. D., Cohen, M., Balaban, V., Woodruff, B. A., Bin, F., Musa, G. J., Mei, L., Cantor, P. A., Aber, J. L., Cohen, P., & Susser, E. (2005). Psychopathology among New York City public school children 6 months after September 11. *Archives of General Psychiatry*, *62*(5), 545–551. doi:10.1001/archpsyc.62.5.545 PMID:15867108

Kar, N., & Bastia, B. K. (2006). Post-traumatic stress disorder, depression and generalised anxiety disorder in adolescents after a natural disaster: A study of comorbidity. *Clinical Practice and Epidemiology in Mental Health*, *2*(1), 17. doi:10.1186/1745-0179-2-17 PMID:16869979

Krebel, M., Clayton, C., & Graham, C. (1996). Child life programs in the pediatric emergency department. *Pediatric Emergency Care*, *12*(1), 13–15. doi:10.1097/00006565-199602000-00004 PMID:8677171

La Greca, A. M., & Silverman, W. K. (2009). Treatment and Prevention of Post-traumatic Stress Reactions in Children and Adolescents Exposed to Disasters and Terrorism: What Is the Evidence? *Child Development Perspectives*, *3*(1), 4–10. doi:10.1111/j.1750-8606.2008.00069.x

La Greca, A. M., Silverman, W. K., Vernberg, E. M., & Prinstein, M. J. (1996). Symptoms of post-traumatic stress in children after Hurricane Andrew: A prospective study. *Journal of Consulting and Clinical Psychology*, *64*(4), 712–723. doi:10.1037/0022-006X.64.4.712 PMID:8803361

Maslow, A. H. (1943). A theory of human motivation. *Psychological Review*, *50*(4), 370–396. doi:10.1037/h0054346

Masten, A. S., & Narayan, A. J. (2012). Child Development in the Context of Disaster, War, and Terrorism: Pathways of Risk and Resilience. *Annual Review of Psychology*, *63*(1), 227–257. doi:10.1146/annurev-psych-120710-100356 PMID:21943168

McDermott, B. M., & Cobham, V. E. (2012). Family functioning in the aftermath of a natural disaster. *BMC Psychiatry*, *12*(1), 55. doi:10.1186/1471-244X-12-55 PMID:22647086

National Commission on Children and Disasters. (2010). *2010 Report to the President and Congress*. Author.

Norris, F. H., Baker, C. K., Murphy, A. D., & Kaniasty, K. (2005). Social Support Mobilization and Deterioration after Mexico's 1999 Flood: Effects of Context, Gender, and Time. *American Journal of Community Psychology*, *36*(1–2), 15–28. doi:10.100710464-005-6230-9 PMID:16134042

Norris, F. H., Friedman, M. J., Watson, P. J., Byrne, C. M., Diaz, E., & Kaniasty, K. (2002). 60,000 disaster victims speak: Part I. An empirical review of the empirical literature, 1981–2001. *Psychiatry*, *65*(3), 207–239. doi:10.1521/psyc.65.3.207.20173 PMID:12405079

North, C. S., & Pfefferbaum, B. (2013). Mental Health Response to Community Disasters: A Systematic Review. *Journal of the American Medical Association*, *310*(5), 507. doi:10.1001/jama.2013.107799 PMID:23925621

Olsson, L., & Barbosa, H. (2019). *Land Degradation—Special Report on Climate Change and Land* (No. 4). Intergovernmental Panel on Climate Change. https://www.ipcc.ch/srccl/chapter/chapter-4/

Perry, B., & Szalavitz, M. (2008). *The boy who was raised as a dog and other stories from a child psychiatrist's notebook: What traumatized children can teach us about loss, love, and healing*. Basic Books.

Perry, R. W. (2018). Defining Disaster: An Evolving Concept. In H. Rodríguez, W. Donner, & J. E. Trainor (Eds.), Handbook of Disaster Research (pp. 3–22). Springer International Publishing. doi:10.1007/978-3-319-63254-4_1

Pfefferbaum, B., Jacobs, A. K., Griffin, N., & Houston, J. B. (2015). Children's Disaster Reactions: The Influence of Exposure and Personal Characteristics. *Current Psychiatry Reports*, *17*(7), 56. Advance online publication. doi:10.100711920-015-0598-5 PMID:25980513

Pfefferbaum, B., Jacobs, A. K., Houston, J. B., & Griffin, N. (2015). Children's Disaster Reactions: The Influence of Family and Social Factors. *Current Psychiatry Reports*, *17*(7), 57. Advance online publication. doi:10.100711920-015-0597-6 PMID:25980512

Pfefferbaum, B., Noffsinger, M. A., Wind, L. H., & Allen, J. R. (2014). Children's Coping in the Context of Disasters and Terrorism. *Journal of Loss and Trauma*, *19*(1), 78–97. doi:10.1080/15325024.2013.791797 PMID:24683315

Pynoos, R., Schreiber, M., Steinberg, A., & Pfefferbaum, B. (2005). Impact of terrorism on children. In *Comprehensive textbook of psychiatry* (8th ed., pp. 3351–3564). Lippencott, Wiliams, and Wilkins.

Quinn, M., Gillooly, D., Kelly, S., Kolassa, J., Davis, E., & Jankowski, S. (2016). Evaluation of identified stressors in children and adolescents after Super Storm Sandy. *Pediatric Nursing*, *42*(5), 235. PMID:29406642

Russoniello, C., Skalko, T., O'Brien, K., McGee, S., Bingham-Alexander, D., & Beatley, J. (2002). Childhood Post-traumatic Stress Disorder and Efforts to Cope After Hurricane Floyd. *Behavioral Medicine (Washington, D.C.)*, *28*(2), 61–71. doi:10.1080/08964280209596399 PMID:12613287

Santiesteban, I., White, S., Cook, J., Gilbert, S. J., Heyes, C., & Bird, G. (2012). Training social cognition: From imitation to Theory of Mind. *Cognition*, *122*(2), 228–235. doi:10.1016/j.cognition.2011.11.004 PMID:22133627

Scrimin, S., Moscardino, U., Capello, F., & Axia, G. (2009). Attention and Memory in School-Age Children Surviving the Terrorist Attack in Beslan, Russia. *Journal of Clinical Child and Adolescent Psychology*, *38*(3), 402–414. doi:10.1080/15374410902851689 PMID:19437300

Shalev, A., & Freedman, S. (2005). PTSD following terrorist attacks: A prospective evaluation. *The American Journal of Psychiatry, 162*(6), 1188–1191. doi:10.1176/appi.ajp.162.6.1188 PMID:15930068

Szalavitz, M., & Perry, B. (2010). *Born for Love: Why empathy is essential and endangered.* Harper Collins.

Tedeschi, R. G., & Calhoun, L. G. (1996). The post-traumatic growth inventory: Measuring the positive legacy of trauma. *Journal of Traumatic Stress, 9*(3), 455–471. doi:10.1002/jts.2490090305 PMID:8827649

Thomas, R. (2005). *Comparing theories of child development*. Wadsworth.

UNICEF. (2007). *The participation of children and young people in emergencies: A guide for relief aBOSTONgencies, based largely on experiences in the Asian tsunami response*. UNICEF East Asia and Pacific Regional Office.

United States Census Bureau. (2022). *Census—Geography Profile*. Retrieved April 10, 2022, from https://data.census.gov/cedsci/profile?q=United%20States&g=0100000US

Ursano, R. J. (Ed.). (2007). *Textbook of disaster psychiatry*. Cambridge University Press. doi:10.1017/CBO9780511544415

Vernberg, E., & Vogel, J. (1993). Part 2: Interventions with children after disasters. *Journal of Clinical Child Psychology, 22*(4), 485–498. doi:10.120715374424jccp2204_8

Wisner, B., Blaikie, P., Cannon, T., & Davis, I. (2004). *At Risk: Natural hazards, people's vulnerability and disasters*. Routledge.

Yule, W. (2006). Theory, training and timing: Psychosocial interventions in complex emergencies. *International Review of Psychiatry (Abingdon, England), 18*(3), 259–264. doi:10.1080/09540260600656134 PMID:16753663

KEY TERMS AND DEFINITIONS

Disaster Management Cycle: The cyclical process aimed at reducing the impact of, responding to, and recovering from disasters. Goals include reduced loss, prompt assistance, and rapid and effective recovery.

Human-Made Disaster: A human-caused hazard, such as school shootings, terrorism, or human conflicts, that causes significant damage or loss of life and overwhelms a community's own capacity and resources to cope. Hazards can be a result of human intent, negligence, or a failure of a human-made system.

Natural Disaster: A natural hazard, such as a tornado, flood, or hurricane, that causes significant damage, loss of life, or economic hardship and overwhelms a community's own capacity and resources to cope.

Chapter 10
Therapeutic Photography

Megan Ribbens
Through Their Eyes, South Africa

ABSTRACT

As the child life profession extends beyond the hospital setting, new opportunities unfold to utilize the profession's strengths of empowering children and families through stressful life experiences. This chapter proposes that therapeutic photography is a fitting and effective tool to be used in any child life setting to promote well-being and describes Through Their Eyes, a child life practice centered on therapeutic photography in a non-traditional setting in South Africa. Differentiations are made between therapeutic photography and phototherapy and therapeutic photography is expounded. The underpinning framework of therapeutic photography with a child life scope of practice is outlined and the therapeutic photography program, Through Their Eyes, is explained. Outcomes give evidence of the ways therapeutic photography programs can connect us to ourselves and to each other, strengthening sense of self, relationships, and family function.

INTRODUCTION

Newly arrived to Abuja, Nigeria in 2007, it was clear, for numerous reasons, this was not the time to engage traditional Child Life work in a medical setting. And yet, the author wasn't at ease simply hanging up her Child Life that she had come to love while working in the specialty clinics at Helen DeVos Children's Hospital in Grand Rapids, Michigan.

Curiously engaging her new context, the author reflected on the essence of who Child Life Specialists (CLS) are and what they have to offer. Both within and beyond the hospital, CLS are champions for children and families. Through their understanding of child development, family-centered care, and expressive play, CLS offer ways to help children and families stay connected to themselves and each other through stressful, challenging life events, create opportunities for expression, and teach coping skills in order to mitigate the long-term effects of stress and trauma. Children, in and out of the hospital setting, need safe spaces to play, reflect, strengthen sense of self, develop emotional literacy, and learn coping skills in order to foster healthy development within challenging life experiences.

DOI: 10.4018/978-1-6684-5097-0.ch010

There was a lot of trial and error implementing different programs in community settings before the author found her niche. In 2011, a Nigerian woman literally knocked on the author's door. "I've had a dream for four years," she explained. "I know adults underestimate what children can contribute to our society. I want to give children a camera so we can literally see what they see. I want to call it 'Through Their Eyes'. The problem is - I'm not a teacher and I'm not a photographer, but my friend told me you could possibly help." Elated to see the Child Life profession fused with the author's favorite hobby of photography, a new journey began to unfold.

In this chapter, the author will define therapeutic photography, outline the underpinnings used for Through Their Eyes therapeutic photography programs, and describe how therapeutic photography aligns within the Child Life scope of practice. The author will explain the current setting in which the program is used, what a Through Their Eyes program entails, and outcomes of the program. Additionally, challenges and future aspirations for therapeutic photography within Child Life will be explored.

BACKGROUND

Therapeutic Photography vs. PhotoTherapy

While one aspect of a CLS's role is to develop and implement expressive, playful activities that are therapeutic in nature to promote healthy development and healing, it is important to distinguish that CLS do not do therapy. Similarly, therapeutic photography and therapy using photography are on opposite sides of a continuum and require important distinctions. PhotoTherapy, as defined by Judy Weiser, is a tool used by trained professionals in formal counseling settings that takes clients through "guided unconscious process work" (Gibson, 2018; Weiser, 2004, p. 35). PhotoTherapy in a counseling setting can include using photos taken by a client, photos taken of a client, self-portraits, family photographs, and "photo-projectives" which involve creating meaning out of taking or viewing photographs (Weiser, 2004). Therapeutic photography does not require a trained counselor or therapist, but it does require clearly defined outcomes for it to be considered therapeutic (Gibson, 2018; Weiser, 2004). These outcomes can promote change and growth at the individual, community, and broader social levels.

Essential Elements of Therapeutic Photography

It is essential to develop a therapeutic relationship with children and their families when working in traditional and non-traditional Child Life settings. Using therapeutic photography as a Child Life practice in a multi-cultural setting within schools, NGOs, and churches has required an emphasis on developing therapeutic relationships. Hallmarks of a therapeutic relationship include building trust and rapport, showing respect, establishing physical and emotional safety, and maintaining healthy boundaries (Association of Child Life Professionals, 2001; Association of Child Life Professionals, 2019). When a safe holding space is created, as described by Winnicott, participants feel safe to explore and express thoughts and feelings (Gibson, 2018).

Therapeutic relationships also require facilitators to align interventions with developmental considerations which honor development levels, emotional states, and cultural beliefs and preferences (Association of Child Life Professionals, 2001; Association of Child Life Professionals, 2020). Additionally, developing a therapeutic relationship requires facilitators to support families, inviting whole family participation and providing education that advocates for and encourages healthy development (Espe-Sherwindt, 2008).

Therapeutic photography is about more than just taking photos. Participants are invited to what Susan Sontag describes as a "set task" around a specific theme, topic, or question to reflect on, interpret, and represent with a photograph (Gibson, 2018). It involves taking photographs, writing narratives about the photograph, talking about a photograph, viewing other people's photographs, and dialoguing, always with the focus on process over product. The photograph serves as a way of objectifying and externalizing the self, strengths and challenges, feelings, and experiences (Gibson, 2018). Photographs create a distance that allows for safe, playful exploration literally at arm's length as the gaze is aimed at the photograph (Freeman et al., 1997).

The photograph that results from the interpretation of the task is then used as a communication tool to elicit reflections that lead to increased self-knowledge and self-awareness, a better understanding of lived experiences, and helps individuals and groups more clearly understand the world around them (Gibson, 2018). Through the therapeutic photography process, individuals are able to literally and figuratively reframe and engage in perspective-taking. Exploring new perspectives through the lens of the camera and taking in new perspectives from others stimulates and promotes important growth, expanding one's horizon of understanding of self, others, and the world (Röttger-Rössler, 2019; Tsirogianni & Andreouli, 2011).

According to Gibson, the three overarching outcomes of therapeutic photography programs aim to increase self-esteem, self-efficacy, and empowerment (2018). No matter the specific task or theme a program is structured around, individuals should leave feeling better about themselves after having gained a greater understanding of self and from the positive feedback participants receive when working in a group. In taking photographs and constructing stories to share about their image, individuals are reminded of their ability to make and produce valuable things which build confidence, restores a sense of control, and increases self-efficacy. Individually, participants are empowered through skill-building which can include photography skills, knowledge regarding healthy development, improved communication skills, or new coping skills. Collectively, social capital is built throughout the duration of the program as relationships are strengthened through group sharing and as photographs and stories are shared beyond the group (Ebersöhn et al., 2014; Nkosi & Daniels, 2007).

While therapeutic photography can be done with individuals, the author has experienced the most benefits from using it with groups. The group process leads to individual and collective benefits. Individuals benefit from self-reflection and personal work, become more present, increase agency as the task requires active participation, and can strengthen connections with supports in their microsystem. Group benefits include receiving positive feedback, feeling less alone, removing stigma from issues, increasing social capital, and the opportunity to learn from their peers. Healthy attachment is fostered as participants practice appropriate boundaries and responsive relationships.

Underpinnings of Through Their Eyes

Even as Through Their Eyes therapeutic photography programs continue to adapt to different geographical locations and contextual needs, the underpinnings over the years have remained consistent. No matter the context or objective of a program, Through Their Eyes programs fall within the Child Life scope of practice, are informed by Bronfenbrenner's socio-ecological model, and utilize the strengths perspective.

Child Life Scope of Practice

Therapeutic photography aligns with the philosophical tenets of Child Life. Photography is a form of play and thanks to the democratization of photography, which has made taking photos accessible and familiar, it is an ideal platform to engage children and families in a safe, non-threatening way (Gibson, 2018). Using the camera to elicit reflection and dialogue on daily life experiences that can encompass stress and trauma is an effective way to playfully promote healthy development and coping. As children walk and "play" with their cameras, they have a sense of control over what photographs are taken and what stories are shared. Existing personal and cultural knowledge are centered while creating a safe space for new knowledge and expression.

Playful Learning

A hallmark of any child life practice is play (Association of Child Life Professionals, 2001; Association of Child Life Professionals, 2020). Through Their Eyes therapeutic photography programs are saturated with play from beginning to end. Each activity within a program, from introducing the theme to practicing photography to storytelling to exhibitions, is guided by the five characteristics of a playful learning experience as defined by the Lego Foundation. Research by the Lego Foundation states "optimal learning through play happens when the activity is experienced as *joyful*; helps children find *meaning* in what they are doing or learning; involves *active*, engaged, minds-on thinking; involves *iterative* thinking; and involves *social interaction* (the most powerful resource available to humans - other people)." (Zosh et al., p.16, 2017).

Therapeutic photography with a Child Life lens prioritizes playful learning as well as playful experiences to promote healthy development and deepen social connections. Engaging in play strengthens our communication skills and attunes us to each other and our environments (Brown, 2009). Beyond play being a familiar and safe way of learning, play promotes healthy development, bridging children to new skills, new neural pathways, self-expression, coping, mastery, and to the unknown (Association of Child Life Professionals, 2020; Brown, 2009).

Family-Centered

Another hallmark of any child life practice, including Through Their Eyes, is family-centered care. Whether working with children or whole family systems, it is essential to center the family as the key support in a child's life (Espe-Sherwindt, 2008). Empowering a child involves empowering the whole family and caregiving system. If we want to empower children and their families, it is essential that we allow for diverse definitions of the family and view families across the entire socio-ecological map, extending beyond the microsystem to the larger societal and historical factors that continue to impact the microsystem (Nkosi & Daniels, 2007; Swick & Williams, 2006)

It is vital to tap into the family system to support a child through any intervention, including participation in therapeutic photography programs. Therapeutic photography programs are primed to support families in the way it fosters enabling and supportive environments that promote nurturing and responsive care (Jamieson et al., 2017). In programs designed for children, child participants can be urged to communicate with and gain support from their family and primary caregivers as they take photographs and complete a task, thus strengthening connections and increasing family knowledge and values throughout the process (Nkosi & Daniels, 2007). Coping tools and information on child development offered to child participants must also be shared with the caregivers who will support the child after the program is completed (Espe-Sherwindt, 2008; Swick & Williams, 2006). Therapeutic photography programs can also be designed for whole family participation (Ribbens, 2020). Engaging in therapeutic photography as a family or caregiver system provides opportunities to better understand each other, show appreciation, increase positive communication, engage in an enjoyable activity together, nurture attachment and responsive caregiving, and learn about and practice strategies to mitigate stress effectively (DeFrain et al., 2010; Mkhwanazi et al., 2018; Ribbens, 2020).

Professional Responsibility

To ensure best practice under the scope of practice as a CLS in the community setting, certification from the Association of Child Life Professionals must be obtained and maintained as a Certified Child Life Specialist (CCLS) (Association of Child Life Professionals, 2020). In addition to maintaining certification, it has been vital to learn from other professionals within the Child Life profession and in the local context of the work. Learning from local professionals, in the author's case Nigeria and South Africa, has invited the author to learn new information, inspect personal bias, and has expanded the author's own horizon of understanding (Tsirogianni & Andreouli, 2011), thus strengthening services and interventions. Another important aspect of providing best practice has been continued learning on the topics of play, child development, global perspectives of the family, and the emerging field of therapeutic photography.

Bronfenbrenner's Socio-ecological Model

Individuals are shaped by a myriad of interconnected influences. "The Nguni proverb *umuntu ngumuntu ngabantu* often translated as 'a person is a person through other persons' captures the interconnectedness invoked by Ubuntu" (Solis et al., 2019, p. 24). DeFrain et al (2010) similarly acknowledged, "Everything that happens to you happens to me. Family strengths research has roots in family systems theories, which argue that family members are inextricably connected with each other" (p. 31).

Beyond our interconnectedness to each other, individuals and families are interconnected with social, political, and historical environments that shape our stories. To solely look to the individual and the family for understanding misses other significant informants. Urie Bronfenbrenner's socio-ecological model beautifully illustrates the contextual nature of how the concentric layers of the meso, exo, macro, and chronoystems inform and affect individuals and families within the microsystem. (Bronfenbrenner, 1986; Swick, 2006). Viewing a child and the family through the scope of the socio-ecological model aligns with the Narrative Therapy approach which separates a person from their problems and acknowledges that the origins of problems can stem from direct and indirect factors coming from communities, society, culture, and history (Bronfenbrenner 1986; Freeman et al., 1997; Phola, 2022).

Underpinning therapeutic photography programs with the socio-ecological model creates opportunities to explore relationships to self, others, our environment, belief systems, values, society, and our histories (Gibson, 2018). These factors shape how we interact with and are impacted by the environments which influence our life story and lived experiences (Bronfenbrenner, 1986). Situating our stories within the context of these diverse influencers helps participants to understand their story in new and different ways (Gibson, 2018). Programming can focus on one specific aspect of the socio-ecological model or could look broadly at the entire model. Participant and contextual needs will determine the most beneficial approach. To safely use the socio-ecological model, facilitators must have an awareness of the wider social issues in which they are working.

Strengths Perspective

The strengths perspective urges an orientation of looking for and building off of individual, family, and cultural strengths. DeFrain et al. assert "not all families are strong, but all families have strengths" (2010, p. 31). Intervention programs that build off of strengths as opposed to pathology or deficits utilize existing protective factors that honor personal and cultural assets (Böök & Mykkänen, 2014; DeFrain et al., 2010; Nkosi & Daniels, 2007). In positioning ourselves with a strengths perspective, we are better postured to extend interventions that "do with" families rather than "do to" families (Benard, 2006).

THROUGH THEIR EYES THERAPEUTIC PHOTOGRAPHY

Setting

Demographics and Realities

South Africa is the current context for Through Their Eyes therapeutic photography programs. South Africa is home to 11 official languages, diverse cultures, rapid urbanization, and is a magnet for migration. While family strengths have been eroded throughout an oppressive history, South African family strengths continue to include displays of resilience and strong cultural values such as Ubuntu, social capital, and indigenous knowledge systems (Nkosi & Daniels, 2007; Ribbens, 2020). Challenges that threaten strong families stem from poverty, over-crowded housing, unemployment, disempowerment, isolation, vulnerability, poor service access and infrastructure, crime, violence, racism, xenophobia, poor health, and the HIV/Aids pandemic (Benjamin & Crawford-Browne, 2010; Cluver et al., 2018; Mkhwanazi, 2018; Nkosi & Daniels, 2007). Benjamin and Crawford-Browne (2010) note children's high exposure to violence, citing that between 67% to 95% of children are exposed to various forms of violence within and outside of the home. These pervasive challenges amplify the effects of toxic stress and continuous trauma which affect the healthy development and functioning of children, adults, and whole communities (Benjamin & Crawford-Browne, 2010; Jamieson, 2017; Van der Kolk, 2014).

South African family structures have distinct differences as compared to Western family structures. Families have experienced much change in both structure and function due to the oppressive apartheid regime that systematically separated families as a form of racial violence, ongoing inequalities, migration, and urbanization (Nkosi & Daniels, 2007). Research studies indicate how these changes have resulted in a decline of parental presence. In 2014, it was reported over 60% of South Africa's children did not live with their fathers; in 2015, it was reported 21% of children in South Africa were not living with either parent (Jamieson, 2017). For children growing up without fathers, there is a 62% higher chance they will experience poverty (Jamieson, 2017).

Needs

Trauma-informed

The author is mindful of the high prevalence of trauma in the current setting of her work, ranging from one-time events to continuous and complex trauma (Benjamin & Crawford-Brown, 2010). While the author does not treat trauma as a CCLS using therapeutic photography, it is paramount to understand the impacts of trauma. Understanding how trauma impedes healthy development and how it shows up in children and families is necessary to build safe and effective programming. Key principles of trauma-informed care include safety, trust, choice, collaboration, and empowerment (Bateman et al., 2013). It is essential to design therapeutic photography programs in community settings with a trauma-informed approach that privileges issues of safety, trust, choice, collaboration, and empowerment to ensure unintended re-traumatization does not occur. Additionally, being trauma-informed equips a CLS for situations when it is necessary to consult with and refer to other professionals who may need to step in to provide additional care that extends beyond the CLS scope of practice.

Research has identified how stress and trauma can lead to disintegration and dissociation (Benjamin & Crawford-Browne, 2010; Siegel, 2015; Van der Kolk, 2014). When the brain must focus on survival, its capacity for other important functions is reduced. Talk therapies have limitations to healing due to dissociation and the way the language center of our brain shuts down (Siegel, 2015; Van der Kolk, 2014). Tapping into the arts is an ideal and culturally-relevant avenue for expression and integration as it moves beyond language (Coleman & Macintosh, 2015; Van der Kolk, 2014). The act of children making photographs in their own community is action-oriented and sensory-based. This somatic process stimulates stories and can bridge children to their words.

Experiencing a loss of control is common for individuals living in situations of toxic stress and continuous trauma (Bateman et al., 2013; Van der Kolk, 2014) Loss of control can leave individuals disempowered and dysregulated, resulting in poor impulse control (Benjamin & Crawford-Browne, 2010). Through Their Eyes participants are reminded throughout the program that they have control over what photographs to take, what is disclosed in their stories and sharing, and have the option to opt-out at any point. The author has never had anyone opt up, but giving that permission reminds participants that they are in control of the process that unfolds.

Another facet of sharing control is the way power is shifted and balanced. Unequal power relations are a hallmark of South African history. Incredible barriers exist due to historical and ongoing unequal distributions of power (Ribbens, 2020). It has been evidenced that photo-based programs, for both therapeutic and research purposes, are effective ways of balancing power relations between facilitator and participants (Böök & Mykkänen, 2014; Gibson, 2018; Röttger-Rössler et al., 2019). However, this balance of power is not automatic and requires intentional program design for power to be truly shared and balanced (Böök & Mykkänen, 2014). It is important to conceive how factors such as relationship building, language, clothing choices, location choice, and seating positions may increase, reduce or redistribute power differentials (Böök & Mykkänen, 2014; Röttger-Rössler et al., 2019).

Cultural Relevance

Healing requires prioritizing people's traditional practices and cultural ways of being (Jamieson et al, 2017; Phola, 2022; Theron & Theron, 2010). Oral storytelling has been a historical strength throughout South African history. Visual storytelling is a culturally appropriate way of engaging communities in

South Africa as it builds on the historical value and protective factor of oral storytelling (Ribbens, 2020). Engaging in therapeutic photography allows participants to tap into personal and collective stories that get beyond the singular stories that can dominate people's lives (Bronfenbrenner, 1986; Phola, 2022). Benard states,

When youth and families are given the opportunity in a small group context – to give voice to their realities and tell their 'stories' – to discuss their experiences, beliefs, attitudes and feelings – and encouraged to critically question societal messages – we are empowering them to be critical thinkers and decision-makers around the important concerns in their lives. (2006, p. 202)

Storytelling and reconstructing stories positions participants to be the experts in their lives and results in empowerment (Gibson, 2018).

While visual storytelling had a cultural resonance in both of the author's contexts in Nigeria and South Africa, it is paramount to assess cultural understandings and beliefs regarding photography before engaging in or offering this type of intervention to children or families. Some cultures do not engage with photography or do not want their image to be taken by a camera. Even within Nigeria where this type of intervention was widely appropriate, there were some people groups that believed your soul was captured when their photo was taken. As a CLS, it is important to assess your cultural context to avoid potential harm or offense through such an intervention. Additionally, it is crucial to train participants in the ethics of taking photographs to ensure they are prepared to understand and respond respectfully if they take photographs of other people. This conversation is an excellent opportunity to build perspective-taking skills and empathy for others in their community.

Evolution of Through Their Eyes

Starting Out

The Through Their Eyes pilot program focused on teaching seven children, ages seven to twelve, five aspects of photography encouraging children to slow down, notice their surroundings, and make meaning from their daily lives. Aspects of photography that were taught included: choosing a point of interest, exploring unique perspectives, filling the frame, using the rule of thirds, and being aware of the light source. The pilot program was designed to test and answer whether children would be interested in a photography program, if it would lead to greater self-awareness, if children would take photographs worthy of printing and exhibiting, and if their photos and titles would captivate the attention of adult audiences. The end result of the pilot program delivered a resounding yes to those questions. The child participants revealed a depth of thought in their self-titled photographs. With permission and active involvement of the participants, the photographs were exhibited at a neighborhood café in Abuja, Nigeria. Adults delighted in their unique perspectives and were challenged by what the children saw and noticed in their community. One viewer was overheard remarking, "You mean children think this way?" while looking at a photograph of garbage in the street titled "Things Could Be Better." It was clear this approach resonated with both children and adults.

Just as Child Life continues to evolve in non-traditional settings, so has Through Their Eyes. Eleven years later, Through Their Eyes therapeutic photography programs continue to contextualize and adapt within schools, NGOs, and churches. Each implemented program has informed the next. Each program has required contextualization due to age, setting and culture, needs of the specific community, length of time, and resources available. What started with teaching five key photographic elements to help children slow down and notice their surroundings in order to document their world and perspectives has evolved into a psychosocial support program to support the healthy development and well-being of children and families that is strengths-based, family-centered, and culturally reflexive. While therapeutic photography is a tool that can be easily incorporated into any Child Life practice, whether in traditional or non-traditional settings, the author has centered her Child Life work in the community around therapeutic photography. Through Their Eyes therapeutic photography has created a safe space to process life experiences and create meaning in order to mitigate the long-term effects of stress and trauma.

Assessment

Assessment within therapeutic photography programs comes at several levels: assessing the needs of the community in order to articulate objectives for a program, assessing the needs of participants throughout a program, and assessing the effectiveness of the program. The first step in any program is identifying a community to work with and listening to the needs assessment from that community. As a white woman from America, the author needs to be cautious when assessing community needs. As a foreigner who represents power and comes with cultural bias, it is not the author's job to assess community needs, which can be influenced by her own cultural lens, bias, and cultural misunderstandings. Assessment of needs to articulate program objectives has required trusting relationships within the community setting where the program will be taking place. For example, if the program is being carried out alongside a school community, the CCLS relies on the school to articulate needs that will direct the formation of the program. It is then the role of the CCLS to develop a play-based, developmentally, and culturally appropriate program to meet those needs. Objectives for the program are co-constructed by the author and local organization.

In assessing the needs of participants, facilitators require a keen understanding and awareness of their professional scope of practice. At times, the therapeutic experience of taking photos, writing about the photos, and sharing about the photos is a catalyst for healing and resolve that mitigates the need for therapy (Gibson, 2018; Weiser, 2004). On the other hand, the catalytic experience can open up deeper wounds that require the attention of a therapist (Gibson, 2018; Weiser, 2004). It is essential to monitor the experience of participants to know when a participant may need the help of other trained professionals who can attend to deeper wounds that are exposed.

In order to provide effective and culturally relevant therapeutic photography programs, it is important to evaluate programs. The author does a self-reflection and reflects with the partner organization to assess if project objectives were met, if the program was developmentally and culturally appropriate, if the timeline was fitting, the strengths of the program, and ways it can be improved going forward. Additionally, participants and their caregivers' complete surveys and/or interviews to provide feedback on their experiences.

Core Program Components

Woven throughout each program is play-based learning, children's literature, reflection, storytelling, and skill-building. Children are taught about photography along with psychosocial skills that correlate with the theme of a particular program. Shaping a playful and safe space for reflection and skill-building creates opportunities for creative expression and growth. Intended outcomes for Through Their Eyes programs change slightly according to the contextual needs, but generally, intended outcomes aim to increase emotional literacy, expand coping skills, make meaning out of life experiences, build stronger connections to the support systems in a child's life (family, teachers, people in the community), deepen self-knowledge and self-awareness, regain a sense of control, and provide a safe space for play for a greater sense of identity, activated agency, and stronger connections.

Once intended outcomes are outlined, research is used to define issues and create pathways for the photographic explorations that will be used. To date, themes and program topics requested by NGOs and schools have included resilience, connection, personal and national identity, child rights, and family strengths through shared enjoyable activities.

Programs are designed to be interactive, engaging the whole body in the learning process in order to increase integrated well-being (Van der Kolk, 2014). Participants play, build, create, practice skills, and actively strengthen relationships with each other. As each photography element is taught, participants venture outside to put that element into practice before learning another aspect of photography. The essential ingredients of play-based learning, the camera, and children's literature are prioritized in order to objectify issues and language, making them safer to explore and easier to understand before connecting to their own lives.

Project logistics and timelines have varied, dependent upon contextual needs and availability of the organization and participants. Program timelines have been both condensed and spread out, fitting within school vacation breaks, weekly school schedules, and on weekends. Some programs have ranged for a two-week span while others have lasted for months. The author prefers small groups in order to ensure each participant is attended to and mentored throughout the program. The number of participants has ranged from a small group of seven to the largest group of 35. While the author has a preference for small groups, at times the final group size has been determined by the local partner entity. Discernment needs to be applied when the number of participants has the potential to compromise the therapeutic benefits of a program. In programs where the participants are many, it is essential to work with trained co-leaders and volunteers to help facilitate small group discussions and for general help in attending to each participant throughout the process.

Through Their Eyes therapeutic photography programs typically follow seven phases.

Phase One: Connect and assess. Connect with a local partner organization in order to build relationships, listen to needs, and co-construct a theme and project timeline. Identify the photographic task and supporting frameworks.

Phase Two: Introduce project. In this phase, it is vital to explain the intended outcomes, explain what is required and gather consent from the local partner, caregivers, and youth participants.

Phase Three: Host workshops. Depending on the specific project, a project could entail one workshop or many. During the workshops, the theme is unpacked through play, photography tips are given and practiced, model and teach new coping skills or developmental concepts, and ideas are brainstormed naming "describing words" and "photo ideas" so participants are equipped to accomplish their task in their home and community.

Phase Four: Mentor. Participants are mentored throughout the duration of each program. One-on-one mentoring as the task is interpreted and accomplished. As participants take photos, it is important to provide ongoing support and check-ins to support their efforts, answer questions, affirm work, and assist with camera problems. This typically takes place in participant homes or at the partner organization.

Phase Five: Gather and print. Cameras and workbooks are collected. A contact sheet of favorite photos is printed for each participant and delivered to participants in order to begin the writing process. If participants have barriers to writing, a family member or facilitator can dictate for them.

Phase Six: Revise and finalize. Drafts of the visual stories are read through in small groups. Final edits are suggested to ensure a clear message is portrayed and understood.

Phase Seven: Exhibit and advocate. Photos and written narratives are printed and exhibit materials prepared. The nature of an exhibition is dictated by project objectives and participant input.

To give an example of the process, the Perfect Square program will be unpacked. A local school noted their students needed to strengthen their resiliency skills, especially before moving on to high school. Dr. Edith Grotberg's Paradigm of Resilience was identified as a tool to guide the program. Grotberg identified when a child can name supportive relationships (I Have), personal attributes and strengths (I Am), and problem-solving ideas or coping skills (I Can), they have a greater chance of bouncing back from setbacks (Grotberg, 1995). The objectives of the program were to strengthen supportive relationships, increase self-knowledge, and articulate known and new coping skills. Play, with rubber bands and string and an inflatable punching bag, helped to define resilience before engaging in either the topic or the camera. Children's literature read throughout the program assisted in understanding perspective-taking. It is reinforced that each participant has a unique perspective and that we can explore different perspectives as we work with camera angles and listen to each other's stories. In this particular program, children's literature was also used to identify what resilience looked like in main characters in stories before naming the participants' own resilience plan. To accomplish their task of creating the visual story of their resilience plan, participants took photos in their home and community to depict the three resilience categories. After identifying their favorite photos with a mentor, participants wrote short narratives to describe each photo.

This program used the photographs in an additional way to remind participants of previous displays of resilience in their lives. Using the children's book *Perfect Square* by Michael Hall, participants took copies of their photographs to cut up, creating their own perfect square, to represent something they've already bounced back from in their lives. Participants were eager to share their resilience plans and perfect squares with their families and friends. The Perfect Square program was implemented in 2016 and again in 2019. Even though both programs had similar intended outcomes, the exhibitions took different shapes due to the needs and desires of participants. The first exhibition was more traditional, featuring printed photographs hung on partitions at an event for the broad viewing by family and friends. The second exhibition involved printing photos and written narratives to put in hand-made books. The resilience plan books were shared within the class and made in such a way that participants could continue to add to their resilience plan as they transitioned to high school.

Advocacy

Advocacy is an important tenet of therapeutic photography and the Child Life profession (Association of Child Life Professionals, 2020; Gibson, 2018). Robust advocacy will be expressed in different forms in order to engage each sphere of a child's ecological map (Bronfenbrenner, 1986). Children, families, and communities are strengthened through direct programming interventions that advocate for and improve family functioning. What is learned through direct interventions can lead to new information which paves the way for advocacy to meet observed and expressed needs.

Educating parents and the community can take place through workshops, campaigns, direct involvement in programs, as well as through photo exhibitions. It is vital that images are displayed alongside the participants' written narratives when exhibiting their work. Images can convey different messages to people due to the way punctum, the emotional connections we have to an image, triggers our own experiences and emotions (Gibson, 2018). With an aim to tell a child's story through an exhibition, it is important that the child's story is clear with image and words to avoid misinterpretation.

While the emphasis of a therapeutic photography program is on the process over the product, exhibiting produced images and written narratives provides participants with a sense of mastery and can strength social capital. Providing an exhibition, no matter its form, creates further opportunities for children to bond with supportive relationships in their lives. Children are empowered as they show off and explain their visual photo stories to family, peers, and other supportive people in their lives, thus strengthening social capital within the family and community. In viewing a child's work, parents have opportunities to attune to their child and gain a deeper understanding. In viewing her child's work in an exhibition, one parent remarked, "I didn't know this is how my child felt." After a long pause, she declared, "I need to spend more time with her because she is changing. And I need to know how." Even if parents and caregivers do not engage throughout the process, exhibitions offer a chance to see and celebrate their child and follow up with new information their visual stories may provide.

Ethics

CLSs have a commitment to demonstrate ethical behavior in their work. As a CCLS using therapeutic photography, the author has a responsibility to only work in areas where she has been trained and to consult with other trained professionals when issues move beyond her scope of practice (Association of Child Life Professionals, 2020). Local play therapists, narrative therapists, and social workers are consulted regularly in the author's work for feedback and referrals. In addition to maintaining certification through the Association of Child Life Professionals, the author completed the Global Consortium for International Family Studies master's degree through the University of Nebraska-Lincoln to better understand families on a global scale. Additionally, in 2022, the author will complete training in the first academic course on therapeutic photography through Robert Gordon University in Scotland.

Consent is sought throughout the duration of Through Their Eyes programs for ethical reasons and as a way of sharing control (Böök & Mykkänen, 2014). Both parents/caregivers and children sign consent forms at the beginning of programs. Before participants go out to take photos in their homes and community, conversations take place about the ethics of taking photos of other people, and consent forms using everyday language are provided should other people be in their photographs. Participants are reminded throughout the program that they are in control of the photographs they take and the stories they share within the group. While some stories are safe to share in the group, they may not feel confident or safe to share them beyond the group. Participants consent to the photographs and stories that are shared in exhibitions.

Realizing participants and their families cannot fully understand what they are consenting to at the beginning of a program, consent is revisited at the end of a program to get permission to share their stories beyond the exhibition (Böök & Mykkänen, 2014). While a participant may give permission to use a photo, they might feel differently ten years down the road. For this reason, when participants give consent to share photo stories, the author does not disclose names in order to keep participants anonymous. Consideration must be given to how long a facilitator has permission to use the photograph, the purpose for which it is used, and the platforms in which it may be shared.

Ownership of a photograph belongs to the participant who took the photo. While participants own their photographs, many Through Their Eyes participants do not have the resources to print their photographs. To honor their work and participation, the author provides printed copies of their final photographs.

Outcomes

The most common reflection received from Through Their Eyes participants has been about the fun factor. The playful nature of the program and the playful nature of taking photos carves out time and space for play, a critical component for contexts where play is threatened due to issues of lack of space, compromised safety, and other pressing physical needs that must be met. The play-saturated programs produce a felt sense of safety that promote connection to self and connection to each other. This sense of safety and connection helps to relieve stress and paves the way for important learning.

Connects Us to Ourselves

The best way to give evidence of the strengthened sense of self is to share examples of photo stories from various programs. Figure 1 shows how one participant used a photo of her reflection in a mirror to reflect on her experience in the program. Her narrative portrays what was learned and how her horizon of understanding expanded as she completed her tasks and as she interacted with others. She wrote,

I loved doing the photography course. I learn new aspects and methods to take better photos, such as the rule of thirds and ways to hold your camera. I had fun and met many different people. When I reflect back on the experience, I realized that by breaking out of my shell, I learned new things about myself.

A fourteen-year-old participant grew up living in different cultural contexts. Figure 2 demonstrates how she was able to use a Lego figure to objectify and externalize her resilience strategies. Through her photo series, she was able to name who supports her, who she is, and what she can do to respond to challenges and setbacks. In naming personal attributes that help her bounce back from setbacks, she took a photo of a Lego army figure that she had carefully tucked into a bush. She titled the photo "A Little Camouflaged – I am Adaptable." Naming her strength to adapt to her surroundings further empowered that strength and led to conversations with her caregivers about how that strength helps her.

Another participant lingered at a park to make his photos for his resilience plan. This twelve-year-old participant observed an eagle flying and patiently attempted to get a photo with the focus on the eagle. As much as he tried, he could not get a photo with the flying eagle in focus. As he sat on the grass attempting time and time again, he made the connection that the blurry eagle represented how he currently felt. Figure 3 shows his final attempt that depicted his inner world. Using tree branches that were in focus to frame the blurry eagle, he realized that the eagle was still soaring even though it was out of focus and possibly unnoticed. He explained that as a second child, he often feels outshined by his older brother and sometimes feels unnoticed. Just like the eagle, he realized that just because he isn't noticed doesn't mean that he isn't flying, soaring with his own talents. Upon this reflection, he titled his photo "Soaring but Unnoticed." Naming this feeling was empowering. It helped him externalize this unnamed internal feeling and unmet need, and urged him to be proud of his gifts and abilities.

Figure 1. Through Their Eyes participant uses a photo of her own reflection to build her narrative of what she learned through reflection. Johannesburg, South Africa. © 2017 Through Their Eyes participant. Used with permission

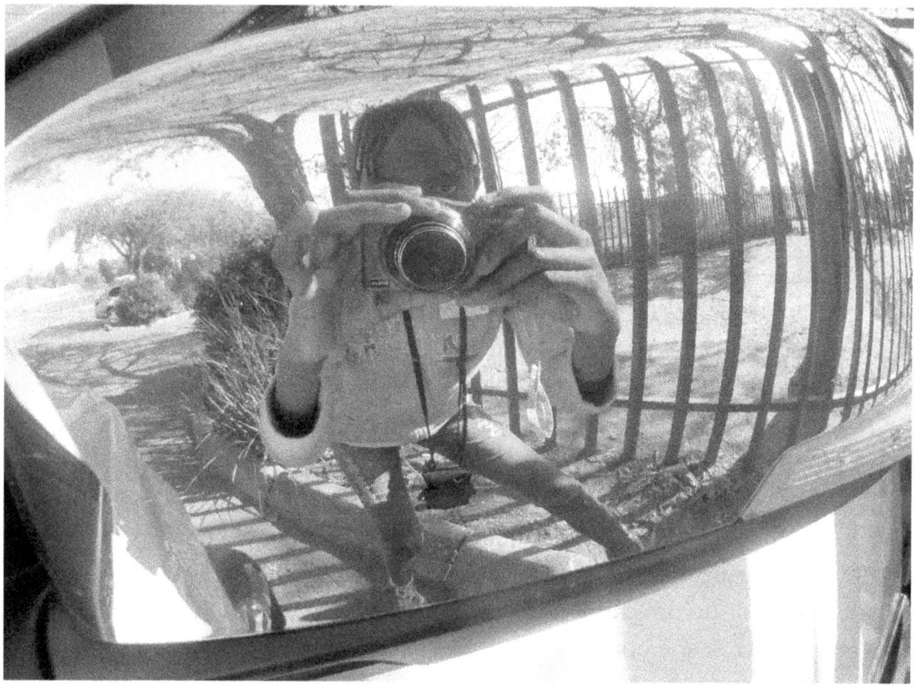

Figure 2. Through Their Eyes participant uses a familiar toy to objectify and externalize her resilience plan. Johannesburg, South Africa. © 2016 Through Their Eyes participant. Used with permission

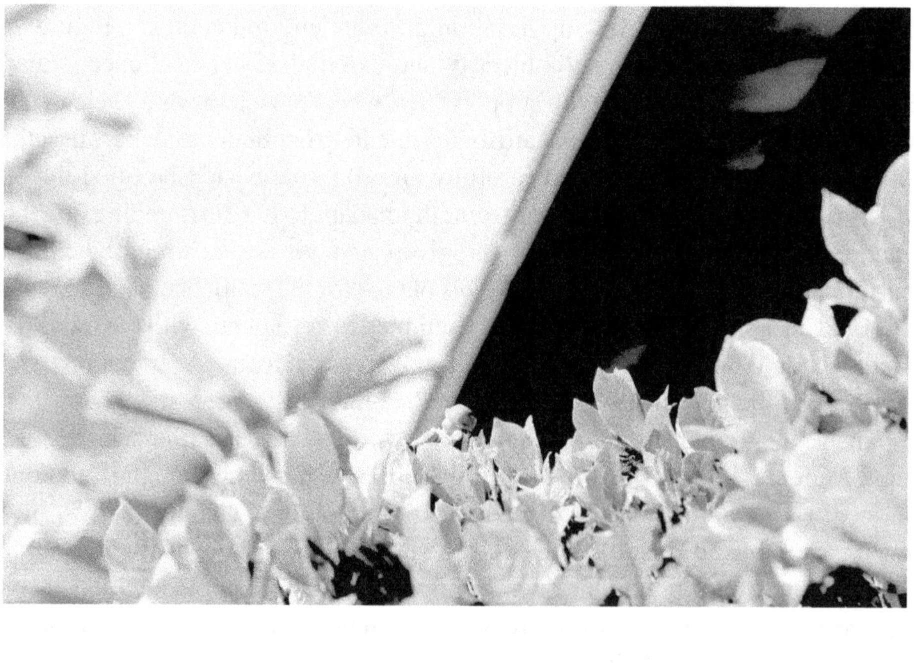

Figure 3. Through Their Eyes participant connects more deeply to his inner world while trying to take the perfect photo. Johannesburg, South Africa. © 2016 Through Their Eyes participant. Used with permission

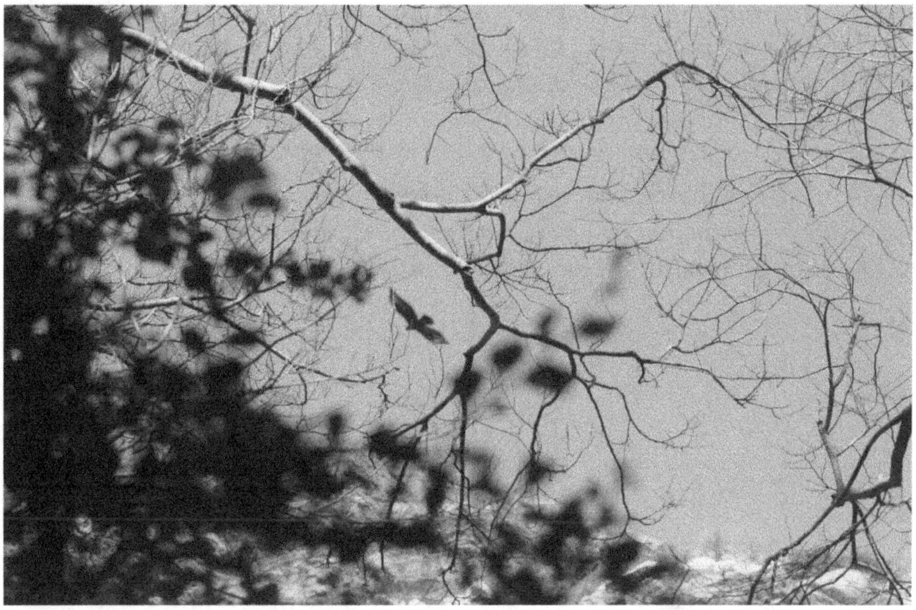

Figure 3 demonstrates how externalizing and objectifying ideas through a photograph has the power to connect us to words and ideas that are difficult to articulate. Between developmental stages, language barriers, taboo issues, and the way trauma impacts our access to words, it can be difficult to feel safe or even have the capacity to explain our thoughts and emotions (Coleman & Macintosh, 2015; Siegel, 2015; Van der Kolk, 2014). Upon reflection on her experience with the Perfect Square program, a twelve-year-old shared "I always had this idea inside of me," pointing to her heart, "but I never knew how to describe it. Taking a picture of the path helped me to describe what was inside."

Connects Us to Each Other

To Relationships, Values, and Beliefs

Therapeutic photography has the power to connect us to our support networks as individuals accomplish program tasks and share their work. The program on the theme of connection was designed using Bronfenbrenner's socio-ecological model (Bronfenbrenner, 1986). Participants reflected on what promotes and hinders connection within self, with others, with God, and with their environment. Images were paired up with narratives that identified what is happening in the photo and how it connected to their life. Most written narratives ended by stating what they will carry forward to promote connection in their lives. Two participants in the connection program used birds to tell stories of what promotes and hinders connection. Figure 4 shows the way one twelve-year-old participant used birds sitting on a fence to explain her view on what promotes connection with others. She wrote,

Two birds are communicating on a fence. I am wondering what they are communicating about. Communication promotes connection with friends. Me and my friends share secrets and we look out for one another. When there are trust issues, we can make an oath to show that they can be trusted. I think with some people having an oath would work. It is wise to try to communicate and helps us avoid fighting, arguing, disrespecting each other, and misunderstandings.

Figure 4. Through Their Eyes participant uses the common object of birds and a fence in her neighborhood to unpack healthy communication and its impact on relationships. Johannesburg, South Africa. © 2017 Through Their Eyes participant. Used with permission

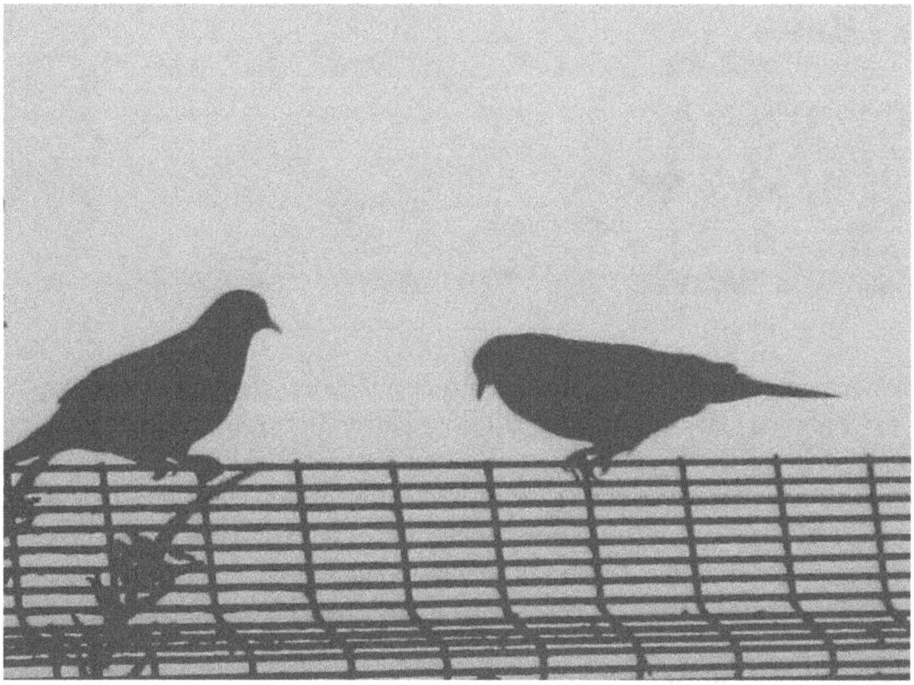

The other narrative focused on what hinders connection. The participant wrote, "The picture shows a bird which is hiding. When you hide from yourself, you won't get to know yourself and others won't get to know you. And you need to know yourself first." Photo stories such as this one are a launching pad for caregivers to continue the conversation, asking the child to name ways they can get to know themselves, and to support continued growth.

Another twelve-year-old participant demonstrated her embodiment of Ubuntu, a cultural value of inclusion, as she reflected on what promotes connection with others. Figure 5 illustrated a common scene and experience of play in informal settlements and townships. She writes, "In my neighbourhood, we play mapakastina with bricks and a plastic ball. When we play a game that everyone likes, it promotes connection because you take turns to play and everyone gets an opportunity to play."

Figure 5. Through Their Eyes participant documents a common and beloved neighborhood game to illustrate how cultural values filter all the way down to games on the street and promote connection. Johannesburg, South Africa. © 2017 Through Their Eyes participant. Used with permission

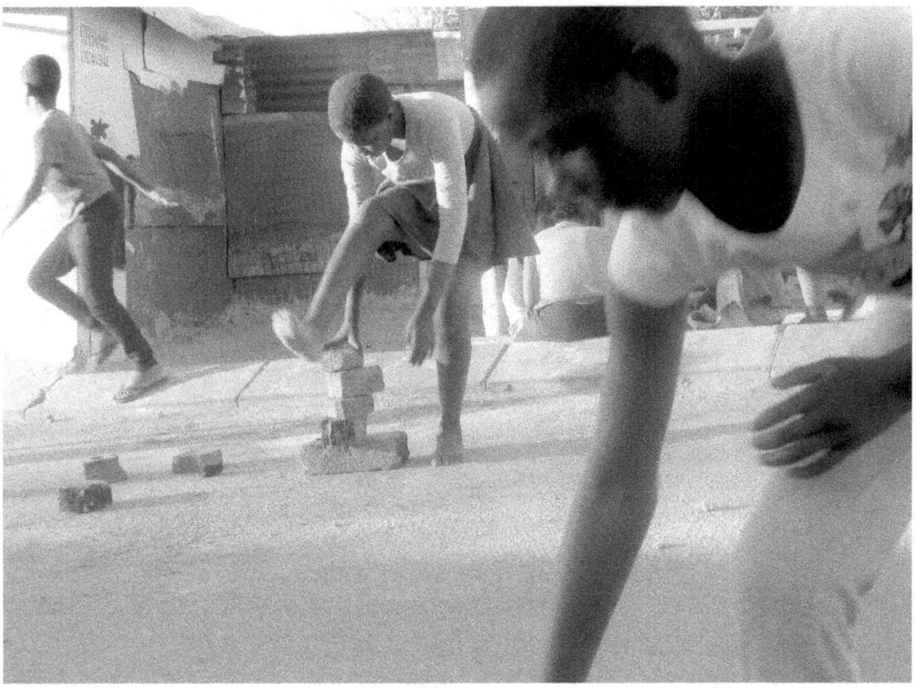

A thirteen-year-old boy was able to describe what disconnects him from others while also naming coping skills for when he feels disconnected. Figure 6 shows the way he used the object of leaves to tell his story. He wrote,

The lower green leaves look like they are shrinking as they go down to the ground even though the leaves are actually all the same size. I feel like I am shrinking when people name-call, bully, or stereotype me. When I start to shrink, it is helpful if my family and friends encourage me.

Figure 7 depicts the physical barriers that keep us from each other. An insightful eleven-year-old participant named the factors that separate us as if she has read Bronfenbrenner herself. Articulating solutions for overcoming these barriers, she wrote,

We are sometimes isolated from others because of either race, wealth, culture, or religion. We have a barrier between others because we aren't eager or curious to find out who they truly are. The way I get curious about people who are different than me is by talking and having a conversation with them.

Figure 6. Through Their Eyes participant uses the everyday object of plant leaves to reflect on how bullying hinders connection and what coping skills he uses in response. Johannesburg, South Africa. © 2018 Through Their Eyes participant. Used with permission

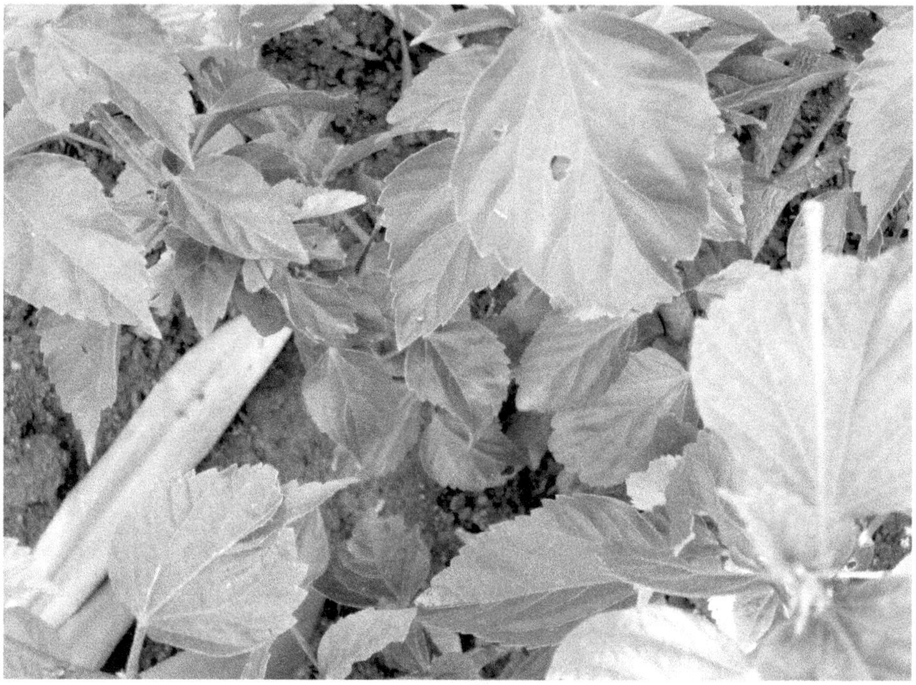

Figure 7. Through Their Eyes participant uses the point of interest of a wall to guide on the barriers that hinder connection in her community. Johannesburg, South Africa. © 2017 Through Their Eyes participant. Used with permission

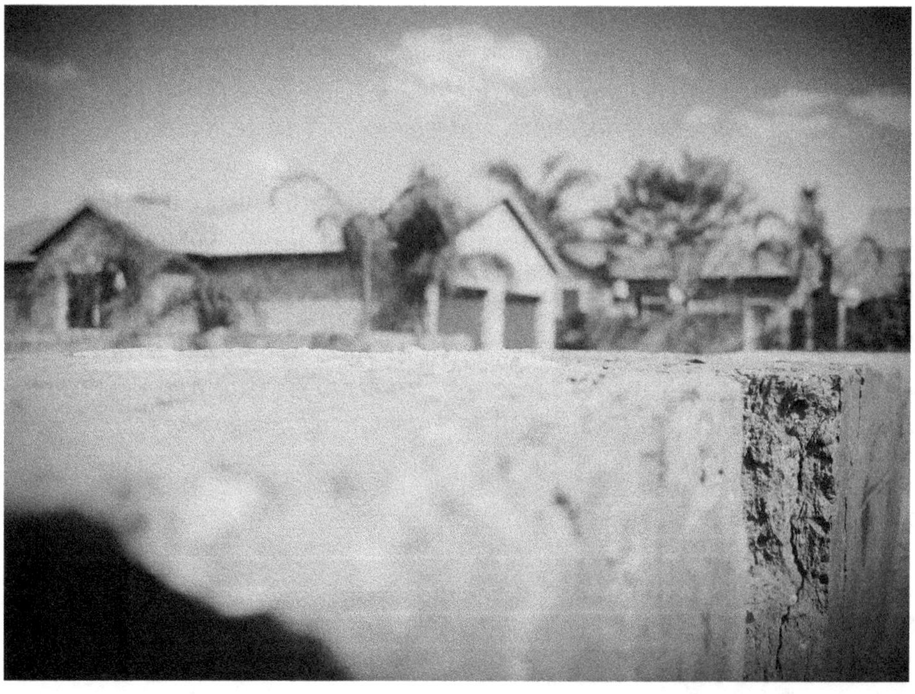

One Nigerian father took an interest in the work his eleven-year-old child was doing at home. He regularly checked in with his son as he gathered images within their community and deliberated on the best titles for his final images. Figure 8 shows the image of freshly hung laundry framed through the hole of a cinderblock. Discussing what this image represented, the father explained to his son, "If you are faithful with small tasks, such as hanging up the laundry, God will bless you with bigger and bigger tasks – but it starts with the laundry." The son concluded his photo should be called "Journey to Stardom." They were both so proud to see that image and title displayed in the exhibition. This photograph and the resulting title gives evidence to the opportunity this process creates for parents to bond and attune, as well as transfer family values and knowledge.

Figure 8. Through Their Eyes participant documented this everyday scene which opened up rich dialogue between father and son, creating an opportunity for the father to transfer values, beliefs and knowledge. Abuja, Nigeria. © 2011 Through Their Eyes participant. Used with permission

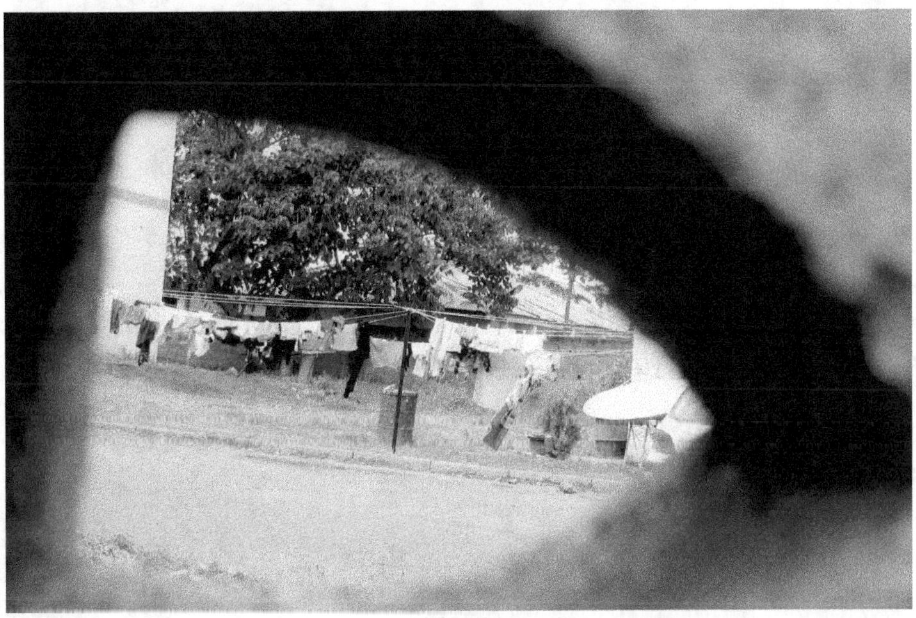

Exhibiting children's work provide additional opportunities to see and celebrate the child and face pain and difficult topics, while also promoting attunement and connection. A great example surfaced in the Perfect Square exhibition. Adolescents displayed their visually depicted "resilience plans" with photographs and titles. Parents, caregivers, and other important people in the participants' lives were invited to their exhibition. One twelve-year-old participant reflected on the loss of her mother during the program. In reflecting on whom supports her, she articulated that she missed her mom, but she still has the support of her father. Figure 9 frames the seasonal purple flowers she came across as she went to make photographs in her community. She remembered that purple was her mother's favorite color. She felt it was a gift from God to have this reminder of her mom every season and titled her photograph, "Always a reminder." Figure 10 documents her sense of empowerment as she proudly explained her photographs and their meaning to her father, together remembering someone special while promoting a further connection between the two.

Figure 9. Through Their Eyes participant was able to remember her mother and take another step in her grief process as she noted the reminders of her mother she has in nature. Johannesburg, South Africa. © 2016 Through Their Eyes participant. Used with permission

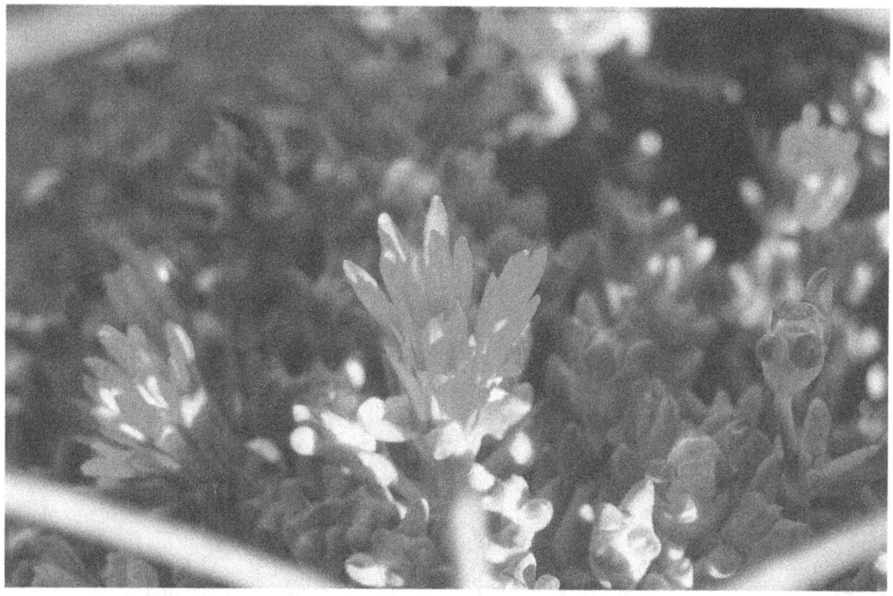

Figure 10. Through Their Eyes participant proudly explains her photographs, stories, and perfect square to her father during an exhibition resulting in empowerment for both child and parent. Johannesburg, South Africa. © 2016 Through Their Eyes. Used with permission

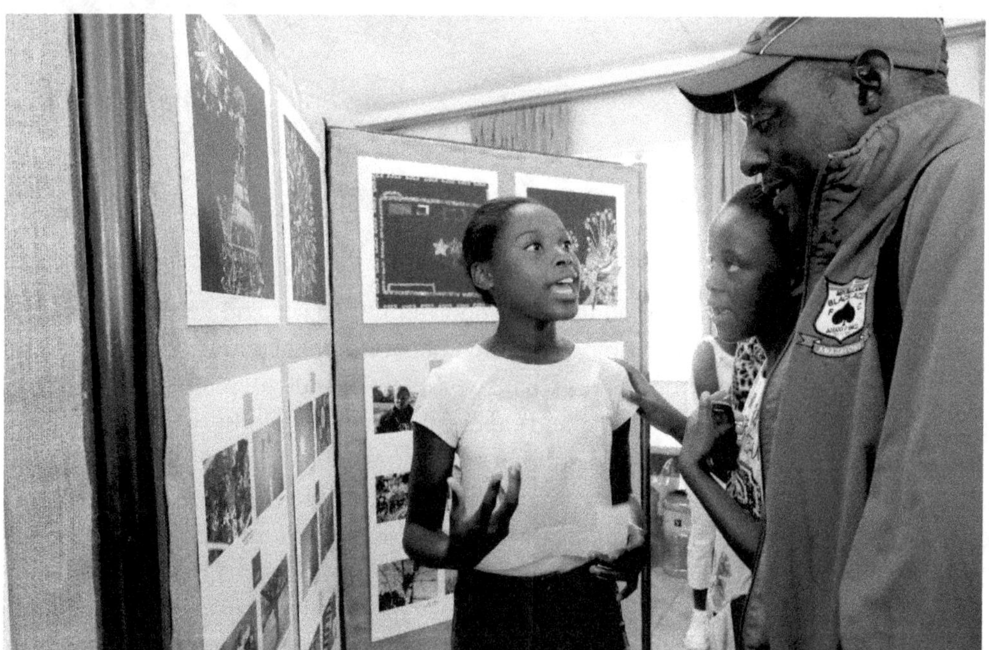

To the CLS or Facilitator

In looking at participant photographs, therapeutic photography facilitators get a literal depiction of a participant's life. Harper notes that photographs used to elicit fall into three categories: inventories depicting people and possessions, current or representations of significant events, and social interactions (Gibson, 2018; Harper, 2002). Similarly, Ulkuniemi articulates that photos are often used to document events/preserve memories, demonstrate unity, facilitate interaction, and build identity (Gibson, 2018). Photographs assist a facilitator to more clearly enter and understand lives outside of their own. When using this with groups, facilitators get a glimpse into the life of a community, be that a physical neighborhood community or a community of individuals working through a similar issue.

Children can easily misconstrue events and problems due to normal stages of development such as egocentrism, magical thinking, or concrete thinking. Likewise, adults can also have misconceptions about a child's world. Assumed understanding can hinder true understanding. The author was reminded of this during a mentoring session with an eleven-year-old participant. Having lived in Nigeria for eight years and South Africa for six years, the author associated razor and electric wires with danger, reminders of the chronic nature of crime and the need to be alert. Figure 11's depiction of razor wire against the sky brought an automatic assumption the child viewed lack of safety as something that hindered connection. In his one-on-one mentor session, he explained quite the opposite. In describing how the razor wire promotes connection in his environment, the participant wrote, "The people use a razor fence to protect themselves from thieves and keep themselves safe in my community. The feeling of safety in my yard allows me to feel connected to my environment." Listening to the participant talk about his photo highlighted the misconception which initially inhibited understanding of the boy's lived experience.

Figure 11. Through Their Eyes participant used razor wire to explain his sense of safety in his community. This photo reminds practitioners of possible misconceptions that can take place when photos and narratives are separated. Johannesburg, South Africa. © 2018 Through Their Eyes participant. Used with permission

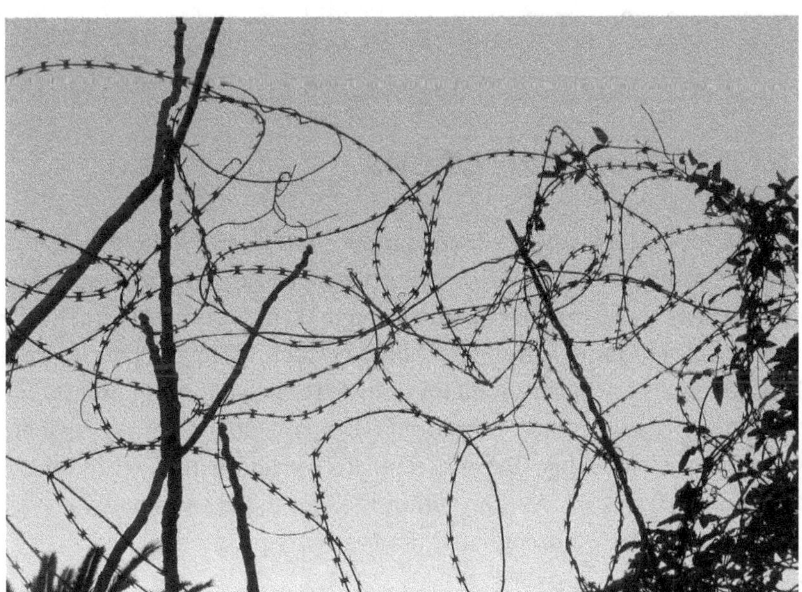

Challenges

While the tool of therapeutic photography is highly effective, it does not come without challenges. One of the biggest challenges is to find ways of balancing power when working with vulnerable or marginalized communities. It takes time to develop trusting relationships that truly distribute power. Rushing this process can lead to artificial stories and a failed therapeutic experience.

Another challenge stems from the combination of the newness of the therapeutic photography field, the relative newness of Child Life in the community setting, and the undeveloped Child Life profession in the author's setting in South Africa. Therapeutic photography is an emerging practice that has yet to define professional standards or scope of practice. Underpinning theories can differ depending on the professional background of the facilitator which makes the assessment of best practice difficult. For many years, the author understood that the approach of using therapeutic photography as a CCLS in the community setting worked, but she didn't have the language to describe why or articulate the right underpinning theories.

Likewise, the newness of CCLS working in the community setting and the unfamiliarity of Child Life in her working context have provided challenges. While always maintaining an identity as a CLS, the author had to let her certification lapse in her early days when living in Nigeria due to poor internet and unstable electricity which impacted access to ongoing training to maintain certification. Improved infrastructure and the advancement of the internet have solved some of those problems, but the author is aware that barriers to the Child Life field still exist in countries without existing or recognized Child Life programming.

Due to undefined therapeutic photography practices and environments where Child Life is still finding its presence, supervision has proven challenging but is not impossible. The author's supervision has primarily come from local professionals within partner organizations and has included play therapists, narrative therapists, educators, and social workers. While local supervision is essential to ensure cultural learning and accountability, it is ideal to also include supervision from the lens of Child Life and therapeutic photography. Connections for both therapeutic photography and Child Life within the continent of Africa are slowly growing. In the meantime, due to the gift of our virtual world, remote supervision in both fields can meet these requirements until local Child Life and therapeutic photography supervision are available.

FUTURE ASPIRATIONS AND DIRECTIONS

Family integration and support have always been an important part of Through Their Eyes programs. In the early days of programming, this looked like parents supporting the process, actively participating in the exhibition, and hopefully moving forward with stronger bonds and attunement. Upon completion of the author's thesis that explored family strengths where both children and parents created visual stories, the author was delighted to see how the participatory, shared experience for parents and children clarified, strengthened, and fostered positive family formation (Ribbens, 2020). South African laws advocate for the family, calling for interventions that strengthen positive relationships within the family and support positive parenting (Gould & Ward, 2015). The author is eager to partner locally and globally to continue to build and implement family-based therapeutic photography programs.

The author is eager to see more CLS, in traditional and non-traditional settings, harness the power of therapeutic photography to promote well-being and healing. As an arts-based initiative, therapeutic photography taps into play-based ways of engaging within an era where the majority of people have a camera in their pocket. This easily-accessible form of art is familiar to the masses. According to Bernard Marr, back in 2018, every minute of the day, 46,740 photos were posted on Instagram and 527,760 photos were shared on Snapchat; every day 300 million photos were uploaded onto Facebook (Marr, 2018). People are familiar with taking and sharing photos, but the audience of social media can increase insecurities and disconnection rather than harness the power of healthy formation and connection. The Child Life profession is primed to tap into this powerful tool, utilizing the camera to promote connection, communication, and healthy formation within the various sectors of society where Child Life is working. Whether in the hospital, classroom, hospice, or courtroom, to name a few, children can document their experiences, name and depict emotions, create resilience plans, depict routines and coping skills, outline their values, explore strengths and challenges - the topics that can be explored within a therapeutic photography intervention are endless.

Implementing therapeutic photography interventions can range from requiring very few to many resources. Resources required for a therapeutic photography program could include the following: cameras, a workbook or something to write reflections in, training materials, materials for printing photographs, and materials for an exhibition. Depending on the resources available to a facilitator, a program can be done with very few resources or could be resource-heavy with all the bells and whistles. While it is wonderful to have printed workbooks, the option to print all the photos, and to create an exhibition with printed photos, these elements are not necessary to have a meaningful and effective intervention. Because taking photographs is such a familiar and accessible tool nowadays, many participants or patients will already have access to a camera or a phone camera. If resources for printing photographs are not available, participants can share photos from their camera or phone. Additionally, virtual platforms can be explored as a way to safely share photos and stories throughout a program and even to exhibit the photos.

CONCLUSION

Berenice Abbott quips, "Photography helps people to see." Sawubona, an isiZulu greeting, translates in English to "we see you." This chapter describes how stress and trauma can hinder healthy development and the ability to see the self and beyond the self. The emerging field of therapeutic photography offers invitations to playfully see, re-see, and re-story. As participants observe their surroundings and make images, they begin to observe the self which results in seeing themselves, their lived experiences, and others in new ways, paving the way for healthy development and stronger families. When situating this powerful tool within Child Life practices, CLS can quickly foster therapeutic relationships and create safe spaces for reflection, learning, and expression in order to prevent long-term effects of stress and trauma.

REFERENCES

Association of Child Life Professionals. (2001). *Mission, values, vision and operating principles.* https://www.childlife.org/the-child-life-profession/values

Association of Child Life Professionals. (2019). *Child life competencies.* https://www.childlife.org/docs/default-source/the-child-life-profession/childlifecompetenciesjune2016.pdf?sfvrsn=2

Association of Child Life Professionals. (2020). *Association of Child Life Professionals position statement on child life in community settings.* https://childlife.org/docs/default-source/aclp-official-documents/updated-governance_position-statement-cl-practice-in-community-settings.pdf?sfvrsn=fa228c4d_10

Benard, B. (2006). Using strengths-based practice to tap the resilience of families. *The Strengths Perspective in Social Work Practice*, 197-220.

Benjamin, L., & Crawford-Browne, S. (2010). *The psychological impact of continuous traumatic stress–limitations of existing diagnostic frameworks* [Paper Presentation]. Continuous Traumatic Stress in South Africa Workshop, Department of Psychology, University of Cape Town, South Africa.

Böök, M. L., & Mykkänen, J. (2014). Photo-narrative processes with children and young people. *International Journal of Child, Youth and Family Studies, 5*(4.1).

Bronfenbrenner, U. (1986). Ecology of the family as a context for human development: Research perspectives. *Developmental Psychology, 22*(6), 723–742. doi:10.1037/0012-1649.22.6.723

Cluver, L. D., Meinck, F., Steinert, J. I., Shenderovich, Y., Doubt, J., Romero, R. H., ... Gardner, F. (2018). Parenting for lifelong health: A pragmatic cluster randomised controlled trial of a non-commercialised parenting programme for adolescents and their families in South Africa. *BMJ Global Health, 3*(1), e000539. doi:10.1136/bmjgh-2017-000539 PMID:29564157

DeFrain, J., Asay, S., & Geggie, J. (2010). Family strengths: An international perspective. In F. Arney & D. Scott (Eds.), *Working with vulnerable families: A partnership approach* (pp. 29–48). Cambridge University Press. doi:10.1017/CBO9780511845376.004

DeFrain, J., & Asay, S. M. (2007). Strong families around the world: An introduction to the family strengths perspective. *Marriage & Family Review, 41*(1-2), 1–10. doi:10.1300/J002v41n01_01

Ebersöhn, L., Sefotho, M., Mampane, R., Loots, T., Omidire, F., Sherman, V., & Nxumalo-Tsebe, T. (2014). *Imbeleko report: Cultivating resourcefulness, not dependency*. Academic Press.

Espe-Sherwindt, M. (2008). Family-centered practice: Collaboration, competency and evidence. *Support for Learning, 23*(3), 136–143. doi:10.1111/j.1467-9604.2008.00384.x

Freeman, J. C., Epston, D., & Lobovits, D. (1997). *Playful approaches to serious problems: Narrative therapy with children and their families*. WW Norton & Company.

Gibson, N. (2018). *Therapeutic photography: Enhancing self-esteem, self-efficacy and resilience*. Jessica Kingsley Publishers.

Gould, C., & Ward, C. L. (2015). Positive parenting in South Africa: Why supporting families is key to development and violence prevention. *Institute for Security Studies. Policy Brief,* 77.

Grotberg, E. (1995). *A Guide to Promoting Resilience in Children: Strengthening the Human Spirit.* Bernard van Leer Foundation.

Marr, B. (2018). How much data do we create every day? The mind-blowing stats everyone should read. *Forbes*, *21*, 1–5.

Mkhwanazi, N., Makusha, T., Blackie, D., Manderson, L., Hall, K., & Huijbregts, M. (2018). Negotiating the care of children and support for caregivers. *Child Fam State, 70.*

Nkosi, B., & Daniels, P. (2007). Family Strengths. *Marriage & Family Review*, *41*(1-2), 11–26.

Oliver, C. (2014). The Fundamentals of Strengths-Based Practice. *Relational Child & Youth Care Practice, 27*(3), 46–50. doi:10.1300/J002v41n01_02

Phola. (2022). *Therapeutic approaches.* Phola – Healing the Nation. https://phola.org/therapeutic-approaches/

Ribbens, M. (2020). *Through Their Eyes: Photo Stories about Family Strengths in Johannesburg, South Africa* [Unpublished master's thesis]. University of Nebraska-Lincoln. https://digitalcommons.unl.edu/cehsdiss/374/

Röttger-Rössler, B., Scheidecker, G., & Lam, A. T. A. (2019). Narrating visualized feelings: Photovoice as a tool for researching affects and emotions among school students. In A. Kahl (Ed.), *Analyzing Affective Societies* (pp. 78–98). Routledge. doi:10.4324/9780429424366-5

Siegel, D. J. (2015). *Brainstorm: The power and purpose of the teenage brain*. Penguin.

Swick, K. J., & Williams, R. D. (2006). An analysis of Bronfenbrenner's bio-ecological perspective for early childhood educators: Implications for working with families experiencing stress. *Early Childhood Education Journal*, *33*(5), 371–378. doi:10.100710643-006-0078-y

Theron, L. C., & Theron, A. M. (2010). A critical review of studies of South African youth resilience, 1990-2008. *South African Journal of Science*, *106*(7), 1–8. doi:10.4102ajs.v106i7/8.252

Tsirogianni, S., & Andreouli, E. (2011). Beyond social cohesion: The role of 'fusion of horizons' in inter-group solidarities. *Papers on Social Representations, 20*(1), 5.1-5.25.

Van der Kolk, B. (2014). *The body keeps the score: Mind, brain and body in the transformation of trauma.* Penguin UK.

Weiser, J. (2004). PhotoTherapy techniques in counselling and therapy—Using ordinary snapshots and photo-interactions to help clients heal their lives. *Canadian Art Therapy Association Journal, 17*(2), 23–53. doi:10.1080/08322473.2004.11432263

ADDITIONAL READING

Al Abdullah, Q. R. & DiPucchio, K. (2010). *The sandwich swap.* Little, Brown Books for Young Readers.

Brown, P. (2014). *My Teacher Is a Monster! (No, I am Not.)*. Little, Brown Books for Young Readers.

Charlip, R. (1993). *Fortunately.* Aladdin.

Cottin, M. (2008). *The black book of colors*. Groundwood Books.

Hall, M. (2011). *Perfect square*. Greenwillow Books.

John, J., & Smith, L. (2018). *Giraffe problems*. Random House Books.

Kostecki-Shaw, J. S. (2011). *Same, same but different. Henry Holt and Company*. BYR.

Munson, D. (2000). *Enemy pie*. Chronicle Books.

Percival, T. (2021). *The invisible*. Simon & Schuster Children's UK.

Rosenthal, A. K., & Lichtenheld, T. (2009). *Duck! Rabbit!* Chronicle Books.

KEY TERMS AND DEFINITIONS

Attunement: Resonating with the inner world and needs of another person.

Continuous Trauma: Trauma associated with living in communities of high levels violence, repeated exposure to violence, and where the person recovering lives with the same on-going threat.

Empowerment: The act of helping others to know they are capable and competent to achieve their goals.

PhotoTherapy: A tool used by trained professionals in formal counseling settings.

Resilience: The capacity to bounce back after setbacks and challenges.

Self-Efficacy: The ability to make and produce things.

Self-Esteem: Feeling good about oneself and believing you can achieve what you set out to do.

Strengths Perspective: A framework of working with people that prioritizes personal and cultural strengths rather than problems or pathology.

Therapeutic Photography: A technique or tool used to promote reflection and that does not require a trained counselor or therapist, but does require clearly defined outcomes to increase self-esteem, self-efficacy, and empowerment.

Ubuntu: An African philosophy that emphasizes the interconnectedness of humanity and way of living.

Section 3
Populations

Chapter 11
Disability

Vanessa Carolyn Andrews
Elizabeth Seton Children's Center, USA

ABSTRACT

The number of children living with a disability is substantial and expanding. Children with disabilities and their families are disproportionately exposed to adverse experiences, increased stress and stigmatization, face more barriers, and are more likely to be diagnosed with mental health disorders. Unfortunately, adequate and specifically tailored professionals, programs, and interventions aimed to enhance resilience, support families, and decrease stigma have not increased proportionately. Certified Child Life Specialists (CCLS) promote coping, validate emotions, and use play-based techniques to build relationships and increase understanding of difficult experiences. By increasing the availability of Certified Child Life Specialists in community settings, children with disabilities and their families will gain additional advocacy, insight, and opportunities to lead fuller, more supported lives.

INTRODUCTION

With advances in science, technology, medicine, and life-saving interventions, children with disabilities, complex medical needs, and comorbid conditions are living longer lives with more specialized interventions. The number of children defined as having a disability has steadily increased throughout the last decade (World Health Organization, 2021). With over two hundred and forty million children and young adults globally categorized as having disabilities (Unicef, 2021) and disability strongly correlating with poverty and inequity (Kuper et al., 2014), Child Life Specialists must expand services beyond the hospital to decrease the risk of trauma and increase access to quality care.

Universally, children with disabilities experience more adverse experiences such as abuse, neglect, and maltreatment (Ammerman, 1997), have challenges with maladaptive behaviors, difficulty communicating their needs, experience more healthcare exposure with less access to quality care (World Health Organization, 2021) and have undermanaged pain experiences (Breau & Burkitt, 2009). Interpersonal relationships can also be challenging due to stigma, isolation, bullying, attachment challenges, and communication barriers. These factors often lead to undesirable and unsafe behaviors, negatively impact mental health, and contribute to lifelong health disparities.

DOI: 10.4018/978-1-6684-5097-0.ch011

Disability-related stressors also affect family members. Caregivers with increasing responsibilities have less time to manage myriad emotions that accompany having a child with a disability. Caregivers must manage additional care, services, behaviors, and educational opportunities and are responsible for ensuring the quality of life for their child. These stressors have been noted in families globally (Olawale et al., 2013; Cheshire et al., 2010; Basaran et al., 2013; Wu, et al., 2017). In order to ensure adequate adjustment for the future, professionals must address the individual and unique needs of siblings. Siblings function better long term when they receive specific interventions to process their experiences.

Advocacy and providing quality care that focuses on strengths and individual needs are essential to optimize functional outcomes, yet barriers remain. Despite the need for interventions, adequate and equitable services have not increased proportionally, and access to quality services is not universally available. These gaps should be considered an opportunity for growth and improvement and can be mitigated with the professional skills of a Certified Child Life Specialist (CCLS).

Child Life Specialists focus on normalizing experiences, supporting and validating emotions, and processing potentially adverse and traumatic experiences while considering the perspective of the individual, family, and culture with a resilience-focused, family-centered lens. Their expertise in play-based interventions and emphasis on the value of building and maintaining relationships allow for unique expression and processing of experiences. This combination of professional scope and individually-tailored interventions is particularly impactful for children with disabilities but is limited to pediatric hospitals and emergency departments where Child Life Specialists primarily practice.

To positively impact the lives of children with disabilities, Child Life Specialists need to focus on meeting the needs of children with disabilities while becoming a standard of care in community settings. Settings include but are not limited to schools, daycares, respite care, outpatient clinics, rehabilitation centers, day programs, and relevant community nonprofits. Additionally, the case for employing Child Life Specialists in young-adult and geriatric facilities is warranted to ensure adults with disabilities continue to receive resilience-enhancing services, particularly regarding potentially traumatic medical procedures, transitions, and other triggers.

This chapter connects the specific needs of those with disabilities and the unique professional scope of Child Life Specialists constructed through theory, evidence-based practice, and case studies.

Specific chapter objectives:

- Discuss the history and evolution of language and models of disability, community, and culture and how this influences care.
- Consider disability-related stressors and disparities for children with disabilities and their families.
- Understand the correlation between stressors and behavior.
- Consider the experiences of children with disabilities and their families through a Diversity, Equity, and Inclusion (D.E.I.) lens.
- Conceptualize the current practices of Child Life Specialists with children who have disabilities.
- Apply successful child life evidence-based practice in hospitals to a variety of broader community settings.
- Contemplate future directions for continued advocacy of the child life profession as a standard of care for children with disabilities in all settings.

LANGUAGE AND TERMINOLOGY

Just as societal perspectives and norms evolve, so does language. Language is culturally influential, shaping our conscious and unconscious beliefs and guiding our responses. Specific language choices have been used in this chapter as described below.

- **Disability** vs. **Special Needs.** While "special needs" continues to be used, a shift towards using the word disability is occurring. Advocates for this shift posit that using any term other than disability further stigmatizes the experience of living with a disability due to passive avoidance of the word. As the National Center on Disability and Journalism (2021) notes, the phrase "special needs" "euphemistically stigmatizes that which is different." In an attempt to both avoid euphemisms and recognize the perspectives of individuals with disabilities, this chapter uses the term disability throughout. However, individuals should always explore language-specific preferences before making assumptions.
- **Person-centered** vs. **Identity-first** language. Conceptually developed in the 80s, person-first language (e.g., an individual with a disability) aims to separate the person from their diagnosis, arguing that an individual is more than their identity (APA, 2020). However, proponents of identity-first language (e.g., disabled person) state that the concept of considering identity second undermines its influential role. Furthermore, when focus deliberately shifts away from identity, it prevents individuals from proudly and unashamedly belonging to their own culture. In other words, insinuating a person should come before their identity forces individuals to disassociate from the very identity which is so influential in their lives, causing further marginalization (Botha et al., 2021). Ultimately, it is essential to embody heightened awareness of both perspectives, and language choice and consideration should be the decision of the individual it affects (APA, 2020). Considering varying perspectives and respecting the inherent choice of the individual, this chapter uses both person-first and identity-first language.
- **Neurodiversity.** Inclusive of autism and other neurologically-based disabilities, the term neurodiverse describes these as a natural continuum and evolution of the brain (Sumner & Brown, 2015).
- **Disability Culture.** Referring to individuals with disabilities as a community with their own norms, history, barriers, and culture honors the community experience and shared identity within that community (Spassiani & Friedman, 2014).
- **Non-speaking vs. Non-verbal.** Increasingly preferred over non-verbal is the term 'non-speaking.' Non-speaking includes individuals who use augmentative technology and other methods of expression exclusive of words and demonstrates that individuals communicate over a spectrum of approaches. Many individuals who do not verbalize exclusively with words feel the term non-speaking is more inclusive of their particular communication method and does not stigmatize them as only being capable of receptive language (NeuroClastic, 2021).

DEFINING DISABILITY

The inherent challenge in defining a population is that it may inadvertently cause further marginalization. Regardless, definitions help draw distinctive boundaries that influence policies, guide the creation of protective laws, and build impactful services. Disability is a vast topic covered by many but singularly defined by few. Globally, definitions vary from broad in scope to narrow in focus. The following definitions are a handful of examples from primarily American organizations. Reviewing each definition informs the direction and creation of further definitions.

Americans with Disabilities Act (ADA). The Americans with Disabilities Act (ADA) defines disability as "a physical or mental impairment that substantially limits one or more major life activities of such individuals; a record of such impairment; or being regarded as having such impairment." This definition excludes mention of specific disabilities, making it one of the broader definitions available (ADA, n.d.).

Center for Disease Control (CDC). The Center for Disease Control defines disability as: "any condition of the body or mind (impairment) that makes it more difficult for the person with the condition to do certain activities (activity limitation) and interact with the world around them (participation restrictions)" (CDC, 2017b). Focusing on a diverse population with a wide range of needs, the CDC explains the effect disability has on everything from cognition to mental health (CDC, 2017b).

World Health Organization (WHO). Offering a global definition, WHO refers to disability as the interaction between individuals with a health condition (e.g., cerebral palsy, Down syndrome, and depression) and personal and environmental factors (e.g., negative attitudes, inaccessible transportation, public buildings, and limited social supports) (World Health Organization, 2021).

Individuals with Disabilities Education Act (IDEA). Concentrating on providing equitable and individually-tailored educational opportunities for children with disabilities, IDEA revolves around creating an Individualized Education Plan (IEP), providing education in the least restrictive environment, involving caregivers and teachers, and ensuring appropriate educational opportunities are provided at no cost to families. IDEA defines disability as "having an intellectual disability, a hearing impairment (including deafness), a speech or language impairment, a visual impairment (including blindness), a serious emotional disturbance (referred to in this part as 'emotional disturbance'), an orthopedic impairment, autism, traumatic brain injury, another health impairment, a specific learning disability, deaf-blindness, or multiple disabilities, and who, by reason thereof, needs special education and related services." (US Department of Education, n. d.).

National Academies of Sciences, Engineering, and Medicine. Pulling from various other definitions of disability, the National Academies of Sciences, Engineering, and Medicine (2018) focuses on the influence of the environment, and the functional limitation(s) has on the ability to participate fully in life events. Specifically, they define disability as "an environmentally contextualized health-related limitation in a child's existing or emerging capacity to perform developmentally appropriate activities and participate, as desired, in society" (p 44).

To be focused yet inclusive, this chapter's perspective on disability aligns with a definition that considers environmental contexts, health-related limitations, and capacity to perform developmentally, as the National Academies of Sciences, Engineering, and Medicine (2018) suggests. Furthermore, though this chapter uses the broad term disability, the focus is primarily on individuals with more severe and limiting forms of disability with intellectual and developmental delays and those considered neurodiverse.

HISTORICAL PERSPECTIVES

While language and definitions unquestionably contribute to a greater understanding of concepts, they must be considered contextually in history. A complete historical overview of disability is beyond the scope of this chapter. However, a brief discussion of the evolution of the models of disability is warranted. These models help shape perspectives while providing a framework through which individuals with disabilities see themselves and, conversely, how society sees them. Understanding these models is essential to delivering culturally-sensitive, individualized, and practical assessments and interventions.

Medical Model of Disability

The medical model posits that something within an individual can, and should, be repaired or changed to improve functioning rather than accepted or accommodated by society (Francis & Silvers, 2016; Shyman, 2016). Focusing mainly on diagnosis for treatment, the medical model seeks to "isolate a set of particular ''facts'' or indices of disability, usually in the form of definable physical or intellectual characteristics, which separates those for whom ''normal functioning'' is attainable without treatment and those for whom it is not" (Shyman, 2016, p.368). While helpful in writing policy and defining treatment, this model can marginalize individuals, increasing the chasm between the disabled and non-disabled (Petasis, 2019).

Social Model of Disability

In contrast, the social model of disability posits that disability lies not within the individual but in society's inability to accommodate and accept atypical functioning, as defined by society (Pestasis, 2019). This shift in the conceptualization of the inherent location (society vs. person) of the disability allows for more significant normalization. The move from fixing individuals to fixing social norms leads to more collectively-focused solutions with a tendency toward systemic change (Dirth & Branscombe, 2017).

Biopsychosocial Model

Balancing medical and societal origins, the biopsychosocial model recognizes that both perspectives influence how impactful, problematic, or challenging a disability will become for the individual (Pestasis, 2019). In this way, interventions should have a medical and social focus to improve health in conjunction with societal norms. Noted is the alignment of the biopsychosocial model of disability with Bronfenbrenner's Ecological Systems theory (1979). Both call attention to and support the individual's experiences being affected by their immediate environment and the larger societal context in which they exist. Given the overlap with the ethics, guiding principles, competencies, and medical/developmental background within the child life profession, this framework will be the primary model through which this chapter views disability.

DISABILITY-RELATED STRESSORS

Societal, organizational, environmental, and attitudinal hurdles add to the challenges children with disabilities face. Family stress, increased trauma, decreased communication ability, sensory issues, and disparate access to play and social opportunities lead to struggles in attachment and peer relationships, negatively influencing overall physical, psychosocial, and mental health. These challenges increase when considered in the context of societal norms, barriers, and expectations that primarily accommodate non-disabled individuals.

Trauma

An estimated 50% of children will experience at least one significant traumatic event in their lifetime (Forkey et al., 2021), and that number is higher for children with disabilities (Santoro et al., 2018; Berg et al., 2019; World Health Organization, 2021). Such trauma may include abuse, neglect, maltreatment, medical trauma, natural disasters, discrimination, and ableism. The experience of trauma can have significant and lasting negative impacts on attachment, building resilience, the stress response, and physical and mental health.

The relationship between physical and mental health has been widely studied (Felitti et al., 1998; Cronholm et al., 2015) and is reciprocal. As physical health and disabilities increase, so does the likelihood of accompanying mental health challenges which in turn affect physical health. In 1998, Felitti et al. conducted the original Adverse Childhood Experiences (ACEs) study. The study found an explicit connection between the number of ACEs (violence, physical, psychological, or sexual abuse, incarcerated caregiver, or caregiver with a mental illness) experienced as a child and incidences of serious physical health problems later in life such as heart disease, lung disease, liver damage, and cancer (Felitti et al., 1998). While the study has been tremendously impactful in promoting trauma-informed care, it lacks diversity. As a result, researchers conducted subsequent, expanded, and more diverse studies with similar findings (Cronholm et al., 2015). Notably, the ACE's study illustrates how adverse childhood experiences impact physical health as an adult. In short, understanding the brain-body connection is vital.

Additional studies have indicated that children with intellectual disabilities are four to five times as likely to have some type of psychiatric disorder than children without intellectual disability (Einfeld & Tonge, 1996), often resulting in unsafe behaviors. Unfortunately, despite the risk factors, access to quality behavioral and mental health interventions remains inadequate (McCarthy & Boyd, 2002).

Medical Trauma

Hospital environments can be particularly traumatic for children with disabilities resulting in suboptimal experiences and maladaptive behaviors (Jensen et al., 2020; Andrews, 2015; Nunez, 2018; Liddle et al., 2018). Additionally, due to the high prevalence of comorbidities, individuals with disabilities experience increased exposure to emergency rooms, specialists, surgeries, and even general medical visits (Schieve et al., 2012), causing children with disabilities more susceptible to experiencing traumatic medical stress. Additionally, higher levels of anxiety can lead to potentially harmful behaviors, further increasing trauma, delaying procedures altogether (Johnson et al., 2012; Behar & Cooper, 2015), and can result in using additional traumatic methods such as sedation and restraint to complete the procedure (McGonigle et al., 2014).

Communication

Many children with disabilities also face challenges communicating verbally and expressively, which attributes to their communication style differing from the traditional verbal exchange. Additionally, due to communication delays, well-intentioned adults may not provide sufficient time to understand the conversation adequately. Children with disabilities often use technology to help them interact and communicate with others. Augmentative or Alternative Communication devices (AAC) are the most commonly used for those with disabilities. From low-tech (Board Maker or Social stories) to high-tech devices (eye gaze and applications for iPads and computers), technology enhances the ability for expression and thereby further increases sense of self and control, which decreases negative or unwanted behaviors (Wang & Barnard, 2004). Unfortunately, reliance on devices or others to communicate has inherent challenges. Technology can be fickle, frustrating, and time-consuming. Professionals and caregivers may not make or have time to allow for this type of communication or troubleshoot when technology breaks down, consequently leading to unreliable or an absence of communication methods and frustration on the part of the individual communicator.

Behaviors

Considering the increased exposure to adverse experiences, challenges in communication and accessibility, and lack of access to appropriate professionals, it is not surprising that children with disabilities exhibit increased maladaptive behavioral patterns such as outbursts, self-injury, sensory-seeking/stimulatory behavior, or aversions, and perceived non-compliance. Behaviors are communicative, and notably, children with disabilities often exhibit undesirable behaviors, particularly when unable to communicate or not being understood. Despite valid origins, these behaviors are often seen as annoyances, described as atypical, or disruptive. Furthermore, behaviors may become unsafe to the individual and others, and staff may implement interventions such as restraints, therapeutic holds, or isolation to maintain safety (Bultas et al., 2016, as cited in Liddle & Sonnentag, 2020). Behaviors can be pain-related, emotionally based, or situationally specific. Regardless of why they occur, behaviors can be seen as maladaptive rather than communicative, and remediation rather than acknowledgment is often emphasized.

Sensory Challenges

Children with disabilities are more likely to have increased challenges with sensory needs and integration (Gupta et al., 2019). Individuals may be hypersensitive or hyposensitive to environments, and sensitivities can come in the form of preferences and aversions for each of the senses. Individuals with heightened sensory needs often have difficulty with sensory integration and organization. Sensory regulation is specifically problematic in medical settings due to the myriad of different sensations surrounding the individual. Additionally, sensory challenges can cause difficulty with daily routines and activities such as teeth/hair brushing, showering/bathing, toileting, and playing resulting in cumulative trauma during everyday experiences. These challenges can further impact the child's ability to integrate into social and academic settings.

Attachment

Attachment forms as infants grow and is dependent primarily on the relationship between a child and their consistent caregiver. Attachment theorists agree that the process is complex and multidirectional and can influence relationships, regulation, and self-identity (Ainsworth et al., 1978; Bowlby, 1969). Children with disabilities, particularly those with an intellectual disability or developmental delay, may experience difficulties with relational behavior and less secure attachment (Hamadi & Fletcher, 2021). At times, the struggle to effectively communicate paired with others' inability to understand can lead to feelings of isolation, incompetence, and helplessness. Caregivers, in turn, may become less responsive to their child's needs which further affects self-esteem (Hamadi & Fletcher, 2021). This persistent pattern negatively affects an individual's ability to develop a secure attachment with caregivers.

Disparities in Play

Children's play is vital to their social, emotional, physical, and sensory development. Play boosts creativity, stimulates learning and imagination, and is critical for developing positive attachment (Ginsburg et al., 2007). Many things factor into restricted play opportunities for children with disabilities. Environmental access, social skills, and toy type can influence the amount and quality of play children experience (Driscoll & Carter, 2009; Ivory & McCollum, 1999). Findings show a significant difference in participation in play between children with disabilities and their non-disabled peers, leading to challenges socially (King et al., 2009 as cited in Barron et al., 2017). Outdoor play environments, such as public playgrounds, often lack accommodations for children with disabilities. These restrictions inhibit full participation and reinforce the notion that children with disabilities should not participate in certain places (Barron et al., 2017). Furthermore, when disabilities affect a child's ability to communicate via language, adults can underestimate or misinterpret the child's ability to play, exacerbating the disconnect between the child and caregiver (Short et al., 2020)

Peer Relationships

Children with disabilities can also face challenges obtaining and maintaining successful peer relationships. Children living at home may be isolated from peers and only have interactions with typically-developing siblings. Inaccessible playgrounds, gyms, or recreational opportunities may further hinder opportunities for social interaction and friendships. However, social inclusion promotes positive peer relationships and can lead to successful outcomes (McGuire & Meadan, 2020). A lack of peer interactions can exacerbate psychosocial difficulties since peers feature prominently in the concept of self and self-esteem. Lastly, bullying trends are higher in children who have physical disabilities or long-term, chronic health issues (Pinquart, 2016) which can reinforce self-esteem challenges and further limit peer interactions.

Socioeconomic Factors

Not only do children with disabilities and their caregivers face inequities due to societal barriers and medically-diagnosed challenges, but further intersectionality exists related to race, culture, ethnicity, and socioeconomic status. Children with disabilities born into families with less financial means may not have equal opportunities for adequate interventions. Finding appropriate and accessible childcare for children with disabilities is another challenge. Families with little to no income may need to forgo work to care for their child and experience higher costs specific to having a child with a disability. Child Life Specialists should explore each of these reciprocal and cyclical relationships, however a comprehensive examination is beyond the scope of this chapter.

Family Systems

The interplay between disability, society, family, and culture is complex, multifaceted, and unique. Family systems are intricate and fundamentally altered when one member has a disability. Stressors that affect a child with disabilities also affect the entire family, which further impacts the child. Frequent appointments, hospitalizations, rehabilitation, comorbidities, financial burdens, and additional care coordination may strain optimal psychosocial functioning. Families may also experience lifelong complex grief and ambiguous loss related to having a child with a disability that requires long-term interventions.

Siblings

Literature on siblings' experiences living with and caring for their brother or sister with a disability varies greatly. While some siblings report positive outcomes (Taunt & Hastings, 2002; Stoneman, 2005; Luijkx, van der Putten & Vlaskamp, 2016), others report feeling anger, embarrassment, fear, anxiety, jealousy, over or under-identification, guilt, and feelings of being responsible for the disability (Meyer & Vadasy, 2008).

Siblings can feel left out, unseen, and overlooked compared to the attention given to the child with a disability. Siblings may also struggle to understand their brother or sister's disability or blame themselves irrationally for the disability (Pearson, 2009). Other factors such as gender, birth order, age, ethnicity, self-esteem, perceived information about disability, and underlying personality can influence how siblings manifest their experiences (Tudor & Lerner, 2015). Additionally, siblings often take on additional care roles to help the family, impacting their sense of self and individual identity.

SUCCESS IN MEDICAL SETTINGS: CHILD LIFE'S ROLE

It is abundantly clear that children with disabilities and their families face multiple challenges and adversities that are complex and interrelated. Prioritizing access to disability-affirming services is essential to mitigate potential long-term effects. Given the increased healthcare encounters children with disabilities face, it is no surprise that Child Life Specialists have proactively recognized these challenges, working towards positive interventions for resolution. Areas of focus include partnering with families, environmental modifications, staff education, communication, play and normalization, and family support.

Partnering with Families

Providing family-centered care has become a staple in pediatrics over the last decade and is often spearheaded by Child Life Specialists. Research has shown that developing relationships with families and recognizing that caregivers are the experts on their child is a successful approach to mitigating negative experiences for children with disabilities (Fraatz, & Durand, 2021). Working towards trusting, supportive, and mutually reciprocal relationships with caregivers and being mindful of continuous communication increase the quality of care and healthcare satisfaction (Bell et al., 2009; Oulton et al., 2019). Family members can help identify triggers, provide helpful child-specific information, and help develop a functional coping plan for success (Jolly, 2012). By communicating this before the procedures, children and staff are less likely to get injured (Johnson et al., 2012), and the procedure is less likely to result in trauma. Additionally, partnering with caregivers to obtain child-specific information can help Child Life Specialists figure out and provide comforting experiences. Providing comforting items or experiences can enhance a child's coping ability (Gariepy & Howe, 2003, as cited in Burns-Nader & Hernandez-Reif, 2016).

Each child or young adult has individual preferences, needs, and fears that, when possible, should be explored before meeting in person. Caregivers of children with disabilities have described the importance of communication with professionals, including obtaining information about their child and their preferences before the procedure or transition (Oulton et al., 2019). Furthermore, caregivers often act as interpreters for their child's needs, emotions, feelings, and experiences. Child Life Specialists play a crucial role in helping advocate for the use of devices to allow children with disabilities, particularly communicative disabilities, the time and space they need to express themselves. Additionally, partnering with professionals like Child Life Specialists who understand behaviors and can help individuals feel understood, can interrupt the negatively reinforced pattern of behaviors that lead to traumatic experiences.

One example of an intervention aimed at including the family perspective in care is the creation of Adaptive Care Plans (ACPs) by the team of Child Life Specialists at Cincinnati Children's Hospital Medical Center. Aimed at addressing the specific sensory, communication, and coping styles of children with disabilities by obtaining caregiver interviews and proactively communicating this to healthcare professionals, ACPs have been instrumental in improving healthcare experiences. After using the ACP, anecdotal reports indicated that children for whom the ACP was implemented experienced less distress and increased coping (Liddle et al., 2018). A follow-up study revealed similar results showing that children diagnosed with ASD experienced greater coping and fewer challenges when implementing an ACP (Liddle & Sonnentag, 2021).

Optimizing the Environment

As previously discussed, children with disabilities often have comorbid sensory challenges that affect their ability to function in overstimulating environments. Unfamiliar smells, sounds, visuals, and tactile experiences can trigger maladaptive emotional responses. Child Life Specialists recognize the importance of being aware of and prepared for these reactions and have implemented changes in hospitals. Indeed, Child Life Specialists have advocated for "sensory-friendly" adaptations to help decrease unpleasant experiences and increase positive coping (Inova Newsroom, 2018). Awareness of saturated sensory areas (beeping, alarms, bright lights, overhead pages, televisions, radios) and potential tactile triggers (gown tags, Band-Aids, pulse-ox monitors) is the first step to alleviating these stressors for hypersensitive individuals. With input from Child Life Specialists, hospitals have taken steps to modify environments resulting in more successful visits and procedures.

Conversely, sensory-seeking individuals cope best when stimulatory options are available. Fidget spinners, sensory carts, adapted toys, and weighted vests all offer positive sensory experiences that induce calming and natural coping. These items provide a favorable exploratory sensory option, and Child Life Specialists can use them as a distraction during procedures. Drake et al. (2012) found that coping kits containing sensory distraction items helped calm patients down while offering positive distractions during treatment.

Staff Education

Studies have shown that increased staff education surrounding disabilities, disability culture, and specific needs of these children increase successful outcomes (Johnson et al., 2012). Hospital staff also report not receiving enough educational support to adequately understand the needs of children with disabilities (Baker, 2008 as cited in Johnson et al., 2012). Child Life Specialists often become valuable sources of educational information to bridge this gap in care. Proficient in communicating many of the above-stated concepts, considerations, and standards, Child Life Specialists offer vital insights that alleviate stressors, normalize behavior, and alter perspectives to be more disability-focused. Consequently, healthcare professionals are more likely to provide sensitive, individualized, and effective care.

Preparation

Adequate preparation leads to success when children experience potentially anxiety-provoking environments. Conversely, staff should also be prepared so they understand the child they will be working with and how to support them. This is especially true for children with disabilities, who have more successful outcomes when expectations are explicit and needs are understood by receiving staff (Glasper, 2017; Liddle & Sonnentag, 2020). To increase preparedness for children with disabilities, Child Life Specialists have developed and implemented various interventions aimed at improving experiences. Pre-operative tours (both in-person and virtual), social stories, specifically tailored preparation books, and adaptive medical play have been instrumental in increasing coping, decreasing behaviors, and mitigating traumatic experiences.

Though specific research with children with disabilities, specifically cognitive or intellectual disabilities, is lacking, Thompson and Stanford (1981) suggest that it is vital to consider delivering information in a way that matches developmental levels and cognitive capabilities. They go on to suggest that research does not indicate a lower age limit for preparation to be beneficial. Inferring from the success of preparing children as young as infancy, even children with severe cognitive and intellectual disabilities benefit from preparation. Child Life Specialists have addressed this in the hospital setting when working with children with disabilities by creating individually tailored preparation books for any potentially triggering or traumatizing event. Crucial for best outcomes is for these stories to be specific, progressive, and accurate, particularly of surroundings and sensory information. For example, a child with acquired anoxic brain injury due to drowning may be triggered by showers, baths, or running water. Creating an individualized preparation book to help the child understand the steps involved in the shower and repeatedly reviewing this prior to showering can help the child regain control over their safety. While reading the story, the child life specialist may pause, saying, 'the nurse is turning on the water; you are safe.' Similarly, the child life specialist may also be present during the shower to provide additional support mirroring the written story.

Play

Play is a "healing modality through which child life practitioners promote growth and development of infants, children, and youth" (Child Life Council, 2002, as cited in Turner, 2009, p23). If play is a child's natural form of communication, and medical experiences and hospitalizations can potentially be sources of trauma, children use play to make sense of these experiences. However, due to lack of access, differing physical capabilities, and variations in play styles, children with disabilities are often afforded fewer opportunities to play. Child Life Specialists in hospital settings recognize these disparities and apply interventions to increase access to play for children with disabilities. Simple modifications and adaptations to toys coupled with scaffolding can help children with disabilities engage in play that is meaningful, effective, and can provide specific information about an upcoming medical test or procedure (medical play). From low-technology (velcro handles) to high-technology (robotics, switch-adapted toys, and adapted video games), Child Life Specialists continue to grow their knowledge about the importance of play opportunities and accessibility for this population. However, research on the effectiveness of adapted play experiences in hospital settings is sparse, creating an opportunity for specialists to expand knowledge in this area.

Medical Play

Medical play, defined as play that includes characteristics such as the use of medical equipment and themes that guide preparation for upcoming procedures in hospital settings, is a foundational skill for Child Life Specialists (McCue, 1988, as cited in Wilkins, 2018). Medical play allows children a sense of control and mastery over their medical journey and helps alleviate fears and misconceptions for children with intellectual disabilities (Weaver et al., as cited in Glasper, 2017). However, most research focuses primarily on doing medical play with neurotypical children, and research on adaptive medical play for disabilities is sparse.

Case Example: Carole is a 10-year-old female diagnosed with extreme prematurity (born at 27 weeks gestation) with an extensive and complicated Neonatal Intensive Care Unit stay followed by continuous medical support at a pediatric long-term care hospital. She is non-speaking, dependent on a wheelchair for mobility, and cannot independently maneuver her wheelchair. Carole communicates primarily with facial expressions, grunts, and other non-verbal noises but is also able to use eye gaze and simple cue cards to make choices. Along with many other routine invasive medical procedures, Carole gets frequent blood draws to monitor sodium levels for a diagnosis of diabetes insipidus. During blood draws, Carole becomes extraordinarily upset when wheeled to the exam room door. She flails her arms, grimaces, screams, and tries to lash out at whoever is near her making it nearly impossible to complete the procedure safely. Attempts at distraction and support by the child life specialist in the clinic were unsuccessful, and staff suggested sedation. Previous attempts at medical play focused on blood draws were frustrating as the medical equipment needed (tubes, band-aids, doll, alcohol swab) was cumbersome for Carole to manipulate, and they often fell to the floor. On a whim, the child life specialist tried adapting medical play before the next attempted blood draw. The child life specialist used soft velcro to help secure the needed items to a tray connected to the top of the wheelchair and added soft fabric handles to the materials for easier manipulation. There was no clear understanding of Carole's ability to participate in, or understand the procedure steps, so the child life specialist presented the items and observed Carole's reaction. As had occurred previously, Carole became very excited upon seeing the objects and immediately tried to grab them. With the support of the child life specialist to open things (band-aid, alcohol swab), Carole proceeded to, in order, reenact the blood draw on the baby doll. Carole repeated this throughout the play session, which lasted 45 minutes. During the next blood draw attempt, the specialist used the doll and medical play items for the procedure (doll gets a tourniquet, Carole gets a tourniquet), and Carole was able to complete the blood draw safely and successfully.

Of note in the case study is adapting medical play for an individual with a disability. Carole's ability to participate in medical play was unknown and therefore overlooked. When the specialist did implement medical play, it appeared unsuccessful due to her inability to manipulate the items (leading to further frustration). With some easy, low-tech adaptations, Carole used play to process her experiences and help her understand the procedure while allowing the child life specialist to gain insight into Carole's understanding of the process. The opportunity for medical play allowed Carole to successfully gain much-needed control over her fear of the procedure. The child life specialist used the doll to demonstrate what steps would be next while offering Carole an opportunity to process the experience. Despite Carole's inability to verbalize her needs, the specialist's ability to presume competence successfully helps Carole navigate the experience with play.

Sibling Support

Having a brother or sister with an illness is a significant stressor (Coddington 1972 as cited in Pearson, 2009). Child Life Specialists play a crucial role in helping siblings understand, process, and make meaning from their experiences, helping them build resilience and develop a sense of self. In the more traditional hospital setting, Child Life Specialists pointedly provide interventions for siblings recognizing their often backseat role in the family dynamic given the attention that inevitably goes to the sibling with a disability. Additionally, Child Life Specialists are often the first professionals to help siblings understand complicated medical equipment, particularly when a sibling becomes disabled after a traumatic accident. Correcting misconceptions about the medical equipment and helping a sibling understand their brother or sister's diagnosis allows the sibling to process the information accurately. Child Life Specialists are often involved in helping facilitate one of the most widely recognized programs to support siblings of children with a disability, Sibshops (Meyer & Vadasy, 2008). Additionally, Child Life Specialists play a vital role in helping caregivers support non-disabled siblings.

In conclusion, Child Life Specialists play an essential role in assisting children with disabilities successfully navigate hospital experiences while minimizing potential trauma. While continued interventions must be applied in the hospital setting, the profession of child life must consider the full context of disability in the lives of children outside the hospital setting. Expanding the child life profession into the community is warranted to support children with disabilities across their contextual experiences.

Care in Outpatient Clinics

As previously noted, children with disabilities use specialized medical services more frequently than their peers. Indeed, medical specialties continue to evolve, and just as with the hospital, there is a high risk for potential trauma due to unsupported invasive and repetitive procedures. Given the percentage of clinic visitors who qualify as disabled and the already proven benefits for all children, hiring a child life specialist in all community clinics should be a standard of care. Only providing trauma-mitigating interventions in hospitalized settings is not enough to effectively prevent medical trauma. Rehabilitation clinics, bracing, Botox, dental offices, and other medical subspecialties would benefit from the knowledge Child Life Specialists contribute.

Additionally, children with disabilities often receive continuous related services such as physical therapy, occupational therapy, and speech and language therapy. While these professionals are excellent at building play into their goals and sessions, it can be more effective and enhance progress to have the additional help of a child life specialist. Child Life Specialists should continuously evaluate the specialty clinics in their community for opportunities for professional involvement to ensure each child is supported across the multitudes of their experiences.

COMMUNITY SETTINGS

Previous publications focusing on child life in community settings neglected the specific needs for services for children with disabilities. This chapter provides insight to assess the needs and provide services to children with disabilities in a variety of settings. The following section highlights a few critical settings Child Life Specialists should consider to most significantly impact children with disabilities and their families beyond the hospital setting.

Schools and Educational Settings

Building on the current movement for schools to become trauma-informed, expanding child life services to school systems in collaboration with school professionals (e.g., applied behavior analysis therapists, special education teachers, counselors) is the most efficient way to ensure continuity of care for children with disabilities in their lives outside the hospital. Child Life Specialists collaborate to provide children with disabilities support for transitions, medical and sensory needs and enhance peer relationships. Offering child life services during the school day also ensures that children, even in rural areas, have adequate preparation, support, and play opportunities when medically related experiences occur (Brown, 2008).

Siblings of children with disabilities are susceptible to adversity and would benefit tremendously from additional support. A school child life specialist can also offer support to siblings of children with disabilities by supporting them individually and supporting their siblings. Peer support groups provide opportunities to process their experience as a sibling with a disability and meet others with similar family dynamics. In these cases, group work can be a powerful tool to help siblings feel less isolated by being able to identify with other members of the group. On an individual level, school Child Life Specialists can provide interventions to assess a sibling's understanding of their brother or sister's diagnosis and implement creative interventions to help process this experience.

Specialized school settings are opportunities for Child Life Specialists in the community to support the most significant number of children with disabilities and their families. The professional scope and skillset of a child life specialist enhance the team of professionals already in place by providing preparation, support, emotional validation, and play in a developmentally appropriate way that further promotes the child's sense of self. Child Life Specialists seeking positions in the school system should also consider schools specifically designed to accommodate children with disabilities.

Lastly, many school-age kids experience trauma both outside the school setting and potentially inside the school walls as well. While professionals are in place to process this trauma, if it is sudden or acute, children who cannot verbally express themselves or their needs may inadvertently not receive services due to immediate attention focusing on typically developing children. Child Life Specialists on staff can be essential contributors to helping children with disabilities process everything from global pandemics to lockdown drills to mass terrorism and violence, especially given the propensity of these events to have a significant impact on children with disabilities and for them to receive fewer interventions. In a medical setting, Child Life Specialists focus on creating a sense of safety, control, and understanding. These same skills can be integral in helping children with disabilities cope during and after traumatic circumstances. Identifying post-trauma triggers and communicating this with teachers and staff is also essential to re-establishing safety for children with disabilities.

Pediatric Hospice

While advances in medical technology have increased the lifespan of children with disabilities, particularly those with medically complex needs and comorbid conditions, life-limiting conditions are still prevalent (Lindley et al., 2016). As previously mentioned, these families also navigate complicated emotions and complex grief while juggling the everyday stress associated with caring for a child with disabilities. Additionally, during end-of-life and palliative care, it is common for families to care for a child at home with the aid of community hospice services. Challenges in pain and symptom management exist as barriers to optimal care at home (Duc et al., 2017). Research shows that families find early introduction to palliative care services beneficial and would recommend early services to others (Liberman et al., 2016). The introduction of child life services early on in the process can be helpful to the family, siblings, and dying child.

Sibling support during end-of-life and palliative care is also essential. One study examining the impact of a sibling death (cancer) on a living brother or sister indicated an increase in anxiety, depression, and substance abuse one-year post-death. Additionally, there is a correlation between the prevalence of these adverse reactions and lack of support at the time of the death (Rosenberg et al., 2015).

Child Life Specialists recognize the caregiver stressors involved in caring for and grieving a child with complex medical needs and disabilities. Child life interventions for palliative care and end-of-life can include but are not limited to memory-making, play, art, and creative experiences directed toward the dying individual or other family members. Child Life Specialists are proficient in providing these services in hospital settings, and the skill easily transfers to community hospice and home.

Adult Care, Nursing Homes, and Geriatrics

While child life services have expanded into areas (namely hospitals) where adults are cared for, interventions primarily focus on children of ill or dying adults. Adults with disabilities and significant cognitive and intellectual impairments also benefit from the skills and interventions of Certified Child Life Specialists. Medical procedures continue into adulthood, and the accompanying stress, trauma, and fear persist. Many of the disability-related challenges in pediatrics continue into adulthood especially given the likelihood that cognition has not changed. As individuals age, medical procedures become more frequent as cognition declines, resulting in increased non-compliance and potential trauma. Already at risk for Post-Traumatic Stress due to a lifetime of exposure to potentially traumatizing medical experiences, adults with disabilities are in dire need of the continued interventions provided by Child Life Specialists.

Adult programs and facilities are often not familiar with the child life profession or, due to the word "child" in the professional title, assume services are only available or appropriate for children. As a result, gaps in service emerge. Additional staffing of Child Life Specialists in areas where young adults with cognitive limitations are integrated would sufficiently mitigate this additional trauma exposure.

Transitions from pediatric to young-adult care can also be challenging. Young adults find themselves surrounded by unfamiliar people, sights, sounds, and smells, which can be triggering. Additionally, there is a lack of appropriate placement for young adults with complex medical needs and severe developmental delays and barriers to inclusion in the community such as transportation, social engagement, and peer support, remain (Hall, 2017). Consequently, the specialized needs of young adults cannot be adequately met due to placement in nursing home settings that are not properly equipped to handle their needs. Since regulatory standards for nursing homes recommend implementing trauma-informed care and practice as of 2019 (CMS, 2019), this presents an excellent opportunity for expanding child life services into young adult and geriatric care. Implementing trauma-informed care often represents a shift in culture for nursing homes and adult care settings, and Child Life Specialists possess the unique skills and academic background to lead this change.

Child Life Specialists consistently evaluate developmental levels when considering children's understanding of concepts. This evaluative process becomes especially imperative when adults need support tailored to a different developmental age. Child Life Specialists can deliver developmentally appropriate information, without infantilizing the individual.

Case Example: Emerson is a 21-year-old male with severe developmental delay due to early childhood non-accidental trauma. Cognitively and developmentally, Emerson functions between a 1 and 2-year-old level. Emerson is dependent on a ventilator and tracheostomy for breathing, a gastrostomy tube for eating, and a specialized wheelchair for mobility and positioning. Emerson depends entirely on others for his play, psychosocial, leisure, and communication needs. While residing in a pediatric setting, Emerson had access to a Certified Child Life Specialist, which was particularly helpful during his tracheostomy changes, where Emerson would become anxious, present with tightened muscles, and become combative with nurses and respiratory therapists. Emerson's child life specialist helped prepare him for tracheostomy changes by arriving five minutes before the procedure, helping him relax with his favorite activity, and explaining the steps of the upcoming tracheostomy change. The child life specialist recognizes that although Emerson cannot express himself verbally, his receptive language is at least partially functioning and he is soothed with calming, gently worded explanations With a progressive relaxation intervention, Emerson's body and muscles relaxed, and as a result, Emerson's tracheostomy changes took less time, were more successful, and were less stressful for both Emerson and the staff involved. When Emerson turned 21, he aged out of his facility and transferred to a nursing home. The new staff, although friendly, did not understand his needs or provide the support he previously received in the pediatric setting. Without this intervention, coupled with previous trauma, Emerson was frightened, combative, and refused to let the respiratory therapists near him for his tracheostomy change. The staff could not understand why Emerson was so upset and told him to "act like a man." Emerson became retraumatized, and the procedure took time and resources to complete. The addition of a child life specialist on staff could have prepared Emerson for the transition and his medical procedure and ensured the most effective and supportive plan of care was in place in his new environment.

FUTURE CONSIDERATIONS

There is strong evidence that "the presence of Child Life Specialists enhances the play behavior of children, increases caregiver-child interactions, reduces the level of negative behaviors exhibited by children, and may facilitate the adjustment of children and their families to a variety of medical settings and conditions" (Thompson & Snow 2009, p 40). Given this, Child Life Specialists should focus on expanding their services to additional settings where they can increase the impact on the disability community. To maintain professionally progressive momentum, Child Life Specialists should continuously evaluate areas for potential growth.

Professional Education

While required child life educational courses focus on child development, death, dying, loss, family-systems, play, and research, certification does not currently require an academic course focused on disability (ACLP, 2019). Many Child Life Specialists report feeling like their educational experience did not prepare them to work with children with disabilities, specifically those who are neurodiverse. Child Life Specialists also say staff in the medical setting feel similarly undertrained (Jensen et al., 2020).

Considering these educational gaps, a required course centered around disability education is strongly recommended for child life professionals. While many Child Life Specialists have effectively created assessments and interventions to improve the experience in the hospital setting, self-motivation rather than an academic requirement is the driver. As a result, despite having a variety of skills that are impactful for children with disabilities and their families, not all Child Life Specialists are prepared for or feel comfortable with working with disability, leading to further inequities in care.

Organizational Partnerships

Nationally and community-based organizations that support children with disabilities and provide services to families in a home setting are optimal starting points for Child Life Specialists to expand their professional reach. Groups such as United Way, Autism Speaks, Dove, Family Voices, and the Partnership for People with Disabilities offer various services to communities, families, and individuals. However, many of these organizations do not have Child Life Specialists. Child Life Specialists interested in supporting children with disabilities within community settings should be aware of these organizations and work towards education and partnership.

Advocates for Disability Culture

Disability culture focuses on the collective experience, language, beliefs, values, and creations of those with disabilities. The essential component of recognizing disability culture is pride rather than shame (Spassiani & Friedman, 2014). This shift is significant when considering the importance of feeling valued by society. Child Life Specialists have an ethical obligation to "maintain an environment that respects variations in culture, age, gender, race, ethnicity, physical ability, sexual orientation, gender identity/expression, religious affiliation, veteran status, and socioeconomic status" (ACLP, n.d.). Child Life Specialists should work towards establishing, supporting, and recognizing disability culture within their practice settings. Since Child Life Specialists are already proficient in building community by connecting children with similar experiences, doing so with children with disabilities in the community would help grow the culture of disability.

Research and Publication

The gap in available research in the child life field is widely recognized, as is research with children who qualify as disabled. Quality literature and studies must be published to continue advocating for the appropriate fit of Child Life Specialists working with children with disabilities. Child Life Specialists should prioritize disability research to recognize value drivers and promote and implement services. Similarly, Child Life Specialists can use their knowledge base to educate caregivers and communities on topics related to the inclusion of children with disabilities and the acceptance of disability culture. When considering the current research gaps, possibilities for future contributions are limitless.

Diversity within the Field

When discussing disability, including the perspective of the individual with a disability is essential. Child Life Specialists should focus on continued partnerships with the disability community to inform perspectives, interventions, competencies, ethics, and guiding principles. To date, this diversification within the field of child life has not been noted and implies consideration for the future.

CONCLUSION

Factors influencing quality of life for children with disabilities are intricate and multidimensional. Views and perspectives on disability will continue to progress as society, laws, and cultures change over time. Additionally, as the number of individuals with disabilities increases and life expectancy expands, community-based services should increase proportionately.

Child Life Specialists provide a unique professional perspective when working with children with disabilities. A background in child development, family-centered care, and a focus on child advocacy and strengths-based assessment and intervention promote optimal psychosocial wellbeing for individuals with disabilities throughout their lifespan.

Boles et al. (2020), in the publication on the value of child life, discuss six evidence-based domains of child life services that contribute to the overall success and value of the child life profession. To conclude, Child Life Specialists should consider their impact in the context of these domains when looking for working models to expand services into the community.

1. **An individualized approach to care.** The diverse range of what is considered a disability and the experiences of those with disabilities and their families warrants a multifaceted, individualized approach to care. Viewing each child's and family's unique experiences, Child Life Specialists build rapport quickly, and individuals feel supported and understood. Additionally, given a child life specialist's focus on individual cultural needs, preferences, and culturally diverse experiences, they can implement meaningful psychosocial interventions to consider diversity, equity, and inclusivity across various settings. Lastly, Child Life Specialists consistently assess strengths by using an approach that recognizes the unique potential each child and family has to build on their successes and celebrate their possibilities, seeing each child through the lens of disability culture, elevating their uniqueness rather than highlighting their differences.
2. **Focus on resilience.** The many challenges individuals with disabilities face across settings they are involved in cannot be ignored. However, Child Life Specialists uniquely reframe this experience to focus on resilience instead of adversity and achievements rather than deficits. This essential reframe allows families and individuals to ponder their journey through a lens of success rather than failure. Additionally, considering this reframe can build confidence, track accomplishments, and contribute to lifelong increases in psychosocial functioning.
3. **Developmentally grounded.** Child Life Specialists demonstrate academic knowledge of child development and family theory allows for a supportive foundation from which they can assess and

provide supportive interventions to those who may deviate from a typical developmental trajectory. This is an essential perspective for children with disabilities who may need adjusted interventions to meet them at their developmental level. In this way, interventions play to developmental strengths rather than highlight deficits.

4. **Trauma-informed.** This chapter previously highlighted the increased risk of exposure to trauma for individuals who are disabled. Considering the multitude of trauma exposures and the value of individualized support, the need for child life services for children with disabilities becomes even more evident. The correlation between adverse experiences and overall physical health is clear, as is the healing power of trauma-informed approaches. In this guise, a trauma-informed child life specialist working with children with disabilities has the potential to positively influence life-long medical and health outcomes while improving overall psychosocial wellbeing.
5. **Relationship oriented.** Relationships are the driver of successful outcomes for children with disabilities. Often the struggle to effectively communicate paired with lack of control, vulnerability, and decreased physical and social skills, leaves individuals with disabilities at risk. One meaningful and effective relationship can positively impact the quality of life while allowing individuals to feel heard and understood. Child Life Specialists build strong therapeutic relationships with children and families that honor the individual, give space for a continuum of communication needs and abilities, and respect the individuality of the family and child.
6. **Play-based.** The benefits of play for children with disabilities, coupled with the lack of access to play, demonstrate play as one of the most critical pieces of knowledge Child Life Specialists possess. Child Life Specialists use their knowledge in child development to adapt play opportunities, increase access to play, and use play to increase effective communication. Play helps children process their experiences (medical and otherwise) as well as provides an outlet for emotional expression. Indeed, few other professionals partnering with children with disabilities and their families possess such diverse, focused, and developmentally informed knowledge.

When considering the versatility, knowledge, and value Child Life Specialists bring to the lives of children with disabilities and their families through these six domains, the need to expand services in the community becomes irrevocably clear. From completing specialized assessments to implementing individualized, strengths-based interventions, Child Life Specialists provide professional, trauma-informed, resilience-focused care that increases advocacy and improves psychosocial functioning. Child Life Specialists must use this professional focus to ascertain and secure positions in non-hospital settings where children with disabilities are supported.

Concurrently, Child Life Specialists and the Association for Child Life Professionals should look towards endorsements of the child life profession as a valued and essential component of disability support systems. Organizations that partner with individuals with disabilities should include recommendations regarding the value of Child Life Specialists in policy statements, research, and legislation.

Over the last decade, the literature has emphasized equal access to quality healthcare for all individuals, and it is time to equally underscore resources that preserve psychosocial wellbeing for children with disabilities. Child Life Specialists are strong professional advocates, ensuring children with disabilities and their families receive services and interventions they need to live fulfilled, resilience-focused and trauma-free lives.

REFERENCES

Ainsworth, M. D., Blehar, M. C., & Waters, E. (1978). *Patterns of attachment: A psychological study of the strange situation*. Lawrence Erlbaum.

American Association of Post Acute Care Nursing. (2019, June 12) *Trauma-informed care. What it is and what and isn't.* https://www.aapacn.org/dns/trauma-informed-care-what-it-is-and-isnt/

American Psychological Association. (2020). *Bias-free language*. https://apastyle.apa.org/style-grammar-guidelines/bias-free-language

Americans with Disabilities Act. (n.d.). *Information and technical assistance on the Americans with Disabilities Act*. https://www.ada.gov/ada_intro.htm

Ammerman, R. (1997). Physical abuse and childhood disability. *Journal of Aggression, Maltreatment & Trauma, 1*(1), 207–224. doi:10.1300/J146v01n01_11

Andrews, V. (2015). Interpreting silent cries. *Child Life Council Bulletin, 33*(4), 8–9.

Association of Child Life Professionals. (2019). *Eligibility Requirements effective 2019*. https://www.childlife.org/certification/becoming-certified/requirements-after-2019

Association of Child Life Professionals. (n.d.). *Child life code of ethics*. https://www.childlife.org/docs/default-source/aclp-official-documents/child-life-code-of-ethics4232ee9c90156ede9dafff00004f030f.pdf?sfvrsn=5327804d_2

Barron, C., Beckett, A., Coussens, M., Desoete, A., Jones, N. C., Lynch, H., Prellwitz, M., & Salkeld, D. F. (2017). *Barriers to play for children and young persons*. De Gruyter Open Ltd.

Basaran, A., Karadavut, K. I., Uneri, S. O., Balbaloglu, O., & Atasoy, N. (2013). The effect of having children with cerebral palsy on quality of life, burn-out, depression and anxiety scores: A comparative study. *European Journal of Physical and Rehabilitation Medicine, 49*(6), 815–822. PMID:24285025

Behar, S., & Cooper, J. (2015). Best practices in the emergency department management of children with special needs. *Pediatric Emergency Medicine Practice, 12*(6). PMID:26118120

Berg, K., Shiu, C., Feinstein, R. T., Acharya, K., Medrano, J., & Small, M. E. (2019). Children with developmental disabilities experience higher levels of adversity. *Research in Developmental Disabilities, 89*(1), 105–113. doi:10.1016/j.ridd.2019.03.011 PMID:30974258

Boles, J., Fraser, C., Bennett, K., Jones, M., Dunbar, J., Woodburn, A., Gill, M. A., Duplechaine, A., Munn, E. K., & Hoskins, K. (2020). *The value of Certified Child Life Specialists: Direct and downstream optimization of pediatric patient and family outcomes*. https://www.childlife.org/docs/default-source/the-child-life-profession/value-of-cclss-full-report.pdf

Botha, M., Hanlon, J., & Williams, G. L. (2021). Does language matter? Identity-first versus person-first language use in Autism research: A response to Vivanti. *Journal of Autism and Developmental Disorders*. Advance online publication. doi:10.100710803-020-04858-w PMID:33474662

Bowlby, J. (1969). Attachment and loss. Vol 1 Attachment. Pimlico: Basic Books.

Breau, L., & Burkitt, C. (2009). Assessing pain in children with intellectual disabilities. *Pain Research & Management, 14*(2), 116–120. doi:10.1155/2009/642352 PMID:19532853

Bronfenbrenner, U. (1979). *The ecology of human development.* Harvard University Press.

Brown, C. (2008). The School Setting. In Child life beyond the hospital (pp. 213-232). Child Life Council.

Burns-Nader, S., & Hernandez-Reif, M. (2016). Facilitating play for hospitalized children through child life services. *Children's Health Care, 45*(1), 1–21. doi:10.1080/02739615.2014.948161

Centers for Disease Control and Prevention. (2020). *Disability and health overview.* https://www.cdc.gov/ncbddd/disabilityandhealth/disability.html

Cheshire, A., Barlow, J. H., & Powell, L. A. (2010). The psychosocial well-being of parents of children with cerebral palsy: A comparison study. *Disability and Rehabilitation, 32*(20), 1673–1677. doi:10.3109/09638281003649920 PMID:20178413

Cronholm, P.F., Forke, C.M., Wade, R., Bair-Merritt, M.H., Davis, M., Harkins-Schwarz, M., ... Fein, J.A. (2015). Adverse Childhood Experiences: Expanding the concept of adversity. *American Journal of Preventive Medicine, 49*(3), 354-361. doi:10.1016/j.amepre.2015.02.001

Dirth, T., & Branscombe, N. (2017). Disability models affect disability policy support through awareness of structural discrimination. *The Journal of Social Issues, 73*(2), 413–442. doi:10.1111/josi.12224

Drake, J., Johnson, N., Stoneck, A. V., Martinez, D. M., & Massey, M. (2012). Evaluation of a coping kit for children with challenging behaviors in a pediatric hospital. *Pediatric Nursing, 38*(4). PMID:22970487

Duc, J. K., Herbert, A. R., & Heussler, H. S. (2017). Paediatric palliative care and intellectual disability- A unique context. *Journal of Applied Research in Intellectual Disabilities, 30*(1), 1111–1124. doi:10.1111/jar.12389 PMID:28836319

Einfeld, S. L., & Tongue, B. L. (1996). Population prevalence of psychopathology in children and adolescents with intellectual disability, II: Epidemiological findings. *Journal of Intellectual Disability Research, 40*(2), 99–109. doi:10.1111/j.1365-2788.1996.tb00611.x PMID:8731467

Felitti, J. V., Anda, R. F., Nordenberg, D., Williamson, D. F., Spitz, A. M., Edwards, V., Koss, M. P., & Marks, J. S. (1998). Relationship of childhood abuse and household dysfunction to many of the leading causes of death in adults. The Adverse Childhood Experiences (ACE) study. *American Journal of Preventive Medicine, 14*(4), 245–258. doi:10.1016/S0749-3797(98)00017-8 PMID:9635069

Forkey, H., Szilagyi, M., Kelly, E. T., Duffee, J., Springer, S. H., Fortin, K., Jones, V. F., Vaden Greiner, M. B., Ochs, T. J., Partap, A. N., Davidson Sagor, L., Allen Staat, M., Thackeray, J. D., Waite, D., & Weber Zetley, L. (2021). Trauma-informed care. *Pediatrics, 148*(2), e2021052580. doi:10.1542/peds.2021-052580 PMID:34312292

Fraatz, E., & Durand, T. M. (2021). Meeting the needs of children with autism spectrum disorder and their families in hospital settings: The perspectives of Certified Child Life Specialists and Nurses. *Journal of Child Life: Psychosocial Theory and Practice, 2*(2). Advance online publication. doi:10.55591/001c.27703

Francis, L., & Silvers, A. (2016). Perspectives on the meaning of "disability.". *American Medical Association Journal of Ethics, 18*(10), 1025–1033. doi:10.1001/journalofethics.2016.18.10.pfor2-1610 PMID:27780027

Gariépy, N., & Howe, N. (2003). The therapeutic power of play: Examining the play of young children with leukaemia. *Child: Care, Health and Development, 29*(6), 523–537. doi:10.1046/j.1365-2214.2003.00372.x PMID:14616910

Ginsburg, K. R. (2007). The importance of play in promoting healthy child development and maintaining strong parent-child bonds. *Pediatrics, 119*(1), 182–191. doi:10.1542/peds.2006-2697 PMID:17200287

Glasper, E. A. (2017). Optimizing the care of children with intellectual disabilities in hospitals. *Comprehensive Child and Adolescent Nursing, 40*(2), 63–67. doi:10.1080/24694193.2017.1309827 PMID:29318949

Gupta, N., Brown, C., Deneke, J., Maha, J., & Kong, M. (2019). Utilization of a novel pathway in a tertiary pediatric hospital to meet the sensory needs of acutely ill pediatric patients. *Frontier Pediatrics, 7*, 367. doi:10.3389/fped.2019.00367

Hamadi, L., & Fletcher, H. K. (2021). Are people with an intellectual disability at increased risk of attachment difficulties? A critical review. *Journal of Intellectual Disabilities, 25*(1), 114–130. doi:10.1177/1744629519864772 PMID:31362566

Inova Newsroom. (2018, April 19). *Understanding sensory processing disorders.* Inova Newsroom. https://www.inovanewsroom.org/expert-commentary/2018/04/understanding-sensory-processing-disorders/

Jensen, E. J., Geisthardt, C., & Sarigiani, P. A. (2020). Working with children with autism spectrum disorder in a medical setting: Insights from Certified Child Life Specialists. *Journal of Autism and Developmental Disorders, 50*(1), 189–198. doi:10.100710803-019-04245-0 PMID:31583622

Johnson, N., Lashley, J., Stonek, A. V., & Bonjour, A. (2012). Children with developmental disabilities at a pediatric hospital: Staff education to prevent and manage challenging behaviors. *Journal of Pediatric Nursing, 27*(6), 742–749. doi:10.1016/j.pedn.2012.02.009 PMID:22465852

Jolly, A. (2012). Handle with care: Top ten tips a nurse should know before caring for a hospitalized child with autism spectrum disorder. *Pediatric Nursing, 41*(1), 11–22. PMID:26281270

Kuper, H., Monteath-van Dok, A., Wing, K., Danquah, L., Evans, J., Zuurmond, M., & Gallinetti, J. (2014). The impact of disability on the lives of children; cross-sectional data including 8900 children with disabilities and 898,834 children without disabilities across 30 countries. *PLoS One, 9*(9), 1–11. doi:10.1371/journal.pone.0107300 PMID:25202999

Liberman, D. B., Song, E., Radbill, L. M., Pham, P. K., & Derrington, S. F. (2016). Early introduction of palliative care and advanced care planning for children with complex chronic medical conditions: A pilot study. *Child: Care, Health and Development, 42*(3), 439–449. doi:10.1111/cch.12332 PMID:27028099

Liddle, M., Birkett, K., Bonjour, A., & Risma, K. (2018). A collaborative approach to improving health care for children with developmental disabilities. *Pediatrics, 142*(6), e20181136. doi:10.1542/peds.2018-1136 PMID:30385639

Liddle, M., & Sonnentag, T. L. (2021). Effectiveness of adaptive care plans for children with developmental disabilities during outpatient clinic appointments. *Journal of Autism and Developmental Disorders, 51*(9), 3028–3038. doi:10.100710803-020-04764-1 PMID:33118074

Lindley, L., Mack, J., & Bruce, D. (2016). Clusters of multiple complex chronic conditions: A latent class analysis of children at end of life. *Journal of Pain and Symptom Management, 51*(5), 868–874. doi:10.1016/j.jpainsymman.2015.12.310 PMID:26747723

Luijkx, J., van der Putten, A. J., & Vlaskamp, C. (2016). "I love my sister, but sometimes I don't": A qualitative study into the experiences of siblings of a child with profound intellectual and multiple disabilities. *Journal of Intellectual & Developmental Disability, 41*(4), 279–288. doi:10.3109/13668250.2016.1224333

McCarthy, J., & Boyd, J. (2002). Mental health services and young people with intellectual disability: Is it time to do better? *Journal of Intellectual Disability Research, 46*(3), 250–256. doi:10.1046/j.1365-2788.2002.00401.x PMID:11896810

McGonigle, J. J., Venkat, A., Beresford, C., Campbell, T. P., & Gabriels, R. L. (2014, January). Management of agitation in individuals with autism spectrum disorders in the emergency department. *Child and Adolescent Psychiatric Clinics of North America, 23*(1), 83–95. doi:10.1016/j.chc.2013.08.003 PMID:24231169

McGuire, S., & Meadan, H. (2022). Social inclusion of children with persistent challenging behaviors. *Early Childhood Education Journal, 50*(61), 61–69. doi:10.100710643-020-01135-4

Meyer and Vadasy. (2008). *Sibshops: Workshops for siblings of children with special needs.* Paul H. Brookes Publishing Co.

National Academies of Sciences, Engineering, and Medicine. (2018). *Opportunities for Improving Programs and Services for Children with Disabilities.* Washington, DC: The National Academies Press. . doi:10.17226/25028

National Center on Disability and Journalism. (2021, August). *Disability language style guide.* https://ncdj.org/style-guide/

NeuroClastic. (2021, August 14). *On Using NonSpeaking, Minimally Speaking, Or Unreliably Speaking Over "Non-Verbal": NonSpeakers Weigh In.* https://neuroclastic.com/on-using-nonspeaking-minimally-speaking-or-unreliably-speaking-over-non-verbal-nonspeakers-weigh-in/

Olawale, O. A., Deih, A. D., & Yaadar, R. K. K. (2013). Psychological impact of cerebral palsy on families: The African perspective. *Journal of Neurosciences in Rural Practice, 4*(2), 159–163. doi:10.4103/0976-3147.112752 PMID:23914092

Oulton, K., Sell, D., & Gibson, F. (2019). Hospitalized children with intellectual disability: Parents as partners in their care. *Journal of Applied Research in Intellectual Disabilities, 33*(5), 917–926. doi:10.1111/jar.12713 PMID:32072753

Petasis, A. (2019). Discrepancies of the medical, social, and biopsychosocial models of disability; A comprehensive theoretical framework. *The International Journal of Business Management and Technology*, *3*(4).

Pinquart, M. (2016). Systematic review: Bullying involvement of children with and without chronic physical illness and/or physical/sensory disability–a meta-analytic comparison with healthy/non-disabled peers. *Journal of Pediatric Psychology*, *42*(3), 245–259. doi:10.1093/jpepsy/jsw081 PMID:27784727

Rosenberg, A. R., Postier, A., Osenga, K., Kreicbergs, U., Neville, B., Dussel, V., & Wolfe, J. (2015). Long-term psychosocial outcomes among bereaved siblings of children with cancer. *Journal of Pain and Symptom Management*, *49*(1), 55–65. doi:10.1016/j.jpainsymman.2014.05.006 PMID:24880001

Santoro, A. F., Shear, S. M., & Haber, A. (2018). Childhood adversity, health and quality of life in adults with intellectual and developmental disabilities. *Journal of Intellectual Disability Research*, *62*(10), 854–863. doi:10.1111/jir.12540 PMID:30117608

Schieve, L. A., Gonzalez, V., Boulet, S. L., Visser, S. N., Rice, C. E., Braun, K. N., & Boyle, C. A. (2012). Concurrent medical conditions and health care use and needs among children with learning and behavioral developmental disabilities., National Health Interview Survey, 2006-2010. *Research in Developmental Disabilities*, *33*(2), 467–476. doi:10.1016/j.ridd.2011.10.008 PMID:22119694

Short, E. J., Schindler, R. C., Obeid, R., Noeder, M. M., Hlavaty, L. E., Gross, S. I., Lewis, B., Russ, S., & Manos, M. M. (2020). Examining the role of language in play among children with and without developmental disabilities. *Language, Speech, and Hearing Services in Schools*, *51*(3), 795–806. doi:10.1044/2020_LSHSS-19-00084 PMID:32402229

Shyman, E. (2016). The Reinforcement of Ableism: Normality, the Medical Model of Disability, and Humanism in Applied Behavior Analysis and ASD. *Intellectual and Developmental Disabilities*, *54*(5), 366–376. doi:10.1352/1934-9556-54.5.366 PMID:27673737

Spassiani, N. A., & Friedman, C. (2014). Stigma: Barriers to culture and identity for people with intellectual disability. *Inclusion*, *2*(4), 329–341. doi:10.1352/2326-6988-2.4.329

Stoneman, Z. (2005). Siblings of children with disabilities: Research themes. *Mental Retardation*, *43*, 339–350. PMID:16131231

Sumner, K. E., & Brown, T. J. (2015). Neurodiversity and human resource management: Employer challenges for applicants and employees with learning disabilities. *The Psychologist Manager Journal*, *18*(2), 77–85. doi:10.1037/mgr0000031

Taunt, H. M., & Hastings, R. P. (2002). Positive impact of children with developmental disabilities on their families: A preliminary study. *Education and Training in Mental Retardation and Developmental Disabilities*, *37*, 410–420.

Thompson & Snow. (2009). Research in child life. In The Handbook of Child Life (pp. 36-56). Charles Thomas.

Thompson & Stanford. (1981). *Child life in hospitals: Theory and practice*. Charles C Thomas.

Tudor, M. E., & Lerner, M. D. (2015). Intervention and support for siblings of youth with developmental disabilities: A systematic review. *Clinical Child and Family Psychology Review*, *18*(1), 1–23. doi:10.100710567-014-0175-1 PMID:25315924

Turner, J. (2009). Theoretical foundations of child life practice. In The Handbook of Child Life (pp. 23-35). Charles Thomas.

Unicef (2021, November 10). *Nearly 240 million children with disabilities around the world, UNICEF's most comprehensive statistical analysis finds*. https://www.unicef.org/press-releases/nearly-240-million-children-disabilities-around-world-unicefs-most-comprehensive

US Department of Education. (n.d.). *About IDEA, Individuals with Disabilities in Education Act. Section 300.8 Child with a disability*. https://sites.ed.gov/idea/regs/b/a/300.8

Wang, K. W. K., & Barnard, A. (2004). Technology-dependent children and their families: A review. *Journal of Advanced Nursing*, *45*(1), 36–46. doi:10.1046/j.1365-2648.2003.02858.x PMID:14675299

Wilkins, C. (2018). Play partners: Incorporating parents into medical play practices. In Handbook of Medical Play Therapy and Child Life: Interventions in Clinical and Medical Settings (pp. 277-295). Routledge.

World Health Organization. (2021, November 21). *Disability and health.* World Health Organization. https://www.who.int/news-room/fact-sheets/detail/disability-and-health

Wu, J., Zhang, J., & Hong, Y. (2017). Quality of life of primary caregivers of children with cerebral palsy: A comparison between mother and grandmother caregivers in Anhui province of China. *Child: Care, Health and Development*, *43*(5), 718–724. doi:10.1111/cch.12464 PMID:28497475

ADDITIONAL READING

Bell, J. L., Johnson, B. H., & McLeod, S. M. (2008). Family-centered care and the implications for the child life practice. In R. H. Thompson (Ed.), *The handbook of child life: A guide for pediatric psychosocial care* (pp. 95–115). Charles C Thomas.

Driscoll, C., & Carter, M. (2009). The effects of social and isolate toys on the social interaction of preschool children with disabilities. *Journal on Developmental Disabilities*, *21*(4), 279–300. doi:10.100710882-009-9142-z

Hall, S. (2017). Community involvement of young adults with intellectual disabilities: Their experiences and perspectives on inclusion. *Journal of Applied Research in Intellectual Disabilities*, *30*(1), 859–871. doi:10.1111/jar.12276 PMID:27456658

Ivory, J., & McCollum, A. (1999). Effects of social and isolate toys on social play in an inclusive setting. *The Journal of Special Education*, *32*(4), 238–242. doi:10.1177/002246699903200404

KEY TERMS AND DEFINITIONS

Complex Medical Needs: Medical conditions that are persistent, prolonged and require extensive medical oversight to manage over time. Complex medical needs often present comorbidly and impact quality of life and activities of daily living.

Disability Culture: The conceptualization of disability being its own culture with a unique history, norms, aesthetics, community, language, beliefs, behaviors and ways of living that specifically pertain to those having a disability.

Neurodiversity: The viewpoint that deviations from what society considers 'typical' neurological functioning, cognition and behavior is common and acceptable. Ranges of functioning occur naturally and should be accepted by society at large.

Neurotypical: Neurological functioning that does not deviate from what society considers as developmentally normal or functional.

Presuming Competence: A strengths-based approach that making the assumption, when working with individuals with disabilities, that despite their potential inability to articulate, speak, or communicate verbally, a basic understanding of what is being said to them (receptive language) is present.

Sensory Avoidant: Avoiding sensory stimuli due to aversion or dislike.

Sensory Integration: The ability to categorize and absorb sensory information in a way that allows for adequate responses and appropriate functioning.

Sensory Regulation: The ability to match arousal responses and states appropriately to the presented environmental stimuli (i.e., quiet voices in a library or dancing at a music hall).

Sensory Seeking: The compulsive need for continuous sensory input to regulate.

Strengths-Based: Conceptualized interventions focused on individual strengths (i.e., what they have and are currently doing positively) and viewing individuals as resilient and resourceful rather than focusing on their deficits, failures, or mishaps.

Trauma-Informed: A model of care that presumes most individuals have experienced and been affected by trauma in the past. Trauma-informed practices seek to understand how the presence of past trauma affects behavior, decisions, health, and relationships.

Chapter 12
Behavioral Health

Angeles Nunez
Holtz Children's Hospital, USA

Bridgette Danielson
Cincinnati Children's Hospital Medical Center, USA

ABSTRACT

The purpose of this chapter is to discuss the developmental and behavioral needs of children and adolescents with mental health concerns and to demonstrate how child life services can be used in a variety of settings both in and out of healthcare. This chapter emphasizes how child life specialists can adapt their skills to meet the needs of the pediatric mental health population, their families, and the interdisciplinary team. Child life specialists can provide psychosocial support to psychiatric patients and families by addressing developmental concerns, identifying emotional and coping needs, and advocating for trauma-informed and family-centered care.

INTRODUCTION

The prevalence of mental health needs has greatly risen over the last decade, thus revealing the glaring issue of lack of support and resources for those affected by psychiatric diagnoses, specifically children and adolescents. Mental health, typically referred to as behavioral health in the pediatric field, is characterized by an individual's level of psychological and/or psychosocial adjustments (Boles et al., 2020). In 2015, the World Health Organization (WHO) predicted that youth psychiatric disorders would rank as one of the five most common reasons for morbidity, mortality, disability, and functional impairment for youth worldwide by the year 2020 (Hunter et al., 2015). Subsequently, in 2021, a national state of emergency in children's mental health was declared by the American Academy of Pediatrics (AAP), the American Academy of Child and Adolescent Psychiatry (AACAP), and the Children's Hospital Association (CHA). At the time, the AAP linked the mental health crisis to the stress from the coronavirus pandemic and the ongoing struggle of racial injustice, both of which exacerbated mental health challenges that youth were already experiencing (AAP, 2021; National Alliance on Mental Illness [NAMI], 2021b). The pandemic

DOI: 10.4018/978-1-6684-5097-0.ch012

resulted in school closures, reduced access to family and friends, reduced access to health care, isolation, and economic pressures, all of which can negatively impact one's mental health (Hudson et al., 2022).

Due to the mental health crisis, there is a growing need to better understand and support the psychosocial needs of these children and their families. Certified Child Life Specialists (CCLS) have the unique skill set to help decrease stress and increase coping amongst children and their family's facing adversity. In this case, that adversity is learning how to cope with and understand one's behavioral health needs as a child or teenager. Certified Child Life Specialists may encounter the behavioral health population both in and out of traditional settings. Coincidentally, children and adolescents with chronic illnesses are at higher risk than their healthy peers for developing a mental illness due to facing more physical, cognitive, social, and emotional challenges (National Institute of Mental Health [NIMH], 2021). However, over the last decade, CCLSs have begun exploring more non-traditional settings such as inpatient psychiatric treatment.

Inpatient psychiatric treatment most commonly occurs in a behavioral health unit within a health care system or a free-standing behavioral health facility. The goals of inpatient psychiatric treatment typically include crisis stabilization, diagnosis, and initiation of appropriate treatment. Prior to discharge, a patient's crisis – defined as the "danger of suicide or homicide, harmful acts to self or to others, or impaired self-care (p. 394)" – is alleviated and proper psychopharmacologic and psychological treatments can continue through outpatient services (Sharfstein, 2009). Common pediatric psychiatric diagnoses include, but are not limited to (American Psychiatric Association [APA], 2013; Pittesenbarger & Mannix, 2013; Sheridan et al., 2015):

- Mood disorders, such as major depressive disorder, anxiety disorder, post-traumatic stress disorder, bipolar disorder, and phobias;
- Developmental disorders, such as autism, attention-deficit/hyperactivity disorder, and learning disorder;
- Externalizing disorders, such as oppositional defiant disorder and conduct disorder;
- Substance-related disorders;
- Eating disorders;
- Personality disorders; and
- Schizophrenia and psychotic disorders.

Youth with mental health concerns often demonstrate self-harm behaviors, aggressive or assaultive behaviors, and/or neurological disabilities (Hazen & Prager, 2017). Some specific behaviors linked to suicidality can comprise of sadness or being withdrawn; trying to harm or kill oneself, or having thoughts of doing so; an increase in risk-taking behaviors; sudden overwhelming fear; severe mood swings; substance use; severe changes in behavior, personality, or eating/sleeping habits; and extreme difficulty in concentrating or staying still (National Alliance on Mental Illness [NAMI], 2015). Externalizing disorders are often associated with negativistic behaviors such as aggression, arguing, behavioral outbursts, screaming, fighting, destruction of property, hostile behavior, threats of homicide, and/or cruelty to animals (Dopheide, 2013; New et al., 2017). It is also common for people with mental illnesses to have auditory or visual hallucinations, cognitive delays, developmental delays, or lower-than-average academic performance (Dopheide, 2013; McLeod et al., 2013).

The skills of a Certified Child Life Specialist can be used to help meet these needs and serve children and adolescents experiencing behavioral health issues. Although behavioral health settings may be considered a non-traditional setting for CCLSs, there are both similarities and differences within child life practice that can be validated and adapted for this population. This chapter will discuss the following in regards to the pediatric behavioral health population: demographics and risk factors, challenges within these settings, and traditional and non-traditional child life services.

Overview of Demographics and Risk Factors

Development and Age

Developmentally, adolescents experience radical and continuous changes in their physical, social, and emotional growth, thus making them more susceptible to mental health concerns. In the pediatric population, behavioral health diagnoses occur most frequently in older school-age children and adolescents, although behavioral concerns can transpire at any age. Typically, 50% of mental health disorders diagnosed over a lifespan begin by age 14 (NAMI, 2021c). Behavioral health issues are the most frequent reason for hospitalization in children ages 10 to 14 and the second most frequent in children ages 15 to 17 (Gallagher et al., 2017). For American youth alone, 20% of children ages 13 to 18 years old currently live with a serious mental illness (NAMI, 2015). Additionally, adolescents may endure increased risk factors due to their age, which include: exposure to adversity; peer pressure; exploration of their identity; media influence; gender norms; lower socioeconomic status; strained relationships with their caregivers; exposure to violence; and risk-taking behaviors (e.g., drinking, drug use, or violence) (WHO, 2021).

Literature also indicates that behavioral health concerns can arise in infants and younger children (Stygar & Zadroga, 2021). Due to foundational emotional and social development throughout infancy and early childhood, one's mental health can be drastically impacted by their environment, especially by their caregivers. Children are more likely to experience behavioral concerns if their caregivers have mental health issues of their own, have a history of abuse or neglect, experience financial stress, or abuse drugs and alcohol (Stygar & Zadroga, 2021). Childhood behavioral issues can cause problems at home and school, when forming friendships, and ultimately with future developmental milestones, thus having potential long-term effects into adolescence and adulthood (Centers for Disease Control and Prevention [CDC], 2021c).

Trauma History

Experiencing trauma puts individuals at risk for behavioral health and substance use disorders (Substance Abuse and Mental Health Services Administration [SAMHSA], 2022). By age 16, more than two-thirds of children have experienced at least one traumatic event, and one in seven has experienced abuse and neglect within the past year. Traumatic events can include (SAMHSA, 2022):

- Psychological, physical, or sexual abuse;
- Community or school violence;
- Witnessing or experiencing domestic violence;
- National disasters or terrorism;
- Commercial sexual exploitation;
- Sudden or violent loss of a loved one;
- Refugee or war experiences;

- Military family-related stressors (e.g., deployment, parental loss or injury);
- Physical or sexual assault;
- Neglect; and
- Serious accidents or life-threatening illness.

Research has shown that traumatic experiences, especially those that occur during childhood, negatively affect development. In the late 1990s, researchers studied the health outcomes of adults who had experienced adverse childhood experiences, commonly referred to as ACEs (Felitti et al., 1998). This study looked at how ACEs (e.g., psychological, physical, and sexual abuse; parental divorce and separation; witnessing domestic violence, and living with an adult experiencing mental illness, substance use/misuse, or incarceration) impacted not only one's physical health, but also their brain development (Felitti et al., 1998). Trauma exposure can lead to biological changes in limbic system functioning, hypothalamic-pituitary-adrenal axis activity, and neurotransmitter-related dysregulation (SAMHSA, 2014). The parts of the brain that process emotions and promote logical reasoning are negatively impacted when a person experiences early and chronic trauma. Early and recurring exposure to trauma has been linked to adverse effects on adolescent self-esteem, the ability to build healthy relationships, school performance, self-regulation, critical thinking, and self-motivation (Hornor et al., 2019). Childhood trauma survivors often experience learning problems, including lower grades and more suspensions and expulsions; increased use of health and mental health services; increased involvement with the child welfare and juvenile justice systems; and long-term health problems (e.g., diabetes and heart disease) (SAMHSA, 2014).

Lesbian, Gay, Bisexual, and Transgender (LGBT+)

There is often fear and stigma associated with identifying as LGBT+. Until 1973, homosexuality was listed as a sociopathic personality disturbance in the Diagnostic and Statistical Manual of Mental Disorders (DSM) (Cabaj, 2022). Youth within the lesbian, gay, and bisexual population are two times more likely to report experiencing persistent feelings of sadness and hopelessness than their heterosexual peers, whereas transgender youth are two times more likely to experience depressive symptoms, seriously consider suicide, and attempt suicide compared to cisgender youth (NAMI, 2022c). Although society has made great strides in the social acceptance of sexual and gender minorities, younger populations who identity as LGBT+ earlier in their lives now may be experiencing more stressors than in previous generations, which can ultimately impact their social relationships and have negative effects on their mental health (NAMI, 2022b). Unfortunately, despite these increased risks, many public settings (e.g. schools, workplaces, housing, and health care) do not have protection for sexual and gender minorities, thus further challenging adequate mental health care (Cabaj, 2022; NAMI, 2022b).

Developmental Disabilities

Children with developmental disabilities may be at a greater risk of encountering the behavioral health setting due to symptoms of their disability. Twenty-four percent of the children and adolescents that are involuntarily committed for psychiatric care have a co-occurring developmental disability and behavioral health disorder (Fahrenwald & Haley, 2021). Children with developmental disabilities are more likely than their peers to experience overstimulation of the limbic system. This manifests as higher levels of anxiety and behavioral outburst occurrences, resulting in noncompliance, self-stimulatory behaviors, and self-injurious behaviors (Fahrenwald & Haley, 2021). Children with behavioral health diagnoses who also experience bereavement and/or trauma may demonstrate uncommon coping styles (e.g. stimming, rocking, spinning, etc.), have increased difficulties with communication or comprehension, and receive a lack of support and understanding from others, further complicating a stay in a behavioral health setting (Hume et al., 2015; Nunez, 2018).

One of the most well-known developmental disabilities is Autism Spectrum Disorder (ASD). ASD can cause significant challenges in an individual's social and communication skills and impact their behavior (CDC, 2021a). According to the CDC (2021a), 83% of individuals with ASD have one or more co-occurring medical or psychological conditions such as ADHD, anxiety, or depression. Recurrent behavioral outbursts are one of the greatest challenges reported by families affected by ASD. For this reason, families may go to the hospital seeking resources and respite or may need to call the police to help with de-escalation (Fahrenwald & Haley, 2021; Siegel, 2018). Other common developmental disabilities may include but are not limited to: intellectual disabilities such as fetal alcohol syndrome disorder; genetic and chromosomal conditions such as Down syndrome and fragile X syndrome; and hearing or vision impairments (CDC, 2021b). Unfortunately, few behavioral health inpatient programs specialize in treatment for ASD and other developmental disabilities. To best support this population, it is important to recognize that every child with a developmental disability is different and can have a vast range of abilities and differences.

Communities of Color

Children and families of low socioeconomic status (SES) and communities of color experience depression and suicidal ideation at higher rates than White middle-class individuals (NAMI, 2022). *Communities of color* refer to any person who is not considered White, such as but not limited to Black, Latino, Alaskan Native, American Indian, and Asian American and Pacific Islander (AAPI). While Black, Indigenous, and People of Color (BIPOC) children are not less likely to be diagnosed with a depression or anxiety disorder, they are less likely to receive treatment. They are also more likely to experience long-term psychological impairments and behavioral and social deficits associated with mental health disorders (Hart et al., 2016; NAMI 2021a). The BIPOC and Latino communities are more likely to experience socioeconomic disparities which may contribute to worse mental health outcomes (Hudson et al., 2022; NAMI, 2021a). Socioeconomic disparities may include poverty, inequitable access to insurance, and exclusion from educational, social, and economic resources (Fahrenwald & Haley, 2021; Hudson et al., 2022; NAMI, 2021a). According to NAMI (2021a), individuals who live in poverty have a higher risk of mental illness and individuals with mental illness have a higher risk of living in poverty. During the coronavirus pandemic, 25% of 18- to 24-year-olds within communities of color reported experiencing suicidal ideation (NAMI, 2021a). The pandemic also furthered already existing disparities in care and resources for specific ethnic and socioeconomic groups, resulting in those families falling behind on bills and/or children spending less time on education (Hudson et al., 2022).

Cultural beliefs, language, mistrust of government services, stigma, and lack of cultural education among medical services are barriers that keep families from seeking mental health services. For example, 63% of BIPOC individuals report they believe a mental health condition is a sign of personal weakness (NAMI, 2021a). Some cultures consider receiving mental health care or therapy as taboo and fear being labeled (NAMI, 2021a). They also reported refusal to obtain therapy due to a sense of pride in their emotions and home life by not wanting to speak about personal or family challenges publicly (NAMI,

2021a). The AAPI community has the lowest help-seeking rate of all ethnic groups and research shows that this community is overall more likely to be misdiagnosed as being "mentally healthy" than White individuals (Hart et al., 2016; NAMI, 2021a). Research shows that a strong sense of ethnic identity is linked to lower suicide rates and resilience in the face of discrimination (Asnaani & Hofmann, 2012; NAMI, 2021a). With this knowledge in mind, therapists who lack competence in specific cultural beliefs may misdiagnose an individual based on a lack of information and how the individual describes their symptoms. The disparities among all of these communities including lack of culturally competent clinicians can lead to a delay or lack of treatment, thus allowing these communities to experience worsened symptoms and a poorer quality of life (NAMI, 2021c).

Challenges and Ethical Considerations

Due to the complex nature of the behavioral health population, there are several special considerations to be aware of, most being the ethical dilemmas that can occur. As noted in the child life community through conferences, social networking, and word-of-mouth, Certified Child Life Specialists appear to be facing challenges when working with the psychiatric population. Many of these challenges may come across as intimidating for healthcare professionals with little to no psychiatric-specific training, especially when working with psychiatric patients in general pediatric settings such as the emergency department (ED) or general medical floors. Therefore, it is important to have an awareness of challenges and ethical considerations in order to provide adequate child life services across all pediatric settings. In an effort to concisely discuss the vastness of potential challenges within psychiatric care, the authors will explore the following topics: stigma and issues faced in general pediatric settings, disparities in care, treatment interventions, social conflicts, as well as staff burnout, and limitations affecting the field of child life.

Stigma and Issues Faced in General Pediatric Settings

Most patients receiving mental health care begin their hospitalization in the Emergency Department (ED) (Field & Shubert, 2010). Throughout 2019 and 2020, there was over a 20% increase in mental health-related pediatric emergency department visits for children and adolescents (NAMI, 2021c). Patients admitted to the ED for psychiatric concerns may inevitably experience a lack of privacy, independence, and control. Patients expressed that they were often met with "stigmatizing attitudes, negative assessments, judgment, and discrimination" (p. 319) and felt "exposed, ashamed, devalued, insecure… or uncomfortable" (p. 319) while discussing their reasons for admission (Carstensen et al., 2017).

From the ED, psychiatric patients may then be moved to any general pediatric floor to wait for medical clearance or to transfer to a psychiatric bed or facility; this process is known as "boarding." According to the Joint Commission, boarding patients in the ED, inpatient medical units, or other temporary locations before proper placement is not recommended to last more than four hours; however, with the national shortage of psychiatric beds during the coronavirus pandemic, patients have endured much longer wait times (Gallagher et al., 2017; Bowden et al., 2022). Boarding can cause stressors for the patients, families, professionals, and hospitals, including delays in receiving immediate and necessary mental health care, loss of medical care to boarding and non-boarding patients, and financial loss (Gallagher et al., 2017; Claudis et al., 2014). During the boarding phase, potentially harmful situations may arise due to a lack of psychiatric education for general health care staff. Staff in "non-psychiatric settings may be less prepared to manage patients' aggressive behaviors than [staff] who practice in psychiatric settings and use de-escalation techniques" (Casey, 2019, para. 4). Research shows that the majority of acts of violence and suicide attempts by patients with mental health concerns occur within the first week of hospitalization, which may be linked to boarding in an unlocked unit with sharp and dangerous medical equipment (Claudis et al., 2014).

Disparities in Care

An observable issue demonstrating disparities in care is how – despite the evident need for behavioral and mental health services – marginalized populations historically have less access to mental health services, are not likely to get necessary care, and receive a lower quality of care in contrast to White individuals (Li et al., 2021). Overall, several BIPOC individuals experience differences in receiving professional help compared to the White population. Other obstacles to receiving adequate care can include the high cost of services and/or insufficient insurance coverage; limited options and/or long wait lists for treatment; lack of awareness of where to go to obtain help; and the social stigma behind mental health care, such as the fear of judgment, especially within younger generations (Wood et al., 2018). Many of these barriers are not related to the cultures behind these populations, but rather how various health care aspects have historically treated minoritized groups (e.g. systemic discriminatory practices and lack of diverse demographics within the workforce) (Li et al., 2021).

Treatment Interventions

Inpatient psychiatric admissions typically include a variety of psychopharmacologic and psychological treatments. There are ethical concerns about whether or not treatment interventions – such as the use of medication, psychotherapy, electroconvulsive therapy, and restraints and seclusion (R/S) (Table 1) – are safe, necessary, and effective.

Table 1. The AACAP (2022) definitions of various psychiatric treatment interventions

Psychiatric Intervention	Definition
Electroconvulsive therapy	A procedure that utilizes brief electrical stimulation of the brain while a person is under anesthesia
Chemical restraints	The use of a drug that is administered to manage a person's behavior in order to reduce their safety risk to themselves or others; these have temporary effects of restricting the person's freedom of movement and are not a standard of ongoing treatment for the person's medical or psychiatric condition
Physical restraints	Any manual, physical, or mechanical device, material, or equipment that immobilizes or reduces a person's ability to move
Seclusion	Involuntary confinement of a person in a room or area that the person cannot physically leave

For example, although research has proven electroconvulsive therapy to be non-harmful and helpful, there is little data regarding its effect on youth "due to historical concern about this treatment approach" (AACAP, 2022, para. 6). Since the early 2000s, there has been an effort within the mental health field to reduce the use of restraints and seclusions (R/S), provide alternative interventions, and recognize how R/S can impact trauma (AACAP, 2022). These interventions are used as a last resort only and in an effort to maintain a safe environment for the person in crisis and those around them. Ultimately, psychiatric treatment choices must be a balance of safety, prevention of harm to those being treated and others in the environment, and use of least restrictive means (i.e., attempting verbal de-escalation before physically intervening in a crisis) (AACAP, 2022). With any treatment, there are always risks and benefits, and it is recommended to youth and their families to weigh the advantages and disadvantages of each option (NIMH, 2009).

Additionally, children and adolescents may not be able to assent to treatment due to their developmental level and/or altered mental status, resulting in their parents or guardians providing consent to treat by proxy. Involuntary commitment for inpatient mental health treatment may cause an issue if youth disagree with their admission, although they may pose a threat to themselves or others. Some states have laws regarding involuntary commitment; the Florida Mental Health Act (more commonly known as The Baker Act) allows law enforcement, mental health professionals, and medical professionals to request a voluntary or involuntary commitment of a person who is in an immediate mental health crisis (University Florida Health, 2022). Such laws can threaten a young person's autonomy, control, and rights. Nevertheless, the AACAP (2022) highly recommends that children should be able to communicate their treatment preferences and should not be excluded from decision-making.

Social Conflicts

Confidentiality, or the act of keeping an individual's information private, can also pose a concern within behavioral health settings. Although protecting a person's privacy is crucial, threats to hurt oneself or others cannot be kept confidential and need to be reported by professionals (AACAP, 2022). The same thought process applies to youth being treated for their mental health in a mental health facility where other peers are admitted for similar concerns. Research shows that social connectedness during pediatric inpatient psychiatric treatment promotes positive identity formation and a sense of group belonging; hospitalized youth who felt like their peers related to them (e.g. similar symptoms, diagnoses, and hospital experiences) reported a sense of validation (Rice et al., 2021). However, if patients are not able to maintain healthy perimeters between themselves and their peers, the social component of pediatric psychiatric group treatment can threaten individuals' boundaries and confidentiality.

Some studies have found that family involvement benefits patients by increasing prevention rates for relapse and reducing hospital stays during adult mental health admissions (Dirik et al., 2017). Conversely, family dynamics such as divorce and single parenthood, socioeconomic adversity, and parents with a history of trauma and/or mental illness have been attributed to suicide in young people and predisposition of mental health diagnoses (Behere et al., 2017). Sibling involvement can play an integral part in family-centered care, yet many siblings of children with mental health needs have a higher rate of having similar psychopathology (Ma et al., 2015). Additionally, foster placements bring unique obstacles of their own such as placing children in developmentally inadequate and problematic homes and difficulty getting assent and consent for interventions (AACAP, 2022). One study demonstrated that 11% of children hospitalized in an inpatient psychiatric unit came from biological families, whereas 89% had some disruption to their family structure (Behere et al., 2017).

Staff Burnout

Lastly, staff burn-out is another issue to consider. According to WHO (2019), burn-out is defined as a "syndrome conceptualized as resulting from chronic workplace stress that has not been successfully managed" (para. 4). As much as 67% of mental health workers experience high levels of burn-out (Morse et al., 2011). Employees with burn-out can experience impaired emotional and physical health and sense of well-being; increased depression, anxiety, and alcohol consumption; and reduced commitment to their workplace. Consequently, employees become less empathic, collaborative, and attentive to their mental health patients, which can ultimately lead to poor treatment decisions (Morse et. al., 2011).

Opportunities Within the Field of Child Life

Certified Child Life Specialists are responsible for maximizing the physical, emotional, social, cognitive, and developmental health and abilities of children as well as minimizing the stress and trauma that children and/or families may experience (ACLP, 2020). The child life competencies illustrate the importance of a CCLS's ability to provide a safe, therapeutic, and healing environment for all youth and families (Child Life Council [CLC], 2014). By assessing potential challenges within pediatric behavioral health settings, child life specialists can explain how the environment affects a child and family's behaviors, identify how to prevent and protect the emotional safety of patients, and promote privacy and confidentiality policies (CLC, 2014) (Table 2).

Table 2. This table explores potential challenges in pediatric behavioral health, the child life code of ethics, and intervention suggestions to mitigate these issues

Challenges	Child life code of ethics principles	Helpful Interventions
Stigma, bias, and/or barriers for receiving adequate mental health care based on demographics and/or circumstances	**Principle 2:** CCLSs have a duty to maintain objectivity, integrity, and competence while exhibiting compassion. **Principle 3:** CCLSs have an obligation to maintain an environment that respects variations in culture, age, gender, race, ethnicity, physical ability, sexual orientation, gender identity/ expression, religious affiliation, veteran status, and socioeconomic status. **Principle 11:** CCLSs recognize that financial gain should never take precedence over the mission, vision, values, and operating principles of the profession.	● Approach children and families with a strength-based and trauma-informed approach. ● Create relationships based on trust and respect. ● Provide services that are free or low cost; utilize donor and/or grant support for funding. ● Celebrate and advocate for all holidays, while knowing that some families may not celebrate any holidays.
Consent to treat and involuntary commitment	**Principle 1:** CCLSs hold a primary commitment to the psychosocial care of the patient and family and uphold the mission, vision, values, and operating principles of the profession.	● Advocate for the best interests of the child and family. ● Provide the child and family with realistic choices to promote a sense of control. ● Encourage a child's autonomy while promoting safety. ● Assess a child's understanding of treatments and ability to assent; share this information with the treatment team.

Continued on following page

Table 2. Continued

Challenges	Child life code of ethics principles	Helpful Interventions
Crossing boundaries and exploiting confidential information between clients and professionals and clients and peers	**Principle 4:** CCLSs respect the privacy of children and families and maintain confidentiality within the standards and requirements of employers, local governing regulations, or private practice standards. **Principle 10:** CCLSs use integrity to assess and amend any personal relationships, social media exchanges, or situations that may interfere with their professional effectiveness or objectivity, or otherwise negatively impact the children and families they serve. Child life professionals ensure the conclusion of their professional role before any personal relationship is permitted to develop with children or the members of families they have served.	● Be aware of a child's history of poor boundaries (e.g. forming close attachments to professionals, asking for personal information, etc.) ● Speak up if another professional is having inappropriate or unhealthy interactions with patients. ● Set the expectation at the beginning of an interaction with the importance of confidentiality. Explain and practice realistic boundaries with youth in one-on-one or group settings. Focus on developmentally appropriate explanations. Have discussions like "What does a healthy relationship with a peer at the hospital look like? With a doctor? With your guardian?"
Controversial treatment interventions	**Principle 8:** CCLSs continually seek knowledge and skills that update and enhance their understanding of all relevant issues affecting the children and families they serve.	● Advocate for do no harm and the best interest of the child and family with the treatment team during rounds or meetings. ● In addition to medical treatment, suggest complementary options such as mindfulness, breathing techniques, or gross motor exertion. ● Use developmentally appropriate education with children and families regarding treatment options (e.g. preparing an adolescent for electroconvulsive therapy). ● Debrief with a child after a restraint or provide emotional support to other peers who may be experiencing trauma from witnessing a crisis.
Complicated family structures and/or relationships	**Principle 2:** CCLSs have a duty to maintain objectivity, integrity, and competence while exhibiting compassion.	● Focus on the strengths within a family system and emphasize family-centered care. ● Collaborate with other disciplines, such as social workers, to understand any family stressors. ● Use broad language when discussing a child's family situation. Instead of, "Tell me about your mom and dad," ask, "Who do you live with at home?" ● Avoid celebrating parent-specific holidays in group settings, such as Mother's Day or Father's Day.
Poor treatment decisions due to staff burn-out	**Principle 1:** CCLSs hold a primary commitment to the psychosocial care of the patient and family and uphold the mission, vision, values, and operating principles of the profession.	● Be aware of the warning signs of burn-out and compassion fatigue in yourself and others. Practice self-care.

CHILD LIFE SERVICES

Research has shown that hospitalization during childhood and adolescence can lead to toxic stress, which can then consequently have adverse effects on an individual's health, well-being, growth, and development (Al-Yateem et al., 2015). When children and adolescents are admitted to a behavioral health setting with mental health concerns, they may not only experience healthcare-related stressors but also personal and environmental problems leading up to their admission (Causey et al., 1998). This population has unique needs that may alter child life approaches and practices. While there is limited evidence-based research regarding Certified Child Life Specialists within mental health settings, there are CCLSs already working with patients with psychiatric diagnoses and/or working in psychiatric settings (Danielson, 2018; Danielson et al., 2019). Certified Child Life Specialists are constantly adapting their interventions to best meet the needs of patients based on several factors including the patient's developmental age, diagnosis, and the setting. Working with the mental health population is within the child life scope of practice; interventions and approaches simply need to be modified as a CCLS would adapt their practice to any other population or setting. The following child life competencies will be discussed and applied to the behavioral health population: assessment, preparation and procedural support, developmental explanations, expressive and normative opportunities, coping and emotional support, and advocacy.

Assessment

Assessment allows Certified Child Life Specialists to determine how much a child or adolescent is at risk for developing negative psychosocial impacts during a stressful event. CCLSs gather information in order to create a care plan that is reflective of a child's development, life experiences, and culture (ACLP, 2018). When a child life specialist is able to assess an individual at their baseline behavior, the child life specialist can evaluate their stress levels and plan and implement appropriate interventions based on their needs. However, what if the reason for a health care admission is due to increased stress levels and unsafe behavior? How do behavioral health settings affect assessment? How can child life specialists best provide adequate services while maintaining safety measures? These are the questions that should be considered with the behavioral health population.

When assessing youth and their families in behavioral health settings, it is important to refer back to the developmental theories that child life practice is based upon with the knowledge that theories should be used more as a guide than a rulebook. Typical theoretical assessment considerations may include: *How do the child's behaviors align with Erikson's Psychosocial Development Theory? According to Vygotsky's Sociocultural Theory, is the child's environment impacting their reason for their admissions? Would Bowlby and Ainsworth make connections between a patient's attachment styles based on their early childhood relationships?* However, development is not black and white, especially when considering a mental health diagnosis. Mental health concerns are usually a "complex interaction between biology, psychology, and environmental factors (NAMI, 2022a, para. 19)." The theories above mainly focused on middle-class Eurocentric and colonialist perspectives that view ill children as "aberrations from the norm" (Koller, 2019, para. 6). CCLSs need to dive deeper into assessment by exploring more modern perspectives, such as the Greenspan Floortime Approach, the Whole Brainchild, Brazelton's Touchpoints Model of Development, the sociology of childhood, early relational health, and implicit bias.

In addition to the theoretical foundation of child life, child life specialists interested in working in behavioral health settings should explore education and training on psychiatry-specific practices. One study showed that nurses in non-psychiatric settings who experienced working with patients with behavioral health concerns had an increased likelihood of facing burn-out and mental exhaustion. However, when those nurses received behavioral health training and education, they reported improvements in their sense of environmental safety, care from their management, communication, and confidence (Casey, 2019). Topics such as psychiatric diagnoses, cultural humility, trauma-informed care, and behavioral interventions may be helpful to pursue before or during work in a behavioral health setting. For example, rather than incorporating cultural competency – which is a finite and fixed approach that focuses on the understanding of all cultures, values, languages, and customs – cultural humility is a lifelong process of commitment to engagement, exploration, self-reflection, and self-critique regarding awareness to and understanding of a patient's cultural background (Li et al., 2021). Certified Child Life Specialists must assess how a patient's presenting problems may be interlinked with their cultural identity in order to treat each patient as a unique individual, to recognize their culture-influenced strengths, and avoid blanket assumptions. Employing a strength-based approach when working with diverse cultures and communities can include culture-specific influences, resources, and coping mechanisms (e.g. faith, social causes, music, etc.) (Asnaani & Hofmann, 2021).

Behavioral health education programs can also be beneficial to child life specialists to strengthen assessments. Courses on mental health first aid focus on identifying, understanding, and responding to signs of mental health and substance use challenges among children and adolescents ages 6 to 18 (Mental Health First Aid, 2022). Other programs such as the Crisis Prevention Institute (CPI) and Therapeutic Crisis Intervention (TCI) can provide more specific crisis intervention education. The goal of CPI is to help the patient "achieve tension reduction at every level of crisis" (p. 8); therefore, if the clinician is able to identify and respond to behavior at an earlier stage, the patient may not escalate into higher crisis levels (CPI, 2020). Similarly, TCI helps to shape adults' responses to children's aggressive behaviors in ways that avoid injury and prevent crises from occurring, focuses on de-escalating potential crises, manages acute physical behavior, and teaches children adaptive coping strategies (Cornell University, 2021). While these trainings may not be required, they can be extremely helpful to gain a better perspective of how to work safely and holistically within this population.

When identifying a patient's developmental strengths, needs, and goals during their mental health admission, child life specialists should still consider the same assessment variables (e.g. child, family, diagnosis, developmental level, etc.). The main difference when working within a behavioral health setting versus a medical setting is that a behavioral health setting typically solely focuses on a patient's psychosocial needs – unless there was an injury or illness in addition to the mental health concerns (e.g. suicide attempt, repercussions of violent behavior, or a chronic illness) which would then warrant a medical admission. Nevertheless, some of the variables that a behavioral health patient exhibits could be heightened compared to patients without mental health concerns. For instance, a history of trauma can impact brain development which may impact one's temperament and affect the way they perceive stress, thus negatively affecting their ability to cope with an inpatient psychiatric admission. By using interventions such as an All About Me sheet (Figure 1), child life specialists can assess a patient's triggers, otherwise known as stressors that can cause behavioral and/or emotional outbursts, ultimately benefiting the assessment process.

Figure 1. This is an All About Me sheet created by a CCLS to assist in the assessment process and to help families better communicate patient needs to staff (Nunez, 2020)

ALL ABOUT ME

My name is ________________ but I like to be called ______________.

I am ___________ years old and I am in the ________ grade.

The people I live with are____.

Some things that I like are: (activities/colors/toys)

1.

2.

Some things I don't like are: (triggers/sensitivities)

1.

2.

I communicate best by: (talking, writing, using pictures/signs): ____________________________________.

Something that scares me in the hospital is ____________________________.

Something that makes me mad in the hospital is ________________________.

Something that makes me sad in the hospital is _________________________.

This is one of my first times in the hospital. Yes or No

Some questions I have about the hospital are:

1.

2.

3.

I might need extra support with: (personal care/medications/eating/drinking) ________________________________

WHEN YOU COME IN I'D LIKE YOU TO TELL ME: <u>YOUR NAME</u>, <u>WHO YOU ARE</u> AND <u>WHAT YOU ARE GOING TO DO</u>

Safety is one of the main concerns when working with and supporting the behavioral health population. Psychiatric settings typically house individuals who demonstrate aggression and self-harm throughout their treatment. Most children ages 3 to 12 years old admitted to a health care setting for behavioral needs exhibit aggressive and combative behaviors with little impulse control, whereas adolescents demonstrate more self-harm and suicidal ideation (Sharfstein, 2009). Therefore, it is pertinent that child life specialists are assessing patients' ability to be safe when implementing services. Some environmental safety measures within a behavioral health setting may include non-breakable windows, break-away shower curtains, absence of clothes hangers and railings, absence of cords and sharp objects, locked unit doors and cabinets, non-tearable blankets, special doors to prevent barricading, and slanted doorknobs or shower heads (Cardell et al., 2009). These features are installed to prevent ingestion of toxic substances, elopement, hanging, self-harm, and/or aggression (Cardell et al., 2009). Additionally, many psychiatric settings limit contraband items due to safety concerns (e.g., sharp objects such as tweezers, glass items, mirrors, dining utensils, and scissors; intentional asphyxiation risks such as shoelaces, belts, long clothing, intravenous tubing, and plastic bags; digestible toxic substances such as nail polish and/or personal hygiene products; and electronic equipment with batteries) (Cardell et al., 2009). Furthermore, mental health settings may include increased levels of surveillance and observation for patients (Reavey et al., 2017). By assessing the safety risk of specific environmental factors, child life specialists can properly provide developmentally appropriate and safe services and materials (Table 2).

Table 2. Every patient has unique needs and settings may vary. As always, CCLSs should consult with their interdisciplinary team before following these suggestions

Low Safety Risk	Medium Safety Risk	High Safety Risk
Games Interactive games: ● I Spy ● 21 Questions ● I'm Going on a Picnic ● Simon Says Card games: ● Uno/Dos ● Skip-Bo ● Phase 10 ● Apples to Apples ● Playing cards **Puzzles** ● Word searches* ● Sudoku* ● Crossword* ● Cardboard jigsaw puzzles ● Matching/memory games **Art Materials** ● Crayons ● Oil pastels ● Coloring books/pages* ● Notebooks/journals* ● Play-Doh (no can) ● Modeling clay ● Sticker scenes ● Origami ● Kinetic sand ● Foam shapes/sticker **Gross Motor Activities** ● Tearing up magazines/paper* ● Peeling glue on hand ● Making slime ● Foam stress balls/Squishies ● Exercise ● Yoga **Other** ● Paperback books ● Foam blocks ● Stuffed animals (without hard body pieces, like eyes; without pockets; without scarves/clothing) *Check for staples	**Games** (Be mindful of small game pieces that can be used for self-harm) ● Candy Land ● Sorry ● Dominoes ● Jenga ● Qwirkle ● Chutes and Ladder ● Connect 4 ● Headbandz ● Checkers ● Chess ● Scrabble ● Guess Who **Art Materials** ● Markers ● Sand art ● Velvet art ● Scratch-off art **Other** ● Hardback books ● Rubik's cube ● Fidget items ● Action figures ● Baby dolls ● Barbie dolls ● Duplo Legos ● Small amounts of Legos ● Plastic animals ● Hot Wheels cars ● Musical instruments (without string)	**Games** ● Most games containing plastic or metal pieces (e.g. Monopoly or Clue) ● Any game referring to topics that could be perceived as inappropriate or triggering (strong language, drug-use, violence related, sexual references) (e.g. Cards Against Humanity) **Art Materials** ● String/yarn/ribbon longer than five inches ● Scissors ● Glue bottles or glue sticks ● Paint brushes ● Pipe cleaners ● Pens ● Colored pencils or lead pencils ● Jewelry craft kits ● Perler/fuse beads **Other** ● Heavy toys (e.g. large plastic vehicles, musical/light-up toys) ● Wooden toys or crafts ● Magazines/books with staples or paperclips ● Access to internet or social media ● Video games, especially anything with cords or CDs ● Electronics, especially cell phones

Group interventions, which are likely to occur in behavioral health units and facilities, can also make assessments more complex. If a child's mental health treatment primarily functions in group settings, a child life specialist may not be able to make a thorough assessment due to less one-on-one time, reduced family interactions, and the risk of breaching confidentiality. This is where observation and professional collaboration can be especially helpful; child life specialists can gather information by simply attending other disciplines' group therapies and observing patients' behaviors. How does a child respond to taking turns, receiving an undesirable answer, or waiting to eat until a group is finished? What non-verbal cues is their body language demonstrating? Interdisciplinary collaboration and co-treatment are also helpful for assessment. The direct unit staff – such as behavioral health staff and nurses – may have more details about a child's behaviors (i.e., coping styles, anxiety levels, and temperament) than their parents or guardians since they are the ones monitoring their day-to-day behaviors during treatment. Co-treatment with other disciplines such as occupational therapy, speech therapy, recreation therapy, music therapy, art therapy, social work, psychologists, holistic health care specialists, and applied behavior analysis (ABA) therapists can improve treatment outcomes and patient and family experiences. While co-treating, child life specialists and other disciplines can work toward a joint goal, such as building rapport, socialization, normalization, and encouraging psychosocial development, and self-expression. During co-treatment, child life specialists can provide distraction and emotional support, promote motivation and compliance, and be an encouraging presence in order to empower confidence in patients.

It is worth noting that, regardless of their behavioral concerns, patients are still children and adolescents. Studies have shown that behavioral health patients encounter similar negative feelings as medical admissions. Behavioral health patients have mentioned frightening and anxiety-provoking experiences such as complying with blood draws, not knowing when they would discharge, and experiencing or witnessing physical restraints (Tally, 2011). Adolescent patients admitted to a psychiatric inpatient unit have expressed feelings of fear, disgust, and confusion when witnessing other peers' unsafe behaviors (Haynes et al., 2011). Due to unfamiliar settings and strict rules, patients have stated that the hospital setting was inflexible, unresponsive to their needs, and restricting, whereas increased observation and surveillance made patients feel "scrutinized and infantilized" (Haynes et al., 2011, p. 152; Reavey et al., 2017). Many patients have expressed feeling that they have little choice and autonomy, that they are disconnected from friends and family, and that their developmental needs such as privacy, independence, and mobility were being unmet (Haynes et al., 2011; Reavey et al., 2017; Tally, 2011). Some patients have even stated that psychiatric hospitalization was viewed as a reinforcement of the stressors that had resulted in their admission (Haynes et al., 2011). All of these factors can affect a patient's mood, affect, and behavior. Child life specialists should be aware of the stressors that are present with mental health admission and how these may impact their ongoing assessment.

Psychological Preparation and Procedural Support

In behavioral settings, patients of all developmental ages may need more psychosocial support than a medical patient, such as increased relationship building in order to gain trust. Patients admitted for psychiatric concerns may experience various unfamiliar and invasive experiences such as painful medical procedures, facility transitions, treatment meetings, and society reentry post-discharge. Due to patients exhibiting behavioral outbursts and an overall lack of coping skills, patients with mental health concerns can greatly benefit from child life specialists providing psychological preparation and procedural support. Procedural preparation alleviates anxieties and fears that impact patient care, allows patients to enhance their coping, and clears misconceptions about their experience (McGee, 2003). Hands-on interventions can be helpful for patients with additional sensory or learning needs as it allows safe and supervised exploration of materials as well as encourages the use of coping skills adapted to their needs and comfort levels (CLC, 2014).

Procedures can be exceptionally stressful for patients in this population due to sensory concerns, mental distress (e.g. hallucinations or delusions), developmental delays, and/or trauma history. Procedures that can be typical in behavioral health settings mostly concern the heart and the brain, and may include: blood draws, electroencephalogram (EEG), electrocardiogram (EKG), magnetic resonance imaging (MRI), and computerized tomography scan (CT). For the mental health population, preparation prior to a procedure allows patients the time to plan and rehearse new coping strategies, work through feelings about past or impending situations, and provide a sense of predictability and autonomy in knowing what to expect during situations that may seem out of their control (Romito et al., 2021). Child life specialists can also provide procedural preparation and support before, during, and after procedures using nonpharmacological pain management techniques including distraction, comfort positioning, medical play, and emotional support.

Components of psychiatric care, such as daily medications, can become another stress-inducing situation if patients do not know how to swallow pills or are unfamiliar with their medications. Studies show that a large percentage of children and adolescents refuse pill or liquid medications and are unable to swallow a standard-sized pill (Ziemer & Tomlinson, 2017). Additionally, trauma can result in consistently high levels of stress hormones, which can negatively affect a patient's ability to cope with a potential threat (Iacona, 2018). Other specific interventions that may decrease the risk of negative responses to medical interactions may include using psychiatric-safe preparation materials and alternative focus options, maintaining a safe distance from patients demonstrating aggression or impulsivity, and spending an extended amount of time with a patient prior to procedures to build rapport. Overall, child life services have been shown to reduce the child's distress and gain cooperation. These services generally require fewer staff to be present in the room, facilitate the safe and effective accomplishment of the medical procedure, decrease parent anxiety, and increase parent satisfaction (Romito et al., 2021).

Prior to being admitted to a behavioral health setting, a unique experience that a child life specialist can support is when a psychiatric medical admission transitions to a psychiatric unit or facility. While waiting in the ED or general pediatric floor, patients may have limited access to resources, are unable to leave their rooms, and are typically placed with a sitter at their bedside. A child life specialist can provide preparation to support this transition to a behavioral health unit/facility which is likely an unfamiliar place with new people and different rules. One way that child life specialists can support this transition is by reaching out to local psychiatric and residential facilities to create preparation books or social stories and gain information to share with patients and families such as photos of the unit/facility, unit schedule, interdisciplinary team members (e.g., psychiatrists or therapists), and visitation hours.

Within a behavioral health setting, patients will likely meet with a therapist and, if appropriate, involve family members to discuss and create treatment goals during and after hospitalization. Patients should be a part of the planning and discharge process in order to allow for autonomy, self-advocacy, and opportunities to plan and prepare for future coping needs. CCLSs can help to advocate for the importance of patient involvement in their plan of care and can support the coping process for the patient and family during the creation of the plan. Preparation for reentry into society is also important for psychiatric patients. This transition can be especially difficult depending on the length of the patient's stay in the psychiatric facility as well as any drastic changes that they may have experienced, such as having limited phone and social media usage, having stricter rules, and returning to inadequate home environments. Child life specialists can provide the opportunity for patients to express themselves and verbalize any concerns about reentry to society while providing emotional support and validation. In preparation for discharge, CCLSs can facilitate activities and discussions regarding coping plans for various settings, like home, school, and their community. These coping plans can be situation- and trigger-based, thus setting the patients up for success in a variety of situations. For example, listening to music as a coping tool may be helpful at home, but not realistic at school; therefore, differentiating between diverse coping tools can assist in reentry into society.

Developmental Explanations

Dealing with a new diagnosis can be overwhelming and confusing, especially if the diagnosis deals with abstract and complex concepts such as mental illnesses. Unlike medical conditions, mental health conditions are usually not as tangible or apparent, which can be difficult for children to understand. However, similar to medical diagnoses, any myths, confusion, and misinformation regarding mental health diagnoses can cause anxiety, strengthen stereotypes, and lead to negative stigma (AACAP, 2017). Certified Child Life Specialists are expertly trained to educate children and their families on various diagnoses by using play-based and developmentally grounded interventions (Boles et al., 2020). By providing mental health diagnosis education, CCLSs are able to minimize fear and anxiety, relieve some uncertainty, increase coping, and provide a stronger sense of control (Johns Hopkins Medicine, 2021).

When approaching the topic of a mental health diagnosis, both the AACAP (2017) and the NAMI (2022a) recommend comparing mental health concerns to those of a physical illness, because essentially, it is a physical illness. A common analogy goes as follows: A child breaks a bone, and that bone cannot be mended by waiting it out, talking to a friend, or taking over-the-counter medicine. The child needs to go to the hospital in order to get professional help, which may include medication or medical treatment. However, with help, the bone will begin to heal, and the child will learn how to live with their new circumstances. That same concept can be applied to a behavioral health concern. Mental health concerns are physical conditions that start with the brain (NAMI, 2022a). The brain controls feelings, thoughts, and behaviors. Everyone feels sad or angry every once in a while, but if those feelings become too big, they can affect parts of lives like school, relationships, and even our physical health; that is when the brain gets too "stressed" and has a hard time dealing with emotions. At that point, professional help needs to get involved. Professional help can include talking to a trained adult like a therapist, taking medicine to help manage emotions, and/or enrolling in programs that help specifically for behavioral health concerns.

Depending on the age of a child, this information should be explained concretely by incorporating physical and visual sensations (NAMI, 2022a). Diagnostic education should include information such as (Johns Hopkins Medicine, 2021):

- An explanation of the diagnosis;
- How various body systems, such as the brain, are involved and are supposed to work/how those systems are not working properly;
- Symptom management and coping with the diagnosis;
- Possible medications, treatment, and hospital admissions; and
- The five senses.

Similar to a traditional medical setting, teaching tools such as books, puppets, visual aids, medical equipment, games, and open dialogue can be used, all while still taking into consideration any safety precautions.

It is important to understand that, because mental illness can severely impact one's emotions, managing the environment and creating a therapeutic space can promote the best outcomes for diagnostic education. As previously discussed, many children affected by mental health conditions have certain psychosocial risk factors (e.g. lower SES and previous trauma) that are associated with lower knowledge of their mental health conditions as well as higher uncertainty for the child and the family, thus leading to an increased need of education (Boles et al., 2020). The AACAP (2017) recommends talking to a child about their mental health when the child feels safe and relaxed while assessing their reactions throughout the discussion. If the child becomes upset or confused, do not hesitate to slow down or pause (AACAP, 2017). Many young people may have questions about their condition based on their developmental understanding. Preschoolers will focus on things they can see or feel, such as crying or yelling; school-age children will ask for more specific information; and adolescents may respond well to open dialogue (AACAP, 2017). Children may feel ashamed or embarrassed about discussing their mental health due to stigma and/or misinformation; therefore, child life specialists should use active listening, reflective statements, and emotional validation when providing education (NAMI, 2022a). By taking a strength-based approach to diagnostic education, child life specialists can focus on the positive attributes of the child, promote a sense of mastery and control, and focus on healthy self-care and coping strategies.

Lastly, child life specialists can also incorporate family and members of the interdisciplinary team into diagnosis education. Family involvement can promote transparency and normalization of a child's mental health diagnosis (NAMI, 2022a). Child life specialists should adequately assess the relationships between the child and family members in order to prevent any stressors associated with familial issues (e.g. family members disagreeing with a diagnosis, abusive caregivers, etc.). By partnering with other disciplines, such as psychiatrists or social workers, CCLSs can complement the knowledge and expertise of these professionals while deciphering any overwhelming or complex information that they may share with the child or family.

Play

Opportunities for play, leisure, and expressive arts are a key component of any young person's life and that does not change within the mental health population. Studies show a link between children with mental health concerns and decreased playtime. Children living in emotionally supportive and stimulating environments are more likely to have positive stress, are more playful, and are more emotionally resilient, while play deprivation is associated with a deficiency in the growth and functioning of key brain regions (Whitebread, 2017). Therefore, child life specialists should encourage play and recreational activities to normalize a mental health setting.

Behavioral health settings can increase the stress levels of children; therefore, play and leisure can be used as coping tools and comfort measures. Safe and developmentally appropriate activities (Figure 2) can be adapted to address the unique needs of patients based on their developmental levels, interests, behavioral conditions, and settings (Child Life Council [CLC], 2014). Developmental play can create trusting relationships with staff, resulting in a greater likelihood of treatment compliance; keep the patient distracted, which provides more structure and less wait time; and give the patients a sense of familiarity (Burns-Nader & Hernandez-Reif, 2016). In a previous study, patients admitted to a hospital for psychiatric concerns labeled staff who were easy to talk to, good listeners, non-judgmental, and reliable as a supportive factor that benefited their admission (Tally, 2011). When staff was able to meet the patient's basic needs, show empathy, actively listen, and validate their feelings, patients were more likely to have an increased sense of belonging, trust, self-expressiveness, and feeling respected (Berg et al., 2017). Normalization of a psychiatric health care setting not only makes the experience more positive for a patient and family but also helps break the negative stigma toward mental illness.

Figure 2. This is a poster created by a Certified Child Life Specialist with the help of an adolescent patient who conducted a slime experiment using different ingredients. The patient had severe suicidal ideation and self-harm tendencies, such as creating skin abrasions with food utensils and broken materials, and needed to be monitored closely for safety precautions. Therefore, the CCLS used low-risk materials (e.g. small amounts of glue, detergent, Model Magic, and lotion) and encouraged the patient to create the slime while the CCLS was responsible for the writing on the poster with the marker. The slime was then locked in a secure cubby with the intention of the patient retrieving it upon discharge

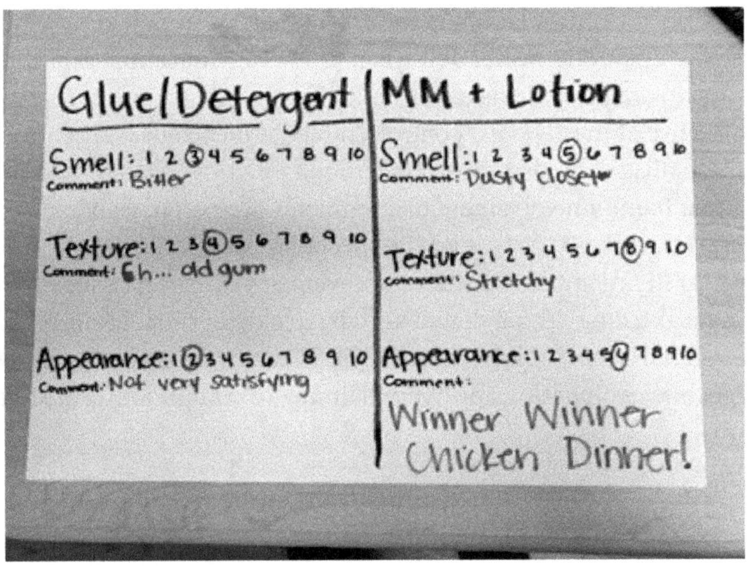

Emotional Support

Patients in behavioral health settings are often experiencing mental distress, are completely out of their element, and are in need of additional coping resources. Hospitalization may "initially exacerbate a young person's difficulties by compromising their autonomy and self-esteem" (Haynes et al., 2011, p. 154). Patients may have a difficult time coping due to fear, anxiety, and lack of preparation for this setting. Depending on the circumstances, arriving at the behavioral health setting may have been sudden or unexpected. Oftentimes, this may be a patient's first time away from their families and/or away from home, potentially resulting in separation anxiety. When a child is experiencing a highly stressful situation, they may have difficulty processing information and complying due to their lack of understanding and heightened emotions.

Behavioral health settings can be chaotic and upsetting; even more so if a patient does not understand why they are there or what to expect. Patients are often already experiencing mental distress or confusion prior to admission and the added distress of this setting can cause more anxiety, fear, and anger. Child life specialists can advocate for a more therapeutic and calming environment to decrease the potential for a traumatic experience. Techniques such as managing the environment and building therapeutic rapport may promote a therapeutic milieu. An example of managing the environment is by creating a safe zone or a sensory room, which is a quiet space away from overwhelming noises that patients can use as needed (Huang-Storms, 2018). Another example is using the One Voice approach; this can be adapted to the psychiatric setting by recognizing that the same techniques used during procedural support can be used during any stressful situation, such as a behavioral crisis (Table 3) (Wagers, 2018). By being aware of patients' triggers, child life specialists can assist patients and staff in behavioral crisis prevention and/or the initiation of the de-escalation process (Huang-Storms, 2018).

Table 3. The One Voice approach is commonly used during procedural support but can be applied to a behavioral health crisis (Wagers, 2018)

One Voice Approach (Wagers, 2018)	One Voice Approach Adapted for Behavioral Health
One voice should be heard during a procedure	● Advocate for one voice to create a soothing environment and to avoid overwhelming a patient further. ● One voice should be heard when a patient appears to be: ● Overwhelmed ● Angry/frustrated/triggered ● Having a behavioral crisis ● Having an anxiety/panic attack
Need parental involvement	● When possible, families should be involved during procedures and behavioral crises. ● If a family is not able to be present, a trusted individual or CCLS should be present to support the patient. ● CCLSs can plan prior to procedures to discuss triggers and coping techniques to best support patients. ● If appropriate, CCLSs can reach out to the family to complete the All About Me sheet (Figure 1) to know how to best support the patient when the family cannot be present.
Educate patient before the procedure about what is going to happen	● Provide education to the patient about procedures and unit policies (i.e. what support staff can provide during the crisis). ● Offer verbal and visual choices.
Validate child with words	● Validate the patient with words and pictures. ● If appropriate, a sticker chart or behavior chart can be created to support activities that are difficult for the patient (e.g. attending groups, eating meals, following the rules, etc.)
Offer the most comfortable, non-threatening position	● When possible, offer choices (depending on age and developmental level, 2-3 choices may be appropriate) such as choice of room, choice of sitting/laying down, and/or choice of coping technique to utilize to begin the calming process.
Individualize your game plan	● Build therapeutic rapport with patients. ● During groups/individual sessions, openly discuss triggers, likes, dislikes, and preferred coping techniques for different situations (e.g. home, school, panic attack, anger, sadness, etc.) ● Include the patient and/or family in the coping plan. ● Offer choices. ● Use of sticker charts/behavior charts.
Choose appropriate distraction to be used	● When appropriate, offer choices. ● Make room modifications when possible (e.g. lights on/off, door open/closed). ● Know the patient's limitations/triggers (e.g. light spinner may trigger a seizure for patients with epilepsy, iPad use may trigger memories of issues with social media).
Eliminate unnecessary people not actively involved with the procedure	● During a behavioral crisis, security officers can be especially triggering. As long as the patient is safe, CCLSs can advocate for extra staff to wait outside the room or out of the patient's eyesight (to be called in if needed).

Coping

Certified Child Life Specialists in psychiatric settings may facilitate therapeutic group sessions or individualized coping interventions. However, it is important to discuss how the therapeutic services that a child life specialist provides are *not* therapy. Child life specialists provide therapeutic opportunities for youth to express themselves in developmentally appropriate and safe ways. Some topics that child life specialists can explore when working with children and youth include coping skills, sense of control, emotional regulation, future goals, self-esteem, grief and loss, positivity, friendship, relationships, honesty, kindness, gratitude, hope, growth/progress, boundaries, diversity and inclusion, connection, and physical/mental health. During these interactions, child life specialists are not analyzing, evaluating, or diagnosing mental health conditions, but rather providing opportunities to reduce stress and anxiety, encourage choice and control, help to maintain self-esteem and confidence, and increase communication and cooperation with peers and authority (Burns-Nader & Hernandez-Reif, 2016; Koukourikos et al., 2015). These optional opportunities allow children to focus on their feelings and emotions related to their mental health needs, the reason for admission, and/or life events (Burns-Nader & Hernandez-Reif, 2016).

An important consideration when providing therapeutic opportunities to the behavioral health population is how group versus one-to-one interactions may affect the services that a child life specialist can provide. Many behavioral health settings primarily function in group facilitated therapies. Group therapy can benefit participants by being a support network and sounding board, helping them realize that they are not alone, and bringing diverse backgrounds and personalities together when problem-solving (Johnson, 2019). However, group settings for children and adolescents can also have challenges. Breaches of confidentiality, poor boundaries between peers, verbal and/or physical altercations, varying developmental levels, and availability of staff support are just a few drawbacks to group interventions. For example, a group of children in an inpatient psychiatric unit could have patients ages 7- to 17 years old with various behavioral health needs. What materials or activities could be provided to address the developmental needs of all of the patients? How might child life specialists adjust their approach to each individual patient while creating an inclusive group environment? Are there themes or topics that might be both concrete and abstract to fit the varying levels of cognitive understanding? With careful assessment and planning, as well as collaboration with staff before interventions, child life specialists can have successful and beneficial group interactions.

While group sessions may be broader and involve patients of various ages and developmental levels, groups can provide opportunities for patients to talk with their peers and learn about new ways to cope while also allowing time for normalization, play, and leisure. However, Certified Child Life Specialists should be prepared if sensitive topics arise during group sessions. Patients may need to be redirected in order to avoid triggering their peers or oversharing. In this situation, patients may benefit from an individual coping skills session in order to validate feelings and teach additional coping techniques (Figure 3).

Based on the child life specialists assessment of the patient, a patient may benefit from a one-to-one session where topics of discussion and activities can be individualized to the patient's needs and all attention can be solely on the one patient. Depending on the patient's safety level, CCLSs may use play and leisure opportunities to help the patient return to their baseline after a crisis or a stressful situation. Coping techniques such as breathing techniques and guided imagery use safe and comforting items to promote calming and distraction. When working with patients who are continuously experiencing stressful situations, using coping techniques that have been successful in the past can improve the patient's understanding of the experience, create a coping routine, and reduce anxiety and the possibility of a behavior outburst (Nunez, 2018). It may be helpful to ask the patient or the family about tools or resources they use at home, such as a first-then board, likes and dislikes, typical behaviors and how they calm down, as well as triggers or sensitivities and how to accommodate them. Child life specialists can also discuss the need for necessary accommodations (e.g., a separate visitation time to decrease overstimulation) (Nunez, 2020).

Figure 3. This is a coping kit created by a Certified Child Life Specialist with the help of a school-age patient. The patient was getting bullied at school and had anxiety and suicidal ideations. The CCLS helped the patient create a coping plan for school and for home focusing on ways to calm and distract self in times of crisis. Together, the CCLS and patient chose empowering words to create positive affirmations and made I-Spy cards with stickers. While in the psychiatric unit the patient was able to use safe materials from the coping kit including their comfort item, stress ball, notepad, crossword, and crayons (without a box). Upon discharge, the patient was able to take the complete coping kit home with the intention of putting some items in their backpack and others in a safe space at home to have easy access to coping items when feeling anxious

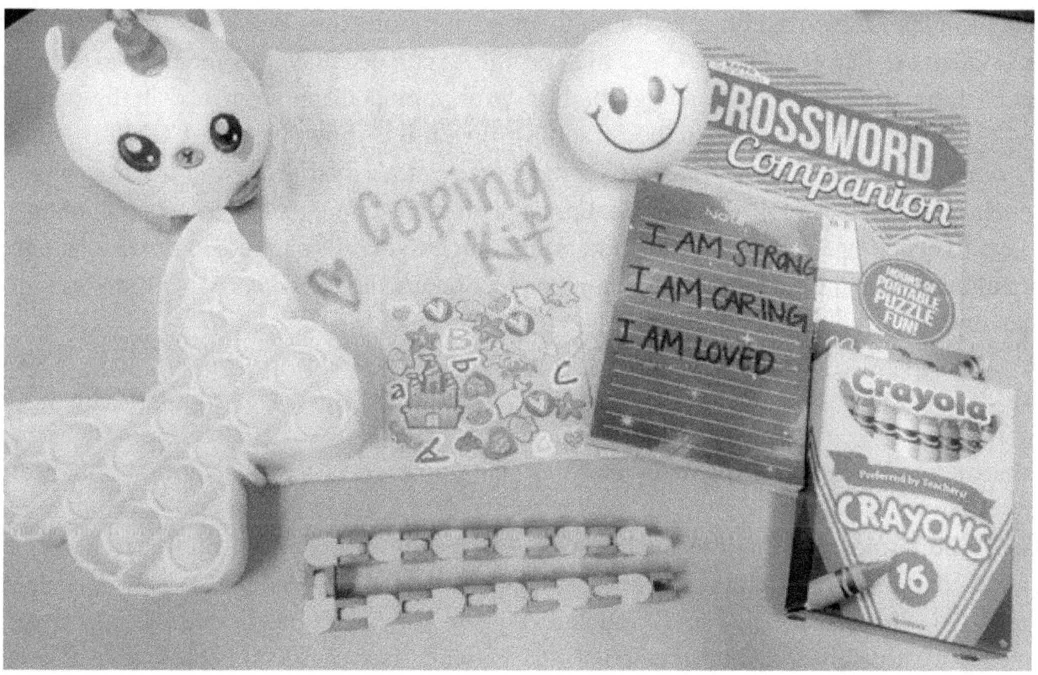

When working with patients in a behavioral health setting whether in a group or one-to-one, it is important to keep safety concerns in mind and to have environmental awareness. It may be helpful to know if the child or adolescent has any behavioral concerns that could affect the safety of the professionals, such as a previous history of assaulting gender-specific individuals, making false allegations against adults, or attempting to have romantic relationships with adults. When preparing to provide services to these children and adolescents, environmental awareness is beneficial. For example, if a child life specialist plans to meet with a patient in a room with a door, having the door open, staying near the exit of the room, and having a staff member remain with the CCLS during the one-on-one can prevent unsafe situations from occurring.

Grief Support

Literature shows that 26% percent of children in the United States will witness or experience a traumatic event before they turn four, while about 4% of children experience the death of a parent and 5% experience the death of a close relative or friend before they turn eighteen (Iacona, 2018; Palmer et al., 2016). Prior to a mental health admission, patients may have experienced bereavement or trauma and may not have healthy coping skills or the knowledge to recognize that they are experiencing grief. Psychiatric admissions may be linked to a patient's grief experience as grief can often lead to major depression, increased anxiety, posttraumatic stress disorder, and social withdrawal (Palmer et al., 2016). Patients may also have experienced trauma in their past or immediately prior to their psychiatric admission (e.g. escorted by police, having a physical altercation, or attempting suicide).

In this setting, Certified Child Life Specialists can provide grief and trauma support with developmentally appropriate interventions and memory-making activities, as well as encouraging opportunities for patients to express their feelings and thoughts regarding previous bereavement or trauma through play, art, and leisure (Brown, 2009). Child life specialists can use play as a medium in which children "manipulate traumatic or anxiety-inducing situations in an attempt to gain control over the event" (Brown, 2009, p. 143). If patients elaborate on their trauma or grief, it is the role of the CCLS to provide active listening, emotional validation, and reflective statements rather than providing treatment suggestions. Furthermore, child life specialists may collaborate with counselors, psychologists, chaplains, and social workers to encourage additional grief and trauma processing for patients in order to avoid crossing professional boundaries. This information can then be documented and shared with the treatment team for further support.

Forensic Interviews

Due to the trauma backgrounds of many children and adolescents with behavioral health diagnoses, forensic interviews, otherwise known as child abuse investigation interviews, are common within this population. The purpose of forensic interviews is to provide evidence for both criminal child abuse investigations and civil child protection proceedings (American Professional Society on the Abuse of Children, 2012). These interviews are conducted by professionals trained in child forensics such as law enforcement investigators and child protective service workers (American Professional Society on the Abuse of Children, 2012). If a child or adolescent is not safe enough to complete the interview outside of a behavioral health setting, some forensic interviews may happen within the same facility. These interviews can be triggering as they likely will address sensitive subjects regarding previous trauma and involve unfamiliar individuals or environments. Although Certified Child Life Specialists cannot prepare a child for the questions that will be asked – that could be considered as tampering with the interview – they can prepare the child for what to expect from the process or how the room/area may look. Before interviews, child life specialists can reassure the child that it is safe to talk to the interviewer about the abuse, provide support through listening and emotional validation, create a coping plan, and prepare the child for tangible aspects of an interview, such as the presence of a recording device. After interviews, if the child feels safe and comfortable, a CCLS can provide a normalizing or stress-relieving activity, such as art, play, or gross motor movement.

Advocacy and Family-Centered Care

Certified Child Life Specialists advocate for family-centered care, an approach to health care in which a mutual partnership is emphasized between patients, families, and health care professionals (Bell et al., 2009). Families often have limited knowledge about the behavioral health setting. During psychiatric admission, caregivers may have unanswered questions about the next steps in care, frustrations with medical and mental health systems, specific fears about inpatient psychiatric treatment, and uncertainty about how to talk to their child about their reason for admission (Bowden et al., 2022). Patients in behavioral health settings often have smaller or more fragile social networks and/or reduced parental or guardian presence. Therefore, partnering with families when possible, can help with mental stabilization (Marcon et al., 2017). Benefits of family-centered care include improvement in medical and developmental outcomes, better responsiveness to the patients' and families' needs, and higher patient and family satisfaction regarding the hospital experience (Bell et al., 2009).

Certified Child Life Specialists provide relationship support by educating about and modeling optimal attachment, enhancing a child's self-advocacy and communication skills, and cultivating understanding and empathy within siblings and peers (ACLP, 2018). By actively listening to the patient to help them address their needs, offering choices, and helping to advocate for the patient, CCLSs establish themselves as safe and trusted support staff. If families are present during any psychiatric admission, child life specialists can provide emotional support, education, and normalization opportunities to caregivers and siblings. If parents are not present, CCLSs can initiate meetings with the family in person or over the phone to introduce child life services and offer any additional support or resources (e.g. sibling support groups, bereavement camps, virtual coping resources, etc.) while advocating for family involvement and family presence when possible. By having an understanding of the family's preferences, child life specialists can encourage and remind the interdisciplinary team about these strategies in order to create a positive experience for the patient and family.

As advocates, child life specialists can be the liaison between the patient/family and the interdisciplinary team, thus creating a child- and family-friendly environment and ensuring concerns are addressed. Child life specialists can help model the importance of family-centered care and can help advocate for open lines of communication by including families in the medical and psychiatric processes (i.e. email, phone, and in-person meetings). Furthermore, part of the role of a Certified Child Life Specialist is to educate families and health care providers on how children communicate and interpret their surroundings. In the psychiatric setting, children need the same support. The literature demonstrates the barriers to appropriate health care not only affect young people diagnosed with psychiatric disorders but also their families and healthcare providers (Romito et al., 2021). Ultimately, CCLSs can share a structured, warm, and compassionate relationship with patients while maintaining professional boundaries (e.g. setting expectations prior to intervention) and being aware of their own self-care needs (e.g. healthy work/life balance, being mindful of personal and professional needs).

CONCLUSION

Childhood and adolescence are critical periods for mental health awareness. There is strong research that links the mental, social, and emotional health of youth to their ability to form relationships, to be able to work, and to their academic achievement (Cornell University, 2021; NAMI, 2022c). Undiagnosed, untreated, or inadequately treated mental illnesses can significantly interfere with a child's ability to continue to learn, grow, and develop; therefore, leading to extensive and long-term delays in social, emotional, and cognitive development (Cornell University, 2021; NAMI, 2022c). Pediatric behavioral health services are an overall underserved population and have a great need for child life services. Due to the needs of pediatric and adolescent patients with psychiatric diagnoses and the nature of child life services, Certified Child Life Specialists should be considered essential members of the multidisciplinary psychiatric team in a variety of settings.

It is recommended that child life specialists be employed in behavioral health settings to support patients and families during this stressful and potentially traumatic time in their lives. Child life services can help to minimize the adverse effects of triggering situations on children and families while teaching lifelong skills that will build resiliency outside of the behavioral health setting. Along with family-centered care practices, child life services have been shown to improve health care outcomes by leading to less anxiety among children and families, reduced length of stay, less analgesic consumption, higher parent satisfaction ratings, and overall improvement of the child's quality of life (Romito et al., 2021). When working with the mental health population, child life specialists can improve health care outcomes by advocating for patients with limited family involvement, encouraging the least restrictive treatment approaches, and providing developmentally appropriate opportunities for self-expression. While this may be considered a non-traditional setting for child life specialists, many interventions are the same and can be adapted for safety considerations. Therefore, child life services need to expand to support vulnerable populations in various settings outside of healthcare. In order to understand the needs of the child life community to best support the mental health population, it may be helpful to survey child life specialists regarding existing gaps in pediatric mental health care through a psychosocial lens. As with other medical disciplines, child life specialists would not only benefit from additional training to better service the mental health population but – with proper education and training – could also provide insight on how to provide adequate psychosocial care for patients and families. Certified Child Life Specialists should conduct and assist in upcoming research bridging the gaps of pediatric and adolescent psychiatric care. With the expansion of child life's psychosocial support, the importance of mental health awareness will be magnified, thus further breaking the stigma and building a more resilient future for youth and their families.

REFERENCES

Al-Yateem, N. B., Issa, W. B., & Rossiter, R. (2015). Childhood stress in health care settings: Awareness and suggested interventions. *Issues in Comprehensive Pediatric Nursing*, *38*(2), 136–153. doi:10.3109/01460862.2015.1035465 PMID:25919580

American Academy of Child and Adolescent Psychiatry. (2017). *Talking to kids about mental illnesses.* https://www.aacap.org/AACAP/Families_and_Youth/Facts_for_Families/FFF-Guide/Talking-To-Kids-About-Mental-Illnesses-084.aspx

American Academy of Child and Adolescent Psychiatry. (2022). *Ethical issues in clinical practice.* https://www.aacap.org/AACAP/Member_Resources/Ethics/Ethics_Committee/Ethical_Issues_in_Clinical_Practice.aspx

American Academy of Pediatrics. (2021). *Declaration of a national emergency in child and adolescent mental health.* https://www.aap.org/en/advocacy/child-and-adolescent-healthy-mental-development/aap-aacap-cha-declaration-of-a-national-emergency-in-child-and-adolescent-mental-health/

American Professional Society on the Abuse of Children. (2012). *Practice guidelines: Forensic interviewing in cases of suspected child abuse.* https://depts.washington.edu/uwhatc/PDF/guidelines/Forensic%20Interviewing%20in%20Cases%20of%20Suspected%20Child%20Abuse.pdf

American Psychiatric Association. (2013). *Diagnostic and statistical manual of mental disorders* (5th ed.). doi:10.1176/appi.books.9780890425596

Asnaani, A., & Hofmann, S. G. (2012). Collaboration in multicultural therapy: Establishing a strong therapeutic alliance across cultural lines. *Journal of Clinical Psychology, 68*(2), 187–197. doi:10.1002/jclp.21829 PMID:23616299

Association of Child Life Professionals. (2018). *Position statement on child life practice in community settings.* https://www.childlife.org/docs/default-source/about-aclp/cbp-on-cl-practice-in-community-settings.pdf

Behere, A. P., Basnet, P., & Campbell, P. (2017). Effects of family structure on mental health of children: A preliminary study. *Indian Journal of Psychological Medicine, 39*(4), 457–463. doi:10.4103/0253-7176.211767 PMID:28852240

Bell, J. L., John, B. H., Desai, P. P., & McLeod, S. M. (2009). Family-centered care and the implications for child life practice. In R. H. Thompson (Ed.), *The Handbook of Child Life: A Guide for Pediatric Psychosocial Care* (pp. 95–115). Charles C. Thomas Publisher, Ltd.

Berg, S. H., Rortvelt, K., & Aase, K. (2017). Suicidal patients' experiences regarding their safety during psychiatric in-patient care: A systematic review of qualitative studies. *BMC Health Services Research, 17*(73), 73. Advance online publication. doi:10.118612913-017-2023-8 PMID:28114936

Boles, J., Fraser, C., Bennett, K., Jones, M., Dunbar, J., Woodburn, A., Gill, M. A., Duplechain, A., Munn, E. K., & Hoskins, K. (2020). *The value of certified child life specialists: Direct and downstream optimization of pediatric patient and family outcomes.* Association of Child Life Professionals. https://www.childlife.org/docs/default-source/the-child-life-profession/value-of-cclss-full-report.pdf

Bowden, C. F., Worsley, D., Pettit, A. R., & Doupnik, S. K. (2022). Caregiver experiences during their child's acute medical hospitalization for a mental health crisis. *Journal of Child Health Care, 26*(1), 123–138. doi:10.1177/13674935211001222 PMID:33787342

Brown, C. (2009). Working with grieving children and families. In R. H. Thompson (Ed.), *The Handbook of Child Life: A Guide for Pediatric Psychosocial Care* (pp. 238–255). Charles C. Thomas Publisher, Ltd.

Burns-Nader, S., & Hernandez-Reif, M. (2016). Facilitating play for hospitalized children through child life services. *Children's Health Care, 40*(1), 1–21. doi:10.1080/02739615.2014.948161

Cabaj, R. P. (2022). *Working with LGBTQ patients.* American Psychiatric Association. https://www.psychiatry.org/psychiatrists/cultural-competency/education/best-practice-highlights/working-with-lgbtq-patients

Cardell, R., Bratcher, K. S., & Quinnett, P. (2009). Revisiting "suicide proofing" an inpatient unit through environmental safeguards: A review. *Perspectives in Psychiatric Care, 45*(1), 36–44. doi:10.1111/j.1744-6163.2009.00198.x PMID:19154238

Carstensen, K., Lou, S., Jensen, L. G., Nissen, N. K., Ortenblad, L., Pfau, M., & Ankerson, P. L. (2017). Psychiatric service users' experiences of emergency departments: A CERQual review of qualitative studies. *Nordic Journal of Psychiatry, 71*(4), 315–323. doi:10.1080/08039488.2017.1288759 PMID:28413938

Casey, C. (2019). Management of aggressive patients: Results of an education program for nurses in non-psychiatric settings. *Medsurg Nursing, 28*(1), 9–21.

Causey, D. L., McKay, M., Rosenthal, C., & Darnell, C. (1998). Assessment of hospital-related stress in children and adolescents admitted to a psychiatric inpatient unit. *Journal of Child and Adolescent Psychiatric Nursing, 11*(4), 135–145. doi:10.1111/j.1744-6171.1998.tb00029.x PMID:10067477

Centers for Disease Control and Prevention. (2021b). *Developmental disabilities.* https://www.cdc.gov/ncbddd/developmentaldisabilities/facts.html

Centers for Disease Control and Prevention. (2021a). *Autism spectrum disorder.* https://www.cdc.gov/ncbddd/autism/index.html

Centers for Disease Control and Prevention. (2021c). *What is children's mental health?* https://www.cdc.gov/childrensmentalhealth/basics.html

Child Life Council. (2014). *Child life services.* American Academy of Pediatrics. doi:10.1542/peds.2014-0556

Cornell University. (2021). *The therapeutic crisis intervention system* (7th ed.). Residential Child Care Project. https://rccp.cornell.edu/downloads/TCI_7_SYSTEM%20BULLETIN.pdf

Crisis Prevention Institute. (2019). *What is nonviolent crisis intervention training?* https://www.crisis-prevention.com/What-We-Do

Crisis Prevention Institute. (2020). *CPI nonviolent crisis intervention training* (2nd ed.). [Participant workbook]. Author.

Danielson, B. (2018, October). *Child life and psychiatry* [Conference presentation]. Great Lakes Association of Child Life Professionals, Cincinnati, OH, United States.

Danielson, B., McEwen, K., & Sullivan, K. (2019, April). *Please see me, I'm sick too: The journey through a mental health care admission* [Conference presentation]. Association of Child Life Professionals National Conference, Chicago, IL, United States.

Dirik, A., Sandhu, S., Giacco, D., Barrett, K., Bennison, G., Collinson, S., & Priebe, S. (2017). Why involve families in acute mental health care? A collaborative conceptual review. *BMJ Open*, *7*(9), e017680. Advance online publication. doi:10.1136/bmjopen-2017-017680 PMID:28963308

Dopheide, J. A. (2013). Recognizing and referring at-risk youth. *The Mental Health Clinician*, *2*(11), 353–361. doi:10.9740/mhc.n145475

Fahrenwald, D., & Haley, J. (2021, September 10-12). *Piecing together autism, baker acts and community inequalities* [Conference presentation]. Florida Association of Child Life Professionals Annual Conference, Orlando, FL, United States.

Felitti, V. J., Anda, R. F., Nordenberg, D., Williamson, D. F., Spitz, A. M., Edwards, E., Koss, M., & Marks, J. S. (1998). Relationship to childhood abuse and household dysfunction to many of the leading causes of death in adults: The adverse childhood experiences (ACE) study. *American Journal of Preventive Medicine*, *14*(4), 245–258. doi:10.1016/S0749-3797(98)00017-8 PMID:9635069

Field, J., & Schubert, C. M. (2010). An examination of emergency department pediatric psychiatric services. *The Journal of Behavioral Health Services & Research*, *37*(4), 412–426. doi:10.100711414-009-9189-8 PMID:19731041

Gallagher, K. A. S., Bujoreanu, L. S., Cheung, P., Choi, C., Golden, S., Brodziak, K., Andrare, G., & Ibeziako, P. (2017). Psychiatric boarding in the pediatric inpatient medical setting: A retrospective analysis. *Hospital Pediatrics*, *7*(8), 444–450. doi:10.1542/hpeds.2017-0005 PMID:28716803

Hanna, M. D., & Rogers, S. (2022). Real or imagined: Racial bias in family assessments. *Child Welfare*, *100*(2), 137–162.

Hart, L., Kelly, C., Kingston, A., Langlands, R., & Masselli, B. (2016). *Mental health first aid USA* [Workbook]. National Council for Behavioral Health.

Haynes, C., Eivors, A., & Crossley, J. (2011). 'Living in an alternative reality:' adolescents' experiences of psychiatric inpatient care. *Child and Adolescent Mental Health*, *16*(3), 150–157. doi:10.1111/j.1475-3588.2011.00598.x PMID:32847238

Hazen, E. P., & Prager, L. M. (2017). A quiet crisis: Pediatric patients waiting for inpatient psychiatric care. *Journal of the American Academy of Child and Adolescent Psychiatry*, *56*(8), 631–633. doi:10.1016/j.jaac.2017.03.022 PMID:28735689

Hornor, G., Davis, C., Sherfield, J., & Wilkinson, K. (2019). Trauma-informed care: Essential elements for pediatric health care. *Journal of Pediatric Health Care*, *33*(2), 214–221. doi:10.1016/j.pedhc.2018.09.009 PMID:30777228

Huang-Storms, L. (2018). *Autism parents seek help for behavioral crises.* Autism Speaks. https://www.autismspeaks.org/expert-opinion/autism-parents-seek-help-behavioral-crises

Hudson, L. (2022). Mental health of children and young people since the start of the pandemic. *Clinical Child Psychology and Psychiatry*, *27*(1), 3–5. doi:10.1177/13591045211072721 PMID:35105247

Hume, K., Regan, T., Megronigle, L., & Rhinehalt, C. (2015). Supporting students with autism spectrum disorder through grief and loss. *Teaching Exceptional Children*, *48*(3), 128–136. doi:10.1177/0040059915618196

Hunter, N. C., Schaefer, M., Kurz, K., Prates, M. O., & Sinha, A. (2015). Individual and organizational predictors of pediatric psychiatric inpatient admission in Connecticut hospitals: A 6-month secondary analysis. *Administration and Policy in Mental Health*, *42*(2), 176–185. doi:10.100710488-014-0558-0 PMID:24879633

Iacona, J., & Johnson, S. (2018). Neurobiology of trauma and mindfulness for children. *Journal of Trauma Nursing*, *25*(3), 187–191. doi:10.1097/JTN.0000000000000365 PMID:29742631

Johns Hopkins Medicine. (2021). *Diagnosis education.* https://www.hopkinsallchildrens.org/Services/Child-Life/Patient-and-Family-Support/Diagnosis-Education

Johnson, B. (2019). *Psychotherapy: Understanding group therapy.* American Psychological Association. https://www.apa.org/topics/psychotherapy/group-therapy

Kerrison, S. A., & Chapman, R. (2007). What general emergency nurses want to know about mental health patients presenting to their emergency department. *Accident and Emergency Nursing*, *16*(1), 48–55. doi:10.1016/j.aaen.2006.09.003 PMID:17198753

Koller, D. (2008). *Child life assessment: Variables associated with a child's ability to cope with hospitalization*. Child Life Council.

Koller, D. (2019). New ways of thinking and doing: A theoretical vision for child life. *ACLP Bulletin, 37*(4). https://www.childlife.org/membership/aclp-bulletin/fall-2019-table-of-contents/new-ways-of-thinking-and-doing-a-theoretical-vision-for-child-life/

Koukourikos, K., Tzeha, L., Pantelidoum, P., & Tsalogidou, A. (2015). The importance of play during hospitalization of children. *Journal of the Academy of Medical Sciences of Bosnia and Herzegovina*, *27*(6), 438–441. doi:10.5455/msm.2015.27.438-441 PMID:26889107

Li, A. S. Y., Lang, Q., Cho, J., Nguyen, V. S., & Nandakumar, S. (2021). Cultural and structural humility and addressing systems of care disparities in mental health services for black, indigenous, and people of color. *Child and Adolescent Psychiatric Clinics of North America*, *31*(2), 251–259. PMID:35361363

Ma, N., Roberts, R., Winfield, H., & Furber, G. (2015). The prevalence of psychopathology in siblings of children with mental health problems: A 20-year systematic review. *Child Psychiatry and Human Development*, *46*(1), 130–149. doi:10.100710578-014-0459-1 PMID:24652033

Marcon, T. D., Girz, L., Stillar, A., Tessier, C., & Lafrance, A. (2017). Parental involvement and child and adolescent eating disorders: Perspectives from residents in psychiatry, pediatrics, and family medicine. *Journal of the Canadian Academy of Child and Adolescent Psychiatry*, *26*(2), 78–85. PMID:28747930

McGee, K. (2003). The role of a child life specialist in a pediatric radiology department. *Pediatric Radiology*, *33*(7), 467–474. doi:10.100700247-003-0900-2 PMID:12819835

McLeod, J. D., Uemura, R., & Rohrman, S. (2013). Adolescent mental health, behavior problems, and academic achievement. *Journal of Health and Social Behavior, 53*(4), 482–497. doi:10.1177/0022146512462888 PMID:23197485

Mental Health First Aid. (2022). *Mental health first aid for youth* [Workbook]. National Council for Mental Wellbeing. https://www.mentalhealthfirstaid.org/population-focused-modules/youth/

Morse, G., Salyers, M. P., Rollins, A. L., Monroe-DeVita, M. M., & Pfahler, C. (2011). Burnout in mental health services: A review of the problem and its remediation. *Administration and Policy in Mental Health, 39*(5), 341–352. doi:10.100710488-011-0352-1 PMID:21533847

National Alliance on Mental Illness. (2015). *Mental health facts: Children & teens* [Infogram]. https://www.nami.org/NAMI/media/NAMI-Media/Infographics/Children-MH-Facts-NAMI.pdf

National Alliance on Mental Illness. (2021a). *Identity and cultural dimensions.* https://www.nami.org/Your-Journey/Identity-and-Cultural-Dimensions/

National Alliance on Mental Illness. (2021b). *Letter to CDC director on child and adolescent mental health.* https://www.nami.org/getattachment/8b6d5549-1d83-431b-92d4-1acd226d720b/2021- Letter-to-CDC-Director-on-Child-Adolescent-Me

National Alliance on Mental Illness. (2021c). *Statement for the record on child and adolescent mental health.* https://www.nami.org/getattachment/7090292f-4cc0-4a54-94a6-bcadefc0620e/Statement-for-the-Record-on-Child-and-Adolescent-M

National Alliance on Mental Illness. (2022a). *How to talk to your child about their mental health.* https://www.nami.org/Your-Journey/Kids-Teens-and-Young-Adults/Kids/How-to-Talk-to-Your-Child-About-Their-Mental-Health

National Alliance on Mental Illness. (2022b). *LGBTQI.* https://www.nami.org/Your-Journey/Identity-and-Cultural-Dimensions/LGBTQI

National Alliance on Mental Illness. (2022c). *Mental health in schools.* https://nami.org/Advocacy/Policy-Priorities/Improving-Health/Mental-Health-in-Schools

National Institute of Mental Health. (2009). *Treatment of children with mental illness: Frequently asked questions about the treatment ofmental illness in children.* https://files.eric.ed.gov/fulltext/ED507899.pdf

National Institute of Mental Health. (2021). *Chronic illness and mental health: Recognizing and treating depression.* https://www.nimh.nih.gov/health/publications/chronic-illness-mental-health#part_6116

New, A., Tucci, V. T., & Rios, J. (2017). A modern-day fight club? The stabilization and management of actively agitated patients in the emergency department. *The Psychiatric Clinics of North America, 40*(3), 397–410. doi:10.1016/j.psc.2017.05.002 PMID:28800797

Nunez, A. (2018). Exploring communication differences: Complications children with developmental disabilities face in medical settings. *ACLP Bulletin, 36*(2).

Nunez, A. (2020). *My child needs to be admitted to the hospital. How can I help them cope with an inpatient stay? How can I explain their needs to the staff?* Autism Speaks. https://www.autismspeaks.org/expert-opinion/my-child-needs-be-admitted-hospital-how-can-i-help-them-cope-inpatient-stay-how-can

Palmer, M., Saviet, M., & Tourish, J. (2016). Understanding and supporting grieving adolescents and young adults. *Pediatric Nursing*, *42*(6), 275–279. PMID:29406651

Pittesenbarger, Z. E., & Mannix, R. (2013). Trends in pediatric visits to the emergency department for psychiatric illnesses. *Academic Emergency Medicine*, *21*(1), 25–30. Advance online publication. doi:10.1111/acem.12282 PMID:24552521

Reavey, P., Poole, J., Corrigall, R., Zundel, T., Byford, S., Sarhane, M., Taylor, E., Ivens, J., & Ougrin, D. (2017). The ward as emotional ecology: Adolescent experiences of managing mental health and distress in psychiatric inpatient settings. *Health & Place*, *46*, 210–218. doi:10.1016/j.healthplace.2017.05.008 PMID:28554098

Rice, J. L., Tan, T. X., & Li, Y. (2021). In their voices: Experiences of adolescents during involuntary psychiatric hospitalization. *Children and Youth Services Review*, *126*, 1–10. doi:10.1016/j.childyouth.2021.106045

Romito, B., Jewell, J., Jackson, M., Ernst, K., Hill, V., Hsu, B., Lam, V., Mauro-Small, M., & Vinocur, C. (2021). Child Life Services. *Pediatrics*, *147*(1), 1–10. doi:10.1542/peds.2020-040261 PMID:33372119

Sharfstein, S. S. (2009). Goals of inpatient treatment for psychiatric disorders. *Annual Review of Medicine*, *60*(1), 393–403. doi:10.1146/annurev.med.60.042607.080257 PMID:18729730

Sheridan, D., Spiro, D., Fu, R., Johnson, K., Sheridan, J. S., Oue, W. A., Van Nes, R., & Hansen, M. (2015). Mental health utilization in a pediatric emergency department. *Pediatric Emergency Care*, *31*(8), 555–559. doi:10.1097/PEC.0000000000000343 PMID:25834957

Siegel, M. (2018). *Help for children with autism and recurring behavioral crises: Part 2*. Autism Speaks. https://www.autismspeaks.org/expert-opinion/help-child-autism-recurring-behavioral-crises-part-2

Stygar, K., & Zadroga, J. (2021). *Infants have mental health needs, too.* Mayo Clinic Health System. https://www.mayoclinichealthsystem.org/hometown-health/speaking-of-health/infants-have-mental-health-needs-too

Substance Abuse and Mental Health Services Administration. (2014). Understanding the impact of trauma. In *Treatment improvement protocol: Trauma-informed care in behavioral health services.* https://www.ncbi.nlm.nih.gov/books/NBK207191/

Substance Abuse and Mental Health Services Administration. (2022). *Understanding child trauma.* https://www.samhsa.gov/child-trauma/understanding-child-trauma /

Tally, M. (2011). Adolescents' perspectives about brief psychiatric hospitalization: What is helpful and what isn't helpful. *The Psychiatric Quarterly*, *82*(2), 121–137. doi:10.100711126-010-9151-1 PMID:20824339

University of Florida Health. (2022). *Baker act.* https://ufhealth.org/baker-act

Wagers, D. (2018). *What is the ONE VOICE approach?* OneVoice4Kids. https://www.onevoice4kids.com

Whitebread, D. (2017). Free play and children's mental health. *Lancet, 1*, 167–169. PMID:30169163

World Health Organization. (2019). *Burn-out an "occupational phenomenon": International classification of diseases.* https://www.who.int/news/item/28-05-2019-burn-out-an-occupational-phenomenon-international-classification-of-diseases

World Health Organization. (2021). *Adolescent mental health.* https://www.who.int/news-room/fact-sheets/detail/adolescent-mental-health

Ziemer, R., & Tomlinson, A. (2017). *Helping kids discover their a-PILL-ities.* https://www.childlife.org/docs/default-source/professional-development/conference/2017-posters/helping-kids-discover-their-a-pill-ities2.pdf?sfvrsn=

KEY TERMS AND DEFINITIONS

Association of Child Life Professionals (ACLP): A nonprofit organization that focuses on supporting and advancing the field of child life nationally and internationally by establishing professional standards, fostering research, and promoting the standards of child life practice and by enhancing the overall professional growth, development, and credibility of the child life profession.

Certified Child Life Specialist: A professional trained in child and family development and psychosocial support that implements stress-reducing interventions in order to improve overall experience.

Coping: The act of overcoming a problem or difficulty.

Emotional Support: Providing validation, encouragement, and reassurance to another person regarding their experiences.

Family-Centered Care: An approach to providing services that focuses on a partnership between the healthcare providers and the family while honoring the families' strengths, expertise, and traditions in the child's care.

Mental Health: The emotional, psychosocial, and developmental well-being that can affect how individuals behave and think.

National Alliance on Mental Illness (NAMI): A national nonprofit mental health organization dedicated to educating, advocating, and listening to help improve the lives of people with mental illness and their families.

Pediatrics: The branch of medical care that focuses on infants, children, and adolescents.

Psychiatry: The medical specialty regarding mental illness diagnosis, prevention, and treatment.

Trauma-Informed Care: An approach to providing services that recognizes the impact that trauma has in a person's past, present, and future; encouraging the need to look at the whole person to provide effective health care services.

Chapter 13
Human Trafficking

Jessika C. Boles
Vanderbilt University, USA

Cheryl Murray Miyamasu
Independent Researcher, USA

ABSTRACT

More than 800,000 children and women are victims of human trafficking each year; they are kidnapped or sold into sex work under the guise of occupational opportunities or the promise of a romantic relationship. The developmental and psychosocial impacts of being trafficked are overwhelmingly challenging for both women and children; thus, there is international need for trauma-informed psychosocial supports that can validate victims' experiences while enhancing coping skills and resilience. Therefore, this chapter will describe the work of a certified child life specialist within a nonprofit aftercare organization in India dedicated to the physical, psychological, and educational support of women who have experienced trafficking. As can be seen, the foundational knowledge, skills, and interventions of a certified child life specialist, when paired with cultural humility and deeply grounded in trauma-informed care, can foster safe and therapeutic relationships while teaching and modeling the lifelong coping skills that are instrumental for ongoing healing.

INTRODUCTION

Suvarna is a 17-year-old female. Hailing from a small village outside of Mumbai, she grew up in poverty as the middle of three sisters. At age 10, widespread drought decimated her family's small crop. So, when a family friend offered to take Suvarna and her sisters into their home in the city, it seemed like an opportunity to improve her current living situation and provide for her aging parents simultaneously. However, when the girls arrived in Mumbai things were not as they seemed, and the family friend was nowhere to be found. Instead, Suvarna and her sisters were met by a brothel owner who clothed them, fed them, and then forced them into sex work to "pay off their debts."*

**Names and details in this chapter have been altered to protect the safety and privacy of those involved.*

DOI: 10.4018/978-1-6684-5097-0.ch013

It is difficult to trace the precise origins of human trafficking, as many cultures have at some point or another employed practices that enslave or exploit other human beings; however, human trafficking remains an international problem even in today's world (Rai & Rai, 2021). Whether called human trafficking, sex trafficking, or commercial sexual exploitation, **human trafficking** is defined as:

Recruitment, transportation, transfer, harboring or receipt of persons, by means of the threat or use of force or other forms of coercion, of abduction, of fraud, of deception, of the abuse of power or of a position of vulnerability, or of the giving or receiving of payments or benefits to achieve the consent of a person having control over another person, for the purpose of exploitation. Exploitation shall include, at a minimum, the exploitation or the prostitution of others or other forms of sexual exploitation, forced labor or services, slavery, or practices similar to slavery, servitude or the removal of organs (United Nations, 2000, p. 42).

Although likely a gross underrepresentation of the true extent of human trafficking practices across the globe, it is estimated that more than 800,000 children and individuals are sold into these various forms of human slavery each year; 80% of these victims will be forced into sex work of some kind (Locke, 2010).

Unfortunately, the human trafficking industry preys upon developmentally and psychosocially vulnerable minor children and adults with very little individual and social resources, perceived or actual power, and marginalized groups (Rai & Rai, 2021). Additionally, the prevalence of human trafficking is greater in underdeveloped countries, areas rife with poverty, and tribal societies living in rural or isolated areas (Dalla & Kreimer, 2017). Despite being able to identify these high-risk groups and areas, human trafficking remains a global issue, likely due to its intersection with other social issues such as corruption, poverty, and immigration. In the United States, those most at risk of sex trafficking are children who identify with minority sexual orientations and gender statuses, who are homeless or have a history of running away from their home environments, have identified mental health needs, are engaged in substance abuse, and have previous experience with the juvenile justice system (Browne-James et al., 2021).

Entry into the human trafficking industry is a traumatic event. Whether the individual has been defrauded into a false romantic relationship, violently kidnapped from their home or community, sold by family members or friends that they once trusted, or lured by the promise of a career opportunity that does not exist, each pathway is fraught with intense emotion, lack of control, a sense of powerlessness, and feelings of helplessness (Dalla & Kreimer, 2017). Moreover, the victim has been extracted from their normative context and community and forced into a host of new environments, situations, and relationships that are unsafe, unpredictable, and externally controlled (da Silva & Sathiyaseelan, 2019). And, whilst working within the confines of coerced servitude, there is little to no access to social support, basic healthcare, mental health resources, or other avenues with the potential to bolster coping and resilience (Dalla & Kreimer, 2017).

Thus, the psychosocial and developmental impacts of human trafficking are multiple, intense, and often unaddressed for long periods of time, if ever. With the knowledge that many are children, adolescents, and young adults from vulnerable backgrounds, there is a collective urgency for and responsibility to locate, rescue, rehabilitate, and support victims of human trafficking in local and global communities. Certified Child Life Specialists (CCLSs), although typically found within pediatric healthcare settings, are psychosocial professionals with the developmental expertise, emphasis on trauma-informed care, and resilience-focused orientation this population needs and deserves as part of comprehensive survivorship care (Boles et al., 2020). However, since little is currently known about child life work in relation to human trafficking, the purpose of this chapter is to describe the first author's direct care and programmatic experiences providing child life services to adolescent and young adult female victims of human trafficking in India. When the mission, vision, values, and scope of the child life role (ACLP, 2022) are applied to the unique developmental and coping needs of children and families in this context, child life services appear to be an under used but valuable support for children and individuals that have experienced human trafficking.

BACKGROUND

Now, standing more than 20 years into the 21st century, CCLSs can be found in most pediatric healthcare facilities in North America – with active expansion of services into five other continents (ACLP, 2022). Much of the work is grounded in the same six domains (see Figure 1 below) foreseen by the play ladies of nearly a century ago, with the addition of decades of empirical evidence demonstrating the wealth of positive outcomes for child and family recipients of child life services (Boles et al., 2020). Integrating seminal theories of child development, family systems, stress and coping, and others, with every decade the child life profession has deepened and strengthened its skills for assessing the multidimensional needs of children and families to provide individualized therapeutic and educational interventions to address those identified needs (Turner, 2018). It is this same cross-theoretical knowledge, practice, and belief in the value of such an approach that can make child life specialists an essential and effective service for children and families affected by human trafficking.

Figure 1. The six domains of child life services
Source: Boles et al., 2020, by permission of the Association of Child Life Professionals©.

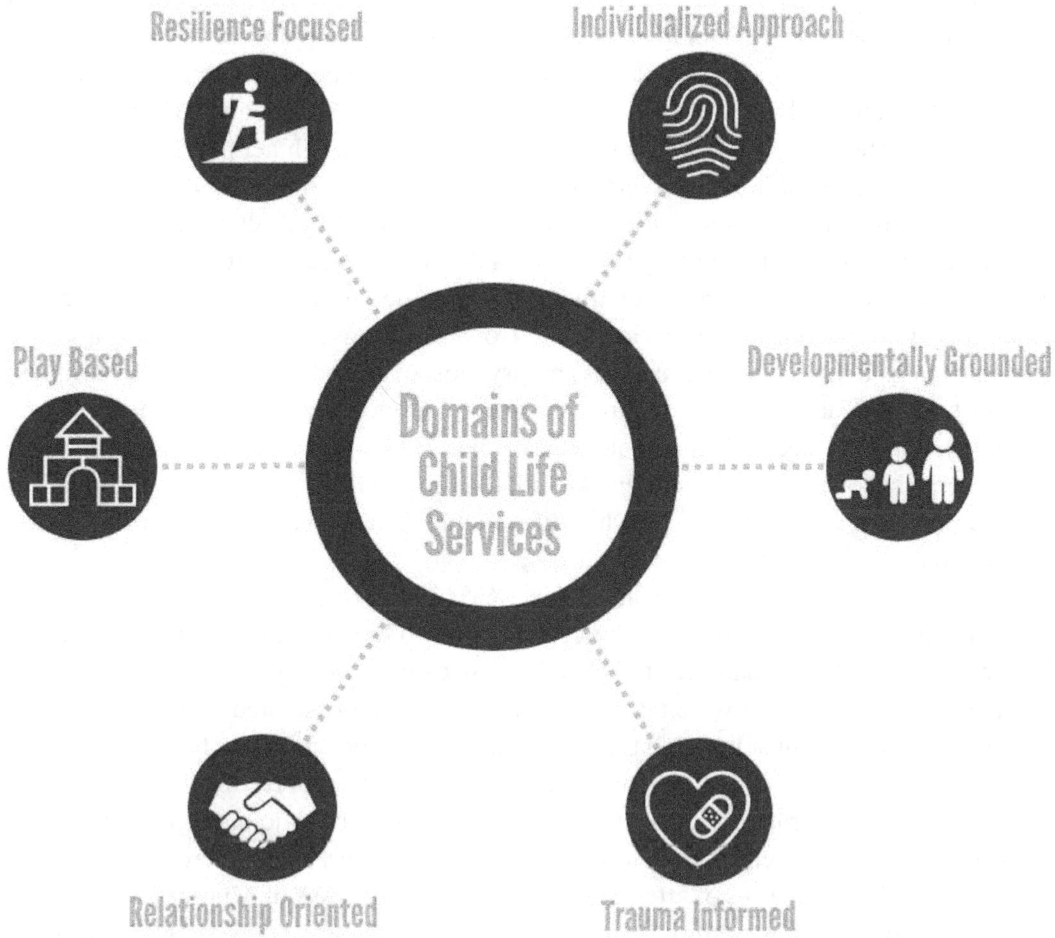

Over the past ten years, child life specialists have become increasingly aware of, invested in, and inclusive of trauma-informed care practices that cultivate emotional safety for both those who have survived traumatic experiences and those at risk of acquiring trauma in specific contexts – most typically, healthcare environments (Stenman et al., 2019). **Trauma-informed care**, as both a principle and a process, is:

...a way of approaching interactions with children and families in which providers remain cognizant of the impacts of trauma while also taking actions to prevent potentially traumatic experiences. In addition, it is the recognition that any event, even one that seems small or non-invasive, can trigger a traumatic response from a child or caregiver. Trauma-informed care, then, is useful and necessary not only in high-risk environments, such as emergency departments or critical care units, but also in general pediatrics clinics and the school nurse's office (Boles, 2017, p. 7).

Trauma-informed care has become a strength and priority of the child life specialist community, and one that is being increasingly recognized in arenas like adult healthcare, school systems, nonprofit organizations, and private practice – many of which are detailed in the chapters of this book. Thus, when the opportunity arose for the author to bring child life services to support survivors of human trafficking, such work not only fit the orientation and skillset of child life specialists in a new and fluent way, but also aligned perfectly with her life-long passion for international travel and service.

From her early teenage years, and by way of introduction through her personal faith community and college coursework, the author felt a connection to the country of India and its vibrant culture, bustling communities, respect for the arts, spiritual belief systems, and the challenges each of those create for under-resourced groups. After earning her master's degree in child life, the author went on to work for several years as a CCLS at a large pediatric hospital in the United States. In this work, she not only provided hospital-based child life services, but also worked closely with the hospital's outpatient specialty clinic teams to help meet the medical and psychosocial needs of underserved communities in the Cincinnati area. She also went on multiple short-term service trips, both international and domestic, working with impoverished and vulnerable populations. Thus, when an opportunity arose to translate the field and work she loved to serve a culture and population she has been passionate about for most of her life, she accepted the opportunity to use child life practice as a mechanism of actionable and sustainable transformation for vulnerable girls and families.

With its name redacted for privacy and safety, XYZ is an organization that provides comprehensive and holistic aftercare to girls who have been rescued from human trafficking in a large, urban area of India. Inclusive of girls who had been trafficked into sex work, pornography, sex slavery, or sold as child brides, the majority of whom were taken from impoverished or isolated communities, XYZ provides healthcare, education, counseling, job training, and community support to help survivors process their experiences in an environment of solidarity, safety, and social support. Specifically, XYZ functions as a bridge to social reintegration for survivors of human trafficking who have graduated from homes for minor girls but could still benefit from systematic education, therapeutic intervention, and social/financial support. XYZ runs a series of aftercare homes in different areas of Mumbai, each with a maximum of six girls at a time and a housemother on duty at all times. House mothers provide direct supervision and support, managing issues or conflicts while also teaching the girls skills like cooking, grocery shopping, cleaning, and maintaining a budget. While living in the homes, all residents participate in regular trauma counseling, coping skills training, and formal education or vocational training to develop a trade that they can use to generate income after they leave the program – depending on the specific goals and interests of the individual girl.

In this region of India, girls who are rescued from trafficking are first placed in government-regulated homes until their case is able to be presented before the child welfare committee. This legal entity is tasked with determining the individual's method of disposition – whether they can be returned to their family and village or require placement in a residential aftercare facility. Some of these aftercare facilities are government run and publicly funded, whereas others are fully or partially private organizations. Minor homes typically serve children under age 18, and there are fewer organizations who serve those ages 18 and older like XYZ (da Silva & Sathiyaseelan, 2019).

Accepting a position as an "Aftercare Intern" at XYZ, the author became the first child life specialist to join a team of social workers, counselors, administrative directors, and support staff in caring for female survivors of human trafficking in Mumbai, India (see Figure 2 below). As an intern, she was asked to review the program's direct and administrative services to identify opportunities for psychosocial service improvements that were trauma-informed and developmentally appropriate. Many times, this involved direct assessment and therapeutic intervention for girls individually and in groups. Community networking, program administration, policy development, and staff education were key elements of her intern role. Throughout this work, her background of knowledge and skill as a CCLS were critical to meeting the girls and staff in a new and foreign culture with humility, an eagerness to learn, and an ability to translate hospital-based interventions into effective means of supporting coping, education, and development in this vulnerable population and setting.

Figure 2. Staff of XYZ

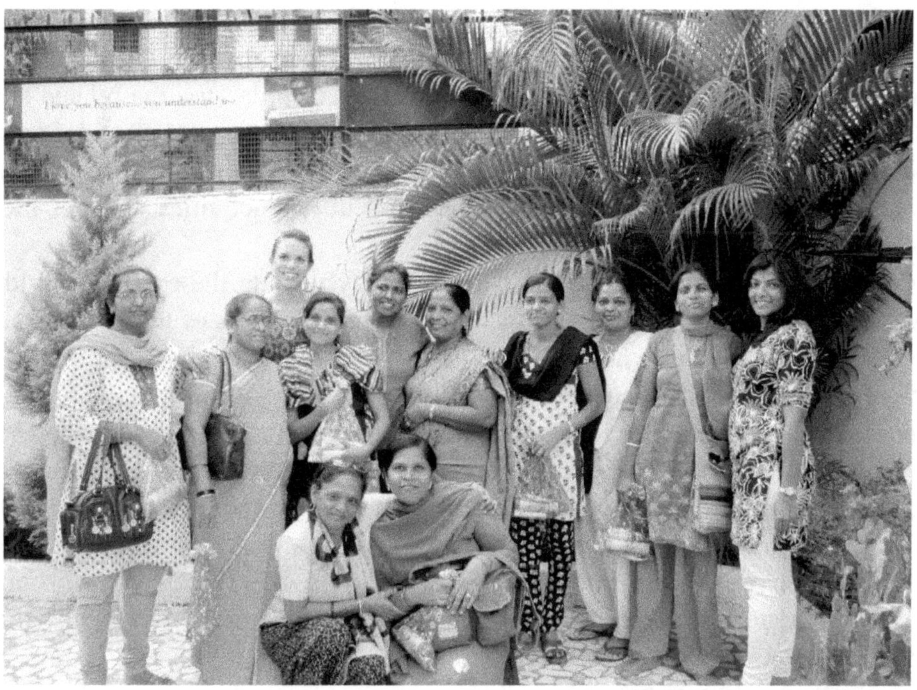

CHILD LIFE SERVICES AND SURVIVORS OF HUMAN TRAFFICKING

Caring for female survivors of human trafficking in a foreign country and culture has many differences from traditional, hospital-based child life work. Despite great alignment in the types of careful assessment and individualized intervention that is needed to cultivate healing and resilience for this population, it is important to translate these practices with a high level of reflexivity and a growth orientation - both of which are critical for nurturing similar strengths, skills, and attitudes in trauma-exposed populations like survivors of human trafficking. Namely, thoughtful preparation for working in this setting should involve cultural humility (and culturally responsive care). **Cultural humility** is a relational stance that attends to how individuals' cultural experiences and identity shape every aspect of their personhood, from their thoughts and feelings to the values they hold and the decisions they make (Foronda, 2020). **Culturally responsive care** refers to a provider's choice to offer and actions that support care that fosters trusting and authentic environments where they seek, respect, respond to, and celebrate the intersectional aspects that make an individual unique; it is, by nature, anti-oppressive, multicultural, and holistic (Kirmayer & Gomez-Carillo, 2019). In approaching survivors of human trafficking in India, obtaining lenses for assessment and intervention such as trauma-informed care and cross-cultural multidisciplinary collaboration cannot be overlooked or under-addressed by child life professionals.

Even years before the internship at XYZ presented itself, the author immersed herself in formal and informal educational opportunities to build on her traditional child life training and skills. Through her college coursework, faith community, and nonprofit organizations, she obtained crucial information about the forms, features, and effects of the human trafficking industry in India's rural and urban sectors. Guided by the philosophy that the realities of the world are far different than one's own experiences, she accumulated ten years' worth of academic study, clinical child life practice, and philanthropic involvement to prepare for the distinct cultural, social, and interpersonal landscape of India. She sought out specialized training in **trauma-focused cognitive behavioral therapy (TF-CBT)**, an evidence-based treatment for individuals diagnosed with post-traumatic stress disorder, trauma-related anxiety and depression, or behavioral problems in response to real or perceived trauma. Offered as a short-term therapy, TF-CBT has three components: increased coping with difficult emotions, learning to tell and process the story of one's trauma, and integrating into post-trauma life and activities with attention to ongoing safety planning (Cohen et al., 2012).

Although providing therapies like TF-CBT are typically outside the scope of child life practice (ACLP, 2022), exploring this approach prior to working with survivors of human trafficking can help child life specialists better anticipate how trauma responses present in children and families, foresee the effects of different approaches and interactions on survivors' sense of safety, and identify adjustments to their communication style to better serve this population. Additionally, the course provided valuable information about child protection policies and mechanisms of action for ensuring children's safety; this aligned well with the author's previous role as a mandated reporter and child life specialist in pediatric healthcare settings. Not only were the tenets of TF-CBT and strategies for child protective work helpful to her direct interventions at XYZ organization, but also for the higher level, culturally humble program development and policy creation the organization operates from even today. Additionally, these principles can easily be mapped onto traditional, hospital-based child life work to enhance outcomes for children and families experiencing illness and injury.

Simultaneously, while seeking out new information and skills to support her upcoming work with XYZ organization as an aftercare intern, the author focused on returning to the child life roots from which she had trained, grown in and hoped to expand in India. It was important at this juncture to reflect on the host of related work experiences she had accumulated, while exploring the new cultural climate into which these skills would need to be adapted. First, she returned to her memories of serving culturally diverse or marginalized groups within the hospital walls. Next, she revisited the binder she once used to facilitate support group programming for children with traumatic injuries and those who had experienced the death of a loved one and envisioned how these resources could be applied to meet the needs of human trafficking victims. She spent two weeks in India receiving extensive culture training before moving to Mumbai. In conjunction with mentors who had both lived and worked both in India and in human trafficking support around the world, the author and her husband had focused time to learn about and learn from those with expansive knowledge of the circumstances and culture in which they would be acclimating. She also connected with mentors who had either lived in India or worked in other organizations with victims of human trafficking. Finally, again reflecting on her experiences of providing preparation for intensive medical procedures, fostering socialization and connection, facilitating emotional expression, and teaching coping skills under the auspices of the child life role, she thought critically about the trauma-informed adjustments and culturally responsive applications that these interventions would require for successful therapeutic use at XYZ.

Integrating into Mumbai

Interning with XYZ organization necessitated an extensive amount of cultural humility, responsiveness, and fluency to serve the organization and its clients with the respect and care they deserved. This meant not only learning about the country and city in which XYZ functioned, but also the social, cultural, and spiritual dimensions of child development and family life in this part of the world. Additionally, being a cultural outsider in this beautiful and complex social world, a commitment to learning and a genuine care for all people affected by the human trafficking industry was critical for building the professional relationships that would support sustainable growth for the organization and the girls it served.

To contextualize this work, it is important to recognize that, unlike the United States, India is still considered an undeveloped country (Dummer & Cook, 2008). Though luxurious skyscrapers are often juxtaposed alongside impoverished slums in its urban centers, most Indian people live in under-resourced conditions in those same cities or in isolated rural communities (Dalla et al., 2020). Despite these challenges, India is also known globally for its distinctive contributions to international art and fashion, the manufacturing, technology, and chemical industries, and elemental resources like iron, steel, and some petroleum-based chemical production (Choudhury, 2020).

Mumbai has a population of 20,961,4762 people, it is often depicted as crowded, bustling, and somewhat loud (World Population Review, 2022). Below this surface glance, however, is a community of people who came to the city with hopes of providing a different or better life for themselves and their families than what might be possible in their rural villages. Unfortunately, the hot and dry climate of Mumbai paired with its significant cultural and structural inequities can make upward social mobility extremely difficult.

The people of Mumbai predominantly practice the spiritual, cultural, and social tenets of Hinduism, which is considered one of the world's five major religions; however, other faith traditions are seen in smaller numbers or in distinctive regions. Hinduism is intricately entwined with the rich and vibrant art, music, and dress that India is known for, yet it also plays a role in how social orders and structures are prescribed and maintained. One of the hallmark tenets of Hinduism is the belief in reincarnation, or rebirth, after death. Depending on the quality and character of the life one has lived, or karma one has accumulated, they can be reborn into a variety of situations and circumstances meant to reflect reward or punishment for their previous choices, actions, and offerings made to the many manifestations of God, or Brahman. Thus, to be born into poverty, disability, or even one's gender is seen to be a result of a past life well or poorly lived, and the favor or lack thereof one has incurred from Brahman (Weightman, 2017).

Partly associated with Hinduism, but also descendant from centuries of indigenous societies and colonization efforts, those in the Western world tend to incorrectly describe India's social organization as the now defunct and outlawed caste system by which it once functioned. The caste system, in its previous decades, was a means by which one could identify their place in society and understand the expectations for and possibilities available to themselves and their families (Gnana, 2018). Certain occupations, marriage traditions, social roles, and religious traditions were seen to correlate with one's accumulation of wealth and resources. These opportunities or lack thereof were interpreted as governed by the karmic cycle and one's experiences in their previous life. Although no longer allowable under the purview of the Indian government, the effects of the caste system can still be seen in some of the country's social functions and issues (Dalla et al., 2020).

Although not specific to India, the human trafficking industry has grown under and been sustained by some of these larger cultural, spiritual, and class-related histories and beliefs. More specifically, beliefs about gender, marriage, sex, and relationships – in conjunction with pervasive poverty and lack of social mobility – all converge to make trafficking a pervasive and challenging issue to address. In many Hindu-based Indian societies, marriage transactions are not only arranged, but also directly shaped by one's gender; for instance, when a daughter is arranged for marriage, her family must pay a large sum of money, or dowry, to the groom's family that is meant to be reflective of the value she will bring to this new union. When a son is married, his family can expect to receive money and resources from the bride's family rather than being expected to offer this form of payment. Thus, women carry a financial cost to their families, whereas men bring opportunities for financial growth. Gender, in some ways, is understood to reflect the karma one attained in their previous life – with greater or more favorable amounts of karma rendering males versus females (Dalla et al., 2020).

Karma, therefore, is seen to affect not only one's social class, but also his or her gender due to the financial gain or deficit one's gender predicts for the family unit. Additionally, marriage and childbearing are viewed as essential achievements in family life, putting great pressure on women and families to make a suitable and feasible match. At the same time, these views on gender, class, and the family cycle work together to generate policies that make being a single female very challenging – such as the inability to access housing as many landlords will not rent to single women (Dalla & Kreimer, 2017).

Gender-specific views on sexual activity are also evident in areas of India. Women are expected to remain celibate until marriage, saving their sexual fortitude for the purposes of procreation once she has been married. In many areas, men, on the other hand, are understood to have sexual needs prior to, and even within marriage, that are best met not by their spouse, but rather by a locally operated brothel. Sex acts that are deemed unnatural or inappropriate to one's wife may be permitted to be performed with sex workers (often from the lower social classes) in exchange for money and goods. Women, however, are forbidden to have sexual contact outside of marriage, making it difficult for women who have experienced human trafficking to reintegrate and be accepted by family and social groups once they have been rescued. In fact, they are often considered unfit for marriage, which perpetuates the cycle of difficulties of single womanhood, lack of resources, and the need for accessible work – which many times is sex work (Dalla & Kreimer, 2017).

For families who may already live with limited resources and anticipate hefty dowries to help their daughters marry successfully, sometimes such pressures require difficult decisions for the good of the larger family. In dire circumstances, a daughter may knowingly or unknowingly be sold into human trafficking to collect enough money to help her sisters someday marry and bear children. With quality education and social mobility only available to those of the higher social classes, families must sometimes make great sacrifices for one to generate opportunities for another (Dalla et al., 2020).

Traffickers prey upon the vulnerable. Many of the girls who are taken into human trafficking are of little economic means, have low education levels, and have few other options. Some will enter violently, abducted from their homes and families and sold to the highest bidder; others will be purchased from their families and friends, or fooled through the promise of needed romantic and financial opportunities to escape the poverty of everyday life. Many times, they know the captors who abduct them, and the girls with whom they are placed in brothels or other settings. Despite the daily trauma of sex work, there is a potential for predictable food and housing that the girls may have lacked in their former homes and villages. However, the risk-to-reward ratio of human trafficking is incredibly unbalanced and detrimental, and a cycle that maintains itself far outside the realm of adequate legal surveillance and control (Dalla et al., 2020).

SPECIAL CONSIDERATIONS WHEN CARING FOR SURVIVORS OF HUMAN TRAFFICKING

Partly a function of the non-Western cultural context, and partly due to the gross amount of physical, psychological, and social-emotional trauma that children witness and experience in the human trafficking industry, there are some ways in which child life philosophies, services, and goals should and *must* be different. First and foremost, assessment must be careful, intentional, and accommodating. Victims of human trafficking will likely not perfectly align with the textbook developmental theories child life specialists are trained to rely upon; additionally, notions of "optimal development" can be difficult to apply to a population that has experienced such chronic and comprehensive trauma. It is important to assess using a specific and individualized lens, rather than applying heuristic models that were generated for white, European, affluent populations with minimal trauma exposure. Additionally, it is important to note that development can be accelerated, halted, and regressed all at once; although she may enter into XYZ around the age of 18, a girl who has been trafficked for several years may present as mature in some ways due to her experiences, but also much younger than her 18 years in other ways. Thus, attending to individual knowledge, behaviors, and cues is especially important when assessing development and coping in this population, much like in traditional child life work but with extra layers of openness to nuance.

An additional domain for assessment that is of utmost importance when working with survivors of human trafficking is that of safety – physical, social, and emotional safety combined. When a girl is rescued from trafficking, she is at high risk of being abducted and returned to her captors, experiencing or enacting aggression and violence to the point of injury, or having her privacy jeopardized in a way that makes the former even more likely (Karandikar et al., 2015). Unfortunately, the Western, hospital-based notion of family-centered care is seldom best in this set of circumstances, as family may either be 1) in accessible due to distance or their whereabouts at the time were unknown, 2) a risk to the girl's safety and privacy by nature of their location or social connections, or 3) the mechanism by which a girl entered trafficking. Families in this sense can be unsafe and unavailable; contrary to hospital-based child life work, but akin to child protection and advocacy work, families should be integrated only if and when the girl is safe and ready for this reconnection.

Also, when working with a diverse population, child life specialists should be especially sensitive to how the socio-political history of the region may affect their ability to gain access, provide care, and do so in culturally responsive ways. In countries like India, there is an extensive history of **colonialism**, or the historical control that has been enacted by white people in attempts to colonize the land and its inhabitants. Although intending to provide support and care, when walking in as a noticeably different-looking person, child life specialists must continually acknowledge how their culture, race, and language will consciously and unconsciously affect their interactions with foreign social groups and structures. Whether one is fluent in the native language, or instead working with trained interpreters day in and out, cultural humility and reflexivity are crucial elements of offering child life care to diverse cultural groups (Bandyopadhyay, 2019).

First and Ongoing Interactions

Like most 15-year-old girls, Veena spent her time building relationships with peers and helping her family with tasks of daily living. One day, an older boy took a specific interest in her, showering her with the types of gifts she was unaccustomed to as a working-class adolescent. They became closer and closer, with Veena confiding her thoughts and feelings to this boy who made her feel important, unique, and loved. Soon, they planned to run away together to his aunt's house, to pursue a life of more stability, privilege, and freedom. When they arrived, he left to ran an errand, promising to return, although he never did. His "aunt" sold her to a brothel where she was raped multiple times a day in exchange for payment. She was physically injured and ill, starving and unhoused, and was drugged or beaten when she did not comply with her pimp or client's requests – all while her whereabouts were unknown to her family and friends. She existed in this painful and abusive cycle for two years, until a police raid brought her into the safety of the legal system, into another aftercare home as a minor, and she was formally placed at XYZ for aftercare.

When a rescued girl first arrives at XYZ for aftercare, an Indian staff member, typically a social worker, completes a full intake assessment on their physical, emotional, psychological, educational, and social needs. There is great variability across the population XYZ serves, as some girls had spent several years prior in a home for minor girls where they received comprehensive services, and others may have only just been rescued days to weeks before their eighteenth birthday. To account for this complexity and variability, multiple staff members contributed their insights, interactions, and observations to the intake assessor's initial findings, resulting in a holistic picture that would form the basis of an individualized treatment plan. Much like in child life assessment practices, a multidisciplinary team-oriented approach to assessment was valued, as well as an understanding of assessment as a continuous and dynamic process rather than a singular task to be completed.

Familiar from her training as a child life specialist, the author observed how the XYZ staff drew from Maslow's Hierarchy of Needs (1943) when assessing and prioritizing the needs of new residents. Maslow's (1943) pyramid-esque representation of human needs kept staff grounded in the primacy of biological needs before more psychological and social-emotional needs can be effectively met. Given the lack of basic provisions the girls had experienced in the human trafficking industry, such as stable housing, food, and control over one's own reproductive system, these were immediate goals for the XYZ team to tackle first. As these became more predictable and stable within the walls of the organization, attention was turned to the girls' next need – per Maslow's (1943) theory – for safety. Though the hospital setting typically leads child life specialists (per their psychosocial role) to emphasize the child's needs for emotional expression and involvement in their care, the first area for assessment and management in XYZ revolved around physical development and instrumental resources.

In terms of physical needs, staff identified what medical needs were present, as they often were, in the form of physical injuries, untreated illnesses, and other physical impairments. Many girls arrived to XYZ having survived not only physical abuse, but also reproductive related procedures such as forced abortions performed by untrained individuals in unsanitary conditions. Some of the girls were also unaware of the extent of these injuries, with some being rendered infertile by these poorly executed procedures. Additionally, many were living in various stages of untreated sexually transmitted illnesses that also needed immediate and effective treatment.

Emotional and psychological needs were gauged through observations of the girl's behavior, demeanor, and verbal cues using a trauma-informed framework. Some arrived ready to engage and participate in group-based activities, whereas others exhibited trauma-related responses and behaviors such as disengagement, retreating, self-isolation, over-sexualized behavior, confusion, difficulty focusing on present tasks, blunted affect, or increased agitation that may have made group participation counterproductive for all involved. Some of these effects could also be seen in the girl's coping efforts, or lack thereof, which helped the team to anticipate which areas needed to be addressed and supported first.

Educationally and developmentally, though the girls were in the same young adult period of development per their chronological age, the influence of trauma and poverty had significant effects on their ability to understand and process information about their experiences and future hopes. Depending on when they were forced into human trafficking, some of the girls had little to no formal education, whereas others may have had the equivalent of almost a high school diploma. Assessing their developmental level and educational level was important not only for intervention planning, but also for grouping the girls with other survivors in the home who may have had similar experiences and were able to process their trauma in more concrete versus abstract ways. XYZ organization has an Educational Coordinator as part of the aftercare team who would ask each girl her educational background, hopes and dreams for education and future employment, and coordinate her educational and vocational experiences to help her achieve those dreams.

Assessment of social needs and supports was essential not only for determining treatment goals, but for also thinking about potential reintegration opportunities. In the author's two and a half years with the organization, only one girl was placed back with her family and village after residing at XYZ. Moreover, cultural barriers associated with surviving human trafficking and single womanhood required extra time and forethought for XYZ staff to identify, build, and sustain partnerships that would give their graduates a chance to secure safe housing, enter educational opportunities, and participate in the social order.

On average, a girl could spend between one to three years with XYZ. During this time, she resided at one of their six aftercare homes, participated in Trauma-Focused Cognitive Behavioral Therapy (TF-CBT), and engaged in group and individual activities to promote therapeutic expression and connection. Individuals received healthcare and educational services as needed (or based on the individual's goals) and experienced the safe and supportive community they could not access while being trafficked. To graduate from the program, each girl needed to meet the following goals: 1) achieve physical and emotional stability, 2) complete her desired level of education or job training, 3) demonstrate practical skills required for independent living (such as navigating public transportation, managing money, locating housing, etc.), 4) obtain a job and a stable form of housing, and 5) identify a source of community support. If a girl required additional time and intervention around these goals, she was welcome to remain at XYZ for additional assessment, intervention, and assistance until she was ready to move forward with reintegration.

SPECTRUM OF CHILD LIFE INTERVENTION

As an aftercare intern with XYZ, the author's role revolved around providing developmentally appropriate education and coping support through individual and group-based activities, while also assessing opportunities for psychosocial service improvement across the organization and in conjunction with the community. All of this was accomplished with the assistance of a native full-time interpreter. Much like hospital-based CCLSs, but also adapted for this specific population and context, her work integrated principles of diagnosis education and preparation with individual/group therapeutic play, normalization, socialization, and coping skills education. Whether helping the home's residents express their developing sense of identity as a trafficking survivor, understand the function and care of their reproductive organs and systems, or identify accessible means of coping with stress and stigma, each individual and group interaction was also an opportunity for staff to model what safe, stable, and trusting human relationships can look like and offer.

Educational Interventions

Many of the girls at XYZ arrived with limited education – both in the sense of formal education, and also informal knowledge about what their bodies needed, experienced, and the healthcare interventions required. Shortly after beginning work with XYZ, a new resident exhibited a deeply distressing overt trauma response during a gynecological exam; the staff member who accompanied her felt challenged by and unequipped to manage this outburst. The author saw this as an opportunity to integrate stress point preparation from her child life skills to help the girls anticipate and understand the gynecological exams and medical interventions they would encounter, while also giving them an opportunity to identify and rehearse the coping skills needed to prevent healthcare from becoming another context of trauma. Using time-tested preparation techniques, and integrating sensory, procedural, and coping skills information, she was able to both enhance coping in XYZ's resident girls, while also extending/modeling the preparation philosophy and skillset to the multidisciplinary team with which she worked.

For example, a young woman arrived to XYZ after several years of forced sex work, genital mutilation, and several ad hoc abortions performed by individuals without medical training. She was initially withdrawn, hesitant to make eye contact, clearly uncomfortable and anxious in the presence of male staff members, and described herself as fundamentally "bad" and "dirty." Given her significant physical injuries and medical history, immediate medical and gynecological assessment and treatment was necessary. However, like most of the girls who came into XYZ, she had virtually no previous experience with healthcare providers, whether for regular preventative care or treatment. Thus, she was just as unfamiliar with the implicit knowledge that healthcare participation requires – such as how to access care and advocate for her individual needs. The author started from the most immediate psychosocial need: stress-point preparation and in-the-moment procedural support. By partnering with an aftercare social worker to support this girl in preparation, describing the sequence of events (with sensory information), the girl was able to learn more about what the physical and gynecological exams would entail; additionally, she was able to identify a supportive staff member to accompany her to the appointment. In conjunction with the staff member, the girl was able to use her preferred coping strategies (deep breathing and closing her eyes), helping her stay present in her body and grounded in the moment, while also attempting to advocate for her needs (primarily for a female provider and with her identified support person present at all times).

Self-advocacy skills were especially challenging to develop in this population given their extensive history of being powerless as a victim of human trafficking. However, their care and coping needs were not unreasonable or unfounded. For example, some girls preferred female medical providers due to their trauma history, felt unsafe being alone with a medical provider, or were unsure how to disclose their medical history (or history of procedures performed by non-medical providers) to a treating physician. Through preparation and procedural support, individual and group work, and individual and staff education, the author's work as a CCLS helped her to assess these needs and cultivate these skills in useful and effective ways for XYZ and the girls it served.

Therapeutic Interventions

Much like in hospital-based child life care, therapeutic art and play activities are a profound medium for promoting normalization, connection, self-expression, and skill development in survivors of human trafficking. This was a significant component of the author's work as an after-care intern at XYZ organization. Armed with her years of experience facilitating support groups for children and families of different needs and backgrounds, and with a full-time interpreter at her side, group activities were an effective format for helping the girls learn to build trust and start to form relationships with the staff and one another. Additionally, they had the opportunities to explore art, games, and music that they had been unable to access during their time in forced sex work. Guitars were purchased for the organization and guitar classes were regularly provided at the vocational center for girls who wanted to learn. All the girls participated in therapies, art classes, and regular life skills sessions. This allowed them the chance to start to identify their specific interests, preferences, and begin to build a positive sense of self and personal identity. Other times, groups revolved around specific education – such as certifications that would expand their future career options, coping skills like journaling, painting, drumming, or guitar, and life skills pertinent to filling out job applications and attending interviews, sex education, and how to interact in certain social settings. Much like in the hospital setting, play activities were also offered to normalize holidays and developmental milestones – such as graduating from XYZ, birthdays, and holidays to inject a sense of normalcy and joy into the hard work that comes with processing multisystemic trauma.

During one particular group activity, the girls discussed metaphors for coping with change, such as the changing colors of fall leaves (see Figure 3 below). Not only was the group an opportunity for the girls to express their feelings about and experiences with change on individual leaves (as part of a collective tree), but also an authentic cross-cultural dialogue about autumn and changing colors as a foreign concept in India where the hot and humid weather only differs across dry and monsoon seasons.

In another group activity, the author facilitated discussion about the use of positive affirmations in times of stress or worry; many of the participants in attendance that day identified that they had never heard positive words about themselves and never thought positive things about themselves before. At the end of the group, the participants had created images and affirmation words to hang in their rooms to remind themselves of their inherent worth and value. Many of the girls took these items with them when they graduated from XYZ, choosing to display them in their new residences as a reminder of the power of positive self-talk.

English language training was also a staple part of XYZ's educational offerings. The information technologies intern crafted a platform that allowed the girls to receive virtual tutoring from native English speakers (see Figure 4 below). Although the most overt goal of these sessions was to build a needed skill in the Indian and international marketplace, these tutoring relationships also gave the girls an opportunity to experience trust and stability in another human relationship. Furthermore, their interactions with the English tutors provided a platform to practice self-advocacy, build confidence in oneself and abilities, and experience a sense of mastery and control that had been absent from their years in the human trafficking industry.

Figure 3. Leaves of Gratitude Activity

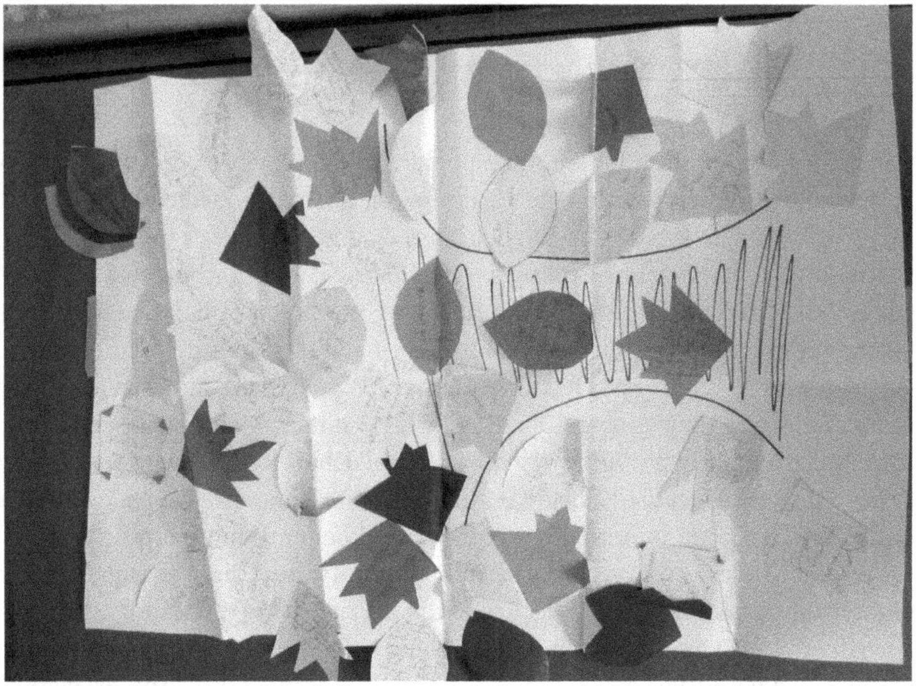

Figure 4. English Language Tutoring

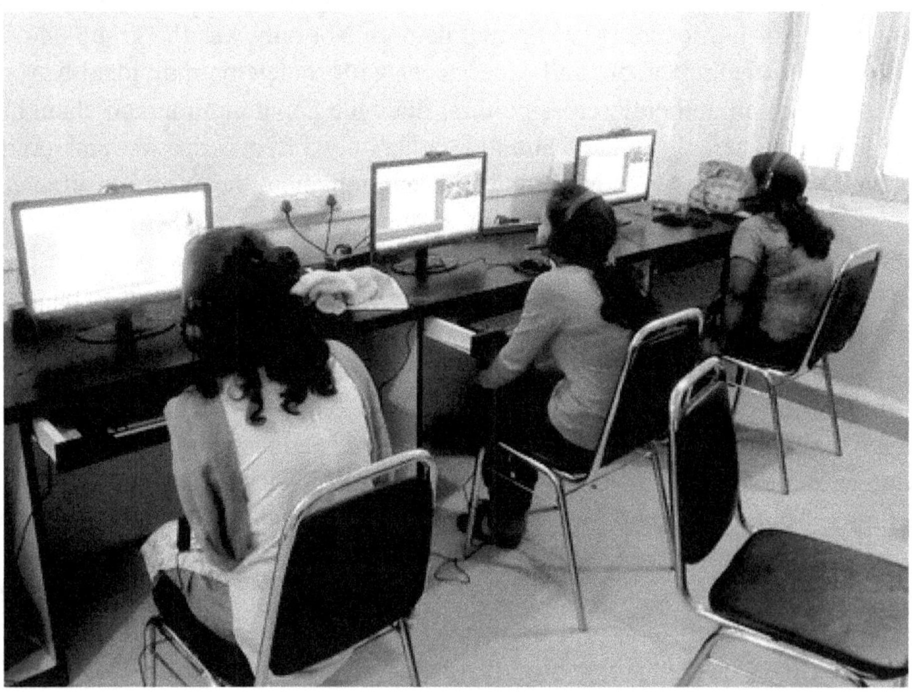

Working with a full-time interpreter was another unique aspect of providing child life services at XYZ; and this was both a notable difference and challenge from the author's previous hospital-based child life work. Although familiar with interpretation services and professionals from her previous hospital-based work, at XYZ, full time translation support was needed in every interaction around the facility and homes. Additionally, in this context the provided interpreter was different from day to day, and their levels of English proficiency were variable from one to the next. Even with interpreter support, the author found it important to keep her communications short, developmentally appropriate, and clear, while avoiding ambiguous English jargon, slang or phrases that would be difficult to translate across cultures. In addition to choosing language carefully to meet the developmental level and needs of the girls, it was also important to think through the interpreter's role as a mediator in that exchange in order to communicate effectively.

While planning and facilitating these groups, many of the same child life skills were necessary in order to attend to complex individual and group dynamics, while also assessing knowledge and development and being sensitive to trauma cues the girls may demonstrate. In addition, with the cultural and language barriers, the author had to maintain an open orientation to understanding the perspectives, experiences, and opinions of the participants in the group. Many of the girls found a sense of confidence and empowerment in teaching her the nuances of mehndi designs (also known as henna ink) or Warli (a traditional Indian drawing style akin to stick figures) or explaining customs and traditions from their home villages and early life.

Twice a year, the team facilitated a camp experience for the girls, complete with opportunities to canoe, hike, complete a ropes course, climb a rock wall, and other traditional camp activities which helped them feel empowered in a new and neutral context while bonding with their peers and staff. Being in a different setting outside the city allowed the girls to experience nature – and their environment – in ways-inaccessible to them during their captivity or even in their lives prior to being forced into sex trafficking (see figure 5). As they worked together to try new things and learned to build trust with their peers and staff, they became more comfortable expressing their fears and finding the internal strength and courage they would need to find resilience. This experience was also powerful for the staff, allowing them to try new activities and experiences themselves, different from the intense and emotional work they did every day.

PROGRAMMATIC SUPPORT AND COMMUNITY COLLABORATION

At a higher administrative level, another function of the author's role was to evaluate the programs, policies, and procedures at XYZ organization from a psychosocial perspective, in the hopes of identifying areas for growth and improvement. Despite her background in child life theory and practice and additional training in trauma-informed care and Indian culture, it was important to approach this component of the role with cultural humility and an emphasis on culturally responsive care practices that the organization could continue to use past the bounds of the author's time-limited internship. Initially, direct care with the residents and collaboration with the staff members provided a foundation and rapport that could be leveraged to generate useful and feasible practice improvements that would benefit all involved.

Figure 5. Outing to Bhushi Dam

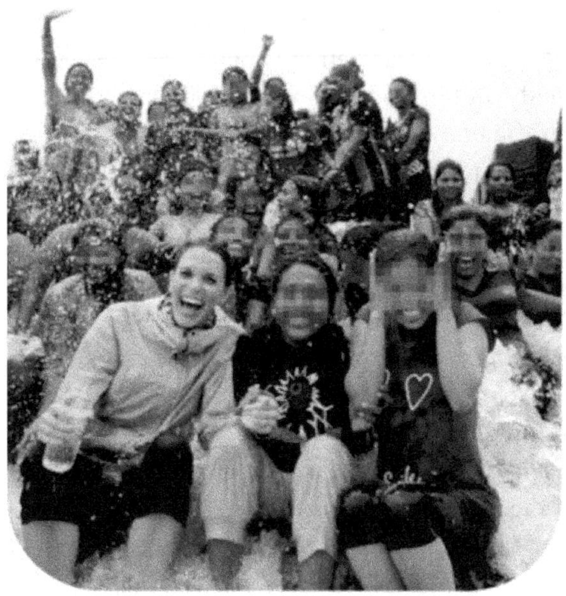

In line with her experiences as a hospital based CCLS, one of the programs the author first helped to implement was guaranteed and consistent female medical help for each girl upon entry to the program. In Mumbai particularly, this was no small feat, as finding an OBGYN who was both female and trauma-sensitive was very difficult. Because of the social stigma surrounding this patient population, very few providers met these criteria and were able or willing to provide care for victims of human trafficking. Eventually, a partnership was established with a local, female OBGYN who both understood and was sensitive to what the girls had experienced; furthermore, she was able to examine and treat these patients with the specialized care and compassion they needed. With this partnership, every girl who entered XYZ was able to receive a thorough medical evaluation so that her medical needs were addressed upon entry.

Recognizing XYZ's small but dedicated full time staff (consisting of administration and finance staff, social workers, house mothers, and an aftercare team), the author assessed the importance of organized programming and policy development to protect and retain these important team members. Given the high level of trauma experienced by the girls, many did not have a solid conception of what a trusting relationship can look like, and how this is formed and practiced with therapeutic professionals. Similarly, the staff who deeply cared for the residents wanted to be constantly and fully available to meet the girls where they were in moments of need or crisis. Providing staff education about the value of clear and consistent boundaries led to collaborative problem solving and the development of a rotating on-call system to support the health and wellbeing of both the resident girls and the multidisciplinary team.

Additionally, staff involvement in group events and celebrations was identified as an opportunity to scaffold the girls' comfort not only with people they did not know well, but specifically with men. As some staff worked solely in the administrative offices and did not have direct contact with the girls, a written policy about involvement in celebrations and special events at the after care homes met two distinct needs: 1) the girls' need to adjust to and feel more comfortable in the presence of vetted men, and 2) the office-based staff's need to witness and participate in the results of their work efforts by engaging with the girls and home-based team members. Additionally, as girls graduated the program, attained gainful and consistent employment, and even married, the author facilitated the creation of a policy to help staff make decisions about when and how to equitably participate in these milestones with former residents while also remaining manageable within the day-to-day responsibilities of the team.

Another key opportunity for growth at XYZ organization was community networking – specifically, building and mobilizing community relationships that were resourceful and sustainable, yet also understanding the needs of the survivors they were serving. In addition to developing a key partnership with the medical community as described above, the author assisted the XYZ staff in building and maintaining relationships with local churches, nonprofit organizations, educational centers, and businesses to obtain needed supplies and help XYZ residents meet the goals that would help them graduate XYZ. Most of the girls arrived to XYZ with few, if any, personal belongings; thanks to community partners, XYZ provides each new resident with a new backpack full of essential items like clothing, undergarments, personal care items, a small purse, water bottle, and even stuffed animals and comfort items. Additionally, local churches and nonprofit organizations became social support centers the girls could rely on after graduation to help them continue their healing journey.

Much like educating community donors about child life services or providing volunteer orientation in the hospital-based setting, the author worked with the XYZ staff in a train-the-trainer model to help them communicate the organization's value and needs in ways that would resonate with donors and volunteers. This outreach not only helped the organization acquire needed supplies and services, but also strengthened relationships with other private and semi-private after care homes in the community to maximize resource use and problem solve in moments of uncertainty. Finally, businesses and educational centers in the area offered opportunities for the girls to learn job skills, gain employment (especially in the hospitality industry), or seek education (often to pursue nursing or social work) depending on the hopes and goals they had identified for themselves.

At one point, the community needed to come together with XYZ to house a rescued girl who had also been diagnosed with leprosy. Although extinct in many parts of the world, leprosy in India still exists and is typically treated with extreme isolation in communities specifically designed for people living with leprosy. Given the highly infectious nature of the disease and the group home model of XYZ, it was imperative to connect with medical providers and other local aftercare homes to identify a best plan of care for a girl who had experienced systematic trauma in the human trafficking industry. By communicating with these other professionals and agencies, more information was gathered about the leprosy disease process, effective treatments, and safe quarantine procedures. Using her CCLS skills, the author was able to translate this medical information into accessible language that the XYZ staff, aftercare house mothers, and girls could understand. This situation not only required collaboration with the team and larger community, but also modeled the importance of effective education in promoting understanding and effective coping for this vulnerable population and the staff that serve them.

In her time at XYZ, the author provided a variety of both formal staff education and informal mentoring/modeling to help the staff better understand the tenets of trauma-informed care and how to apply these in their work setting. Although all the staff were highly engaged in and passionate about this population, some had no training or education in trauma-informed care. Knowing this and reflecting on the importance of cultural humility for the success of these efforts, rarely was education a unilateral delivery of content from the author to the staff, but rather a dialogue of collaborative problem solving that could identify culturally appropriate and responsive solutions. In these ways, the author's experience with communicating complex concepts to children and families in the healthcare setting was well suited for helping the staff reflect on, understand, and apply trauma-informed care practices as the girls processed their extensive traumatic histories while anticipating eventual reintegration into Indian society.

One of the most important elements of this staff- and policy-directed work was always retaining and exercising cultural humility. For instance, in the United States, productivity and efficiency are high values even in healthcare settings where vulnerable children and youth are served. Conversely, relationships are of the utmost importance in Indian culture. Thus, orienting staff education around their primary cultural drive for and investment in relationships was much more appropriate and effective than the professional development sessions or skills assessments more prevalent in the United States. Therefore, the author dedicated the first six months at XYZ to building relationships and understanding the history and dynamics of its dedicated staff members, rather than exacting change. Then, as areas of opportunity emerged, a strong foundation of mutual trust was already established, and individualized conversations over tea breaks or organic office chats led to team-driven and sustainable improvements. By refusing the tendency to approach as a "white savior" with some illusion of "all the answers," and instead holding a mindset of wanting to truly help the staff who were living this work day-to-day, the author was able to use the philosophy of "meeting people where they are" to help XYZ meet its identified and prioritized goals as smoothly as possible.

Also, to this end, the author spent significant time in her role at XYZ providing staff support to ensure that they could continue providing the incredibly intense services its resident girls needed. Noticing how the housemothers, aftercare staff, and administrative staff worked tirelessly to achieve the goals of the girls and the organization, the author implemented and facilitated a variety of group supervision sessions and training to ward against burnout and secondary trauma. At times, the group sessions revolved around topics such as self-care, positive coping skills, and therapeutic boundaries, simultaneously building their trust with one another and enhancing the staff's perceived support network. Additionally, throughout her time at XYZ, the author regularly participated in individualized counseling via Skype both to normalize the value of seeking support, and to remain as emotionally engaged and healthy as possible along the way.

OUTCOMES

Much like traditional, hospital-based child life services, it is difficult to measure the outcomes of this relational and process-oriented work with individuals from such varied backgrounds, experiences, and personal characteristics. Additionally, with the author's work being deeply woven into XYZ's multidisciplinary mission and approach, it is challenging to identify which components of child life services in this setting may have contributed to each girl's personal journey and successes. Perhaps it is more useful to evaluate each girl's experiences individually, noting how her needs, coping skills, and abilities to participate in normative social interactions may have grown or changed during her months or years at XYZ.

Quantitative trauma scales or quality-of-life measures are limited in their ability to assess the extent of the experiences that survivors of human trafficking may have and benefit from at XYZ. However, anecdotally, there are stories like Veena's. Deceived into forced sex work by a persuasive romantic partner, she spent years being physically, sexually, and emotionally abused, coming to believe that she was not worthy of love or happiness. However, after three years at XYZ, Veena learned English, participated in individual and group counseling and life skills training, and began building trusting relationships with the housemothers and girls in her home. She finished her college degree and went on to get her master's degree in social work, with a desire to help those who had likewise survived the trauma of human trafficking. Upon leaving XYZ, she became a social worker at a non-governmental agency serving survivors of human trafficking.

Five years after completing her tenure at XYZ and returning to the United States, the author returned to Mumbai. While visiting, the author returned to the organization to spend time with the staff and interact with the girls receiving the services they helped establish and enhance. While there, the staff hosted a reunion with twenty human trafficking survivors whom the author supported during her service in Mumbai who had graduated from the program. The experience was indescribable; the same girls who had entered the organization traumatized, withdrawn, and in pain were now holding jobs, completing higher education programs, married, and having children. In fact, the author held the new baby of a girl with whom she had worked for several years. Witnessing the transformation and healing her work had helped to effect in this way was overwhelming, just as the epidemic of human trafficking is as well. But, in that visit, it was evident that the XYZ program – with its trauma informed and culturally responsive care – can help to bring life and hope to the other side of unimaginable trauma.

Even years after that brief return to Mumbai, XYZ enjoys continued success even today as it mobilizes multidisciplinary, evidence-based, and person-centered care to equip female survivors of human trafficking for reintegration into society. With the author's child life training and experiences in hospital-based service, she was able to leave the organization changed in various ways – from the acquisition of a dedicated physician for XYZ's residents, to stronger policies and understanding of child protection and therapeutic boundaries for the staff. In the wake of her internship, girls at XYZ continue to benefit from expanded community partnerships, educational and vocational opportunities, and trauma-informed individual and group interventions. The vocational center she helped established remains in place today, as well as the therapeutic outings and field trips the girls experience during their time at XYZ. Now, she remains on the organization's board of directors, frequently hearing stories of challenge, growth, and ultimately success both for the organization and for the individuals it serves. Although the prevalence of human trafficking in India remains largely unchanged, the staff and community partners of XYZ continue to improve their abilities to identify, assess, treat, and advocate for those who have been globally abused and silenced.

FUTURE DIRECTIONS AND NEEDS

Unfortunately, human trafficking is a global issue, taking place in and across most every corner of the world. As the effects of human trafficking ripple outwards from survivors to their families, communities, and social systems, psychosocial providers – especially CCLSs – must understand and be cognizant of the risk factors associated with being trafficked, the array of traumatic experiences survivors have accumulated, and the effects of and outcomes associated with trafficking to better identify and serve this vulnerable population. Only with international and integrative efforts can the epidemic of global trafficking be adequately addressed.

Specifically in the United States, much work is needed and being undertaken to better identify and support child victims of human trafficking. Often referred to as domestic minor sex trafficking (DMST) in North America, healthcare facilities have noted that up to 90% of child victims have never been seen by a healthcare provider at some point in the five years prior to their rescue – and less than half of these providers documented any concern for the youth's safety or involvement in sex trafficking (Ertl et al., 2020). These encounters primarily took place in emergency departments and involved children who already demonstrated high prevalence of sexual assault, running away from home, involvement in the juvenile justice system, or being rejected from private and/or government homes (Albright et al., 2020; Browne-James et al., 2021; Ert et al., 2020). Thus, many child victims of human trafficking go unnoticed and untreated even in one of the world's most developed and wealthy countries. And, when systemic racial biases, provider discomfort and lack of training, and the inaccessibility of healthcare for most children and youth without involved and knowledgeable caregivers are factored in, CCLSs have a responsibility to keep their eyes and ears open, assessments gear turning, and advocacy skills ripe and ready for use on behalf of vulnerable populations such as this.

As the author's experiences at XYZ highlight, there is tremendous opportunity for the application of child life theory and practice in service of human trafficking victims and their families and communities – whether across international and cultural lines, or in local clinics or emergency departments. Just as preparation, coping skills education, socialization opportunities, and therapeutic activities foster resilience in children with healthcare needs, so too can these interventions be mapped onto trauma-informed care in settings like XYZ with girls who have experienced human trafficking and forced sex work. With intentional knowledge acquisition, skill development, and both reflective and reflexive practice, CCLSs can provide high quality psychosocial care adapted for victims of human rights violations, like human trafficking, on a global stage. As CCLSs build, maintain, and model the sanctity of and safety that human relationships can hold and provide, it is possible to enhance self-esteem and self-worth despite repeat and overwhelming trauma. With multidisciplinary collaboration and multisystemic interventions, CCLSs can help support the development of adaptive coping skills that victims of human trafficking can use in future contexts of their ongoing growth and recovery efforts.

CONCLUSION

Achal arrived to XYZ just after what would have been her 18th birthday. Growing up in a large family in the slums of Mumbai, she never expected a big house, nice things, or even a lucrative career opportunity. However, she did not expect that her parents would be tricked into selling her into forced sex work, instead of the housing and job opportunity they had been promised. At first she was angry, then she felt nothing as she was beaten, raped, and drugged day after day, year after year. It was unexpected when she and her underage coworkers at the brothel were found and liberated during a scheduled raid. After living in another aftercare home until she was 18, she arrived to XYZ in physical and emotional pain, with limited family, friends, or resources to draw on. Three years later, she left with a high school diploma, a full-time job at a local communications company, and a network of supporters in her new neighborhood. She knew her worth now, could draw on her new coping skills (such as journaling and playing the guitar) to combat intrusive thoughts or distressing memories, and found a home where she felt safe and strong.

Children and adults who have been trafficked accumulate traumatic life experiences that most people can only imagine, and that research has only recently begun to understand. When developmental and coping processes are known to be compromised or at risk, and resiliency factors are low and difficult to access, trauma-informed, developmentally grounded, and individualized psychosocial support is an integral dimension of comprehensive care after trafficking. Therefore, CCLSs are uniquely poised to harness the expansive power of play, the creative arts, and education to begin to dress the many physical and psychosocial wounds incurred by these experiences – whether in children, adolescents, or adults.

At the same time, it is important to transfer and adapt child life skills and interventions to new populations and contexts with a growth orientation, cultural humility, and the flexibility required to assess and meet the patient- and family-centered goals of a new cultural and institutional context (or distinctive population). Furthermore, should the opportunity arise to combine one's child life training and experiences with personal passions – such as international travel and service – the potential to positively impact on vulnerable communities exponentially increases. Should such a possibility emerge, then, proceed with both passion and caution, confidence and humility, an eagerness to teach and to learn, and a willingness to meet people, families, and cultures both exactly where they are, all the while envisioning where they could be and what they could achieve with the right individually tailored supports.

ACKNOWLEDGMENT

The authors would like to thank Keana Gonzales for her contributions to this chapter, as well as the many women and girls whose experiences with human trafficking informed this chapter.

This work received no funding from any agency in the public, commercial, or not-for-profit sectors.

REFERENCES

Albright, K., Greenbaum, J., Edwards, S. A., & Tsai, C. (2020). Systematic review of facilitators of barriers to, and recommendations for healthcare services for child survivors of human trafficking globally. *Child Abuse & Neglect, 100*, 104289. doi:10.1016/j.chiabu.2019.104289 PMID:31787336

Association of Child Life Professionals. (2022). *Standards of clinical practice*. Retrieved from: https://www.childlife.org/docs/default-source/aclp-official-documents/4-standards-of-clinical-practice.pdf?sfvrsn=893e8c4d_2

Bandyopadhyay, R. (2019). Volunteer tourism and "The White Man's Burden": Globalization of suffering, white savior complex, religion and modernity. *Journal of Sustainable Tourism*, *27*(3), 327–343. doi:10.1080/09669582.2019.1578361

Boles, J. C. (2017). Trauma-informed care: An intentional approach. *Pediatric Nursing*, *43*(5), 16–18.

Boles, J. C., Fraser, C., Bennett, K., Jones, M., Dunbar, J., Woodburn, A., Gill, M., Duplechain, A., Munn, E., & Hoskins, K. (2020, January). *The value of Certified Child Life Specialists: Direct and downstream optimization of pediatric patient and family outcomes* (Full report). Retrieved from: https://www.childlife.org/docs/default-source/the-child-life-profession/value-of-cclss-full-report.pdf?sfvrsn=5e238d4d_2

Browne-James, L., Litam, S. D. A., & McRae, L. (2021). Child sex trafficking: Strategies for identification, counseling, and advocacy. *International Journal for the Advancement of Counseling*, *43*(2), 113–125. doi:10.100710447-020-09420-y PMID:33432250

Choudhury, R. G. (2020). Distinctive marketing strategies of different industries in India. *The Business & Management Review*, *11*(2), 13–18. doi:10.24052/BMR/V11NU02/ART-02

Cohen, J. A., Mannarino, A. P., Kliethermes, M., & Murray, L. A. (2012). Trauma-focused CBT for youth with complex trauma. *Child Abuse & Neglect*, *36*(6), 528–541. doi:10.1016/j.chiabu.2012.03.007 PMID:22749612

da Silva, I. M., & Sathiyaseelan, A. (2019). Emotional needs of women post-rescue from sex trafficking in India. *Cogent Psychology*, *6*(1), 1631584. doi:10.1080/23311908.2019.1631584

Dalla, R. L., & Kreimer, L. M. (2017). "After your honor is gone…": Exploration of developmental trajectories and life experiences of women working in Mumbai's red-light brothel districts. *Sexuality & Culture*, *21*(1), 163–186. doi:10.100712119-016-9388-4

Dalla, R. L., Panchal, T. J., Erwin, S., Peter, J., Roselius, K., Ranjan, R., Mischra, M., & Sahu, S. (2020). Structural vulnerabilities, personal agency, and caste: An exploration of child sex trafficking in rural India. *Violence and Victims*, *35*(3), 307–330. doi:10.1891/VV-D-19-00048 PMID:32606215

Dummer, T. J., & Cook, I. G. (2008). Health in China and India: A cross-country comparison in a context of rapid globalization. *Social Science & Medicine*, *67*(4), 590–605. doi:10.1016/j.socscimed.2008.04.019 PMID:18554766

Ertl, S., Bokor, B., Tuchman, L., Miller, E., Kappel, R., & Deye, K. (2020). Healthcare needs and utilization patterns of sex-trafficked youth: Missed opportunities at a children's hospital. *Child: Care, Health and Development*, *46*(4), 422–428. doi:10.1111/cch.12759 PMID:32037615

Foronda, C. (2020). A theory of cultural humility. *Journal of Transcultural Nursing*, *31*(1), 7–12. doi:10.1177/1043659619875184 PMID:31516091

Gnana, S. R. (2018). Caste system, dalitization and its implications in contemporary India. *International Journal of Sociology and Anthropology*, *10*(7), 65–71. doi:10.5897/IJSA2017.0713

Karandikar, S. A., Gezinski, L. B., & Kaloga, M. E. P. (2015). *Health Care Among Sex-Trafficked Women and Girls in India*. Retrieved from: https://www.gahts.com/publications/ecjl9xjsxz95fhg-gns5a-7wc46-ksfe5-8pbkw-j7g9t-6pp2j-p6rf4-7xkhm-ssxlb-whxwr-7rd83-98ben-tawpp-3bhct-ww5eb-y7f5t-xs585-zaaff-m272e-96gr3-xxa77-pz4p4-4pse3-kzrd2-z67jx-ma9re-estlf

Kirmayer, L. J., & Gómez-Carrillo, A. (2019). *Culturally responsive clinical psychology and psychiatry: An ecosocial approach*. Hogrefe.

Kolb, E. (2019). 75,000 people per square mile? These are the most densely populated cities in the world. *USA Today*. Retrieved from: https://www.usatoday.com/story/news/world/2019/07/11/the-50-most-densely-populated-cities-in-the-world/39664259/

Locke, R. A. (2010). *Rescued, rehabilitated, returned: Institutional approaches to the rehabilitation of survivors of sex trafficking in India and Nepal* (Doctoral dissertation, University of Denver). Retrieved from: https://digitalcommons.du.edu/cgi/viewcontent.cgi?article=1377&context=etd

Maslow, A. H. (1943). Dynamics of personality organization. *Psychological Review*, *50*(5), 514–539. doi:10.1037/h0062222

Rai, R., & Rai, A. K. (2021). Nature of sex trafficking in India: A geographical perspective. *Children and Youth Services Review*, *120*, 105739. doi:10.1016/j.childyouth.2020.105739

Stenman, K., Christofferson, J., Alderfer, M. A., Pierce, J., Kelly, C., Schifano, E., Klaff, S., Sciolla, J., Deatrick, J., & Kazak, A. E. (2019). Integrating play in trauma-informed care: Multidisciplinary pediatric healthcare provider perspectives. *Psychological Services*, *16*(1), 7–15. doi:10.1037er0000294 PMID:30431310

Turner, J. C. (2018). Theoretical foundations of child life practice. In R. H. Thompson (Ed.), *The Handbook of Child Life* (2nd ed., pp. 34–54). Charles C. Thomas Publishers.

United Nations Office on Drugs and Crime. (2000). *United Nations convention against transnational organized crime and the protocols thereto*. Retrieved from: https://www.unodc.org/documents/treaties/UNTOC/Publications/TOC%20Convention/TOCebook-e.pdf

Weightman, S. (2017). Hinduism. In J. R. Hinnells (Ed.), *A New Handbook of Living Religions* (pp. 261–309). Wiley. doi:10.1002/9781405166614.ch5

World Population Review. (2022). *Mumbai Population 2022*. World Population Review. https://worldpopulationreview.com/world-cities/mumbai-population

ADDITIONAL READING

Albright, K., Greenbaum, J., Edwards, S. A., & Tsai, C. (2020). Systematic review of facilitators of, barriers to, and recommendations for healthcare services for child survivors of human trafficking globally. *Child Abuse & Neglect*, *100*, 104289. doi:10.1016/j.chiabu.2019.104289 PMID:31787336

Association of Child Life Professionals. (2021). *Position statement on child life practice in community settings*. Retrieved from: https://www.childlife.org/docs/default-source/about-aclp/cbp-on-cl-practice-in-community-settings.pdf

Bandyopadhyay, R. (2019). Volunteer tourism and "The White Man's Burden": Globalization of suffering, white savior complex, religion and modernity. *Journal of Sustainable Tourism*, *27*(3), 327–343. doi:10.1080/09669582.2019.1578361

Boles, J. C. (2017). Trauma-informed care: An intentional approach. *Pediatric Nursing*, *43*(5), 16–18.

Boles, J. C., Fraser, C., Bennett, K., Jones, M., Dunbar, J., Woodburn, A., Gill, M., Duplechain, A., Munn, E., & Hoskins, K. (2020, January). *The value of Certified Child Life Specialists: Direct and downstream optimization of pediatric patient and family outcomes* (Full report). Retrieved from: https://www.childlife.org/docs/default-source/the-child-life-profession/value-of-cclss-full-report.pdf?sfvrsn=5e238d4d_2

Dalla, R. L., & Kreimer, L. M. (2017). "After your honor is gone...": Exploration of developmental trajectories and life experiences of women working in Mumbai's red-light brothel districts. *Sexuality & Culture*, *21*(1), 163–186. doi:10.100712119-016-9388-4

Dalla, R. L., Panchal, T. J., Erwin, S., Peter, J., Roselius, K., Ranjan, R., Mischra, M., & Sahu, S. (2020). Structural vulnerabilities, personal agency, and caste: An exploration of child sex trafficking in rural India. *Violence and Victims*, *35*(3), 307–330. doi:10.1891/VV-D-19-00048 PMID:32606215

Finigan-Carr, N. M., Johnson, M. H., Pullmann, M. D., Stewart, C. J., & Fromknecht, A. E. (2019). A traumagenic social ecological framework for understanding and intervening with sex trafficked children and youth. *Child & Adolescent Social Work Journal*, *36*(1), 49–63. doi:10.100710560-018-0588-7 PMID:31929679

Foronda, C. (2020). A theory of cultural humility. *Journal of Transcultural Nursing*, *31*(1), 7–12. doi:10.1177/1043659619875184 PMID:31516091

Karandikar, S. A., Gezinski, L. B., & Kaloga, M. E. P. (2015). *Health Care Among Sex-Trafficked Women and Girls in India*. Retrieved from: https://www.gahts.com/publications/ecjl9xjsxz95fhg-gns5a-7wc46-ksfe5-8pbkw-j7g9t-6pp2j-p6rf4-7xkhm-ssxlb-whxwr-7rd83-98ben-tawpp-3bhct-ww5eb-y7f5t-xs585-zaaff-m272e-96gr3-xxa77-pz4p4-4pse3-kzrd2-z67jx-ma9re-estlf

Maslow, A. H. (1943). Dynamics of personality organization. *Psychological Review*, *50*(5), 514–539. doi:10.1037/h0062222

Mukherjee, M. (2020). Featured counter-trafficking program: Arpan. *Child Abuse & Neglect*, *100*, 104152. doi:10.1016/j.chiabu.2019.104152 PMID:31519409

Singh, S., & Kometiani, M. K. (2019). Use of the expressive art therapies to bring healing from the trauma of commercial sexual exploitation in Kolkata, India. In *Art Therapy Treatment with Sex Trafficking Survivors* (pp. 139–161). Routledge. doi:10.4324/9780429469671-7

Wallace, C., Lavina, I., & Mollen, C. (2021). Share our stories: An exploration of the healthcare experiences of child sex trafficking survivors. *Child Abuse & Neglect*, *112*, 104896. doi:10.1016/j.chiabu.2020.104896 PMID:33434686

KEY TERMS AND DEFINITIONS

Colonialism: Historical colonization or control of indigenous populations by larger, often European American, conquerors and settlers. In India, remnants of colonialism are seen in how the political structure is still organized and the underdevelopment of its cities, forces, and trade markets.

Cultural Humility: A relationship stance that acknowledges how individuals' cultural experiences and identity impact their personhood, from the things they think and feel to the decisions they make about things like healthcare.

Culturally Responsive Care: A provider's intentional orientation towards and efforts to offering care that specifically fosters environments that seek, respect, respond to, and celebrate the intersectional aspects that make an individual unique; it is, by nature, anti-oppressive, multicultural, and holistic.

Human Trafficking: The luring, transportation, and sale or receipt of persons, typically using abduction, extortion, deception, and physical or relational force. Victims of human trafficking are typically forced into sex work or other types of systematic abuse and servitude in exchange for payment, which they are told is necessary to alleviate their "debts" and purchase their "freedom."

Trauma-Informed Care: An approach to care interactions that seeks to understand the impacts of previous trauma on individuals' current functioning, while also working to minimize the potential for additional trauma in those care interactions. Trauma-informed care has six components: 1) safety, 2) transparency and trust, 3) peer support and self-help resources, 4) collaboration and shared goals in care, 5) extending choice and control wherever possible, and 6) awareness of confounding issues related to culture, history, gender, and other identity facets.

Chapter 14
Transgender and Gender Expansive

Adrianna Ortega
Caterpillar Child Life, USA

Christy French
Cohen Children's Medical Center, USA

ABSTRACT

This chapter focuses on using the child life competencies to support transgender/gender expansive children and their families. The chapter highlights challenges families face and addresses the important support they need, helping families identify coping skills and model peer interactions related to gender identity. Additionally, it is intended to provide child life specialists with foundational knowledge about gender identity which will guide and influence their work when they support children who are transgender or gender expansive.

INTRODUCTION

Imagine a five-year-old who was assigned male at birth, but has explained time and time again that he loves "girl things." His preference for all things pink and sparkly is accepted by his family. They reassure him that girls and boys play with all sorts of toys, he can choose whatever toys he likes, and they will always love him. The five-year-old is a smart, creative, kind-hearted, cooperative child and a wonderful older brother.

Then the five-year-old starts kindergarten and struggles to make friends. He isn't interested in playing with the boys, and the girls think that it's strange that a boy wants to play princesses. The five-year-old becomes more and more aware that he is "different" from his classmates. With this increased awareness comes great anxiety and loneliness; the once happy, secure child slowly disappears. This child comes home in tears, begging not to go back to school. He begins to have difficulty sleeping, and for the first time in his life he is beginning to have massive tantrums almost daily. He starts asking his par-

DOI: 10.4018/978-1-6684-5097-0.ch014

ents, "What is wrong with me? I hate myself! I hate this world!" His parents have a feeling that all of this is related to their child's gender expression, but avoid the complicated possibility. Then one night, crying in his mother's arms, the five-year-old states, "I wish that we could go to Disney World and meet a Fairy Godmother and ask her to turn me into a girl. It's too hard to live like this." The parents must face reality and recognize their child may be transgender.

The statistics on suicide within the transgender community terrify these parents. They know every year transgender people are assaulted and killed based on their identity. They fear their child and family may be rejected and harmed. They are consumed with anxiety. How will our extended family react? How will our community respond? What will our coworkers think? What does the future hold for our transgender child and family?

These are just a few of the many questions and fears parents may ask upon discovering their child is transgender/gender expansive. Unfortunately, there are limited resources for young children and families trying to better understand gender identity. Parents may search the internet for helpful information, but when one's child suffers with gender dysphoria, often what a parent seeks most is someone who can guide them through their unique journey. They need someone who knows their child, who understands child development, gender identity, and who can provide individualized care. Such specific psychosocial, developmental support can be difficult to find, even in large metropolitan areas. However, child life specialists armed with knowledge regarding gender identity have the clinical skills to fill this unmet need in any setting.

In 2019, applying supported evidence and personal experience, a child life specialist and mother of a transgender child created Caterpillar Child Life, a non-traditional child life practice that helps meet the needs of young transgender/gender expansive children. Caterpillar Child Life provides individual and group support to children, parents, and siblings navigating transgender/gender-expansive identity. Using play, education, expressive arts, coping techniques, and connections with peers, Caterpillar Child Life helps transgender/gender expansive children thrive despite the many challenges stacked against them. This chapter highlights the common needs of this population, resources available, and how Certified Child Life Specialists (CCLS) can serve this unique population. Additionally, the chapter provides specific information needed to best support transgender/gender expansive children and their families.

SERVING AN AT-RISK POPULATION: TRANSGENDER/GENDER EXPANSIVE CHILDREN AND THE ROLE OF CHILD LIFE

Identifying Risk Factors

People who are transgender have been recognized all over the world in different cultures for centuries. A brief list includes the third gender of Greece in 380 B.C., eunuchs of biblical times, the muxe of Mexico, the hijras of South Asia, and the two spirit indigenous people. However, despite transgender people existing across cultures for centuries, transgender/gender expansive children continue to have their identities questioned, judged, and rejected. In the United States, transgender youth have alarming rates of suicidal ideation. In a national survey conducted in 2021, the Trevor Project (2021) found that 52% of transgender and non-binary youth seriously considered attempting suicide within the previous year, and 20% of those polled had attempted suicide within the previous year. The same study found that 77% of the transgender and non-binary youth had experienced a significant level of anxiety, and 70% experienced depression. Nearly half of those that polled stated that they wanted support or counseling, but did not receive it. It can be assumed transgender individuals face similar adversity worldwide where there is discrimination against gender non-conforming individuals.

In addition to depression and anxiety, eating disorders have a high prevalence within this population. Individuals "living in an incongruent cognitive state where their physical body is in conflict with their self-perceived identity", or in conflict with social and cultural expectations, may develop an eating disorder. The emphasis on body shape in a person struggling with gender dysphoria and in a person struggling with an eating disorder suggests there may be some overlap (Couturier et al., 2015).

Transgender youth are nearly three times as likely as their cisgender peers to restrict eating, almost nine times as likely to use diet pills, and seven times more likely to use laxatives to control their weight (Guss et al., 2016). To protect LGBTQ+ youth, provide appropriate support and services, and eliminate mental health disparities, it is essential for clinicians to assess risk factors creating disproportionate numbers of adverse outcomes (Vance and Rosenthal, 2018).

A survey conducted by the National Center for Transgender Equality surveyed adults who identify as transgender about their experiences in restrooms (James et al., 2016). The survey results demonstrated that 59% of the transgender participants have avoided bathrooms in the last year because they feared confrontations in public restrooms at work, school, or in other places, 31% avoided drinking or eating within that year so that they would not need to use the restroom, and 8% reported having a kidney infection, urinary tract infection, or another kidney-related medical issue from avoiding restrooms in the last year. While this survey was conducted with adults, transgender youth have also reported self-restricted eating and drinking while at school because they unable to use bathrooms aligning with their gender identity. Some schools do not have gender neutral bathrooms or do not understand gender identity, and sometimes students are simply scared to be outed or bullied. Consequently, they are at risk to develop significant health problems as described from the survey (Rosen, 2022).

Most major medical associations support the use of current evidence-based clinical gender-affirming care. This includes the American Academy of Pediatrics, The American Academy of Child and Adolescent Psychiatry, The American Medical Association, and the Pediatric Endocrine Society (Simon, 2022). These associations also state that gender-affirming care, including puberty suppression and hormone therapy for transgender children should be seen as lifesaving care. In addition, there are numerous studies that show that the use of a youth's preferred pronouns and name significantly lowers the risk of depression and suicidal ideation. One final study indicated that transgender youths between the ages of 15-21 had 71% fewer symptoms of severe depression if permitted to use their chosen name at school, at home, at work, and with friends (Russell et al., 2018).

Parents of transgender/gender expansive children are increasingly aware of these risks and are recognizing a need for guidance in preventing anxiety, depression, eating disorders, and other mental health concerns. CCLS are well equipped to fill the role. They possess knowledge regarding healthy development and trauma prevention, which is critical to supporting this vulnerable population. They recognize the intersection of gender identity and mental health and anticipate additional psychosocial stressors of co-occurring conditions. It is clear CCLS can help children and families navigate the potentially stressful experience of having a transgender/gender-expansive child.

CLINICAL KNOWLEDGE AND SKILLS

Upon review of the Official Documents of the Association of Child Life Professionals one will find the seven competencies around the care of children, youth, and families (ACLP, 2019). In the private practice setting, each of these competencies, along with competencies in the areas of professional responsibility, education and supervision, research fundamentals, and administration, can be applied to work with children who are transgender/gender expansive. The table below will highlight how the first seven competencies relate to working with this population.

Working with this population requires comprehensive knowledge and ongoing research on gender identity. Typically, children are assigned male, female, or intersex at birth; the infant's gender corresponds with the genitalia. However, research shows children do not begin to form gender identity until the age of three or four (Rafferty, 2022), and some evidence reveals gender identity begins to present as early as two years of age (Brill and Pepper, 2008). For many children, their gender identity aligns with their sex assigned at birth, referred to as cisgender. For other children, female or male does not fit. The child may begin to verbally express wanting to be the opposite gender or say they "feel" like the opposite gender. Children expressing a combination of genders may be described as gender creative, gender expansive, gender fluid, gender nonconforming, or gender variant. The term non-binary is also used to express gender identity outside of the finite, dual category of female or male.

Transgender is an umbrella term encompassing those whose gender identities or gender roles differ from those typically associated with the sex they were assigned at birth (Human Rights Campaign, 2022). In this chapter, transgender and gender expansive are recognized as synonymous. It is also important to know that the term "transgender" is an adjective and *not* a noun. Cisgender, another adjective, is used to describe people whose gender identity does align with their sex assigned at birth. As one learns more about gender identity it becomes clear that gender is not a binary. Gender should be thought of as a spectrum, a range of identities derived from an internal sense of self. Gender can also be fluid, changing in different settings (Rafferty et al., 2018). To get a better understanding of the spectrum of gender identity, gender expression, and how these differ from sex assigned at birth and sexual attraction, one can refer to the Gender Unicorn infographic that has been created and shared by Trans Student Educational Resources (2021).

This infographic can be particularly helpful when working with younger children. It provides a more concrete example of gender and sexuality. How a child life specialist presents the infographic will depend on the developmental level of the child, as well as the individual needs of the family. For instance, some families may be experiencing a situation where their child has gender dysphoria. This is when psychological distress results from an incongruence between one's sex assigned at birth and one's gender identity. The *Diagnostic and Statistical Manual of Mental Disorders* (American Psychiatric Association, 2013) defines gender dysphoria in children as a marked incongruence between one's experienced/expressed gender and assigned sex at birth, lasting at least 6 months, as manifested by at least six of the following:

- A strong desire to be of the other gender or an insistence that one is the other gender (or some alternative gender different from one's assigned sex)
- In boys (assigned sex), a strong preference for cross-dressing or simulating female attire; in girls (assigned sex), a strong preference for wearing only typical masculine clothing and strong resistance to the wearing of typical feminine clothing
- A strong preference for cross-gender roles in make-believe play or fantasy play

- A strong preference for the toys, games, or activities stereotypically used or engaged in by the other gender
- A strong preference for playmates of the other gender
- In boys (assigned sex), a strong rejection of typically masculine toys, games, and activities and a strong avoidance of rough-and-tumble play; or in girls (assigned sex), a strong rejection of typically feminine toys, games, and activities
- A strong dislike of one's sexual anatomy
- A strong desire for the physical sex characteristics that match one's experienced gender

The Gender Unicorn helps the child and the family comprehend that gender expression is entirely different than one's assigned sex at birth or sexuality. Equipped with this knowledge comes acceptance, and when a child feels accepted the dysphoria tends to dissipate.

The infographic also helps CCLS explain to parents the nuances of gender and sexuality. Many individuals see gender and sexuality as one and the same, but they are not synonymous. Definitions of gender, sex, and sexual orientation can be found under key terms in the appendix of this chapter. When working with transgender/gender expansive children, it is important to note the difference between **gender identity and gender expression. Gender identity** is one's deeply felt internal sense of who they are. As mentioned earlier, infants have no concept of identity at birth, gender identity evolves over time. In early childhood, a parent might hear, "I have a boy body, but a girl heart" or "I'm a girl on the outside, but a boy on the inside." Later, a school-age child or adolescent might have more sophisticated language and communication skills to convey their identity. As an emerging adult and beyond, gender identity continues to unfold. **Gender expression**, on the other hand, is the way in which an individual expresses themselves on the outside. Gender expression includes the individual's chosen hairstyle, clothing, accessories, mannerisms, preferences, and outward appearance. An example would be a child assigned female at birth, who says they are a girl, but presents in a more typically masculine fashion; people often refer to a girl who has a masculine gender expression as a "tomboy." While a child's gender expression may be indicative of their gender and/or their sexuality, one's gender identity and gender expression are not always the same. What is important to convey is gender expression does not define a child. Children go through several stages of development and evolve over time. It is also important to note that gender identity does not always remain fixed, even in adulthood.

The language of gender in the U.S. is vast, complicated, and continually developing. Entire books are written on this subject matter and this chapter only includes a small portion of what is needed to best serve this vulnerable population. To receive a better understanding of gender identity and gender expression it is recommended that child life specialists continue to educate themselves through current articles, books, conferences, specialized training, and independent studies. *The Transgender Child: A Handbook for Families and Professionals* (Brill & Pepper, 2008) is an excellent place to begin. Additional resources and readings can be found at the end of this chapter.

SAFETY

When working with this population several factors must be considered to ensure the safety of the child life specialist and the clients. Due to violence and hate crimes directed towards transgender individuals and communities, it is critical to determine what to share with the general public. If working in a private practice, having a P.O. box protects the exact location of the office. The practice's website and marketing materials may include the P.O. box, but the practice's actual location might remain concealed, only to be shared with prescreened clients.

CLINICAL SUPERVISION

One final variable to be considered when starting a private practice is clinical supervision. It may be challenging to find a certified child life specialist with expertise in gender-related topics. The ACLP has stated, in the Standards and Guidelines for Child Life Practice in Community Based & Non-Traditional Settings, that a child life specialist has the professional responsibility to seek supervision to enhance professional development, enhance reflective skills, and ensure that ethical standards are maintained. The ACLP suggests that this supervision meeting should be, at minimum, 60 minutes on a monthly or bi-monthly schedule (ACLP, 2020). In the event one is unable to find supervision with a CCLS possessing such a specific skill set, it may be best to seek supervision with an alternative professional who has expertise in working with transgender/gender expansive children and families.

BUILDING CLINICAL RELATIONSHIPS

Assessment

When a family first contacts the child life specialist it is likely through the website, email, or a referral. The child life specialist then contacts the potential client/family to assess their specific needs. An initial phone screening enables the child life specialist to gather information, like the child's age, stressors, the family's overall needs, and to explain the role of the child life specialist. This preliminary call will determine if services are appropriate. It is critical that the child life specialist explains their role and how it differs from other types of therapeutic and mental health support. If the child life specialist deems a family's needs fall outside the scope of child life, the child life specialist should provide a referral and appropriate resources. However, if services are found suitable, an intake can be scheduled. The intake can take place in person, over the phone, or virtually, provided there is a method for parents to sign legal documents giving consent for services. At the time of intake, the child life specialist would explain to the parents, once again, the scope of practice and the services provided by a child life specialist. Additionally, the child life specialist may share more information about their education, background, and what qualifies them to provide this type of support to families. The child life specialist should also discuss fees for the types of support available (for example, parent consultations, individual child sessions, sibling sessions, and group support). The client would then provide additional information, supplementing the child life assessment of needs and potential therapeutic services. Below is a list of questions to consider during intake:

- Why is the family seeking services?
- How well versed are the parents in the language and concepts of gender identity?
- Are there any signs of stress in the child connected to their understanding of traditional gender norms and their own developing gender identity?

- Are there any signs of gender dysphoria and if so, what are they?
- How are the parents coping with the exploration of gender identity?
- How does the child typically deal with challenges and stressors?
- What conversations have taken place between the child and parents regarding gender?
- What other needs and major stressors is the family experiencing as their child explores, transitions, and changes their gender identity or gender expression?
- What are the child's strengths?
- Does the child have any special needs or accommodations?
- What kind of support system does the family and child have? How supportive are friends, family, and the school community?

Depending on the answers given by parents during the intake, the next step is to create a plan for support. The child life specialist may use the following questions to internally process and make recommendations:

- Do the parents need guidance and education?
- Does the child need a safe space to explore their gender identity with the child life specialist?
- Does the child need to enhance or develop coping skills?
- Does the child need to create a plan to share their gender identity with friends and classmates?
- Do siblings need support in dealing with the changes in their family?

The child life specialist should collaborate with the parents to determine what services would be most beneficial. Services can include parent consultations, individual child sessions, family sessions, group support for the transgender/gender expansive child, peer support for parents, sibling support, or a combination of these modalities.

Plans and Interventions

After assessing the needs of each patient and family, the CCLS will share with the parents on what services might be appropriate. Services might include:

- Providing emotional support for the child
- Engaging the child in therapeutic play and expressive opportunities
- Facilitating interventions to help the child cope and adjust to certain social settings
- Providing developmentally appropriate explanations

Some common areas of support for parent guidance and consultation include:

- Providing general information on healthy development, gender identity, gender expression, and gender dysphoria
- Helping parents identify signs of stress in their child and tools to support coping
- Educating parents on how to speak to children about gender identity using developmentally appropriate language
- Helping parents prepare for transitions (e.g., medical, social)

- Advocating for the parents to follow their child's lead (e.g., preferred pronouns, clothing, name changes)
- Preparing parents for conversations with family, community, and peers
- Empowering parents to advocate for their child's needs within all settings (e.g., school, extracurricular, medical)
- Helping parents acquire information about gender rights and legislation
- Providing emotional support to parents
- Providing comprehensive resources (book, blogs, podcasts, conferences, websites, etc.) and referrals (e.g., organizations, support groups, other professionals)

All information should be discussed with the parents prior to working with the child. Given that these topics may be sensitive, this will ensure that parents and the child life specialist are on the same page in terms of how and when to share specific information with the child. Once this is determined, the CCLS might begin by providing developmentally appropriate definitions of gender identity and gender-related vocabulary and topics. The child life specialist might also choose to incorporate bibliotherapy using children's books about gender identity (see references). Equally important, the CCLS must discuss issues of privacy and disclosure to preserve the child's autonomy. Emphasis should be placed on how gender identity is personal; it should be the child's choice when, how, and with whom information is shared. Depending on the private practice location, the political climate of the area, as well as the social culture, the CCLS might further explore how to share the child's gender identity safely. Ultimately, it is the child life specialist's professional responsibility to identify effective communication skills to support a child and family, identify values related to sociocultural diversity, and provide a safe, therapeutic, healing environment (ACLP, 2019).

Specific Preparation

If the child is approaching puberty the child life specialist can provide developmentally appropriate explanations for biological or medical information received from a medical professional. The CCLS would assess understanding, provide developmentally appropriate descriptions, and clarify misconceptions.

In addition to medical preparations, the CCLS can prepare the child for other social situations that transgender children face. The CCLS can educate children about different aspects of social transitions and help children think through potentially difficult conversations related to their gender identity. Role-playing can be used to practice having conversations about why they are changing their appearance, name, or pronouns. Through role-play, children and adolescents can also gain mastery over how to respond to situations of harassment, bullying, or inquisitive peers who are curious about the changes that they are witnessing in their friend.

Expressive Art Activities

Child life specialists can also use expressive arts to support transgender/gender expansive clients. Expressive art activities can help this population express their feelings about their identity and strengthen resilience. The private practice should be well stocked with art supplies, including a variety of mediums to explore different themes. Some common prompts may include:

- Your family, friends, and support systems
- The best, worst, scariest, exciting, challenging part(s) of your world
- How your life would be different if your gender was different
- Your favorite things
- What you want to be and do when you grow up
- What you see when you look in the mirror

The activities should be open-ended. If the child does not complete the work, they can always bring it home, or if the private practice has storage space the artwork can be kept for the next session.

Another expressive art activity is creating affirmation bracelets. The child life specialist can provide a variety of charms or beads for the child to select, reflecting positive characteristics such as creativity, kindness, strength, and intelligence. An alternative would be to create an affirmation bracelet out of craft supply slap bracelets. These blank slap bracelets can be purchased from craft websites. Using a permanent marker, the child writes positive affirmations on the slap bracelet. For more ideas on expressive art, activities refer to the additional reading section at the end of this chapter.

Coping Tools

Another role of the child life specialist is to teach coping skills to deal with stressful situations. Children who are transgender/ gender expansive will potentially experience a great deal of stress. Common triggers for elevated stress include: the time of their transitions (social and/or medical), gender dysphoria, puberty, and unsupportive school environments. The child life specialist can help by providing a developmentally appropriate description of stress and help children identify what that stress feels like in their own bodies. The child life specialist can then help the child identify specific coping strategies. Strategies might include deep breathing, guided meditation, music, and physical exercise. The child life specialist should encourage the child to practice these coping strategies during individual sessions, group sessions, at home, and in other settings, like school.

Feelings activities often used in the hospital or at camps may also be modified to serve clients in terms of coping, and another great tool is the concept of "bucket filling." The child life specialist could begin by reading "Have You Filled a Bucket Today?" and then engage the child or the group in the activity. The activity requires providing the child or children with a small craft bucket, paints, paper, and markers, and then suggesting to fill the bucket with compliments to a specific person (most likely the client). It might be beneficial to have parents and the child life specialist write compliments on small pieces of paper to help fill the child's bucket too!

Finally, it may be worth considering items that have magical or wish-fulfilling themes such as a magic lamp, a wishing well, a fairy godmother, and superhero toys to help the child express themselves, but at a minimum the practice should possess manipulatives, a punching bag, a doll house, fidgets, and other general items for stress relief.

Therapeutic Play Opportunities

As in any other setting, play is essential to the developing child. For a child life specialist working with children who are transgender there are several types of play that can be very useful. A private practice serving transgender/gender expansive youth should have a play area that contains gender-neutral furniture and toys. The overall environment should feel inclusive and welcoming. The play space should specifically offer dramatic play opportunities. Offering a variety of costumes and accessories will allow children to explore gender roles openly and safely. The child life specialist's role will be to follow the child's lead using the child-centered play techniques of tracking, reflecting, and encouragement. Using this technique returns control to the child and helps build self-esteem and confidence. The play area should also have dolls representing different gender identities, ethnicities, and abilities. If possible, finding male and female dolls with a variety of clothing and accessories will allow children to explore gender expression using the dolls. Paper dolls with a wide variety of clothes might also provide a chance to try out different outfits, and puppets allow a child to create explore characters that might cross traditional gender norms. The child may be more comfortable expressing themselves through the dolls or the puppets. Essentially, the child is able to explore their gender through play before openly transitioning.

The child life specialist should also have medical play materials available. Medical play can be implemented in preparation for hormone blockers, which pubescent children will receive through monthly injections or a surgically placed implant. Older adolescents who have stopped the use of puberty blockers will begin to receive hormone treatment which is also administered through regular injections or a surgical implant. Teenagers approaching eighteen years old, may begin exploring gender-affirming surgeries as well.

Other materials that can be incorporated into play and therapeutic interventions would include card games, board games, and physical games. Just as child life specialists have become adept at modifying games to suit the therapeutic needs of a child in the healthcare setting, these games can be modified to provide therapeutic benefits to children exploring their gender identity. For example, a game of Uno can be modified with questions about gender identity, feelings, and coping skills. Candy Land can be modified to include questions about identity, self-esteem, self-confidence, and team building. Likewise, games that already have a therapeutic purpose such as Emotions Bingo or The Pronoun Game can also be purchased and incorporated into sessions. Ideally, the practice should have a wide variety of games that can be used with children of varying ages.

Lastly, there are also several excellent books about gender identity, gender expression, feelings, and coping skills that can be used to support play themes (see references).

Sessions and Groups

Individual sessions should be structured differently for children of different developmental levels. Play-based groups may begin with a check-in, an icebreaker, and then a therapeutic activity. Therapeutic activities may include art, bibliotherapy, games, and role-play followed by child-led play. Children in the groups may be the only child in their class (and perhaps the only child in their school) that identifies as transgender/gender expansive. The opportunities to create bonds with children that have similar experiences is valuable.

Simultaneously, parents may meet for a peer-led support group. Parents will have an opportunity to bond over shared experiences, offer support to one another, share resources, and celebrate each other's successes. In addition, family social events that includes parents, the transgender/gender-expansive child, and their siblings can be useful to encourage community-building through shared experiences.

Evaluation

It is the professional responsibility of the CCLS to continuously evaluate the effectiveness of services rendered. There are many ways to document interventions, it is up to the person running the private practice on how they would like to document their visits. The CCLS should review evaluations during clinical supervision.

ADVOCACY AND BEYOND: THE FUTURE OF SUPPORTING TRANSGENDER/GENDER CHILDREN AND FAMILIES

With increased awareness, more parents are seeking support and ways to embrace their children's gender identities. There is a significant need to increase psychosocial, developmentally appropriate services for this population and CCLS are well-suited for the role. This chapter has demonstrated exactly how to establish a private practice serving transgender/gender expansive children and families. However, other platforms exist. Child life advocacy and support for transgender youth can be applied in other areas. A child life specialist could could work on developing non-profits dedicated to serving transgender/gender-expansive children and families or perhaps look into filling school-based roles focused on supporting transgender/gender expansive youth. CCLS can also share knowledge and expertise about working with this population at conferences, in webinars, articles, books, and on social media. There are numerous ways to support the development, health, and well-being of transgender/gender expansive youth.

CONCLUSION

In the Child Life Code of Ethics and in the ACLP's recent commitment to diversity, equity, and inclusion, the ACLP has been clear that child life specialists must serve *all* children (ACLP, 2020); this includes children who are transgender/gender expansive. Child life specialists, dedicated experts in development, family-centered care, and cultural competency, coupled with comprehensive knowledge of gender and sexual orientation, are well equipped to create safe spaces promoting awareness, resilience, and connection (ARC FAMILY, 2020).

REFERENCES

ACLP. (2019, November). *Child life competencies*. ACLP Official Documents. Retrieved April 11, 2022, from https://www.childlife.org/docs/default-source/aclp-official-documents/child-life-competencies_november-2019-updates.pdf?sfvrsn=d33e8c4d_2

ACLP. (2020, January). *Child life code of ethics*. ACLP Official Documents. Retrieved April 11, 2022, from https://www.childlife.org/docs/default-source/certification/child-life-code-of-ethics.pdf?sfvrsn=2

ACLP. (2020, November). *Community based standards and guidelines*. ACLP Official Documents. Retrieved April 11, 2022, from https://www.childlife.org/docs/default-source/aclp-official-documents/community-based-standards-and-guidelines_final-approved.pdf?sfvrsn=c7d1864d_2

American Psychiatric Association. (2017). Diagnostic and statistical manual of mental disorders: Dsm-5 (5th ed.). APA.

ARC Family. (2020). *Child Life & ARC*. Retrieved August 4, 2022 from https://www.arcfamily.org/child-life-arc

Brill, S. A., Pepper, R., & Puttonen, M. (2011). *The transgender child: a handbook for families and professionals*. Post Hypnotic Press.

Couturier, J., Pindiprolu, B., Findlay, S., & Johnson, N. (2015). Anorexia nervosa and gender dysphoria in two adolescents. *International Journal of Eating Disorders*, *48*(1), 151–155. doi:10.1002/eat.22368 PMID:25421316

Guss, C. E., Williams, D. N., Reisner, S. L., Austin, S. B., & Katz-Wise, S. L. (2016). Disordered weight management behaviors and non-prescription steroid use in massachusetts transgender youth. *The Journal of Adolescent Health*, *58*(2), S102–S103. Advance online publication. doi:10.1016/j.jadohealth.2015.10.217

James, S. E., Herman, J. L., Rankin, S., Keisling, M., Mottet, L., & Anafi, M. (2016, December). *The report of the 2015 us transgender survey*. The National Center for Transgender Equality. Retrieved April 10, 2022, from https://transequality.org/sites/default/files/docs/usts/USTS-Full-Report-Dec17.pdf

Rafferty, J. (2022, May 11). Gender Identity Development in Children. *Healthy Children*. Retrieved from https://www.healthychildren.org/English/ages-stages/gradeschool/Pages/Gender-Identity-and-Gender-Confusion-In-Children.aspx

Rafferty, J., Yogman, M., Baum, R., Gambon, T. B., Lavin, A., Mattson, G., Wissow, L. S., Breuner, C., Alderman, E. M., Grubb, L. K., Powers, M. E., Upadhya, K., Wallace, S. B., Hunt, L., Gearhart, A. T., Harris, C., Lowe, K. M., Rodgers, C. T., & Sherer, I. M. (2018). Ensuring comprehensive care and support for transgender and gender-diverse children and adolescents. *Pediatrics*, *142*(4), e20182162. doi:10.1542/peds.2018-2162 PMID:30224363

Rosen, D. (2022). *GLSEN. Gender-neutral Bathrooms Are Radical, but Not How You Think*. Retrieved from https://www.glsen.org/blog/gender-neutral-bathrooms-are-radical-not-how-you-think

Russell, S. T., Pollitt, A. M., Li, G., & Grossman, A. H. (2018). Chosen name use is linked to reduced depressive symptoms, suicidal ideation, and suicidal behavior among transgender youth. *The Journal of Adolescent Health*, *63*(4), 503–505. doi:10.1016/j.jadohealth.2018.02.003 PMID:29609917

Simon, B. (2022, March 1). *Medical association statements supporting trans youth healthcare and against discriminatory bills*. GLAAD. Retrieved April 11, 2022, from https://www.glaad.org/blog/medical-association-statements-supporting-trans-youth-healthcare-and-against-discriminatory

The Gender Unicorn. (2021, February 7). Trans Student Educational Resources. Retrieved April 10, 2022, from https://transstudent.org/gender/

The Trevor Project National Survey. (2021). The Trevor Project. Retrieved April 10, 2022, from https://www.thetrevorproject.org/survey-2021/

Vance, S. R. Jr, & Rosenthal, S. M. (2018). A closer look at the psychosocial realities of LGBTQ youth. *Pediatrics*, *141*(5), e20180361. doi:10.1542/peds.2018-0361 PMID:29661942

ADDITIONAL READING

Baldacchino, C., & Malenfant, I. (2014). *Morris micklewhite and the tangerine dress*. Groundwood Books.

Brill, S. A., & Kenney, L. (2016). *The transgender teen: a handbook for parents and professionals supporting transgender and non-binary teens*. Cleis Press.

Brill, S. A., Pepper, R., & Puttonen, M. (2011). *The transgender child: a handbook for families and professionals*. Post Hypnotic Press.

Duron, L. (2013). *Raising my rainbow: Adventures in raising a fabulous, gender creative son*. Broadway Books.

Ehrensaft, D., & Menvielle, E. (2011). *Gender born, gender made: raising healthy gender-nonconforming children*. The Experiment.

Ehrensaft, D., & Spack, N. (2017). *The gender creative child: pathways for nurturing and supporting children who live outside gender boxes*. Simon & Schuster Australia.

Gonzalez, M. (2017). *Gender wheel: A story about bodies and gender for everybody*. Reflection Press.

Hall, M. (2018). *Red: A crayon's story*. Library Ideas, LLC.

Herthel, J., Jennings, J., & McNicholas, S. (2014). *I am jazz!* Dial Books for Young Readers, an imprint of Penguin Group (USA) LLC.

Human Rights Campaign. (2022). Retrieved August 4, 2022, from https://www.hrc.org/resources/get-the-facts-about-transgender-non-binary-athletes

Jennings, J. (2017). *Being jazz: My life as a (transgender) teen*. Ember.

Kilodavis, C., & DeSimone, S. (2012). *My princess boy*. CNIB.

Newman, L., & Mola, M. (2017). *Sparkle boy*. Lee & Low Books Inc.

Pessin-Whedbee, B., & Bardoff, N. (2017). *Who are you? The kid's guide to gender identity*. Jessica Kingsley Publishers.

PFLAG. (2022, April 3). Retrieved April 11, 2022, from https://pflag.org/

Prismic. (2019). *Gender spectrum website*. Gender Spectrum. Retrieved April 11, 2022, from https://www.genderspectrum.org/

Storck, K. (2018). *Gender identity workbook for kids: a guide to exploring who you are*. New Harbinger Publications.

Thorn, T., & Grigni, N. (2019). *It feels good to be yourself: A book about gender identity*. Henry Holt and Company.

Transgender Law Center. (2022). Retrieved August 4, 2022, from https://www.transgenderlawcenter.org

TransYouth Family Allies. (2017). Retrieved April 11, 2022, from http://www.imatyfa.org/

Welcoming Schools. (2022). Retrieved August 4, 2022, from www.welcomingschools.org

KEY TERMS AND DEFINITIONS

Assigned Sex at Birth: The sex (male or female) assigned to a child at birth, based on the child's external anatomy. Also referred to as birth sex, natal sex, biological sex, or sex.

Cisgender: An adjective that describes people whose gender identity matches their assigned sex at birth.

Gender: Complex relationship between physical traits and one's internal sense of self as male, female, both, or neither (gender identity), as well as one's outward presentation and behaviors (gender expression).

Gender Creative: Another term for gender expansive, gender non-conforming, or nonbinary.

Gender Dysphoria: Distress experienced when a person's assigned sex at birth does not align with their gender identity. Gender dysphoria can range from mild discomfort to unbearable distress. The intensity, frequency, and triggers of gender dysphoria can vary widely from person to person and change over time as one transitions socially, medically, and legally.

Gender Expansive: Refers to a person with a wider, more flexible range of gender identity and/or expression than typically associated with the binary gender system. Often used as an umbrella term when referring to young people still exploring the possibilities of their gender expression and/or gender identity.

Gender Expression: Refers to the external appearance of one's gender identity, usually expressed through behavior, mannerisms, clothing, hairstyles, and voice. A person's gender expression may or may not conform to socially defined behaviors and characteristics typically associated with being either masculine or feminine.

Gender Fluid: Refers to a person who does not identify with a single fixed gender or has a fluid or unfixed gender identity. People that are gender fluid may move between genders depending on the setting, the day, or who they are with. They experience gender as something that is dynamic and changing rather than static.

Gender Identity: Our deeply held, internal sense of self as masculine, feminine, a blend of both, neither, or something else. One's gender identity can be the same or different from their assigned sex at birth.

Gender Nonconforming: A broad term referring to people who do not conform to the traditional expectations of their gender, or whose gender expression does not fit neatly into a category. While many also identify as transgender, not all gender non-conforming people do. The term Gender Expansive and Gender Creative can also be used in place of Gender Nonconforming.

Intersex: One of the three categories that someone can be assigned at birth (male, female, or intersex). People may be assigned intersex at birth due to a variety of differences in their sex traits and reproductive anatomy. There is a wide variety of difference among intersex variations, including differences in genitalia, chromosomes, gonads, internal sex organs, hormone production, hormone response, and/or secondary sex traits. Intersex has more to do with biology than it does with gender, therefore many (and some would say most) people who are intersex do not identify as transgender.

Nonbinary: An adjective that describes a person who does not identify exclusively as a man or a woman. Non-binary people may identify as being both a man and a woman, somewhere in between, or as falling completely outside these categories. While many also identify as transgender, not all non-binary people do. Non-binary can also be used as an umbrella term encompassing identities such as agender, bigender, genderqueer or gender-fluid, gender nonconforming, or gender-expansive.

Transition: A series of processes that some transgender people may undergo to live more fully as their true gender. This typically includes social transition, such as changing name and pronouns, medical transition, which may include hormone therapy or gender-affirming surgeries, and legal transition, which may include changing the legal name and gender marker on government identity documents. Transgender people may choose to undergo some, all, or none of these processes.

- **Legal Gender Transition:** Legal steps that can be taken by a transgender person to live more fully as their true gender identity. This may include a legal name change or legal change of their gender marker on the birth certificate, passport, driver's license, and other government identification.
- **Medical Gender Transition:** Medical steps that can be taken by a transgender person to live more fully as their true gender identity. These steps might include the use of puberty blockers, hormone therapy, and/or gender-affirming therapies.
- **Social Gender Transition:** Social steps that can be taken by transgender people to live more fully as their true gender identity. These steps might include changes in their physical appearance, clothing, name, and/or pronouns.

Sex: In the United States, individuals are assigned "female" or "male" sex at birth, based on physical attributes and characteristics. This assumed physical dichotomy of sex is itself belied by a variety of naturally occurring conditions.

Sexual Orientation: Describes an individual's enduring physical, emotional, romantic, and/or spiritual attraction to another person. Gender identity and sexual orientation are not the same.

Transgender: An adjective describing people whose gender identity does not align with their assigned sex at birth. It can be used as an umbrella term for people whose gender identity and/or expression is different from cultural expectations based on the sex they were assigned at birth. Being transgender does not imply any specific sexual orientation. Transgender individuals also can be described as gender creative, gender expansive, or gender non-conforming.

Chapter 15
Adoption

Catherine J. Howe
Southern Adoption Agency, USA

Laura F. Weber
Missouri State University, USA

ABSTRACT

A Certified Child Life Specialist (CCLS) has the knowledge, skills, and clinical training that is essential to work in the field of infant adoption. Child Life Specialists working as infant adoption specialists promote emotional support, education, and coping for the biological parent(s) and families who want to adopt a child. Using the competencies to ground the work, Child Life Specialists focus on the therapeutic relationship, attachment, and bonding while also understanding grief and loss experienced by the biological parent(s). This chapter also examines how socioeconomics, varying cultures, ethnicities, and trauma histories can affect the adoption process.

INTRODUCTION

Adoption is extremely prevalent within the United States and across the globe. In 2019, 25,000 private domestic adoptions and 66,087 adoptions through foster care were reported in the United States alone (Koh et al., 2020). While the numbers are impressive, each adoption is unique and impacts the biological parent(s), adoptive families, and children directly involved and the individuals supporting them. In order to meet the needs of those involved, adoption takes many forms, including domestic private adoption, international adoption, foster care to adoption, embryo adoption, surrogacy, and family adoption. Within each context are social, emotional, and legal aspects that affect the children, the biological, adoptive, and foster families, and the public and private entities involved in the adoption process. This chapter will solely focus on private domestic infant adoption.

There are myriad reasons families choose to pursue infant adoption. Some choose adoption due to infertility, loss, or medical reasons that make it impossible to carry a child to term. Others may choose adoption as an alternative way to grow a family (Fallon & Goldsmith, 2013). Regardless of why families choose infant adoption, adoption agencies have an obligation to complete thorough evaluations that assess

DOI: 10.4018/978-1-6684-5097-0.ch015

the fit, needs, and emotional responses of those seeking to adopt an infant. When a biological parent(s) decides to select adoptive parents to care for their infant, a unique connection is formed, often referred to as an adoption triad. An adoption triad consists of the biological parent(s), adoptive parent(s), and child (Foli et al., 2013). Each adoption triad member presents with individual physical and emotional needs that must be addressed through guidance, social and emotional support, and therapeutic intervention as they enter and continue their adoption journeys (Foli, 2012). Although this chapter focuses on private domestic infant adoption, there may be similarities to other types of adoption.

The purpose of an infant adoption specialist is to educate, support, advocate, and provide ongoing care to biological parents, adoptive parents, and children. This chapter will demonstrate how Certified Child Life Specialists (CCLSs), in the role of an infant adoption specialist, use their competencies to provide family-centered care and support to the entire adoption triad during the adoption process (Association of Child Life Professionals, 2020b). The needs of the infant, biological parents, and adoptive parents and the supportive child life interventions will be addressed in each phase of the adoption process.

PRE-ADOPTION

Biological Parents

Biological parent(s) may reach out to adoption agencies when unexpectedly pregnant and unsure of their next step. A large majority of biological mothers in contact with adoption agencies are subject to challenging circumstances such as childhood trauma, socio-economic hardships, abusive relationships, or addictions (Clutter, 2017). Representing multiple demographics, biological mothers may be as young as 11 up to the age of 45, of diverse cultural backgrounds, single, married, in a same-sex relationship, incarcerated, homeless, employed, unemployed, and may possess varying levels of education. Biological mothers may also have varying levels of support from the biological father, family, and friends. Along with other factors, the level of support the biological mother receives may contribute to her adoption decision. Some biological mothers may feel that adoptive parents will provide a more stable home and a better life for their child compared to what they could provide at the time (Clutter, 2014). No matter the rationale, their decision should be respected and supported fully.

"CCLSs have a duty to maintain objectivity, integrity, and competence while exhibiting compassion," which allows them to create a comfortable and non-judgmental environment in which the biological parent(s)' adoption decision is respected and upheld (ACLP, 2020a, p. 1). The Child Life Code of Ethics outlines additional principles which guide a CCLS's work regardless of their job title (ACLP, 2020a, p. 1). A CCLS's comprehensive assessment skills would suit them for the role of infant adoption specialist. Maintaining promises and adhering to professional boundaries is another characteristic of CCLSs that applies to the role of infant adoption specialist. Biological parent(s) may have a history of relationships full of broken promises. It is imperative that clients feel safe and know that every conversation will be kept confidential, a reassurance that may first require trust between the biological parent(s) and the infant adoption specialist.

After contacting an adoption agency and establishing trust, the biological parent(s) meet with an infant adoption specialist to discuss potential options regarding their pregnancy. One essential goal of child life practice in community settings is to "assess coping responses and psychosocial needs of children, families and their support systems" (ACLP, 2018, p. 2). Infant adoption specialists use their initial meeting with the biological parent(s) to build rapport, develop trust and complete a comprehensive assessment. This assessment includes a mother's age, health, socioeconomic status, racial background, past trauma, available resources, birth fathers' engagement, and family/peer support. Food, clothing, and shelter are provided to biological parent(s) if needed. Available resources vary by state, dependent on governmental support and legislation. Following an initial meeting and assessment, the infant adoption specialist develops a plan of care and provides support based on the biological parent(s) individual needs and decisions to continue with the adoption process. An essential role of the infant adoption specialist is to support the biological mother in disclosing decisions to her extended family and the identified biological father. Careful consideration must be taken if the biological mother is in an abusive or potentially dangerous relationship with the biological father.

Encouraging participation in healthy habits and prenatal care during pregnancy is an additional role of the infant adoption specialist. Developing healthy habits during pregnancy is vital as infants are particularly vulnerable to the adverse effects of stress, malnutrition, and harmful substances such as alcohol and illegal drugs in utero. Prenatal care support may involve assisting biological mothers in finding an obstetrician (OB), providing transportation to appointments, preparing for and emotional support during prenatal care treatments, and providing comfort when receiving concerning medical information. Discussing the level of involvement the biological parent(s) hopes to maintain with the infant and adoptive parents post-adoption is also an important aspect of support during this time period. This can promote a sense of control for biological parent(s) in a time when they may have no sense of control over the future.

Grief may take place at any stage during the adoption process, prior to (anticipatory grief) and even years beyond placement, therefore, infant adoption specialists continue to assess the biological parent(s) coping as they may experience and process grief. An infant adoption specialist's knowledge and training in the field of grief and loss assist the biological parent(s) in managing emotions and identifying effective coping mechanisms to process grief. Common coping mechanisms include journaling, writing a letter for their unborn baby to read in the future, or creating a photo book to document the pregnancy and adoption process. Biological parent(s) seeking adoption services often experience considerable stressors and intense emotions during pregnancy. Infant adoption specialists provide a nonjudgemental space for listening. Often taking place between other supportive responsibilities such as car rides to and from OB appointments, over lunch, or in doctor's office waiting rooms, infant adoption specialists validate the biological parents' feelings, concerns, and experiences. Regardless of if the biological parent(s) chooses to pursue an adoption plan, the infant adoption specialist still offers support to the biological mother through her birth journey and after the baby is born. Of utmost importance, still, is the infant adoption specialist's obligation to respect the biological parents' decision regarding their unborn baby. Only then may the infant adoption specialist determine resources that may benefit the biological parent(s), including referrals to baby basics and parenting classes.

Adoptive Parents

Families pursuing infant adoption need the guidance and support of an infant adoption specialist at each step of the process, much like the biological parent(s). During the pre-adoption process, an infant adoption specialist evaluates the adoptive parents' readiness and prepares them for the responsibilities of parenthood while providing emotional support. Once adoptive parents' applications are approved, the adoption agency proceeds with a home assessment. This intensive step of the adoption process involves background checks, individual and joint interviews, a home safety inspection, and adoption education training which details the social, legal, and emotional aspects of adoption, the necessary cultural considerations when adopting an infant of a different racial or ethnic background, the impact of prenatal care on development through the lifespan and fostering a positive adoption triad relationship. If the home assessment concludes with approval, adoptive parents will determine their preferences in adopting an infant to assist the infant adoption specialist in providing appropriate adoptive parent profiles from which a biological mother may choose. When a match between biological parent(s) and adoptive parents is made, a meeting may occur to establish trust and discuss the terms of the adoption, including the frequency of pictures and updates being exchanged and the possibility of visitation between the infant and biological parent(s). In infant adoption, a biological mother voluntarily consents to the termination of her parental rights before a judge or by signing a written consent. Putative fathers, meaning any possible biological fathers, are given notice of the adoption plan and can choose to sign a consent or assert their parental rights. If the biological mother is married, then her husband is termed the legal father, even if he is not the biological father. It is important to note that adoption laws regarding voluntary or involuntary consent of biological and legal parents vary by each state. A child is not adoptable until the rights are terminated of all biological and legal parent(s). Once an adoptive family successfully completes their post-adoption supervisory period, their adoption will be finalized, and they are decreed to be legal parents of the infant.

Infant adoption specialists use their skills to support adoptive parents, beginning with a thorough explanation of the adoption process's social, emotional, legal, spiritual, and financial aspects. Providing appropriate expectations ensures adoptive parents make an informed decision to continue with the adoption process.

A CCLS's understanding of child development and family systems supports a thorough and careful home assessment (ACLP, 2020a, p. 1). Individual and joint interviews during the home assessment allow the CCLS to assess each adoptive parent's ability to care for an infant, not only at the time of placement but throughout the infant's life, to discern the coping responses and psychosocial needs of the adoptive parents and assess their support systems (ACLP, 2018).

Preparation is key to providing guidance and support to prospective adoptive parents during the pre-adoption process. Bergsund et al. (2018) suggest that adoptive parents must be prepared for adoption before a child is added to their home. Receiving information, acquiring parenting tools, listening to other adoptive families share their adoption stories, and gaining insight about children with special needs is helpful to adoptive parents during the pre-adoption process (Bergsund et al., 2018). CCLSs are prepared to provide expertise in areas regarding, but not limited to, "growth and development across the lifespan, family systems, grief and loss, and psychological preparation and preventative support for significant life experiences'' while integrating evidence-based research into conversations with adoptive parents (ACLP, 2018, p. 3). This enables infant adoption specialists to prepare adoptive parents for conversations with siblings surrounding the addition of an adopted infant to their family and possible sibling responses. Bergsund et al. (2018) also suggest discussions on attachment and child development as helpful preparation for adoptive parents in navigating new experiences as their adopted and biological children grow.

Further, infant adoption specialists facilitate discussions with adoptive parents to determine their adoption preferences, considerations include the race and mental health status of the biological mother and father and the infant's health and exposure to substances during pregnancy. These factors may impact the infant's development through the lifespan and the relationship between the infant and his or her adoptive family. Helping adoptive parents understand the magnitude, and potential reality of adopting an infant with a different racial background from themselves, developmental delay, or possible health concerns provides an opportunity for infant adoption specialists to deliver information in a way the adoptive parents can best understand while creating space for the intense emotions that information may evoke. Additionally, it is important for both parties to understand the permanent commitment they are making. Adoption is not a one-time event but an ongoing relationship with a child who will experience their own gains and losses (Foli et al., 2013).

It is likely that an infant adoption specialist will mediate initial and subsequent meetings between biological parent(s) and adoptive parents once a match has been made. The first encounter between the biological parent(s) and adoptive parents is the beginning of a journey in which trust is built. When siblings are involved, an infant adoption specialist may provide play opportunities, offer developmentally appropriate explanations to correct misconceptions, or create a safe space to express emotions regarding the adoption. CCLSs skilled in leading conversations that cultivate a safe and trusting environment provide an opportunity to assess siblings' understanding of the potential adoption. Following a home assessment, preparation for the adoption, and meeting with a biological parent(s), infant adoption specialists continue to provide support and guidance throughout the adoption process.

HOSPITAL EXPERIENCE

Infant delivery and care are important parts of the adoption process. With new life comes the responsibility to meet the infant's physical and emotional needs, a task easier said than done when the needs of the adoption triad must also be taken into account. If a newborn is unexpectedly admitted into the neonatal intensive care unit (NICU), additional support is needed as biological and adoptive parents may experience additional uncertainty, fear, anxiety, and loss of control that are layered on top of the mix of emotions already being felt regarding the adoption process (Craig, 2019). Overall, the hospital journey provides rewarding and sometimes bitter-sweet experiences for both biological parent(s) and adoptive parents. Biological parent(s) are often preparing to say goodbye to their newborn infant. In contrast, adoptive parents must balance their joy and excitement with respect for the biological parent(s)' grieving process. An infant adoption specialist provides ongoing support for the adoption triad through what often feels like a "roller coaster of emotions" and acts as a liaison between the adoption triad and the medical staff.

Biological Parents

Choices regarding hospital location, medical decisions, and level of adoptive parent involvement at the time of birth are decided by the biological mother. An infant adoption specialist's presence may be valuable in providing support during labor, delivery, and postpartum care. After the birth, the biological parent(s) are encouraged to spend as much time with their infant as desired to promote a secure attachment between the biological parent(s) and infant while transitioning into the care of the selected adoptive parents.

A CCLS's extensive training and experience in healthcare settings make them uniquely suited to provide support throughout delivery and postpartum care. Certified Child Life Specialists understand the need for psychological preparation for potentially traumatic events to reduce stress and increase coping while also responding to misconceptions about treatment, pain, and care. Certified Child Life Specialists provide honest and accurate information regarding the biological mother's hospital experience, including sensory information. A CCLS's ability to describe and practice coping methods with a biological mother is another characteristic that demonstrates their fit for the position of an infant adoption specialist.

Further, Certified Child Life Specialists have experience remaining calm and focused during procedures and unlikely medical circumstances that could occur, such as an emergency Cesarean section. Their experience in healthcare settings allows CCLSs to interact with healthcare staff efficiently and effectively while constantly advocating for the biological mother's best interest. A Child Life Specialist's training in grief may facilitate conversations and encourage emotional expression regarding the biological parents' impending loss. A CCLS practicing trauma-informed care understands the importance of considering previous loss, abuse, or trauma when navigating interactions with the biological mother. Finally, their experience in healthcare settings and knowledge of child development may make CCLSs uniquely suited to support the biological parent(s) in the event their infant is admitted to the NICU, where strict infection control guidelines and intimidating medical equipment are commonplace.

Adoptive Parents

While the adoptive parents' presence and level of involvement during the hospital experience is ultimately decided by the biological mother, an infant adoption specialist may be required to mediate interactions between the biological parent(s) and the adoptive parents. Involving and collaborating with hospital staff may ensure these interactions are productive and positive and the needs of both parties are met. If an infant the parents are hoping to adopt is admitted into the NICU, an infant adoption specialist can prepare the parents for what they may feel, see, and hear, so they will know what to expect as they visit the newborn in the unfamiliar environment.

CCLSs are trained to "understand the unique perspectives of children and families and their support systems and have the ability to advocate their needs to others" (ACLP, 2018, p. 1). This allows the CCLS to mediate interactions effectively and respectfully among the biological parent(s), adoptive parents, and their support systems. As mentioned previously, a CCLS's experience in healthcare settings may improve collaboration with hospital staff in meeting the needs of all parties involved. A CCLS's ability to navigate stressful events and subsequent emotions provides direction to adoptive parents looking for guidance when interacting with and supporting the biological parent(s). "CCLSs establish relationships with children and their families that address their vulnerability and foster positive coping" (ACLP, 2018, p. 1). CCLSs may share coping methods with adoptive parents to reduce stress as they wrestle with the possibility of the biological parent(s) changing her mind and choosing to parent her infant (Fallon & Goldsmith, 2013).

POST-ADOPTION

Biological Parents

As stated previously, in infant adoption, a baby becomes available for adoption when the infant's biological mother has voluntarily terminated her parental rights, and all biological father(s) rights have been terminated during the legal process. Following this, the adoptive parents assume permanent, legal guardianship of the infant after their successful completion of the post-placement supervisory period. During the post-adoption period, infant adoption specialists support the biological parent(s) through possible court hearings, bereavement, and resources to promote a healthy and productive life following adoption placement.

Biological mothers may experience tremendous grief on the day of their court hearing to relinquish parental rights (Clutter, 2017). In the weeks and months following the adoption, biological mothers may experience intense bouts of grief and seek intervention and support. Clutter (2014) explains that biological mothers may fixate on projects or alternative facets of life as a coping mechanism. During the first year, mothers' grief experiences might include depression and guilt, along with anxiety, sleep difficulties, and lowered self-worth (Brodzinsky & Smith, 2014). Biological mothers may keep their adoption decision from family and friends if she assumes their disapproval or lack of support, adding a supplementary dimension to their grief (Clutter, 2014). A CCLS is trained to provide opportunities that enhance coping, mastery, self-expression, and resilience (ACLP, 2018, p. 1). CCLSs possess the knowledge and skills to support grieving individuals regardless of their loss. Integrating their background in trauma-informed care allows CCLSs to consider previous losses the biological mother has experienced to provide individualized support. Memorialization and legacy building represent two interventions commonly implemented in traditional child life settings that infant adoption specialists may use to support bereaved biological parent(s). For instance, infant adoption specialists may engage biological parent(s) in creating a scrapbook documenting the day of the infant's birth or establishing a tradition to mark the infant's birthday to help with legacy building. The counseling and support infant adoption specialists provide to biological parent(s) extends far beyond adoption placement. In fact, Clutter (2014) suggests support should be available to biological mothers for a lifetime as adoption is not a singular event, and biological mothers grieve differently. Biological mothers often find solace and healing given time and appropriate support (Brodzinsky & Smith, 2014; Clutter, 2014).

Following the adoption placement, infant adoption specialists may use their assessment skills to understand the needs and goals of the biological mother as she moves forward. Resources typically provided to biological mothers include education opportunities, employment options, support in forming healthy relationships, drug, and alcohol treatment, and opportunities to share their adoption experience with others (Clutter, 2017). A biological mother may feel her adoption experience provided an opportunity for maturity and personal growth and may wish to continue that journey (Clutter, 2014).

Adoptive Parents

Adoptive parents commonly undergo a post-placement supervisory period to evaluate the infant's development, safety in the home, recent healthcare experiences, the adoptive family's coping, attachment with the infant, and level of engagement. Including and acknowledging sibling responses to the infant's placement and adjustment is vital in producing a comprehensive evaluation. The post-placement supervisory period involves interviews and questioning to understand both current circumstances and feelings regarding the placement of the infant in the adoptive parent's home and encourages behavior that will support secure attachment and positive development for all family members. Possible evaluative questions are listed below.

- How does each parent interact with the infant?
- Can the parent comfort and soothe the infant when crying?
- Does the parent appear attached to the infant?
- Does the infant maintain eye contact?
- Does the infant respond positively to each parent?
- Is the infant meeting developmental milestones?

During the post-adoption supervisory period, adoptive parents provide a monthly photograph and written report detailing the infant's health, parental coping, and parental joys and concerns. Documented developmental delays as a result of prenatal or hereditary factors may incite referrals to additional agencies to support the infant and adoptive family. Following a successful evaluation period, adoptive parents are permitted to finalize the adoption. Infant adoption specialists may attend court with the adoptive family for the finalization hearing to signify the support they have offered throughout their adoption journey. Adoptive parents will receive an amended birth certificate with the infant's given name and the adoptive parents listed as legal parents.

The Certified Child Life Specialist's comprehensive assessment skills accurately depict the infant's safety in his/her new home and the adoptive family's adjustment to the infant's placement during the post-placement supervisory evaluation. CCLSs' vast understanding of attachment theory allows them to determine each adoptive parent's level of attachment with the infant and encourage behaviors that will further promote secure attachment, such as skin-to-skin contact. As stated previously, a CCLS's knowledge and training in grief and loss may even be valuable to adoptive families during the post-adoption process. Adoptive parents may experience feelings of grief and loss in the post-adoption process if they are unable to make an immediate connection with the infant following placement. Holding an adopted infant may bring previous losses to light if adoptive parents never had the chance to hold their expectant infant. Adoptive parents may also experience grief as their newly placed infant grows and ask questions regarding their adoption story or biological family. A finalized adoption does not mark the end of challenging experiences and emotions children and families will endure. However, a CCLS's dedication to cultivating resilience provides adoptive families with the knowledge and tools they need to create a healthier and more fulfilling life.

Fostering Secure Attachment

Infants, unable to care for themselves, are dependent on caregivers to provide for their needs (Thompson, 2018). The continuous process of responding to infant needs begins at birth and lasts throughout a child's life (Hoffenkamp et al., 2012). According to Erikson's theory of Psychosocial Development, infants are in the stage of Trust vs. Mistrust. Their needs must be met on a consistent basis enabling them to trust the world. Continued unmet needs create general feelings of mistrust (Thomas, 2005, p. 91). Accurately responding to needs provides the basis for a newborn to feel safe and secure. Infants inherently attach to another human being, and it is an important process (Young, 2013). As described by Bowlby and Ainsworth, attachment theory indicates that attachment is a continuous process that impacts future relationships throughout a child's life (Young, 2013). The cycle of healthy attachment begins the moment an infant is born. When an infant expresses a need by crying, the caregiver, if present, responds by meeting this need. If met appropriately, the infant feels relief and soon learns that calling their caregiver results in being cared for. If this cycle persists, a healthy attachment is supported, and trust is built between the infant and caregiver (Thompson, 2018). The attachment cycle occurs hundreds of times in the first weeks of life and continues still, stimulating the infant's brain with each caring interaction (Purvis et al., 2007). Attachment is vital for newborns and adoptive parents unable to bond during pregnancy. Adoptive parents should understand that attachment connection are gradually formed (Fallon & Goldsmith, 2013). Whether the meeting between biological parent(s) and adoptive parents takes place within hours or months of the infant's birth, infant adoption specialists work to initiate and facilitate meaningful interactions between the newborn and adoptive parents to promote strong attachment. Understanding how an attachment is formed is crucial to both the infant and the adoptive parents (Fallon & Goldsmith, 2013). As adoptive parents respond to the needs of the infant, the infant gains trust. Although this cycle begins at birth, an infant may be affected by feelings their biological mother experiences during pregnancy.

A mother's choice for adoption should be respected and supported (Bergsund et al., 2018; Clutter, 2020). One way of advocating for the biological mother is supporting her choices immediately after the baby is born. After the infant is born, hospital staff give the biological mother the option to keep the newborn in her room, send the newborn to the nursery, or send the newborn directly to the adoptive parents if they are staying in another hospital room. Additional considerations include whether the biological mother will give the adoptive parents time alone with the newborn or time altogether as the biological mother continues to bond with the infant. While respecting the biological mother's wishes is important, early moments spent with adoptive parents provide the foundation for healthy attachment with the infant.

An infant will experience an immediate or gradual loss of connection with the biological mother depending on the level of engagement after delivery. Bonding between the infant and the biological mother is not only healthy but aids in the biological mother's coping prior to the release of the infant for adoption. As the biological mother spends time bonding with the baby during pregnancy, so has the baby bonded by hearing her voice and learning her scent. These sensations are familiar to the newborn, providing a feeling of safety and security (Fallon & Goldsmith, 2013). Therefore, adoptive parents need to begin bonding with the baby as soon as possible in order to mitigate a break in attachment. Although infants experience a loss of connection with their biological mother, the negative impact on attachment is lessened when adopted at a young age (Fallon & Goldsmith, 2013).

Since the infant has known the care, sound, and touch of the biological mother, it is paramount that adoptive parents recognize that infants placed in their care will experience loss and need time to adjust to the rhythms, voice, and touch of the adoptive parents (Halverson, 2018). An infant adoption specialist preparing both the biological parent(s) and adoptive parents promotes co-regulation as each learns the others' cues and comforting techniques (Halverson, 2018). In time, the infant will learn the adoptive parents' scent, voice, touch, and emotional connection. According to Fallon and Goldsmith (2013), infants are born with a natural ability to bond and acclimate, which is enhanced in healthy environments. Infant adoption specialists provide education to help the adoptive parents regard feedings, changing, and comforting the baby as opportunities to foster attachment between them. Not all adoptive parents will feel an immediate bond with their adopted infant; bonding between the two may be gradual (Swartz et al., 2012). An infant adoption specialist providing continued support to the adoptive parents may suggest holding, feeding, soft touch, talking in a calm voice, swaddling, and skin-to-skin contact as ways to promote bonding once home with the infant (Barker et al., 2017; Flacking et al., 2012). Infant adoption specialists are also available to listen to any fears or concerns the parents are experiencing regarding the baby or the relationship with the biological family.

ADOPTIVE PARENT AND BIOLOGICAL PARENT RELATIONS

It is possible that the biological parent(s) will be involved in ongoing visitation with the infant placed for adoption. The level of involvement adoptive parents wish to maintain with biological parent(s) post placement is made clear in adoptive parent profiles. This may play a part in whom biological parent(s) choose as their adoptive parents. Once chosen, the adoptive parents and biological parent(s) often sign an agreement regarding the frequency of pictures and updates that will be provided as well as possible visitation arrangements with the adoptive family and the child. This is often termed a semi-open or open adoption, meaning the biological parent(s) has varying degrees of communication and face-to-face contact with the adoptive family throughout the child's life. Some open adoptions evolve into a relationship similar to that of an extended family (Clutter, 2014). In fact, mothers who placed their infant for adoption experience improved psychological healing and joy when they were involved in an open adoption (Rezaei et al., 2019; Clutter, 2014). Biological fathers also may desire to be a part of the ongoing relationship with the adoptive family and the infant and reported positive emotional health when given the opportunity to be involved in an open adoption (Clutter, 2020). Helping the adoptive and biological family navigate their relationship is an additional responsibility of an infant adoption specialist. An infant adoption specialist provides guidance for the adoption triad members and mediates relationships between the adoption triad to promote trust and create boundaries that benefit each triad member (McLaughlin et al., 2013). As all relationships ebb and flow within the adoption triad, adoptive parents may doubt their parenting abilities while biological mothers imagine what it would be like to parent their biological child. (Clutter, 2014). Building trusting relationships between adoption triad members and creating appropriate boundaries may prevent misunderstanding and disagreements and provide support to each member.

DISRUPTED ADOPTION PLACEMENT

On occasion, a biological mother changes her mind after adoption placement and chooses to parent her infant, or a biological or legal father asserts their legal rights. This may occur anytime after a biological parent(s) chooses adoptive parents until all parental rights have been terminated. If the biological parent(s) decides to keep custody of her infant, adoptive parents may experience intense feelings of grief and loss. An infant adoption specialist provides support for bereavement and connects adoptive parents with other adoptive families and resources. If the infant has already been placed in the adoptive parents' home, they are often given the choice to bring the infant back to the agency office or have agency personnel retrieve the infant from their home. The biological mother then picks up her infant from the adoption agency. Albeit a challenging situation for all involved, adoption specialists must empathize with and provide support for the adoptive parents and the biological parent(s) likely experiencing a mix of emotions.

THE LIFE-LONG JOURNEY

Adoption is a continuous relationship and permanent commitment to a child. Infant Adoption Specialists continue to provide support to each member of the adoption triad indefinitely and as needed. A major part of this continued support includes providing guidance for adoptive parents as their infant grows into a child and then an adolescent. Adoptive parents are encouraged to share their adoption journey and unique story with their adopted child and his or her siblings as early as possible using developmentally appropriate tools and language. Through each developmental stage, an adopted child comes to new realizations inspiring new and more complex questions surrounding the adoption. While questions surrounding one's adoption may be posed infrequently, adoptive parents should provide their adopted child(ren) with freedom and encouragement to express their questions relating to adoption and birth family candidly. Adoptive parents often contact their infant adoption agency once their adopted child has expressed interest in or disclosed specific questions about the adoption and birth family. Again, a

CCLS may be uniquely suited for the role of infant adoption specialist due to the extensive knowledge of child development and family theory. Infant adoption specialists support adoptive parents in providing developmentally appropriate explanations to the questions children ask regarding their adoption. In addition, they facilitate activities that promote positive family relations and provide opportunities for mastery, reframing, and emotional expression with an adopted child.

MULTI-RACIAL ADOPTION

Multi-racial adoption impacts a child's development throughout the lifespan. Identifying with a different race than that of your adoptive parents or family presents a multidimensional and complex circumstance. Multi-racial adoption is not solely about skin color, but the culture(s), perspectives, and opportunities associated with that skin color which should be introduced early in the adopted child's life and reiterated often using developmentally appropriate language. Adoptive parents should celebrate their adopted child's race and provide opportunities for them to be surrounded by others who share the same race through diverse schools, community gatherings, religious organizations, extracurricular activities, etc. Not only should adopted children be surrounded by others who look like them, but also learn about their race and culture through mentors of the same background. Adoptive parents must prepare for comments, questions, and potential disapproving looks while out in the community with their adopted child. Occurrences like these may happen more frequently when the adopted child's skin tone is drastically different from their adoptive parents (Weller, 2019). Infant adoption specialists are qualified to provide education and resources to adoptive parents as their infant grows, including multi-racial support groups, linking them to other families experiencing multi-racial adoptions, and providing educational resources on cultural histories, hair and skincare, and how to handle offensive interactions regarding race. This support begins during pre-adoption and continues through the adopted child's adolescence. There may be an increased need for support during various developmental stages (Heiden-Rootes et al., 2019). The support given to family members involved in multi-racial adoptions promotes inclusion and cultural consciousness on behalf of the child and the adoptive parents and fulfills commitments detailed in the Association of Child Life Professional's Position Statement on Diversity, Equity, and Inclusion (ACLP, 2020b).

ETHICAL CONSIDERATIONS

Infant adoption specialists have state guidelines that they must adhere to regarding work with biological mothers, adoptive parents, and children. Adoption includes emotional, social, and legal implications. As infant adoption is confidential, infant adoption specialists must be discreet both in the office and the field. Biological parent(s) may meet with agency staff in an office or public location. However, documents must be kept covered, and specialists should avoid presenting any identifiers that indicate the meeting is for an adoption. If an infant adoption specialist comes into contact with a biological parent(s) or adoptive family in the future, they should avoid acknowledgment unless approached first. When addressed in the community, infant adoption specialists should neither confirm nor deny former clients' involvement with the adoption agency. These advisories align with Principle 4 of the Child Life Code of Ethics, which states, "CCLSs respect the privacy of children and families and maintain confidentiality within the standards and requirements of employers, local governing regulations, or private practice standards"

(ACLP, 2020a, p. 1). Additionally, each party commonly permits disclosure, and an adoption provider is responsible to keep everything else in a confidential file. Most adoption records are confidential and continue to be without a court order, including all case notes written.

In order to assure an adoption is ethical and within a biological parent(s)' legal rights, the biological parent(s) must never be forced or coerced into making a voluntary adoption decision. This could cause issues and setbacks in a legal adoption case. Therefore, infant adoption specialists must provide support no matter the biological parent(s) adoption decision. Infant adoption specialists should take every precaution never to pressure nor coerce biological parent(s) into placing their infant for adoption.

CONCLUSION

Although this chapter has discussed private domestic infant adoption, there are other types of adoption where a CCLS could use their knowledge and skills in assessment and intervention. These other areas include foster care to adoption, international adoption, embryo adoption, surrogacy, and family adoption. Like in infant adoption, many social, emotional, and legal factors encircle each of these. From foster care to adoption, the children range in age between birth and eighteen. Some children may have experienced multiple foster home placements and have experienced physical or emotional trauma. A CCLS may work with the child to develop coping skills or educate adoptive parents using trauma-informed care. Children adopted internationally are usually older infants or children and may have medical needs. These adoptive families often seek assistance in order to help their children acclimate to a new culture and language. Though the role of CCLS may shift with each form of adoption, all are possible avenues for child life services to be integrated into the community.

REFERENCES

Association of Child Life Professionals. (2018). *Association of child life professionals position statement on child life practice in community settings.* https://www.childlife.org/ docs/default-source/aclp-official-documents/cbp-on-cl-practice-in-community-settings_deireviewed.pdf?sfvrsn=62b5834d_2

Association of Child Life Professionals. (2020a). *Child life code of ethics.* https://www.childlife.org/docs/default-source/certification/child-life-code-of-ethics.pdf?sfvrsn=2

Association of Child Life Professionals. (2020b). *Position statement on diversity, equity, and inclusion.* https://www.childlife.org/docs/default-source/aclp-official-documents/statement-on-diversity-equity-and-inclusion.pdf?sfvrsn=c4d0864d_2

Barker, J., Daniels, A., O'Neal, K., & Van Sell, S. L. (2017). Maternal-newborn bonding concept analysis. *International Journal of Nursing & Clinical Practices*, *4*(229). Advance online publication. doi:10.15344/2394-4978/2017/229

Bergsund, H. B., Drozd, F., Hansen, M. B., & Jacobsen, H. (2018). Pre-adoption training: Experiences and recommendations from adoptive parents and course trainers. *Children and Youth Services Review*, *95*, 282–289. doi:10.1016/j.childyouth.2018.11.008

Brodzinsky, D., & Smith, S. L. (2014). Post-placement adjustment and the needs of birthmothers who place an infant for adoption. *Adoption Quarterly*, *17*(3), 165–184. doi:10.1080/10926755.2014.891551

Clutter, L. B. (2014). Adult birth mothers who made open infant adoption placements after adolescent unplanned pregnancy. *JOGNN*, *43*(2), 190–199. doi:10.1111/1552-6909.12280 PMID:24502258

Clutter, L. B. (2017). Open adoption placement by birth mothers in their twenties. *The American Journal of Maternal/Child Nursing*, *42*(6), 345-351. doi:10.1097/NMC.0000000000000370

Clutter, L. B. (2020). Perceptions of birth fathers about their open adoption. *The American Journal of Maternal/Child Nursing*, *45*(1), 26-32. doi:10.1097/NMC.0000000000000591

Craig, J. W. (2019). The neonatal intensive care unit (nicu): Self-efficacy of caregiving and the lived experience of parents post-nicu discharge. *Neonatology Today*, 25-31.

Fallon, A. E., & Goldsmith, B. L. (2013). *Theoretical contributions to the understanding of parent-child bonding in adoption. In Working with adoptive parents: Research, theory, and therapeutic interventions.* Wiley.

Flacking, R., Lehtonen, L., Thomson, G., Axelin, A., Ahlqvist, S., Moran, V. H., Ewald, U., & Dykes, F. (2012). Closeness and separation in neonatal intensive care. *Foundation Acta Pædiatrica*, *101*(10), 1032–1037. doi:10.1111/j.1651-2227.2012.02787.x PMID:22812674

Foli, K. J. (2012). Nursing care of the adoption triad. *Perspectives in Psychiatric Care*, *48*(4), 208–217. doi:10.1111/j.1744-6163.2012.00327.x PMID:23005588

Foli, K. J., Schweitzer, R., & Wells, C. (2013). The personal and professional: Nurses' lived experiences of adoption. *The American Journal of Maternal/Child Nursing, 38*(2), 79-86. doi:10.1097/NMC.0b013e3182763446

Halverson, K. K. (2018, March 6). *How infants grieve: A guide for new adoptive parents*. Adoption.com. https://adoption.com/how-infants-grieve-a-guide-for-new-adoptive-parents

Heiden-Rootes, K., Miller, B., & Moore, R. (2019). Cultural socialization in transracial adoption: Adoption support, multicultural experiences, perceptions of discrimination, and positive feelings toward racial minority groups. *Adoption Quarterly*, *22*(4), 247–264. doi:10.1080/10926755.2019.1627447

Hoffenkamp, H. N., Tooten, A., Croon, M. A., Braeken, J., Winkel, F. W., Vingerhoets, A. J. J. M., & van Bakel, H. J. A. (2012). The impact of premature childbirth on parental bonding. *Evolutionary Psychology*, *10*(3), 542–2012. doi:10.1177/147470491201000311 PMID:22947677

Koh, E., Hanlon, R., Daughtery, L., & Linder, A. (2020). *Adoption by the numbers*. National Council for Adoption. https://adoptioncouncil.org/themencode-pdf-viewer-sc/?tnc_pvfw=ZmlsZT1odHRwczovL2Fkb3B0aW9uY291bmNpbC5vcmcvY29udGVudC91cGxvYWRzLzIwMjIvMDUvQWRvcHRpb24tYnktdGhlLU51bWJlcnMtTmF0aW9uYWwtQ291bmNpbC1Gb3ItQWRvcHRpb24tMjAyMi5wZGYmc2V0dGluZ3M9MTExMDEwMTExMDAxMDAxMDAwMCZsYW5nPWVuLVVT#page=&zoom=page-height&pagemode=thumbs

McLaughlin, A. M., Feehan, R., Coleman, H., & Reynolds, K. (2013). Negotiating openness a qualitative study of adoptive parents' experience of contact in open adoption. *Canadian Social Work Review, 30*(1). https://www.researchgate.net/publication/260087431_Negotiating_openness_A_qualitative_study_of_adoptive_parents'_experien ce_of_contact_in_open_adoption

Purvis, K., Cross, D. R., & Sunshine, W. L. (2007). *The connected child: Bring hope and healing to your adoptive family*. McGraw Hill.

Rezaei, S., Pastrana, L., Brown, K., & Lancaster, A. (2019). Openness in adoptions satisfaction and psychological outcomes among birth mothers. *Adoption Advocate, 133*, 1-8. www.adoptioncouncil.org

Swartz, A., Brabender, V., Shorey, H. S., & Fallon, A. (2012). The maternal-bonding trajectory for mothers who adopt young, international children: A qualitative analysis. *Journal of Social Distress and the Homeless, 21*(3&4), 138–167. doi:10.1179/105307812805100171

Thomas, R. M. (2005). *Comparing theories of child development* (6th ed.). Thompson Wadsworth.

Thompson, R. (2018). *The handbook of child life: A guide for pediatric psychosocial care*. Charles C. Thomas.

Weller, M. R. (2019). "I Guess They're All Real Moms Then": Constructing Motherhood Through Language in the Adoption Community. *Adoption Quarterly, 22*(4), 265–283. doi:10.1080/10926755.2019.1675836

Young, R. (2013). The importance of bonding volume. *The International Journal of Childbirth Education, 28*(3), 11–16.

KEY TERMS AND DEFINITIONS

Adoption: To legally take into one's family and raise as one's own child.
Adoption Triad: The biological parents, adoptive parents, and child.
Postnatal: The period following the birth of a child.
Prenatal: The period between conception and birth.
Putative Father: The alleged father of a child.

Section 4
Frameworks

Chapter 16
Private Practice

Korie Leigh
Marian University, USA

Shani Thornton
Child Life Mommy Private Practice, USA

ABSTRACT

Many seasoned child life specialists begin to think about expanding their role to serve different pediatric populations and/or settings. This chapter will focus on child life specialists building and sustaining a private practice within the community. Topics will include the need for service, executing a business plan, building community partnerships, and staying within the ethical and professional boundaries as a Certified Child Life Specialist. Additionally, case studies that describe assessments, preparation, developmental explanations, interventions, expressive arts, and play are included. Examples of business documents to help guide child life specialists interested in starting a private practice within their community are also included.

INTRODUCTION

The Certified Child Life Specialist (CCLS) in private practice operates uniquely. As community practitioners, these specialists seek to build a referral network and work individually with children and families in the community. In this chapter, the word client will be used to describe a child, parent, or family that works with a child life specialist.

It is estimated that 32 million U.S. children live with a chronic illness (Bethell et al., 2011), and more than three million children are hospitalized in the U.S. annually (Pediatric Hospitalization, n.d.). Although children with chronic illnesses experience hospitalization, treatments can often be provided through outpatient care. Children of adult patients are also impacted by a loved one's illness, affecting their overall mental wellness (Wittenberg et al., 2013). With six out of ten U.S. adults having a chronic disease and four out of ten having two or more medical conditions, families can benefit from psychosocial and emotional support in their communities (CDC, 2022).

DOI: 10.4018/978-1-6684-5097-0.ch016

Certified Child Life Specialists bring a multifocal lens with expertise in child development, family systems, and skills to provide psychosocial and emotional support for families coping with stressful events. According to the 2018 ACLP Member Survey, over 6,000 child life specialists are certified. However, not all are employed or work in a hospital-based setting (ACLP, 2018). Once patients are discharged, they may have very little to no contact with a child life specialist. As a result, there is a significant gap in service to support families once they leave the healthcare setting. The Association of Child Life Professionals (ACLP), formally known as the Child Life Council (CLC), has stated that community involvement has long been a part of a CCLS's role due to the natural fit between the needs of the community for educational services and the skills that a specialist has to offer (CLC, 2006). Whether a child has an acute or chronic illness, has a loved one that is ill, struggles with understanding emotion, or has experienced the death of someone close to them, there is a continued need for education, preparation, normalization, and validation. Children and families challenged by situations that affect their ecological system and development continue to need ongoing support.

Child life specialists working in private practice recognize the need for service. As they assess their community for additional supports that are in place, such as bereavement centers and wellness programs, they begin to build their practice, filling in gaps of service. Their practice begins to develop using their experienced skill set, a niche for a particular population, and collaborating with community agencies, such as schools, nonprofits, and healthcare programs.

Child life programs in healthcare settings are free with no billing code, meaning the institution does not bill insurance for child life services. Without an established billing code, payment for child life services becomes a challenge for CCLSs working in private practice. Many private practitioners will charge families directly and offer a superbill that families can submit to their insurance in hopes of full or partial coverage. A superbill is a paid invoice with an itemized list of services the client has received. Child life specialists are committed to providing health equity and support to communities (ACLP, n.d.). For families unable to pay the fee for service, specialists may offer a sliding scale or pro bono. Specialists can also apply for grants or contractual work with community agencies to support families without billing them directly.

Child life specialists in private practice may work individually with clients, in a group setting offering support groups or coaching, and offer consultation and professional outreach support to organizations and businesses. No matter the clinical area of focus, it is essential to work within the ethical scope of child life practice.

SETTING

Office

Child life specialists in private practice often provide services in either an office space or a client's private home. The benefits of office space include increased control over environmental factors (e.g., materials, design, predictability, and privacy). The office space should include various developmental toys, games, activities, art materials, culturally inclusive children's books, and dolls of various skin tones. There should be room for a child to explore and manipulate items on the floor and at a table. The room may also include a sitting section for teens and adults. The office space will allow the child life specialist to create a work environment separate from home. This can help to establish healthy work boundaries and self-care.

In-Home

Child life specialists may also provide sessions in the client's homes. Working within the client's home helps clients feel at ease due to familiarity while also providing the child life specialist an opportunity to assess clients in their normative environment. The child life specialist can observe and assess family operations, dynamics, and relationships in a more naturalistic setting through in-home services. This is useful in creating effective interventions to best support their needs. Additionally, there may be benefits logistically for clients as it alleviates transportation needs and further disruptions in routines.

SCOPE OF PRACTICE

Child life specialists must stay within their scope of practice when serving clients (ACLP, 2020). Working within a traditional hospital-based program offers a strong foundation and boundaries to help specialists stay within their scope. Many hospital-based programs have a clinical ladder system that includes upper management, collaboration and communication with other medical departments, and reflective supervision. Specialists working in private practice have a smaller foundation of support. They may be a sole proprietor, essentially a one-person program. They may align with other specialists to create a small private practice or partner with licensed social workers, creative art therapists, nutritionists, and marriage and family therapists to form a private practice.

Overview of the Importance of Assessing and Staying within the Scope

Child life specialists are required to stay within their scope of practice and follow the professional and ethical boundaries of a Certified Child Life Specialist. According to the ACLP *Position Statement on Child Life Practice in Community Settings*, "when the needs of children, families, and their support systems extend beyond the scope of practice, it is the ethical responsibility of the child life specialist to make recommendations for and referrals to additional services (ACLP, 2018)." For example, it has been suggested that the CCLS and registered play therapists work in conjunction with one another on cases to enhance the delivery of care (Lerwick, 2019). Child life specialists can also help to fill the gap in service with these organizations and be of service through collaborative work.

Collaborations within the Community

Building a referral network within the community is essential. According to the official documents of the ACLP, principle six states, "Certified Child Life Specialists provide services within their competencies and make appropriate referrals with due regard for the professional competencies of other members of the health care team and the community within which they work" (ACLP, 2020). Thus, establishing a trusting partnership with other professionals, organizations, and nonprofits helps a specialist expand their practice. Assessment of the community's needs and resources and collaborative efforts creates trusting partnerships with medical and dental providers, hospice agencies, funeral homes, and nonprofits serving bereaved families. As a result, new referrals and developments continue to expand as partnerships grow within the community.

Continuity of Care and Collaboration with Other Professionals

The referral network can also provide collaborative efforts when working with clients. For example, specialists may work with a client's school counselor to discuss struggles and strategies to support them in both settings. The specialist can also work with other mental health providers, physicians, dieticians, and other professionals to create a cohesive treatment plan to best support the client's needs. The client's caregivers should sign a HIPAA release form to allow health information to be shared between the specialist and other providers. This legal document allows private information to be shared and discussed between two parties.

Specializing in a Specific Clinical Area

The private practice child life specialist may focus on a particular population, such as grief and loss, specific diagnosis or medical experiences, or general child development and coping with stressful events. Child life specialists specializing in bereaved families can offer that support in private practice. They have the flexibility to create an individualized treatment plan that may include support during end-of-life hospice care, preparation for a funeral or memorial services, grief support, parent coaching, and collaboration with school and other community organizations that work with families. Child life specialists could also offer grief groups for different developmental age groups and caregivers. With their deep knowledge, experience, and training, child life specialists can provide workshops on grief topics to caregivers, educators, community members, and professionals in various settings.

Child development is another area of expertise of a child life specialist. CCLSs can use this knowledge to collaborate with community organizations that serve children in various settings. The collaborative approach may involve leading training workshops for those professionals. For example, a child life specialist may work with a family dental office to educate their team on strategies to better connect with pediatric patients and make their dental care experience positive. The specialist can empower the team with education and coping strategies and make suggestions to create an inviting space for families.

The child life specialist may also connect with a preschool and conduct workshops for teachers and parents. Sharing information and strategies to support children through new experiences that could be stressful for the family, such as having a new sibling, divorce, or pet loss, are examples of this collaboration. In addition, the child life specialist could collaborate with community organizations, such as schools, nonprofits, and churches, to provide services to larger audiences using a virtual platform.

Filling Needs in the Community Using Market Research

Conducting a needs assessment of a community using market research is an ideal way to identify the needs within that community and begin targeting a specific population. An area of business development that is often overlooked is engaging in market research before beginning to work with clients. Market research is a way for a business owner to understand the ideal client's needs, desires, and interests (McQuarrie, 2015). In addition, a complete market research analysis will help the CCLS learn how to price services. Pricing services are unique to each practitioner based on skills, location, and population services.

Undertaking market research allows the CCLS to know the client, what keywords they use when they describe their issue, what keywords are put into an internet search to find providers, and most importantly, what price point they are willing to pay to work with a professional. Conducting market research will require a few steps. The following is a revised process from *The Market Research Toolbox 4th edition.*

First, identify the ideal client population and identify the gatekeeper to that population. For example, the gatekeeper will be the primary caregiver if working with children. The child life specialist would want to interview the parent or guardian and not the child to obtain this market research information.

Second, develop a list of questions that will yield rich data to analyze. The data, in this case, are the words used by the client. Think of this step as conducting a qualitative study. Ask open-ended questions that will provide depth. Some questions might include *What words do you type into Google when you have tried to find someone that can help with the problem? How do you describe the problem that you are seeking help with? How much are you willing and able to pay for your child to work with someone that can help them?*

Third, after having conducted at least five interviews with the ideal client, analyze the data looking for themes. For example, if every person interviewed stated that they couldn't afford anything over $90, the Certified Child Life Specialist would want to consider that when setting the fee. Analyzing the data will provide a starting place to ensure the right population is targeted with the correct language to meet the ideal client's unique needs.

Modalities often used in Child Life Intervention

Play

Play is a central component of a child's development. According to The American Academy of Pediatrics (Romitio, 2021), play is crucial to a child's social, emotional, and cognitive development. It is even more critical during adversity or stress points in a child's life. Child life specialists have a core competency in play and can assess, facilitate, and promote play opportunities (ACLP, 2016). Child life specialists in private practice create play opportunities for children in unique ways. Some specialists have an office space designed as a play and creative arts room. Some provide in-home services and set up a space to play in the family's common area or even the backyard. Child life specialists can also meet in community spaces, such as a local park, school, or church. When they meet a client for the first time, they incorporate play to build a rapport and assess their needs. They use play to prepare them for new experiences, gain mastery, and process information.

A typical play technique that child life specialists use in private practice is child-centered play. Child-centered play has been defined as a "theoretically grounded and evidence-based intervention that recognizes the relationship between therapist and child as the primary healing factor for children who are experiencing emotional and behavioral challenges" (Landreth & Ray, 2019, p.18). The child can play with open-ended materials in various ways, while the specialist's job is to connect and reflect on what the child is saying or doing. Their role is to be present with the child without judgment or agenda. When this occurs, the child is empowered, and their developmental capabilities are released for self-exploration, and self-discovery, resulting in constructive change (Landreth, 2002, p. 60). This technique can create a therapeutic relationship and help promote healing, empowerment, and resiliency.

In the following sections, various case studies highlight different aspects of clinic practice. Following many case studies will be questions that are aimed to help guide the process of learning how to practice as a child life specialist in a community-based setting. In addition, these questions are helpful for those studying in an academic setting or those wishing to apply their critical thinking skills to possible scenarios they may encounter if working as a private practice child life specialist.

Case Example

The CCLS received a referral from a contracted hospice agency. During the phone intake, the mom informed the specialist that her mother had recently moved into her home with her husband and two small children (a 3-year-old daughter and an 18-month-old son). Her mom was diagnosed with terminal cancer. She explained that she did not think child life services would be beneficial because "How do you talk to a toddler about cancer and dying?" The CCLS explained the role and provided education on how children process illness and loss. The mother agreed and was open to services.

*The CCLS met with *Katie (pseudonym) and her brother, Charlie (pseudonym), every other week for four months. The goal was to provide a safe space to explore and play using child-centered play techniques. The specialist typically brought the same leading toys (dollhouse, medical play kits, people figurines, and animal finger puppets) and added a new toy, book, or art activity each session to the supply bag. For the first few months, Katie would play themes of caretaking. For example, she would place bandages on the "Grandma" and say things like, "Aww, you sick? I help you feel better. All better, Grandma." then she would kiss the doll.*

As Katie's grandmother's illness progressed and she transitioned into an active dying stage, Katie's play themes slightly changed. The CCLS observed her act out the dolls to be crying and taking "sick grandma" to the hospital while the others would comfort one another.

After Katie's grandma died, the specialist added a sand tray to the activity bag and observed Katie's play themes evolve. Katie would play out the same storyline of the grandma becoming sick, crying, and going to the hospital. Then she would bury the figurines in the sand and dig them out. She would say, "Oh no, I can't see you. I will help. Thank you, Mommy, for helping me." She had themes of coming and going, disappearing, burying, rescuing, and caretaking.

During these sessions, the specialist used the child-centered play technique reflecting Katie's play with empathetic responses. The CCLS let Katie lead the play and did not take control. As a result, Katie could continue to process all these real-life challenges through the safest and most natural way, play.

Questions to guide clinical practice or academic preparedness:

- ***What materials and play items would you need to purchase to provide child-centered play opportunities in your practice?***
- ***What is your comfort level with engaging in child-centered play techniques?***
- ***If you plan to include child-centered techniques in your practice, how would you advocate for such interventions to a family that is not familiar?***
- ***How can you use child-centered play to inform your assessment and care plan for a client?***

Expressive Arts

Expressive arts include modalities such as movement, visual arts, music, writing, and nature (Knill, Levine, & Levine, 2005). While Certified Child Life Specialists are not licensed expressive arts therapists, they do use modalities that allow children to experience therapeutic benefits through the process of creating art.

Incorporating therapeutic art with children and teens provides a safe metaphor for expression. The use of creative arts enhances the creation of personal meaning as the child's unique imprint is embedded in the work (Edgar-Bailey & Kress, 2010). Child life specialists in private practice tailor interventions to support the client's form of expression.

Neurological and developmental importance. Expressing emotions is vital for a child's development. Brain development encompasses the interaction between biology and experience; therefore children's social and emotional experiences play a critical role in the growth of the brain's architecture (Housman, 2017). Children and adults want to feel validated and witnessed, especially when facing life's stressors. Big emotions can take over their bodies and minds and impact how they adjust and cope.

Case Example

A pediatrician referred Anne (pseudonym) a ten-year-old girl to the child life practice after a recent wellness visit. The pediatrician ordered a blood panel to rule out some issues that may be causing Anne not to grow at a developmentally appropriate rate. Anne has a massive fear of needles and verbalizes her fear to her mom and pediatrician.*

In the first session, the goal was to provide education and preparation to Anne for an upcoming blood draw. The child life specialist wanted her to understand how the body functions, specifically the heart and blood. The specialist also provided education on how the brain operates and involuntary physiological responses to threats. There was a discussion about the steps involved in the blood draw and a specific coping plan was created to suit her needs.

Anne went for her blood draw the following day and completed it successfully without any additional trauma or anxiety. The CCLS met with her a few days later for a post-procedural session. The goal was to provide Anne with an expressive art activity to help strengthen her resilience over her needle fear. The CCLS provided Anne with a large white canvas. The CCLS asked her to keep the middle of the canvas blank and choose different colored markers to write or draw images representing her fears. Anne quickly grabbed a marker and began to draw. She wrote, "I hate needles." The CCLS provided validation of her feelings and normalized that many children and adults do not like them. The CCLS then asked if there were other worries that she may have. She added, "bugs, the dark, snakes, and spiders." When she was done, the CCLS asked her to think of empowering words or a mantra that she could tell herself. After a few minutes of brainstorming, the CCLS had her write the words down in the middle of the canvas. She wrote, "I am brave. I am strong. I am beautiful. I am smart." The CCLS then had her cover the mantra with painter's tape.

The CCLS wanted to incorporate an expressive art activity that would strengthen her resiliency, so syringe painting was introduced. Anne picked paint colors placed in medicine cups and then squirted them on the canvas. She could manipulate the syringe and become more comfortable with it in a non-threatening manner. This provided her with mastery and control. She covered the words representing her fears and the mantra protected by painter's tape.

Later that day, the CCLS instructed her to remove the painter's tape to reveal her mantra. It was a powerful piece of art with her strength in the center and the splattered paint covering her fears around it.

Questions to guide clinical practice or academic preparedness:

- ***When introducing a creative expression intervention to a client, how can you ensure it is developmentally appropriate?***
- ***What are some other expressive arts interventions you might provide?***
- ***How can you assess if an expressive arts intervention is appropriate for the needs of your client?***

Child Life Services in Private Practice

Assessment

Assessing the fit and scope of a referral is arguably the most critical point of contact with any new referral. Ensuring that intake forms cover vital areas not only protects the business owner but protects the family from seeking support from a professional that is not trained to meet their needs. The following case example highlights the importance of a robust intake process.

Intake Assessment

Before working individually with a child, the family fills out an intake form and meets with the child life specialist for an assessment session. The intake form is the first point of entry. Intake forms will be unique to each private practice and should reflect questions based on the area of specialty and services available. However, basic information such as demographics, contact information, and reason for referral can be found on all intake forms. If the family discloses any information that deems a need for services not within the scope of child life practice, the child life specialist can provide them with an outside referral to meet their needs.

Comprehensive Psychosocial Assessment

The second point of entry is the assessment session. During this time, the child life specialist meets with the primary caregiver to further assess their goals for working together and the background which brings them to seek child life services.

Case Example

**Erica (pseudonym) is a single mother of two children under the age of six. The initial referral came through the local play therapy practice stating, "mother wants help with child's tantrums." Initially, the referral appeared to fit the scope of practice supporting families' ability to understand their child's behavior during times of stress and uncertainty. The Covid-19 pandemic had begun only three months prior. Thus, the timing of this referral also appeared to fit the circumstances of the CCLS's scope of practice. Erica provided brief responses on the initial intake form, sometimes in one-word answers, and left many questions blank. Nothing on the intake form indicated that this family would not benefit from working with a Certified Child Life Specialist. After this initial intake, the CCLS held an assessment session with the mother. During the assessment session, after asking many questions surrounding the origins of the tantrums, Erica disclosed that her children had witnessed a very traumatic event and had been diagnosed with PTSD. Erica was desperate to find 'therapy' for her children. The assessment session finished with the child life specialist providing validation and emotional support to Erica and her wish to find help for her children. A brief psycho-educational session ensued regarding how to support her children in developmentally appropriate ways. The child life specialist worked closely with Erica to refer her back to the play therapy center to begin work with a trauma-informed play therapist.*

Questions to guide clinical practice or academic preparedness:

- ***How would you handle this situation?***
- ***What questions do you think should be included on an intake form to potentially capture referrals that are outside your scope?***
- ***Who will be on your referral list when a family comes to you outside your scope of practice?***
- ***How might reflective supervision aid in your experience of providing support to this family?***

Preparation

Child life specialists are competent in providing education and preparation that is developmentally appropriate (ACLP, 2016). Child life specialists working in a traditional hospital setting commonly focus on medical preparation for a procedure, treatment, or new diagnosis. Similarly, CCLSs in private practice may also work with children preparing for medical experiences. Often, a specialist in private practice will educate the family on child life services available in the hospital but can also provide the preparation service to deepen the learning process. Three components are used to prepare children for new experiences. These include using developmentally appropriate language, opportunities for emotional expression, and building trust with caregivers (Koller, 2007). In addition, there is often a rush within the hospital environment, with intense energy and constant interruptions; child life specialists in private practice can set aside time to create an individual preparation and coping plan to best serve the client's needs. Parents and caregivers can also be part of these preparation sessions as they will help to implement them during the medical appointment.

Child Life Developmental Competency

Child life specialists' skills encompass understanding life's stressors on a child's development. Using theory and research, child life specialists provide education and preparation in the developmentally appropriate language to support children and teens. Using developmentally appropriate explanations is critical in helping children understand what they will experience. Child life specialists address what will occur and why, incorporating the five senses to help children deepen their learning (Koller, 2007).

Case Example

The child life specialist in private practice had been working with a family for about six months with the primary referral of grief support. The mother experienced two traumatic pregnancy losses in the third trimester. Her two living children, aged six and eight at the time of our initial work together, were struggling with grief and understanding how to make sense of these losses.

*During the 6-month mark of working together, a crisis emerged with 8-year-old *Paul (pseudonym). Paul had begun experiencing a sudden onset of auditory and visual hallucinations, joint pain, fatigue, headaches, and a sudden increase in anxiety in the form of panic attacks. The clinical assessment at the time was for the family to have Paul receive medical services and to start working with a licensed therapist. As the family sought a medical diagnosis and worked with a clinical psychologist for Paul's needs, the CCLS continued working with the family to address grief-related challenges.*

During this time, the sessions also included parent coaching, where the child life specialist helped the parents learn how to advocate for Paul. Sadly, the doctors they were seeing kept dismissing Paul and his symptoms. The child life specialist helped empower the parents to ask questions, research specialists, and connect to other families struggling with similar challenges in seeking a medical diagnosis.

At the 8-month mark of working together, the family had a diagnosis; PANDAS that originated from untreated Lyme disease. Paul underwent medical treatment and continued to see the psychologist. However, due to the rapport they built, Paul began to ask the child life specialist questions about Lyme disease and PANDAS, why he was hearing and seeing things that were not there, and how to make it stop. After consulting with the clinical psychologist, the child life specialist began to work with Paul to help him understand Lyme disease and PANDAS. The specialist also explained, what happens in the brain when we hear and see things we know are not there, and how to use stress relieving techniques when anxiety is high.

During the duration of work together, the child life specialist and Paul looked at virtual models of the brain to understand what parts help people see and hear. Together, they discovered what parts of the brain are active when one feels anxiety, and they looked at the spirochete called borrelia burgdorferi to understand Lyme disease. Finally, a coping plan was created that included breathing techniques, guided relaxation, and a stress plan that his whole family could be a part of. Finally, during the last few weeks of work together, Paul created an All About Lyme and PANDAS book. Paul wrote this book to help other children understand and cope with these chronic conditions. Paul is now being interviewed for a documentary being made about PANDAS.

Questions to guide clinical practice or academic preparedness:

- ***When consulting with another clinician, what forms and paperwork would you need before you talk with the provider?***
- ***At what point, in this case, would you have considered transitioning care altogether?***
- ***Is there any place where you feel the scope of practice was outside child life services?***

Life Transitions

In a private practice setting, the child life specialist uses this transferable skill set to translate challenging concepts so the client will understand using simple concrete language and various teaching modalities, such as visuals, books, videos, and play. Some common explanations that specialists will address are medical/dental procedures, visiting a loved one in hospice, becoming a new sibling, moving to a new home, and death and dying.

Death and Dying

Preparation is not limited to medical intervention or education but covers any new experiences a child or teen may have. Many specialists in private practice will also prepare children for other common experiences, such as the arrival of a new sibling, relocation to a new home, and memorial services. In addition, child life specialists prepare children to say goodbye to a dying loved one or prepare them for a funeral service. Death and dying are very much part of our lives, however, North American culture tends to avoid this topic. Alongside socio-cultural trends that have removed death from everyday life, many adults endorse attitudes of shielding children from the reality of death (Longbottom & Slaughter, 2018). Child life specialists are skilled in helping all family members navigate the life cycle and prepare children for these experiences. According to the American Academy of Pediatrics (Romito, 2021), child life specialists can help siblings, for example, to have a voice that is respected and honored in the family about a loved one's terminal prognosis and death.

Case Example

The Certified Child Life Specialist was referred to work with a family after tragically losing their toddler in an accidental home death. The parents also had a 6-year-old son who witnessed his sibling's death and the chaos that quickly followed with emergency services arriving at his home. During the intake and assessment with the mom, the CCLS found out the family would have an open casket for a private family viewing and a large mass ceremony open to friends and family the following day. The funeral service was to take place five days after the intake appointment.

The goal for the first in-person child life session would be to build rapport and educate the 6-year-old on the cause of death of his sibling, address any misconceptions, prepare him for the funeral service, and facilitate a memory-making activity. The CCLS created a preparation book for this new experience using developmentally appropriate tools and language. The CCLS included what a funeral service was, the people attending, how they may behave, photos of the church, and a social story of what he will experience using his five senses. The specialist also offered coping strategies and choices that could make him feel more comfortable, including having a point person to take him outside if he becomes overwhelmed.

After the in-person session, the CCLS met with his mother to discuss the themes and assess his developmental understanding of the death and coping needs. The specialist also provided the mother with developmentally appropriate language to use while they continued to prepare him for the funeral service.

The child and family had a precise preparation and coping plan to serve their needs best. The CCLS met with the family a few days after the funeral service. The family explained that their son not only attended the viewing and service without any anxiety but he also placed the memory-making items he had created next to his sibling's casket. He then, on his own, raised his hand to speak in front of the large audience at the mass. He spoke from his heart about his love for his sibling and the memories he will forever cherish.

This case study demonstrates that child life competencies of preparation were used. The child understood what would be occurring, his role and his choices to help him cope.

Questions to guide clinical practice or academic preparedness:

- ***Could other preparation goals have been made?***
- ***Could the child life specialist also attend the service to provide support? Why or why not?***
- ***What follow-up interventions would you facilitate at the next appointment?***

Coping Support

Supporting clients in coping with life stressors is certainly a transferable skill of the child life specialist. In a community-based setting, the same principles of stress and coping theory (Lazarus & Folkman, 1984) apply to the assessment process. Mainly, that coping refers to an individual's cognitive/behavioral responses (both verbal/nonverbal and active/passive) resulting from their perceptions of stressors and self-perception (Fraser et al., 2020). However, the primary threat to coping in a community setting may not be illness or hospitalization. Instead, the threat to coping may stem from normal developmental stressors in a child's life, such as loss or life transitions. Therefore, the private practice child life specialist may assess and provide coping strategies for life events surrounding separation, life transition, relationship building, and generalized emotion regulation. The community-based CCLS then teaches, models, and facilitates adaptive coping skills that can be applied to many facets of a child's life.

Case Example

The CCLS was referred to work with a family after their dog traumatically died by accident. The family went on an afternoon drive with their dog on a hot summer day. When they returned home, they all went inside, thinking that another family member had also brought the dog in with them. It was not until hours later that they realized the dog was not inside. They ran to the car, but it was too late. The dog died from heat exhaustion.

*During the intake with the father, he expressed his concerns for his two older children, ten-year-old, *Jeff and 12-year-old, *Henry (pseudonyms). He stated they had witnessed the traumatic event and were having a "difficult time." He explained that they were both not sleeping well, Jeff was tearful throughout the day, and Henry was angry and withdrawn.*

The CCLS provided individual telehealth support to the boys. During the session, the CCLS observed that they were struggling and coping very differently from each other. Jeff verbalized his story and cried on and off. He shared the trauma of witnessing his dad scream in terror when he found the dog. He expressed a tremendous amount of grief and guilt. He was also able to express that his dog was a "peacekeeper" to the family. The family was already struggling with the ups and downs of the pandemic shutdown and a recent move. The family had experienced many losses, and their dog was a big part of their coping outlet.

Henry did not share his story of what occurred that day. Instead, he would share his story starting from the following morning after the loss. He explained that he woke up thinking that his dog was asleep at the foot of his bed, but then he would realize that she was not there and that the "nightmare" was real and not a dream. Henry shared that he felt incredibly lonely, isolated, and angry.

Over the next several weeks, the CCLS educated the kids on trauma and grief, facilitated therapeutic outlets for expression, and taught healthy coping strategies. During that time, the CCLS observed Jeff cope with his loss through tinkering, creating, reading, crying, and talking to his mom and the child life specialist. Henry had a more difficult time coping. He would look for control by being authoritative towards his younger brother, arguing with his parents, and becoming explosive in his behavior. He admitted his difficulty accepting the loss as an accident and felt tremendous guilt and shame. The CCLS continued to work closely with Jeff and provided sporadic support to Henry. However, he required more support from an in-person therapist at his school.

Questions to guide clinical practice or academic preparedness:

- ***What tools can you use to assess how a child is coping?***
- ***Consider the limitations of telehealth sessions; what might be some barriers to assessment in this environment?***
- ***What policies and forms would you need to speak with the school therapist?***

Advocacy

While building therapeutic relationships with clients, child life specialists can assess their psychosocial and emotional stressors, coping strategies, and other services or support they may need. Concurrently, specialists can advocate on the client's behalf or teach the client advocacy skills. Advocacy helps empower children and families to participate actively in their healthcare experiences (Fraser et al., 2020). As per the ACLP Child Life Competencies, the fifth child life competency is "the ability to support infants, children, youth, and families in coping with stressful events." (ACLP, 2019). At the heart of this competency is advocacy. Specialists within the hospital setting advocate for parental presence, developmentally appropriate play, pain management, and encourage children to have autonomy in their medical needs.

Specialists working in private practice continue to help clients advocate for themselves. For example, while they provide support to a family coping with a loved one's terminal prognosis, they may also advocate additional support for children at school. In addition, they can educate teachers and school administration on the impact of illness and grief and how they can best support the student during this traumatic and stressful time.

Case Example

*The child life specialist was working with 12-year-old, *Lily (pseudonym), diagnosed with Crohn's disease and juvenile rheumatoid arthritis. The specialist received the referral from her mother, who explained that Lily had needle fear related to her weekly immunosuppressant injections.*

During the first two sessions, the CCLS could assess some other struggles that she was coping with. Lily said she missed a lot of school due to not feeling well or having outpatient infusion treatments. She stated that only two of her friends knew about her diagnosis and the rest of her friends and classmates were unaware. The CCLS asked her what she tells her peers when she is late to school or unable to attend in person. She explained that she made up stories such as going to the dentist or sleeping in by accident. Lily also spoke about the importance of doing well in academics. She explained that she sometimes struggles with the workload and does not want to disappoint her teachers by not completing the assignments on time.

The CCLS spoke with Lily about her goals of doing well in school and her comfort level in explaining her diagnosis to her closer peers. The specialist also spoke to Lily, and her mother about implementing an educational 504 plan to support her medical needs. Within a few weeks, the school administrators, teachers, and Lily's parents met to have the 504-document created. As a result, Lily had accommodations that included shortened assignments, extra time for exams, and extensions on her classwork. In addition, she would no longer be penalized if she turned in late work.

The CCLS observed Lily and her mother coping much better in the next session. They expressed that the stress load had decreased immensely, and Lily stated that she was feeling much "happier." The specialist was able to teach both Lily and her mother to advocate for her needs and find a better way to manage her stress.

Questions to guide clinical practice or academic preparedness:

- ***Can other communication and advocacy support be done between the client and school settings?***
- ***How familiar are you with a 504 plan? How might you learn more about this option for the children you work with?***
- ***What does advocacy mean to you? Write your advocacy statement and compare it to your practice- can you integrate your definition into your clinical practice? Why or why not?***

CLINICAL SUPERVISION AND SELF CARE

Child life specialists are subject to burnout and compassion fatigue. Vicarious trauma can quickly occur as they help families cope with life's stressors. Burnout and compassion fatigue can lead to emotional exhaustion, depression, frustration, and a sense of loss in one's achievements; in healthcare providers, this can adversely affect patient care (Kase, Waldman, and Weintraub, 2018). In 2008, the ACLP created a position statement on clinical supervision. It states that regular, ongoing clinical supervision is needed to provide opportunities to process, decrease compassion fatigue, promote the growth and development of child life specialists, and ensure that competent care is provided to patients and families (Brown et al., 2008).

Committing to reflective supervision decreases the potential of burnout and compassion fatigue (Dehlin & Lundh, 2018). Supervision facilitates self-care activities and strengthens healthy boundaries working in private practice. Reflective supervision by an experienced specialist or psychotherapist is paramount to the child life specialist in private practice. According to the *Clinical Supervision Position Statement of the Child Life Council,* clinical supervision enables individual practitioners to develop knowledge and skills, assume responsibility for their practice, and is central to the ongoing process of professional growth and learning (Brown et al., 2008). There is an added layer of responsibility to supporting families in the community in the utmost ethical and professional manner as a CCLS. Working in a hospital environment or an extensive program with multiple child life specialists, individuals can collaborate, process, and work through challenging cases as a team or in one-on-one supervision. Working as a sole proprietor in private practice is like working in a one-person child life program at a hospital. There is not that extra cushion of support built in. Scheduling reflective supervision is crucial in ensuring that the specialists stay within their scope of practice, process cases, and continue to grow professionally.

According to the *Standards and Guidelines for Child Life Practice in Community Based and Non-Traditional Settings*, it is recommended that an experienced Certified Child Life Specialist provide supervision to a specialist in a community-based setting (ACLP, 2020). It can take time to educate and build trust within a community on the services a child life specialist can provide. Often, the referrals for possible clients are meant for the scope of a licensed mental health provider. Child life specialists may be eager to take on some of these clients as they fall into a gray area within their scope. Child life specialists may have the skills and training to work with those in a particular manner, such as preparation for transitions, but CCCLs need to be clear when clients need to be referred to a mental health provider, not a child life specialist. Reflective supervision will help a child life specialist have a sounding board for those gray area referrals.

BUSINESS

Developing a business plan is a helpful strategy to undertake before starting a private practice. The benefits of creating a business plan include having a firm understanding of the business structure being created, having a budget for expenses, and understanding where the financial burden exists within the business.

The first part of a business plan is to identify what kind of business structure will exist. The two most common options are a) starting as a sole proprietor or b) incorporating as a Limited Liability Company (LLC). There are benefits and limitations to both. The chart below provides a snapshot of the difference between the two. In choosing the type of business, one must also adhere to local, state, and federal guidelines for tax filing. Regardless of business structure, setting aside a certain percentage of income for tax filings will be important. It is strongly recommended to work with a seasoned tax professional.

Table 1. Pro and con list LLC or sole proprietor

LLC: Pro	LLC: Con
LLC allows members to manage the company. This will allow the LLC member to hire someone who has more business experience to operate it. This can be helpful for day-to-day business operations.	LLC is more complex when starting up. It may require hiring a registered agent, drafting an Operating Agreement, and obtaining an EIN (Employer Identification Number) for tax purposes.
LLC offers variation business models that can be chosen to fit a member's needs. For example, single member- LLC, general partnership, and series LLC.	LLC has a higher upfront cost. You must file state paperwork and file annually. Besides paying personal federal, state, local, and the self-employed version of FICA taxes, you might also be required to pay State Business Taxes and Unemployment Taxes.
LLC protects your personal assets and finances, including homes, cars, and bank accounts. This means that LLC members aren't personally liable for the company's actions.	LLC does have limits. There could be possibilities that your personal assets are not fully protected. For example, if a member does not fully separate personal and business transactions.
Sole Proprietor: Pro	**Sole Proprietor: Con**
Sole proprietorship is relatively easy and straightforward to start. There is not much paperwork, except for county or state requirements of licenses and/or permits.	Sole Properties are not eligible for equity building grants or accessing a business line of credit or loan.
Sole proprietorship allows you to begin working immediately, and you are entitled to all the profits you make	Sole proprietorship does not provide you with financial protection, and you are responsible for all the liability.
Sole Proprietors are not required to pay taxes on the total amount of your sole proprietorship's income. Instead, you'll only pay taxes on the profit of your business.	Sole proprietorship is nearly impossible to sell or transfer to another individual if you die or decide to stop running the business.

*Information gathered from Wang (2022) and Wood (2020).

Business Forms

Some basic business documents need to be created and looked over by a legal representative. Having an intake form is essential in gathering information about the client. Include sections about contact information, family member involvement, demographics, the reason for services, and the client's strengths, hobbies, and struggles.

Creating a client agreement form can also protect a private practitioner's business. Include information about informed consent, description of services, service fees, late or missed appointments, HIPAA, and hold harmless clauses. A hold harmless clause is a legal agreement between the client and practitioner that prevents one party from being liable to the other if there are injuries or damages. Practitioners may also create a photo and video release for educational and marketing purposes. If the practitioner offers phone or telehealth services, creating informed consent for technology-assisted support should also be included.

Marketing and Social Media

There are several ways to market a private practice within the community. A straightforward and affordable way is through social media. According to Pew Research (2021),72% of Americans use social media. Setting up a business account on various platforms with consistent information can help. Having a logo, vision statement, business, and contact information listed will help followers understand the service available. There needs to be engagement with social media to reach a large audience and establish relationships. Sixty-eight percent of consumers agree that social media enables them to interact with companies (Cover, 2021). This includes liking, sharing, commenting, and sending private messages. When followers receive comments back, that helps to strengthen social engagement.

Creating new content or sharing other's social media content must connect to the business and vision statement. This will help followers understand the private practice focus. An algorithm for social media platforms can confuse new business owners, especially when marketing is not their expertise. Tailoring strategies to fit the vision and goals of practice requires researching reliable websites or following marketing influencers. Many companies can help new business owners create and share content on social media for free or a small fee with their upgrade packages. It is a learning curve with social media, and it is constantly changing.

There are excellent networking opportunities that can also happen through social media. Connecting with similar professionals, nonprofits, and business owners can help expand social media presence. Collaborating on projects, such as blog posts, podcasts, live social media meetups, and face-to-face events, are all valuable tactics. These connections can turn into partnerships, scaling them to the level that works for business. In addition, specialists can learn about resources that benefit their practice, such as grants, donations, and contractual work.

Child life specialists can also use social media to bring awareness to the services they provide and the field. The ACLP vision statement includes the professional responsibility to continue educating, training, and collaborating with individuals, disciplines, organizations, and communities to support children and families (ACLP, 2001). Sharing content created by the specialist and other resources will help reach a larger audience. Health care professionals also use social media for personal and professional use. It is estimated that 70% of U.S. healthcare organizations use social media (Ventola, 2014). Providing education of the child life professional through social media will help the local community understand the value of child life work within the private practice setting while reaching a regional and possibly global community, increasing awareness of the field.

Fees and Finances

The final part of the business plan includes creating an operating budget of anticipated expenses. There will be upfront costs, long-term costs, and client-specific costs. Upfront costs include everything necessary to get the business off the ground. These costs might include fees to file for an LLC and hiring an attorney to review the agreement forms, marketing, and materials. Long-term costs are considered costs that will incur yearly, regardless of how many clients the business serve. These might include website maintenance, marketing materials, and office rent. Client-specific costs may include art and play materials for specific age groups or client needs. The business plan's fourth part is obtaining liability insurance and clinical supervision. The fifth part of the business plan is to create a networking and marketing plan. Identify who the primary stakeholders and gatekeepers are in the community and begin to introduce child life services to them.

Child life specialists must follow the ACLP *Standards of Clinical Practice* for appropriate documentation and confidentiality (ACLP, 2020). In addition, specialists working in the community will need to consider how to document and communicate on HIPAA-compliant platforms to adhere to the *Child*

Life Code of Ethics (ACLP, 2020). There are several platforms available for specialists to choose from. Weighing out the pros and cons for each will help in the decision-making for their business plan.

Figure 1. Flowchart of business preparation steps

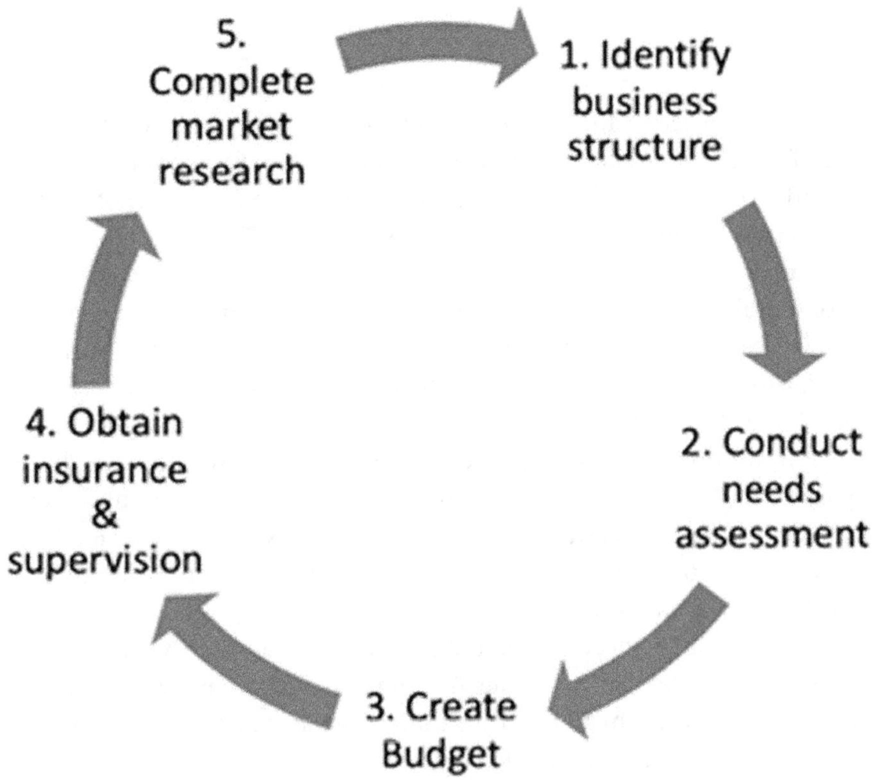

When determining the fee structure, it is essential to consider various aspects.

- *Your client:* Whom will you be working with? What is their primary concern or need?
- *Geography:* Where do you plan to practice? Consider whether you live or work in a major city or a rural setting. What is the gross household income for people that live in your area?
- *Like-services:* What do similarly educated professionals charge in your area?
- *Location of service:* Will you be traveling to work with the client in their home or meeting in a central community space? How far are you willing to travel? Will there be additional costs for mileage outside of your central zone? If renting a space, consider the overhead costs associated with your business budget.
- *Creating content:* If you are creating content that will be presented to a community organization, you need to consider the time and effort that will be given. The service fee may not just include an hourly rate for the actual presentation but the preparation time associated with it.

Other aspects include the training, education, and professional years of experience in the field. For example, a CCLS with six years of experience and a bachelor's may have a different fee than a CCLS with over fifteen years of experience and a master's. Additionally, consider if child life specialists are traveling with bridge tolls, gas costs, and parking fees and providing all materials for in-home sessions, renting an office space, or conducting sessions virtually. All aspects contribute to the overall cost it takes to run the business.

Billing

Given that the profession of child life is not yet a billable service in the United States, many private practice specialists find it challenging to bill insurance companies for the services provided. Therefore, some specialists will provide a superbill to clients when insurance is not accepted. A superbill is a paid invoice with an itemized list of services the client has received. The superbill will have the child life specialist's contact information, National Provider Identification (NPI), the service that was provided using Current Procedural Terminology (CPT) codes, and the total amount the client paid. The National Provider Number is a ten-digit number used to identify the health care provider in HIPAA standard transactions. Specialists can apply for an NPI number at the National Plan and Provider Enumeration System (Applying for an NPI Number, 2020). Current Procedural Terminology (CPT code) are medical codes that healthcare professionals use to describe diagnoses, services, medical procedures, and administrative purposes. (American Medical Association, n.d.). The CCLS must, however, use caution when using a CPT code. The CPT code should not be confused with diagnosing. As the CCLS is not a professional who diagnoses or treats medical or mental health conditions, it is advised not to provide a diagnosis code on billing documents.

Some specialists have found success in getting families reimbursed when fees are paid through a Health Savings Account or Flexible Spending Account offered by many insurance plans. Still, most specialists bill on a fee-for-service model with a sliding scale fee structure. This means that families pay the specialist directly for the services and cannot receive reimbursement from their health insurance plan. Child life specialists may also do contractual work with an organization for services. They can provide the service to the family referred by the organization and then bill the organization directly. Grants have also been used in the community to pay for services and not charge families directly.

Budget

Many child life specialists who start a practice must supplement their income in other ways. Some will continue to work within a hospital or take a part-time adjunct teaching job. Saving money to stay afloat and pay bills is a priority while laying the foundation to launch a practice. It can be a challenge to think about what the budget of a business will be. There are so many things to consider. Looking through the provided checklist will help with creating the budget.

Typically, some of the more costly items in the budget are renting office space, supplies, travel, reflective supervision, and childcare for those who have children. However, there are ways to manage the budget to fit needs effectively. For example, job supplies such as art and play materials do not have to be brand new. A child life specialist can gather many of these supplies by reaching out to friends and family, local community programs, garage sales, and social media marketplaces. Local pediatric offices may also donate medical and dental supplies.

Child life programs in the hospital are typically also on tight budgets, so having that experience will help to navigate this new business venture. Many hospitals rely on donations from nonprofits. These nonprofits have a mission to support pediatric patients and families coping with illness or hospitalizations. Many of these same organizations are also happy to support child life programs within the community. Contacting and educating them can be another opportunity to gain supplies for clients and help bring awareness to their nonprofit within the community. As the practice continues to grow, the budget will also begin to expand. It may have more income flowing making it possible to invest back into the business. There may be more money to purchase new supplies or invest in professional development.

Some things that should not be skipped in planning are liability insurance, adequate HIPAA-compliant documentation, and reflective supervision. These all fall under the ethical and professional standards of being a Certified Child Life Specialist. Child life specialists must follow the ACLP *Standards of Clinical Practice* for appropriate documentation and confidentiality (ACLP, 2020).

Behind the Scenes

Much like in a hospital setting, the private practice child life specialist has numerous behind-the-scenes responsibilities. In a hospital setting, people only see the play and interventions. They do not see charting, team meetings, toy cleaning, budgeting, and volunteer supervision. Private practice operates in a very similar way. Below are some examples of the breakdown of private practice's visible and hidden responsibilities. Remember, each child's life specialist's experience in private practice will be different. Therefore, the examples below should not be taken as prescriptive.

Example 1

The Certified Child Life Specialist (CCLS) has been practicing for more than seventeen years and has been in private practice for twelve. This CCLS holds advanced degrees and certifications, including a doctorate. The CCLS practices online and holds other responsibilities outside of the practice. A full caseload for the CCLS is 10 to 12 clients. The CCLS does not spend any time on social media; instead, she focuses on presenting and publishing.

Example 2

The Certified Child Life Specialist has been practicing for more than fifteen years, has been in private practice for seven, and holds an advanced degree and certifications. The CCLS provides in-home child life services, leads workshops within the community, and contracts with local agencies to support clients. The CCLS also presents to child life students regionally and nationally and has a solid social media presence.

Table 2. Full caseload example: The following is a week's glance of two Certified Child Life Specialists when the caseload is full

Responsibility	Example 1 Hours Per Week	Example 2 Hours Per Week
Direct client work	10	8-10
Indirect client work (charting, session prep, ordering materials, supply cleaning, driving).	5-6	10-12
Payment spreadsheet, budgeting, and scheduling	1	3
Networking with community agencies	0	1
Referral contact and follow up	2-3	1-2
Presentation preparation & content creation	2	1
Publishing work	1	1
Social media and marketing	1-2	4-5
Reflective supervision, continued education, collaborative work	2	2
Total Hours Per week	27 hours, only 10 of direct client work	37 hours, only 8-10 of direct client work

Table 3. Low caseload example: The following is a week's glance of two Certified Child Life Specialists when the caseload is low

Responsibility	Example 1 Hours Per Week	Example 2 Hours Per Week
Direct client work	4	6
Indirect client work (charting, session prep, ordering materials).	2	6-8
Payment spreadsheet, budgeting, and scheduling	1	2-3
Networking with community agencies	5	4
Presentation preparation & content creation	5	3
Publishing work	6	2
Social media and marketing	2	6-7
Reflective supervision, continued education, collaborative work	2	3-4
Total Hours Per week	27 hours, only 4 are direct client work	37 hours, only 6 of direct client work

FUTURE OF CHILD LIFE IN PRIVATE PRACTICE

There is exponential growth each year in the child life profession, with new specialists becoming certified and entering the field. There has also been more awareness of the scope of practice and the transferable skills that child life specialists have to serve in community settings. Child life specialists have begun to push out of their typical role within the hospital setting and fulfill the large gap in service within the community. Ideally, Certified Child Life Specialists should be available in every community. Having a child life specialist collaborate with community organizations, such as school districts, bereavement centers, and free-standing pediatric facilities, will continue to fill a significant gap in service to best support the needs of children and families. It will also create job opportunities and bring greater awareness to the child life profession. Lastly, as the United States continues to expand and improve the healthcare system, we may soon see a time when child life services can be reimbursable through insurance providers.

Table 4. Supplemental materials private practice checklist: Use the checklist below to help organize your practice before you take on clients

Item	Check off when complete.
County & State Requirements for having a business (Business license)	
Liability Insurance	
Intake Form(s)	
Client Agreement/Policy Form(s)	
Photo Release & Consent Forms	
HIPAA Compliant Documentation	
HIPAA Release Form	
Budget	
Reflective Supervision	
Fee Structure (slide scale)	
Billing & Payment Options	
Supplies	
Travel Cost	
Physical or Virtual Office	
Sole Proprietor, LLC, Business Ownership	
Marketing & Outreach	
Website, Business Cards	
Continued Education & Training	
Child Life Certification	
Full Time or Part Time	
Phone, email	

REFERENCES

American Medical Association. (n.d.). *CPT® overview and code approval.* Retrieved March 25, 2022, from https://www.ama-assn.org/practice-management/cpt/cpt-overview-and-code-approval

Applying for a National Provider Identifier number. (2020). *Comphealth.* Retrieved March 25, 2022, from https://comphealth.com/resources/national-provider-identifier-npi/

Association of Child Life Professionals. (2001). *Mission, values, vision, and operating principles.* https://www.childlife.org/docs/default-source/the-child-life-profession/mission-vision-values.pdf

Association of Child Life Professionals. (2016). *Child life competencies.* https://www.childlife.org/docs/default-source/aclp-official-documents/child-life-competencies_november-2019-updates.pdf

Association of Child Life Professionals. (2018). *2018 ACLP member survey*. https://www.childlife.org/docs/default-source/default-document-library/aclp-2018-year-in-review.pdf?sfvrsn=454cb24d_4

Association of Child Life Professionals. (2020). *Child life code of ethics.* https://www.childlife.org/docs/default-source/aclp-official-documents/child-life-code-of-ethics4232ee9c90156ede9dafff00004f030f.pdf?sfvrsn=5327804d_2

Association of Child Life Professionals. (2020). *Standards and guidelines for child life practice in community-based and non-traditional settings.* https://www.childlife.org/docs/default-source/aclp-official-documents/community-based-standards-and-guidelines_final-approved.pdf

Association of Child Life Professionals. (n.d.). *Position statement on diversity, equity, and inclusion.* https://www.childlife.org/docs/default-source/aclp-official-documents/statement-on-diversity-equity-and-inclusion.pdf

Bethell, C. D., Kogan, M. D., Strickland, B. B., Schor, E. L., Robertson, J., & Newacheck, P. W. (2011). A national and state profile of leading health problems and health care quality for U.S. children: Key insurance disparities and across-state variations. *Academic Pediatrics, 11*(3), S22–S33. doi:10.1016/j.acap.2010.08.011 PMID:21570014

Brown, C., Mattera, G., Millar, T., Palm, S., & Rode, D. (2018). *Clinical Supervision Position Statement of the Child Life Council.* https://citeseerx.ist.psu.edu/viewdoc/download?doi=10.1.1.690.7183&rep=rep1&type=pdf

Centers for Disease Control and Prevention. (2022, January 24). *Chronic diseases in America.*https://www.cdc.gov/chronicdisease/resources/infographic/chronic-diseases.htm

Child Life Council. (2006). *Guidelines for the development of child life programs in health care settings* (4th ed.). CLC.

Cover, L. (2021, August 18). 7 statistics that prove the importance of social media marketing in business. *Sprout Social.* https://sproutsocial.com/insights/importance-of-social-media-marketing-in-business/

Dehlin, M., & Lundh, L. G. (2018). Compassion fatigue and compassion satisfaction among psychologists: Can supervision and a reflective stance be of help? *Journal for Person-Oriented Research, 4*(2), 95–107. doi:10.17505/jpor.2018.09 PMID:33569136

Edgar-Bailey, M., & Kress, V. E. (2010). Resolving child and adolescent traumatic grief: Creative techniques and interventions. *Journal of Creativity in Mental Health, 5*(2), 158–176. doi:10.1080/15401383.2010.485090

Fraser, C., CCLS, C., & Munn, E. K. (2020). *The Value of Certified Child Life Specialists: Direct and Downstream Optimization of Pediatric Patient and Family Outcomes.* Academic Press.

Housman, D. K. (2017). The importance of emotional competence and self-regulation from birth: A case for the evidence-based emotional cognitive social early learning approach. *International Journal of Child Care and Education Policy, 11*(1), 1–19. doi:10.118640723-017-0038-6

Kase, S. M., Waldman, E. D., & Weintraub, A. S. (2018). Compassion fatigue, burnout, and compassion satisfaction in pediatric palliative care (P.C.) providers in the U.S. *Pediatrics, 142*(1). Advance online publication. doi:10.1542/peds.142.1MA7.672

Knill, P. J., Levine, E. G., & Levine, S. K. (2005). *Principles and practice of expressive arts therapy: Toward a therapeutic aesthetics*. Jessica Kingsley Publishers.

Koller, D. (2007). Preparing children and adolescents for medical procedures. *Child Life Council Evidence-Based Practice Statement,* 1-13.

Landreth, G. L. (2002). *Play therapy: The art of the relationship*. Brunner-Routledge.

Landrethh, G. L., & Ray, D. C. (2019, September). Child-centered play therapy. *Play Therapy, 14*(3), 18–19.

Lazarus, R. S., & Folkman, S. (1984). *Stress, appraisal, and coping*. Springer Publishing Company.

Lerwick, J. (2019). An Exploration of the Roles of Certified Child Life Specialists & Registered Play Therapists in the United States. *International Journal of Pediatric Research, 5*, 49. doi:10.23937/2469-5769/1510049

Longbottom, S., & Slaughter, V. (2018). Sources of children's knowledge about death and dying. *Philosophical Transactions of the Royal Society B: Biological Sciences, 373*(1754). doi:10.1098/rstb.2017.0267

McQuarrie, E. F. (2015). *The market research toolbox: A concise guide for beginners*. Sage Publications.

Pediatric Hospitalization. (n.d.). *Connecticut Hospital Association.* Retrieved March 6, 2022, from https://cthosp.org/advocacy/quality-and-patient-safety/patients-guide-to-quality-hospital-care/pediatric-hospitalization/

Pew Research Center. (2021). *Social media fact sheet.* https://www.pewresearch.org/internet/factsheet/social-media/

Romito, B., Jewell, J., Jackson, M., Ernst, K., Hill, V., Hsu, B., Lam, V., Mauro-Small, M., & Vinocur, C. (2021). Child life services. *Pediatrics, 147*(1). Advance online publication. doi:10.1542/peds.2020-040261 PMID:33372119

Ventola, C. L. (2014). Social media and health care professionals: Benefits, risks, and best practices. *P&T, 39*(7), 491–499. https://www.ncbi.nlm.nih.gov/pmc/articles/PMC4103576/ PMID:25083128

Wang, A. L. (2022, February 10). *What is an LLC? Pros and cons of a limited liability company*. Nerdwallet. https://www.nerdwallet.com/article/small-business/starting-successful-llc#benefits-of-an-llc

Wittenberg, E., Saada, A., & Prosser, L. A. (2013). How illness affects family members: A qualitative interview survey. *The Patient-Patient-Centered Outcomes Research, 6*(4), 257–268. doi:10.100740271-013-0030-3 PMID:24142495

Wood, M. (2020, December 16). *The advantages and disadvantages of sole proprietorship*. Nerdwallet. https://www.nerdwallet.com/article/small-business/advantages-of-a-sole-proprietorship

KEY TERMS AND DEFINITIONS

Advocacy: A strategy to help empower children and families to participate in their healthcare experiences.

Business Plan: The process of identifying the type of business that will be operated, creating budget, and understanding the financial responsibility as it relates to taxes and liability.

Child-Centered Play: Therapeutic play technique that supports a child through nonjudgmental, unconditional positive regard and empathy.

Clinical Supervision: Enables individual practitioners to develop knowledge and skills, assume responsibility for their practice, and is central to the ongoing process of professional growth and learning.

Comprehensive Assessment: The second point of entry when working with a client. More detailed information including history and background of presenting problem is gathered from the primary caregiver

CPT Code: Current Procedural Terminology are treatment codes for medical services and procedures that medical providers use for uniform documentation.

Expressive Arts: The use of modalities such as movement, visual arts, music, writing, and nature targeted to address the specific non-verbal, social emotional needs of clients.

Hold Harmless Form: A contract between the practitioner and client that protects the practitioner from the potential liability of injury or damages.

Intake Assessment: The first point of entry when working with a client. Each is unique to the private practice and should reflect questions based on the area of specialty and services available.

Limited Liability Company: Self-employed business that protects individual of personal assets.

Market Research: A process undertaken by the business owner to understand their ideal client's needs, desires, and interests by setting fees and offering target services within a community.

NPI Number: National Provider Identifier is a ten-digit number HIPAA requires of medical professionals providing services.

Private Practice: Self-employed private practitioner serving clients.

Referral Network: A collaborative effort among outside agencies that provide clients to the private practice.

Reflective Supervision: Targets specific issues within clinical practice and seeks to decrease the potential of burnout and compassion fatigue by focusing on the supervisee's emotional experiences in clinical work.

Scope of Practice: The ethical standards to practice within a set of clinical parameters specific to the training and skills of a child life specialist.

Sole Proprietor: Self-employed business owner that can keep all profits after taxes.

Superbill: A paid invoice with an itemized list of services the client has received.

Chapter 17
Virtual Platforms

Katie Taylor
Child Life On Call LLC, USA

ABSTRACT

Americans spend large portions of their day online. Data shows that there are more than 245 million internet users in the U.S. alone. This data, combined with what we observe in healthcare trends, including tele-med and other virtual options, demonstrates the need for child life services to be available online. This chapter explores the various ways child life specialists can use their skills to support children and families using digital tools. Embracing technology and exploring innovative approaches will only enhance and validate the field of child life.

INTRODUCTION

There has been a dramatic increase in the use of digital tools that can enhance, replace, or reinforce typical interactions that were once only possible when meeting in the same physical space. There are more than 4.66 billion internet users worldwide (Lambert, 2022).

The trend of people spending much of their time online demonstrates the need for Certified Child Life Specialists (CCLSs) to comply with the changing world and adapt their services to include virtual settings and online platforms. Digital habits provide an opportunity to increase awareness about the psychosocial needs of children and families and an opportunity to spread awareness about the child life profession.

As the child life profession integrates into the ever-changing and fast-paced world of digital resources, the field can look for new ways to diversify and expand the child life specialist's skill set. There has been dramatic growth in digital resources and programming. Audio stories, specifically podcasts, have grown in popularity due to their accessibility and affordability. In 2017, the number of podcast listeners in the United States was about 46 million. In 2022, the number has doubled to almost 88 million (Statista, 2022). Within the field of child life, blogs, social media posts, videos, and websites that address the needs of children and families affected by illness and healthcare have been on the rise. Examples include websites and online tools maintained and published by hospitals, child life specialists, and other child life community organizations. The child life profession originated within hospitals and has adapted to expand to community settings. The same expansion mindset can be applied to virtual platforms. Increased

DOI: 10.4018/978-1-6684-5097-0.ch017

awareness of the child life profession in digital media has created an opportunity to bring exposure to the field. This chapter will describe various virtual methods and online tools that Certified Child Life Specialists could use while staying within their scope of practice as defined by the Association for Child Life Professionals Standards of Clinical Practice (*Standards of clinical practice chapter 4*, n.d.). Throughout the chapter, patient is used when referring to children in hospital settings, and client is used when working with children in the community, including virtual spaces.

BACKGROUND

As a result of the Covid-19 pandemic, new, virtual-based opportunities arose that were modeled after existing programs like music therapy. These new opportunities opened up new possibilities for research in those fields. Nonprofit organizations successfully integrated telehealth into their programming by providing additional online services for children of adult patients in conjunction with their established in-person support. Many, like Project Sunshine, have continued with virtual programming, offering video calls facilitated by volunteers promoting play and normalization activities during hospital stays (projectsunshine.org). Another organization, JoyRx, supports children's emotional needs through the use of music, offering online jam sessions, lessons, or mini concerts with musicians (joyrx.com). Finding new opportunities for child life specialists to learn about and use the virtual tools available to expand their practice grows each day.The focus on technology and its effect on our society's ability to communicate and interact has become a crash course in finding answers to the question: How do virtual interventions work? Are they successful?

According to a study in a New York City intensive care unit among those who lost their loved ones, remote family visits to intensive care units evoked feelings of happiness, joy, gratitude, and relief (Sasangohar et al., 2021). Neurological music therapists used telehealth and found they could transfer their services effectively from in-person to telehealth for all domains (sensorimotor, cognitive, and communication), especially when caregivers were involved (Cole et al., 2021).

Providing services virtually expands child life specialists' ability to reach more than just patients and families who walk through the doors of hospitals or other community-based settings. This dramatic growth in scope can meet the needs of more diverse groups of families who benefit from child life services.

One currently underserved population of pediatric patients that could benefit from virtual child life services is those who are diagnosed with a chronic condition but seldom hospitalized for their diagnosis. In 2013, only five percent of children with asthma were hospitalized. (CDC, 2013). This statistic sheds light on the enormous opportunity for child life services to meet the psychosocial needs of children and families affected by chronic illness who are rarely hospitalized. Every child deserves emotionally safe care, and technology affords this opportunity (Every child deserves emotionally safe care, 2021).

Child life interventions directly intended for children and families, like promoting positive coping, providing medical education, and evidenced-based preparation techniques can all be provided virtually. Online interventions expand a spectrum of diverse opportunities, from customized interventions to more general education. Examples of online interventions and uses are a child life specialist using telehealth to prepare a patient for an upcoming medical procedure, facilitating a virtual visit to a classroom to talk about a classmate's diagnosis, or a parent receiving tips from a child life influencer using social media to provide education. Expanding child life services to digital platforms increases the integration of family-centered care practices in meaningful ways. The stress of diagnosis can negatively impact caregivers, who are susceptible to the negative effects of high levels of burden and psychological morbidity (Newman et al., 2019). A public health journal published findings on the role of internet-based digital tools in reducing social isolation and addressing support needs among informal caregivers. The findings suggested that internet-based digital tools can be a cost-effective and convenient way to develop programs that help unpaid caregivers form communities, gain support, and access resources. Service providers can also leverage digital tools to deliver support to caregivers within online communities (Newman et al., 2019). Child life specialists with training and clinical experience working with children and families in hospitals have an opportunity to fill gaps in service by transferring skills from in-person to online (Newman et al., 2019).

DIGITAL PLATFORMS

Podcasts

One area child life specialists have expanded is podcasts. One out of every three podcast listeners in the US says they enjoy tuning in to podcasts to learn new things, gain inspiration, be entertained, or follow the news. Child life specialists have also branched out into this medium (Statista, 2019).

Each year, unique podcasts related to the field grow in popularity, demonstrating how child life services are expanding and exploring new audio mediums. Many podcasts share platforms and basic technology yet are diverse enough to generate interest in a wide range of topics that are relevant to the field. The following is a small sample of podcasts that are related to the child life field.

Table 1. Topics and podcast titles

Topic	[Audio Podcast] Title
Amplifying young adult and adolescent experiences during cancer treatment	Children's Hospital of Philadelphia. *AYA Cancer Chat: Life Interrupted* Penn State Health. *Life on Pause*
Parent and caregiver experiences in having a child with illness, disease, or a medical diagnosis	Cheney, M. *The Rare Life* Given, C. *Mindset for Medical Moms* Kozar, R. *Living with Scanxiety* Parks, E. *Once Upon A Gene* Taylor, K. *Child Life On Call*
Parents with children who have special and sensory needs and/or Autism Spectrum Disorder (AS)	Dawkins, G., *The Parenting Cipher* Hall, M., *Markeisha Hall Podcast* Patay, J., *We Are Brave Together* Ryska, K., *The Special Needs Mom Podcast*
Child Life Professionals	Association for Child Life Professionals., *#childlife* Lowry, G. Porter, R *Coping Kit for Everyday Life* Lewin, J., *Child Life Wild Life Podcast* Jones, A., *Child Life Cooperative* Taylor, K. *Child Life On Call*

A child life specialist must first identify a need for a podcast before creating one. Child life specialists may want to use podcasts to connect with others who share their interest in using podcasting to help children and families, especially caregivers who struggle with finding others going through similar experiences (Family Caregiver Alliance, 2012). Child life specialists might also be interested in helping educate people about the field of child life and inform them about opportunities available in the field. Podcasting allows professionals in the field to share their knowledge and expertise while providing an opportunity to connect with others who may be interested in the profession.

Social Media

Social media platforms provide child life professionals with a way to share their knowledge, education, and experiences with others they might not otherwise meet. Social media offers a platform that helps build community, connection, awareness, and understanding inside and outside hospitals. Child life specialists using social media engagement are educating healthcare users and professionals about ways to support children and families during healthcare experiences by sharing ideas, programs, educational opportunities, and strategies reaching far beyond the medical center's walls.

Online Networking and App Development

Online platforms that specifically target children who face illnesses and hospitalizations have been developed to reduce social isolation and foster connection among these individuals. Two examples of organizations that offer such services are Upopolis.com, which provides a safe, fun, and secure environment for young people to connect with each other and their peers who are going through similar experiences and Get Your Play On(line) which provides virtual play opportunities using video tutorials. Both these examples of websites provide an online space for children and families to engage in a safe environment.

Child life specialists are currently using digital media resources such as tablet-based preparation books and kid-friendly apps for distraction and normalization during interventions. Child life specialists have been involved in the development of apps that support the psychosocial needs of children and families. For example, Simply Sayin', created by the child life team at Phoenix Children, is an educational app using sensory language to explain medical conditions, treatments, and procedures. Child Life on Call LLC has developed a mobile app that helps support and empower parents of children who are hospitalized. The app provides information on how to best communicate with medical staff, how to cope with the stress of hospitalization, and how caregivers can advocate for their child's care. The app also includes a directory of care team members and resources for families to empower caregivers to support their child through a hospital stay.

ACCESS AND EQUITY

There are both benefits and challenges of using telehealth-type technologies with children and families within and outside the hospital setting. Families living in internet deserts or those coming from low socioeconomic backgrounds may be at a higher risk of not having access to telehealth services than others. Not all patients have access to or use devices, cellular data, or internet services necessary to engage in virtual visits (American Medical Association, 2020). Patients with Medicaid or Medicaid waiver insurance coverage were less likely to have access to these tools than those with commercial health plans (Webber et al., 2022).

In 2021 millions of households across America, disproportionately among minority groups, rural areas, and poor households, lacked reliable and accessible internet connectivity (Fourteenth, 2021). Data indicates that 80% of White adults in the US report having a broadband connection. Among Black and Hispanic respondents, it was 71% and 65%, respectively. (*Internet/broadband fact sheet*, 2021). Poor internet connections in remote rural areas cause difficulties for families making online visits or accessing information on the web. Because of this, child life specialists must consider diversity, equity, and inclusivity factors that may affect virtual interventions. Other challenges include family comfort with technology, the ability to problem solve technical difficulties, and the potential impact on therapeutic relationships (Kraus et al., 2022). However widespread and available digital tools may be, child life specialists must consider how technology access, use, and acceptance varies within families. Some children and their parents don't feel comfortable using technology, have not used virtual tools before, and may be hesitant to use them. Broadband adoption is important for households' ability to successfully use digital tools like telehealth (Seidemann & Barboza, 2021).

Child life specialists should ensure that their materials are inclusive and accessible to people with disabilities and developmental variations, including recording videos and providing closed captions, using chat boxes to share information, and adjusting visits to meet family's needs. Child life specialists should adapt the technology to meet the needs of individuals and families instead of increasing existing disparities in public health (Beaunoyer et al., 2020).

TELEHEALTH

Child life specialists provide a safe, therapeutic environment for people of all ages (Official Documents, Child Life Competencies, 2019). Child life specialists must create virtual environments that are safe, therapeutic, and healing. Digital access enables the CCLS to meet parents where they live rather than in an unfamiliar location. Hospitalized patients who experience a loss of control by being in an unfamiliar environment suffer from some negative consequences. These negative consequences are lessened if the patient's family stays in his/her home environment (Williams et al., 2008). Disruptions in the home that may impact a virtual child life session are similar to those experienced by child life specialists when healthcare professionals enter the room. Child life specialists should be proactive in developing plans with families to solve technical issues.

Other clinical and medical practitioners, including physicians, nurses, and psychotherapists, successfully use virtual options for interventions with children and families (Schniering et al., 2022). Online therapy between children, adolescents, and therapists has been shown to be effective in treating various mental and behavioral health needs (Schueller et al., 2017). Telehealth is now increasingly used to expand the geographic reach of health care services and improve access to care. Factors such as convenience and efficiency, among others, have been identified by patients as important reasons for using telehealth (Gajarawala & Pelkowski, 2021). Child life specialists have previously experienced challenges with in-person support groups or working with patient siblings because child life specialists do not always have the resources to accommodate family barriers like travel, childcare, and work schedules. There are several benefits to using telehealth to communicate between patients and their providers, including no transportation times or costs, decreased need for childcare, online chat functions, same-day appointments, increased accessibility to specialists, decreased wait times, and sometimes even improved patient health (*Advantages of telemedicine for patients*, n.d.).

ASSESSMENT IN THE ONLINE ENVIRONMENT

The Association of Child Life Professionals states that child life specialists evaluate the developmental and psychological needs of infants, children and youth, and their families (Association of Child Life Professionals, 2017). According to The Handbook of Child Life: A Guide for Pediatric Psychosocial Care (2018), child life specialists need to know how to gather information from a variety of sources to assess child growth and development, family systems, and the potential impact of stress and healthcare experiences. A child life assessment involves asking questions about the family and their past experiences, identifying developmental needs, and determining ways to help children feel comfortable during potentially stressful situations. Assessments are usually done through conversation with and observation of the child and family. Tools like the Psychosocial Risk Assessment in Pediatrics (PRAP) developed by Cincinnati Children's Hospital Medical Center (2013) and the Stress Potential Assessment Model (Gaynard et al.,1990) help child life specialists determine needs, interventions, and resources (p.40). Observing children at play and observing their responses to stressful events such as illnesses, separation from loved ones, or unfamiliar healthcare professionals helps child life specialists collaborate with multidisciplinary teams to develop plans of care.

Assessments in virtual environments may look different, but the goals, skills, and knowledge used are the same. Child life specialists rely on their professional assessment and decision-making skills to determine which technologies and delivery methods best meet the needs of children and families and keen observation skills during virtual sessions to assess the needs and goals of the child and family.

Assessment is key to a successful virtual meeting. Initial information gathering can be completed by phone, using a survey, and email. Child life specialists can look to child life specialists working in private practice and fields such as music therapy (*COVID-19 resources - telehealth considerations and resources*, n.d.), online counseling, and play therapy to adapt documents for virtual services. These documents include but are not limited to informed consent, confidentiality agreements, waiver of liability, virtual practice guidelines, and include statements regarding that child life services are not a replacement for psychotherapy from a licensed professional. For example, Child Life on Call, a podcast that interviews families with special healthcare needs, uses a document that guests complete prior to meeting with the host. Using this document, the host of Child Life on Call talks with potential guests to assess the readiness of those wanting to share their stories. This helps to learn guests' intentions and goals regarding what they want to share publicly and the type of support they will need. Similarly, when planning a telehealth visit with children, talking with parents prior to a virtual session leads to a better understanding of needs, expectations, and supports in the home that is vital to a successful virtual intervention.

TRAUMA INFORMED CARE

Trauma-Informed Interventions involve an empathetic, compassionate approach to recognizing and addressing the impact of trauma on individuals, their families, communities, and society (Goddard, 2021). Involving families in the process of setting up a secure and trustworthy environment for online interaction is key to providing safe, consistent, and supportive spaces. To ensure that children and families feel safe using a virtual environment, child life specialists must provide predictability, structure, and an opportunity for adaptation. Regularly connecting with and receiving feedback from parents and children helps the child life specialist assess the unique ways in which the child and family process information and support their children. Similar to a clinical setting, for a patient to assent or a family to consent, they must understand information regarding diagnosis, treatment, and care (Bester, Cole, and Kodish, 2016). Medical and psychosocial staff, including child life specialists, must adapt language and presentation to fit the needs of the family to increase understanding and obtain informed consent. Building rapport and establishing relationships is an important component of any intervention for a child life specialist, regardless of the environment. Due to topics discussed during virtual interventions, clients and caregivers may feel overwhelmed. Creating a plan of care to address those moments empowers children and families. Discussion with older children, teens, and caregivers regarding different levels of comfort with certain topics, signs of stress and discomfort, and what resources and support are available during and post-sessions lead to the development and use of coping tools. Encouraging the natural role of the family as supportive, ongoing, and those who know their child best empowers children, teens, and caregivers to advocate for themselves and their children (Gaynard et al., 1998). Encouraging parental involvement in care decisions improves child symptoms and increases positive parenting practices (Ashcraft et al., 2019).

PATIENT AND FAMILY CENTERED CARE

Patient-and Family-Centered Care practices are to support patients' and families' ability to take an active role in their own care (Institute for Patient and Family Centered Care, 2022). Child life specialists' use of technology promotes collaboration among patients and families and helps them gain greater control over their lives. Considering parents' beliefs and attitudes about online learning is equally important. How parents feel about the use of online tools can influence the quality and quantity of online learning opportunities and experiences (Erdogan et al., 2018). For example, when used for therapeutic interventions, patients who received speech therapy with their mothers showed a significant improvement in language skills than those who did not receive speech therapy with their mothers (Pamplona, 2000). Therefore, child life specialists must attend to caregiver buy-in and include caregivers in discussions and involvement throughout the treatment plan to increase the success of an intervention.

For example, a child life specialist is consulted to conduct a virtual support session for a family whose youngest daughter was given a new diagnosis. After completing the assessment, the child life specialist begins the intervention and suggests a personalized e-book. The child life specialist and parent(s) collaborated to create an e-booklet for the child, recognizing that this tool can lead to better learning experiences for younger children (Huang, 2012). Working together, the CCLS and parents provided psychosocial support and developmentally appropriate information about complex diagnoses, treatment, and hospitalization in a format that was familiar to the child, created by those who know the child best and grounded in research. See *figure 1*.

The graphic in figure 1 shows two pages of a storybook with text and pictures.

Figure 1. Caregiver collaboration tool for parent-led discussion with the child

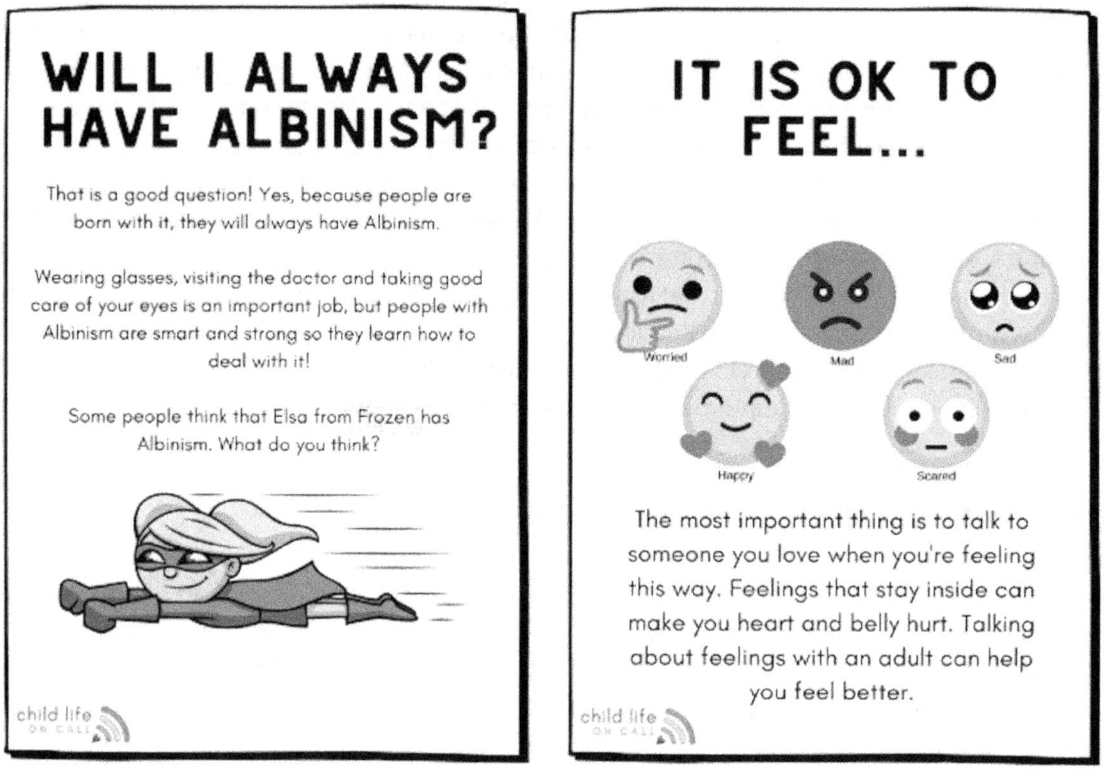
WILL I ALWAYS HAVE ALBINISM?
That is a good question! Yes, because people are born with it, they will always have Albinism.
Wearing glasses, visiting the doctor and taking good care of your eyes is an important job, but people with Albinism are smart and strong so they learn how to deal with it!
Some people think that Elsa from Frozen has Albinism. What do you think?
IT IS OK TO FEEL...
Worried
Mad
Sad
Happy
Scared
The most important thing is to talk to someone you love when you're feeling this way. Feelings that stay inside can make you heart and belly hurt. Talking about feelings with an adult can help you feel better.

Child life services provides a multidimensional lens that focuses on both patients and their families, which is an essential part of resilience building ("Value Proposition Statement", 2020). When planning for virtual visits, CCLS must consider the lived experiences, cultural backgrounds, values, and beliefs of families (Institute for Patient and Family Centered Care, 2022) Virtual visits have the capacity to be more flexible and accommodating around work schedules, school hours, and the needs and activities of other children. Using a "parent empowerment" approach found that children's progress is accelerated when parents feel heard and cared for (Sherred, 2019).

Recent hospital protocols in response to Covid-19 restricted patients' social networks from visiting them in healthcare settings. This limitation of visitors in health care settings caused people to adapt by using video calls or conferencing applications (Hugelius et al., 2020). By April 2020, there were 300 million people who used Zoom™ every day, compared to just ten million in December 2019 (Vailshery, 2022). Child life specialists recognized a need to find innovative ways to continue family support and connection. Pre-pandemic NICU settings have used cameras to allow caregivers to watch babies when they were not able to be with them (Epstein, 2017). Additionally, live and recorded music has been used to support bonding and attachment between parents and babies during their absence. Child life specialists recognizing the importance of these opportunities to connect children with their families expanded upon them during the pandemic in innovative ways to help children and families thrive.

An example of this during a virtual visit is when a mother described that "Face Timing grandma" was the highlight of her child's daily routine. Recognizing the importance of the grandmother's relationship, the CCLS integrated virtual visits between the child and the grandmother as part of the child's coping plan for upcoming medical procedures.

Follow-up is equally important in virtual spaces as in traditional healthcare settings providing summaries of the visits, discussing any developmental concerns, and recommending additional resources when necessary. Because the child life specialist cannot physically check in with families or patients, providing a follow-up phone call, post email, or document that reinforces what was discussed, a review of skills, coping tools, and practice guides reinforce patient and family-centered care goals of information sharing, collaboration, and participation (ipfcc.org, 2022).

COMPONENTS OF A CHILD LIFE VIRTUAL SESSION

Rapport

Rapport building remains the same regardless of location. A common way of building rapport with children is by asking them open-ended questions about things they are interested in or things that are important to them (Myers & APSAC (American Professional Society on the Abuse of Children), 2010). Child life specialists use familiar games, puzzles, books, and coloring with children to help establish rapport. While these techniques typically require shared physical space, they can be adapted using whiteboards, online games, and spinners.

Child life specialists must also recognize the importance of choice and control in the online setting. Some families may need more time before allowing others to view their homes. Allowing the patient or family to keep their video off and only use the voice feature in virtual settings can effectively promote control, choice, and comfort with the platform.

Play

Play is essential to development because it contributes to children and youth's cognitive, physical, social, and emotional well-being (Ginsburg et al., 2007). Play can be used as a vital tool to assess and create developmentally appropriate interventions that support the child's ability to cope (Burns-Nader & Hernandez-Reif, 2014). In addition, play is how children cope. Child life specialists have used technology long before the most recent COVID-19 pandemic to support, educate and provide play opportunities that normalize the hospital environment, teach children about diagnoses, and support coping during procedural interventions (Burns-Nader, Joe, and Pinion, 2017). Play is childhood's most prominent and powerful adaptive modality (Yogman et al., 2018). Integrating play with technology is a practice that is currently being used by CCLS in traditional and community settings. Internet-, mobile-, and tablet-based apps are used to promote a sense of normalization, offer opportunities for alternative focus, and help build rapport. Play provides child life specialists with opportunities for continued assessment while deepening relationships and determining a plan of care for children and families (Turner, 2009). During virtual interventions facilitating play offers opportunities for purposeful rapport building, ongoing assessments, unbiased feedback, and adaptability. See *figure 2* as an example of a Google Slides room used for introductions, assessment, and rapport building. Examples of well-known, transferrable play activities include online games like Connect 4, I-spy, reading a book through the computer, and many others. Creating a plan beforehand and having multiple options for relationship building and conversation starters create opportunities to build rapport through play.

The graphic in figure 2 shows a virtual classroom with a CCLS avatar.

Figure 2. Interactive child life virtual room using google slides

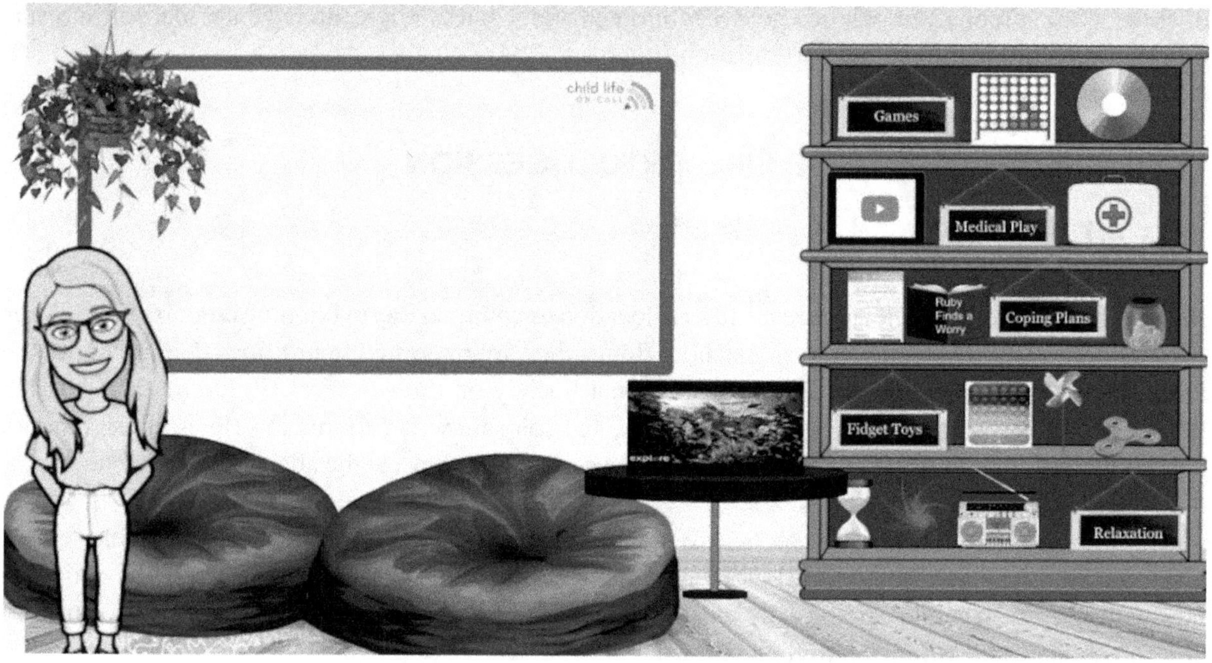

Preparation

Psychological preparation for medical procedures is an important job function of the child life specialist. It is estimated that between 50% and 75% of children develop some degree of preoperative anxiety (Eijlers et al., 2019). Some recognized risk factors for developing preoperative anxiety include age, temperament, previous medical experiences, and caregiver anxiety (William, 2007). The process of preparing children for medical procedures involves providing them with developmentally appropriate information, encouraging their questions and emotional expressions, and forming a trusting relationship with a healthcare provider (Child Life Council, 2009).

Using online video platforms for preparing a medical procedure is similar to doing so in a traditional environment. It is important for child life specialists to consider each patient's individual needs when using technology to provide preparation to reduce anxiety and improve coping skills for children (Osborne, 2018). Videos showing families in unfamiliar environments and audio depicting sounds from recorded medical equipment are often integrated into practice by child life specialists. While not in a shared space (e.g., a patient hospital room), the camera can show, teach, and describe sensory experiences. Screen sharing and screen mirrors can support these same techniques for virtual services.

Hands-on preparation with medical material, an effective practice of the child life specialist (Romito, 2019), is possible during virtual preparation if there is enough time and planning. Child life specialists are resourceful, using household, inexpensive materials and recyclables to create therapeutic activities or educational opportunities. Giving children choices about materials, activities, and surroundings can help children understand more about illness, treatment, and hospitalization (Wigfield et al., 2016).

Before an intervention, the child life specialist creates a plan to present the material in an online setting. An example of this would be an apprehensive eight-year-old struggling to cope with vaccinations. The CCLS recreating the experience online uses screen sharing technology to show the child the room where they would get vaccinated, allowing the child to interact with the image by clicking on the different parts of the room to access information, demonstrate coping strategies, identify roles and dismantle misconceptions. Child life specialists provide children with accurate developmentally age-appropriate explanations while supporting the use of coping tools in a non-threatening environment. See *figure 3.*

The graphic in figure 3 shows a gymnasium with two chairs and a table.

Figure 3. Interactive child life preparation room using google slides

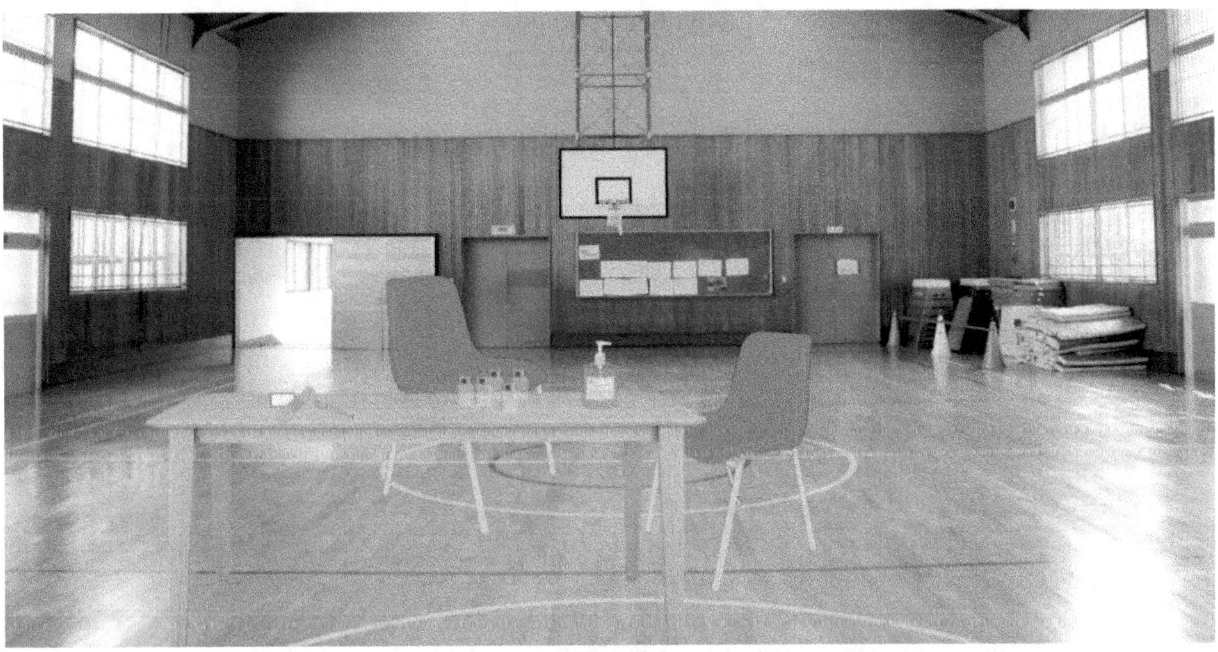

During the pandemic, many child life programs looked to enhance existing virtual programs and develop their own content for hospitalized children. Many institutions held video calls with patients and family members, recorded videos of child life specialists playing games, created medical models from everyday materials, and taught coping strategies to decrease anxiety. They offered virtual musical sing-alongs and explained why a doctor wears personal protective equipment, all in an effort to find innovative ways to continue to educate, prepare, and support children and families during the pandemic and beyond (Murcia, 2020).

Expressive Arts

Expressive arts use various modalities to help children express themselves, understand their feelings, and validate their own experiences. Expressive therapies include art, music, dance, movement, drama, poetry, creative writing, play, and sandbox therapy within psychotherapeutic, counseling, rehabilitative, or health care services (Hoffman, 2016). Children who participate in expressive art activities often experience improved mental health and increased social support (Malchiodi, 2005). These same benefits can exist when using virtual platforms to provide child life services.

Music, literature, and art may be used to enhance an intervention by providing additional means for patients to express their feelings and emotions. On the screen, collaboratively, the child life specialist and the patient can search through music, creating a playlist that promotes coping and calming. Artistic software such as Nathan Friend's (nathanfriend.io) enables the user to create images by drawing a spiral graph. Scrapcoloring.com is great for younger children exploring colors together, and Toytheater.com offers an assortment of art tools that allow for expression, exploration, and curiosity. These programs supported by a CCLS offer children opportunities to explore, express, and identify feelings through art and music.

Coping

Child life specialists are resilience-oriented and aim to promote coping abilities by providing different experiences for children (Boles et al., 2020). Engaging parents in the process is critical to encourage and optimizing patients coping plans and promoting resilience.

Visualizing potential coping skills during virtual visits helps children learn better by enhancing their learning processes (Shabiralyani et. al., 2015). The interactive virtual office (image 2) offers several well-known fidgets or relaxing options on the shelves to encourage deep breathing, develop visualizations, and progressive muscle relaxation. Each item on the image's shelf is a link to a website that can be accessed directly from the virtual office, providing more information and application. With the support of the CCLS, the child and/or their parents can discuss what works best for the child and practice using them. Practicing with the child life specialist supports the therapeutic relationship by increasing involvement and decision-making in the child's own healthcare.

Another tool used to promote coping is digital whiteboards. A whiteboard can be used for drawing, writing, and playing word games such as hospital Pictionary and word jumbles using medical terminology connected to the child's illness or hospitalization. Tools like these normalize the experience, provide choices, and teach new information. Using the digital whiteboard, child life specialists can ask children and adolescents to create lists specific to each child's experience, like "what I can control" or "what I can't control." They can create lists of questions to be asked of the health care team, supporting a child's sense of control and mastery over his/her own body. Maintaining an adaptive, inquisitive, and investigative outlook can help child life specialists find creative and appropriate tools for their patients. Existing tools already being used by other professions (e.g., teachers and counselors) can be used and adapted for supporting the child life specialist's virtual practice. The CCLS also encourages the child or teen to consider the use of these newly developed skills in other settings when interacting with new and unfamiliar environments and people.

SPECIAL CONSIDERATIONS

Pricing

The child life specialist should receive fair and adequate pay for services regardless of the environment. Market research should be conducted before developing products and services, and include pricing, user motivations, and access. Child life specialists should also consider their own years of experience, education, and training. It is also important to consider the costs and budget of starting and maintaining a virtual private practice or providing consulting for an organization or health care facility.

There is little research or preexisting information at this time that can guide the CCLS in creating a profitable and valuable online service. With the goal to serve families facing medical struggles, the cost may be considered a barrier for some families. This fact does not diminish the value of virtual interventions but is important to consider when creating non-discriminatory services.

As part of the discovery phase, the CCLS should research practitioners in their area providing similar services (e.g., life coaches, fitness trainers, and mindfulness coaches). All are health-focused, and most offer services online not typically covered by insurance. Payment methods can be fixed rates or more flexible depending on family needs, circumstances, and the comfort of the CCLS. One option is to have the client pay what they are able, which allows the CCLS, especially in the beginning, the opportunity to find a median number to begin charging for services. Another approach is creating a sliding scale for families or having a fixed rate based on the number of sessions with the ability to adapt to unique family circumstances as they surface.

Professional Boundaries

Virtual child life services have unique and challenging boundary issues. Digital platforms appear to have fewer restrictions due to a lack of connection to physical boundaries and time constraints. Using digital platforms often means child life specialists can meet families anytime rather than the typical 9-5. When "work" is in your home, it is harder to delineate professional and personal space. Establishing boundaries for oneself not only supports self-care, prevents burnout, and is also important to developing a therapeutic relationship with families. To maintain professionalism and boundaries, child life specialists could consider using neutral and non-identifiable images in the background setting of the screen. This can be easily achievable by using the virtual background options often given on platforms like Zoom™ or by setting up the camera so that there is a blank and un-distracting wall behind the child life specialist. Child life specialists can look to the Code of Professional Ethics by the Association of Child Life Professionals on topics like social media relationships with families (*Child Life Code of Ethics*. n.d.).

Therapeutic Relationships

Therapeutic relationships thrive when boundaries are set and followed from the beginning. Boundaries are established not only for the benefit of the child life specialist but also for the safety of the therapeutic relationship with the family. Collaborating with families amplifies their voice. Telepsychology has developed a list of best practices that could be adapted for use by child life specialists working in virtual spaces with children and families. Drum and Littleton (2014):

1. Maintain professional hours and respect the timing of sessions.
2. Ensure timely and consistent feedback and manage excessive communications.
3. Ensure a private, consistent, professional, and culturally sensitive setting.
4. Ensure privacy of non-clients and prevent unintentional self-disclosures.
5. Ensure that telecommunication technologies are used to convey professionalism.
6. Model appropriate self-boundaries.
7. Ensure privacy of the therapist's work.
8. Use professional language and consider alternative interpretations.
9. Ensure competence in the practice of telepsychology.

Abuse and Neglect

Being able to "see into '' children's homes offers a view into their lives that may indicate the child or other family members may be experiencing abuse or neglect. Although outside of the scope of this chapter, it is important to note that child life specialists are state-mandated reporters and should know when and how to make a report of abuse or neglect and what support services are available to the children and families after a report has been made.

CONSENT CHARTING AND PRIVACY

Whether a child life specialist is hosting a podcast, posting to social media, or providing therapeutic interventions using digital platforms, child life specialists must ensure the privacy of children and families by upholding the standards set by the entity they work for, local governing regulations, and private practice standards. Child life must specialists follow Principle 4 of the Code of Professional Ethics by the Association of Child Life Professionals "Certified child life specialists respect the privacy of children and families and maintain confidentiality within the standards and requirements of employers, local governing regulations, or private practice standards" (*Child Life Code of Ethics*. n.d.). Getting consent to use images, sharing someone's story, and establishing a safe space are paramount for children and families to feel free to express fears, worries, and concerns.

Child life specialists must adhere to HIPAA-compliant policies and securely store private health information, chart notes, and correspondence. Platforms such as Google and SimplePractice offer encrypted HIPAA-secure options and use a secure email server to store and share initial assessments, intake forms, signed consents, chart notes, and ongoing evaluations with the client. It is ultimately the responsibility of the CCLS to ensure these practices are upheld.

FUTURE CONSIDERATIONS

Child life specialists can use technology to provide services to families remotely. Still, there are many other ways in which the field could grow and expand online. With life increasingly being lived online, there is also an increase in professional interactions within the child life field on social media platforms like LinkedIn, Instagram, Twitter, and Facebook. Meeting regularly has become easier because there are no geographical limitations. Social media enables professionals to develop meaningful relationships through online communication. There are now community groups for parents online through Facebook and other sites, and there is indeed a role for child life specialists in helping facilitate and support these groups.

Child life specialists are already using online tools like tablet-based preparation books, pictures, and apps for distractions and normalization. Research looking into the benefits of online, video, and virtual tools used by child life specialists to understand efficacy and impact and provide insight by examining coping, comprehension, and relationship building are essential.

CONCLUSION

A child life specialist's job is to support and promote the well-being of children and families during challenging life events. As more families integrate online tools into their daily lives, the field has an opportunity to meet each other and families beyond their local geographical location. Not exploring options, challenging ourselves, and investigating new strategies to support families and each other is a missed opportunity. Embracing technology and exploring innovative approaches will only enhance and validate the field of child life.

REFERENCES

Advantages of telemedicine for patients. (n.d.). Chiron Health. Retrieved August 8, 2022, from https://chironhealth.com/definitive-guide-to-telemedicine/telemedicine-info-patients/advantages-telemedicine-patients/

American Medical Association. (2020, August 7). *Why so many patients still can't connect to doctors via telehealth.* Retrieved October 10, 2022, from https://www.ama-assn.org/practice-management/digital/why-so-many-patients-still-can-t-connect-doctors-telehealth

Ashcraft, L. E., Asato, M., Houtrow, A. J., Kavalieratos, D., Miller, E., & Ray, K. N. (2019). Parent empowerment in pediatric healthcare settings: A systematic review of observational studies. *Patient, 12*(2), 199–212. doi:10.100740271-018-0336-2 PMID:30328069

Association of Child Life Professionals. (2021). *Child Life Professional Data Center.* https://www.childlife.org/resources/for-child-life-specialists/child-life-professional-data-center

Beaunoyer, E., Dupéré, S., & Guitton, M. (2020). COVID-19 and digital inequalities: Reciprocal impacts and mitigation strategies. *Computers in Human Behavior, 111.*

Bester, J., Cole, C. M., & Kodish, E. (2016). The limits of informed consent for an overwhelmed patient: Clinicians' role in protecting patients and preventing overwhelm. *AMA Journal of Ethics, 18*(9), 869–886. doi:10.1001/journalofethics.2016.18.9.peer2-1609 PMID:27669132

Burns-Nader, S., & Hernandez-Reif, M. (2014, October 6). Facilitating play for hospitalized children through child life services. *Children's Health Care, 45*(1), 1–21. doi:10.1080/02739615.2014.948161

Burns-Nader, S., Joe, L., & Pinion, K. (2017). Computer tablet distraction reduces pain and anxiety in pediatric burn patients undergoing hydrotherapy: A randomized trial. *Burns: Journal of the International Society for Burn Injuries, 43*(6), 1203–1211. doi:10.1016/j.burns.2017.02.015 PMID:28318748

Child Life Council. (2009). Preparing Children and Adolescents for Medical Procedures. *Child Life Council Evidenced-Based Practice Statement.* https://www.childlife.org/docs/default-source/research-ebp/ebp-statements.pdf?sfvrsn=6395bd4d_2

Childlife.org. (n.d.a). Retrieved August 8, 2022, from https://www.childlife.org/docs/default-source/aclp-official-documents/child-life-code-of

Childlife.org. (n.d.b). Retrieved August 8, 2022, from https://www.childlife.org/docs/default-source/research-ebp/ebp-

Cincinnati Children's Hospital Medical Center. (2013). *Psychosocial Risk Assessment in Pediatrics.* https://praptool.com/

Cole, L. P., Henechowicz, T. L., Kang, K., Pranjić, M., Richard, N. M., Tian, G. L. J., & Hurt-Thaut, C. (2021). Neurologic Music Therapy via telehealth: A survey of clinician experiences, trends, and recommendations during the COVID-19 pandemic. *Frontiers in Neuroscience, 15*, 648489. doi:10.3389/fnins.2021.648489 PMID:33897362

COVID-19 resources - telehealth considerations and resources. (n.d.). Retrieved August 7, 2022, from https://www.musictherapy.org/about/covid19_resources_telehealth_considerations_and_resources/

Drum, K. B., & Littleton, H. L. (2014). Therapeutic boundaries in telepsychology: Unique issues and best practice recommendations. *Professional Psychology, Research and Practice, 45*(5), 309–315. https://doi.org/10.1037/a0036127

Eijlers, R., Utens, E. M. W. J., Staals, L. M., de Nijs, P. F. A., Berghmans, J. M., Wijnen, R. M. H., Hillegers, M. H. J., Dierckx, B., & Legerstee, J. S. (2019). Systematic review and meta-analysis of virtual reality in pediatrics: Effects on pain and anxiety: Effects on pain and anxiety. *Anesthesia and Analgesia, 129*(5), 1344–1353. https://doi.org/10.1213/ANE.0000000000004165

Epstein, E. G., Arechiga, J., Dancy, M., Simon, J., Wilson, D., & Alhusen, J. L. (2017). Integrative review of technology to support communication with parents of infants in the NICU. *Journal of Obstetric, Gynecologic, and Neonatal Nursing, 46*(3), 357–366. doi:10.1016/j.jogn.2016.11.019

Every child deserves emotionally safe care. (2021, February 9). Emotional Safety Initiative. https://emotional-safety.org/

Family Caregiver Alliance. (2012, September 21). *Caregiver isolation and loneliness.* https://www.caregiver.org/news/caregiver-isolation-and-loneliness/

Gajarawala, S. N., & Pelkowski, J. N. (2021). Telehealth benefits and barriers. *The Journal for Nurse Practitioners: JNP, 17*(2), 218–221. https://doi.org/10.1016/j.nurpra.2020.09.013

Gaynard, L., Wolfer, J., Goldgerger, J., Thompson, R., Redburn, L., & Laidley, L. (1990). *Psychosocial care of children in hospitals: A clinical practice manual for the ACCH child life research project.* Association for the Care of Children's Health.

Ginsburg, K. R., American Academy of Pediatrics Committee on Communications, & American Academy of Pediatrics Committee on Psychosocial Aspects of Child and Family Health. (2007). The importance of play in promoting healthy child development and maintaining strong parent-child bonds. *Pediatrics, 119*(1), 182–191. doi:10.1542/peds.2006-2697

Goddard, A., Janicek, E., & Etcher, L. (2022). Trauma-informed care for the pediatric nurse. *Journal of Pediatric Nursing*, *62*, 1–9. https://doi.org/10.1016/j.pedn.2021.11.003

Hoffmann, B. (2016). The role of expressive therapies in therapeutic interactions; art therapy - explanation of the concept. *Trakia Journal of Science, 14*(3), 197–202. doi:10.15547/tjs.2016.03.001

Huang, Y.-M., Liang, T.-H., Su, Y.-N., & Chen, N.-S. (2012). Empowering personalized learning with an interactive e-book learning system for elementary school students. *Educational Technology Research and Development, 60*(4), 703–722. doi:10.1007/s11423-012-9237-6

Hugelius, K., Harada, N., & Marutani, M. (2021). Consequences of visiting restrictions during the COVID-19 pandemic: An integrative review. *International Journal of Nursing Studies*, *121*(104000), 104000. https://doi.org/10.1016/j.ijnurstu.2021.104000

Internet/broadband fact sheet. (2021, April 7). Pew Research Center: Internet, Science & Tech. https://www.pewresearch.org/internet/fact-sheet/internet-broadband/?menuItem=3109350c-8dba-4b7f-ad52-a3e976ab8c8f

Isikoglu Erdogan, N., Johnson, J. E., Dong, P. I., & Qiu, Z. (2018, May 28). Do Parents Prefer Digital Play? Examination of Parental Preferences and Beliefs in Four Nations. *Early Childhood Education Journal*, *47*(2), 131–142. https://doi.org/10.1007/s10643-018-0901-2

Kraus, E. J., Nicosia, B., & Shalowitz, D. I. (2022). A qualitative study of patients' attitudes towards telemedicine for gynecologic cancer care. *Gynecologic Oncology*, *165*(1), 155–159. https://doi.org/10.1016/j.ygyno.2022.01.035

Lambert, S. (2022, January 14). *Number of internet users in 2022/2023: Statistics, current trends, and predictions*. Retrieved September 23, 2022, from https://financesonline.com/number-of-internet-users/#:~:text=There%20are%20currently%20about%204.66,90%25%20as%20of%20January%202021

Malchiodi, C. (2005). Using art activities to support trauma recovery in children. *Trauma & Loss: Research & Interventions*, *5*(1), 8–11.

Murcia, J. (2020). *Child life specialists begin using telemedicine to reach hospitalized children during COVID-19*. Retrieved August 7, 2022, from https://connect.uclahealth.org/2020/04/03/child-life-specialists-begin-using-telemedicine-to-reach-hospitalized-children-during-covid-19/

Myers, J. E. B. & APSAC (American Professional Society on the Abuse of Children). (2010, June 16). *The APSAC Handbook on Child Maltreatment* (3rd ed.). SAGE Publications, Inc.

Newman, K., Wang, A. H., Wang, A. Z. Y., & Hanna, D. (2019). The role of internet-based digital tools in reducing social isolation and addressing support needs among informal caregivers: A scoping review. *BMC Public Health*, *19*(1), 1495. https://doi.org/10.1186/s12889-019-7837-3

Osborne, C. N. (2018). A child life perspective: The role of technology in preoperative preparation and distraction. The University of North Carolina at Charlotte.

Pamplona, A. Y. M. C. (2000). Active participation of mothers during speech therapy improved language development of children with cleft palate. *Scandinavian Journal of Plastic and Reconstructive Surgery and Hand Surgery, 34*(3), 231–236. doi:10.1080/02844310050159800

Sasangohar, F., Dhala, A., Zheng, F., Ahmadi, N., Kash, B., & Masud, F. (2021). Use of telecritical care for family visitation to ICU during the COVID-19 pandemic: An interview study and sentiment analysis. *BMJ Quality & Safety*, *30*(9), 715–721. https://doi.org/10.1136/bmjqs-2020-011604

Schniering, C., Einstein, D., Kirkman, J., & Rapee, R. (2022). Online treatment of adolescents with comorbid anxiety and depression: A randomized controlled trial. *Journal of Affective Disorders, 311*, 88–94.

Schueller, S. M., Stiles-Shields, C., & Yarosh, L. (2017). Online treatment and virtual therapists in child and adolescent psychiatry. *Child and Adolescent Psychiatric Clinics of North America*, *26*(1), 1–12. https://doi.org/10.1016/j.chc.2016.07.011

Seidemann, J. S., & Roxanna Barboza, R. (2021). *Rural imperatives in broadband adoption and digital inclusion.* Retrieved October 10, 2022, from https://www.ntca.org/sites/default/files/documents/2022-03/src-whitepaper-broadband-adoption-and-digital-inclusion.pdf

Shabiralyani, G., Hasan, K. S., Hamad, N., & Iqbal, N. (2015). Impact of Visual Aids in Enhancing the Learning Process Case Research: District Dera Ghazi Khan. *Journal of Education and Practice*, *6*(16), 226–233. https://doi.org/https://eric.ed.gov/?id=EJ1079541

Sherred, L. (2019, August 31). *Does online speech therapy work as well as in-person therapy?* Expressable. Retrieved September 23, 2022, from https://www.expressable.com/learning-center/online-speech-therapy/does-online-speech-therapy-work-as-well-as-in-person-therapy

Standards of clinical practice chapter 4. (n.d.). Retrieved August 8, 2022, from https://www.childlife.org/docs/default-source/the-child-life-profession/standardsofclinicalpractice.pdf?sfvrsn=2

Statista. (2021, January 8). *Leading reasons for listening to podcasts in the U.S. 2019*. Retrieved October 10, 2022, from https://www.statista.com/statistics/610691/main-reasons-listening-to-podcasts-us/

Statista. (2022, February 23). *Number of podcast listeners in the United States 2017-2024*. Retrieved October 10, 2022, from https://www.statista.com/forecasts/1123105/statista-amo-podcast-reach-us

Turner, J. C., & Fralic, J. (2009). Making explicit the implicit: Child life specialists talk about their assessment process. *Child and Youth Care Forum*, *38*(1), 39–54. https://doi.org/10.1007/s10566-009-9066-x

Vailshery, L. S. (2022, August 11). *Zoom daily meeting participants worldwide 2020*. Statista. Retrieved September 23, 2022, from https://www.statista.com/statistics/1253972/zoom-daily-meeting-participants-global/

Value Proposition Statement. (n.d.). *Default*. Retrieved August 8, 2022, from https://www.childlife.org/the-child-life-profession/value-proposition-statement

Webber, E. C., McMillen, B. D., & Willis, D. R. (2022). Health care disparities and access to video visits before and after the COVID-19 pandemic: Findings from a patient survey in primary care. *Telemedicine Journal and E-Health: The Official Journal of the American Telemedicine Association, 28*(5), 712–719. doi:10.1089/tmj.2021.0126

What is PFCC? (n.d.). Retrieved August 8, 2022, from https://www.ipfcc.org/about/pfcc.html

Wigfield, A., Gladstone, J., & Turci, L. (2016). Beyond cognition: Reading motivation and reading comprehension. *Child Development Perspectives, 10*(3), 190–195. https://doi.org/10.1111/cdep.12184

William, L. I., Lopez, H. C., & Lee, V. (2007). Effects of preoperative therapeutic play on outcomes of school-age children undergoing day surgery. *Research in Nursing & Health, 30*(3), 320–332.

Williams, A. M., Dawson, S., & Kristjanson, L. J. (2008). Exploring the relationship between personal control and the hospital environment. *Journal of Clinical Nursing, 17*(12), 1601–1609. https://doi.org/10.1111/j.1365-2702.2007.02188.x

Yogman, M., Garner, A., Hutchinson, J., Hirsh-Pasek, K., Golinkoff, R. M., Baum, R., Gambon, T., Lavin, A., Mattson, G., Wissow, L., Hill, D. L., Ameenuddin, N., Chassiakos, Y. L. R., Cross, C., Boyd, R., Mendelson, R., Moreno, M. A., Radesky, J., Swanson, W. S., ... Smith, J. (2018, September 1). The Power of Play: A Pediatric Role in Enhancing Development in Young Children. *Pediatrics, 142*(3). https://doi.org/10.1542/peds.2018-2058

KEY TERMS AND DEFINITIONS

Blog: Written content shared on the internet.
Podcast: Media shared through audio format.
Telehealth: Healthcare provided online using software.
Virtual: Online or Internet-based software.

Chapter 18
Nonprofits

Melissa Hicks
Wonders & Worries, USA

Meredith Cooper
Wonders & Worries, USA

ABSTRACT

This chapter will guide the reader through the development and growth of a community-based nonprofit organization with a sustainable approach to the initial core values. This chapter serves as an informed roadmap for clinicians interested in pursuing the development of their own nonprofit. Working with children of adult patients will serve as the backdrop to highlight the concepts of the development and trajectory of the organization; the extrapolation of the process and skills to other populations will be addressed. The longitudinal experience of Wonders & Worries has afforded the organization the opportunity to learn many lessons and develop solid evidence-based practices in relation to clinical offerings coupled with overall organizational growth and strength. This chapter will provide the concepts, examples, and guidance to encourage sustainable child life programming in a variety of community settings supporting children and families.

INTRODUCTION

There is a multitude of significant life challenges affecting children within the community that can be supported through a community-based nonprofit agency. Certified Child Life Specialists (CCLS) often possess the clinical skills to address these support needs. However, they may not have the background knowledge, experience, and business acumen to start a nonprofit organization.

This chapter uses and expands on the growth and development of Wonders & Worries; a nonprofit agency initially highlighted in Beyond the Hospital (Cooper & Hicks, 2008). Wonders & Worries is a Texas-based nonprofit agency providing support to families coping with parental illness. The focus of this chapter will be on evidence-based practices and the sustainability of a nonprofit over time.

Case examples from Wonders & Worries will be shared to provide a frame of reference for consideration for those seeking to develop a unique organization to meet the needs of their community. The process

DOI: 10.4018/978-1-6684-5097-0.ch018

from conception and initiation to sustainability well into the future is highlighted. Critical questions for the reader to consider regarding goals to begin formulating action steps are shared throughout the chapter.

HISTORY OF WONDERS AND WORRIES

The founders connected in the Spring of 1999 to initiate the creation of Wonders & Worries. The needs assessment and qualitative experience of an unmet need and emerging research documenting the validity of this need provided the catalyst for the inception of Wonders & Worries. From the initial phone conversation, the two realized they shared a vision and deep awareness of the need for child life support for children when it was the parent who had the illness. This innovation and vision in the professional community of child life provided great insight into children's current and future needs. At the time of the development of this program, child life services focused on a child and their family who encountered the healthcare environment. The two founders met, beginning with an evaluation of the need to initiate a community-based organization.

The first step in this process was determining if the entity would be a private practice with associated fees or a nonprofit that did not charge client families for services. The founders determined to focus on the creation of a nonprofit largely due to the recognition that most families with a serious diagnosis had financial uncertainty, often with an increase in financial burdens. The founders' desire to have services accessible to all propelled this business model. Furthermore, the established professional contacts and resources between the two founders were significant to this nonprofit's beginning and ongoing development.

Fortuitous timing and an established professional relationship allowed Wonders & Worries to have a significant initial funder to launch this dynamic model. The initial Wonders & Worries business was small, with just two employees. The two founders worked out of one office and performed all the functions of the nonprofit, from program delivery to community outreach of services and paying bills. The funding allocated was 30 hours of work a week for both child life specialists. Through the development of the nonprofit, the skills needed to initiate, maintain, and grow a nonprofit were identified.

Over time additional employees were hired as funding and needs grew. Office locations expanded and grew both to reach different segments of the population (e.g., bilingual services) and ease commute times for client families. At this time, this community-based nonprofit has grown from a two Certified Child Life Specialist woman-owned and run nonprofit organization to a nonprofit organization that has over 7 physical sites, multiple employees, and dozens of Wonders & Worries providers throughout the United States. The initial budget upon inception was $120,000 per year and is now well over one and a half million dollars annually. Most noteworthy in 2022 is that over 13,000 individuals have been served since the inception of Wonders & Worries in 2001.

NEEDS ASSESSMENT AND CHILD LIFE RATIONALE

Why begin a community-based nonprofit? How does an individual initiate services and make them successful? This question often results from recognizing an unmet need in the community. Three components of a multifaceted needs assessment are: identifying an unmet need, having the skills to meet the need, and having the personal drive and passion to take action. These three things are required to begin the journey to creating a nonprofit agency.

The first component in the needs assessment process is to thoroughly analyze the data related to the needs of the population and communities intended to serve. It is imperative for the organization's success with funders, referring professionals, and the community at large to have validated research documenting the needs the organization is seeking to meet. This in-depth assessment requires setting aside time early and continuing to dedicate a portion of the organization's time to continue maintaining knowledge of the current research. Access to the most recent journals of academic works may be difficult but very important as a resource to accomplish this. When documenting the evidence-based need, one must include landmark studies in addition to the most current data. This concept of research and evidence to support the need for services will be addressed at several points throughout this chapter.

A community-based assessment is essential to establishing needs and gaps in services and supports a solid process for how proposed services will fulfill an unmet need. This thorough assessment of the community support landscape will identify gaps in services. This point will be crucial when seeking funding as it can be difficult to procure funding for services that are a duplication of already existing support.

The next component is to think about and clearly articulate why a CCLS is uniquely qualified to meet the needs identified in the community-based assessment. There are many skills that a Certified Child Life Specialist possesses that can be readily translated to a community-based setting. There are supporting documents and publications to review and ascertain which competencies of a CCLS are most relevant to the clinical services that will be offered and the client population who will be served (Association of Child Life Professionals, 2019; Hicks, 2008; Hicks & McCue, 2018). When considering the rationale for the nonprofit, it is essential to align the child life specialist's skills with the community's specific needs.

Child life specialists possess strong knowledge of growth and development across the lifespan and awareness of potentially stressful situations for a child, teen, or adult. This is often the unique expertise and competencies the Certified Child Life Specialist brings to a new or existing community-based agency. Armed with this knowledge, the child life specialist can proactively offer play and therapeutic interventions either directly to a child or through parent or family consultation. This preventative evidence-based model is unique within many settings. Programs that seek to be preemptive in nature, especially within the medical arena, are only recently emerging and being offered. Often personnel in adult medicine, including social workers and other mental health workers, have limited knowledge of children's growth and development and the overall effect on their emotional wellbeing. They may not be equipped with the tools to offer support to a parent, family member, or child who is often confused or scared within the stressful situation of a parent's diagnosis of a serious illness. Therefore, they welcome the support of professionals with clinical expertise in that arena. Many more transferable skills are highlighted throughout this publication. When establishing a nonprofit, it will be most important to align those competencies and skills to meet the needs of the population served. (For specific information on the established competencies of a Certified Child Life Specialist, refer to the Association for Child Life Professionals Official Documents found at www.childlife.org).

One exercise to help visualize this needs assessment is to create a simple chart that lists the needs of the population to be served along with the competencies a CCLS possesses to meet those needs. In the example below, a simple template is shared to help frame thoughts surrounding the needs of the proposed service population coupled with the competencies, knowledge, and skills of a Certified Child Life Specialist, indicating they are uniquely and proficiently qualified to meet the need. As highlighted in Figure 1 below, it is also important to reflect on aspects of clinical practice for additional education and training to maintain ethical delivery of services. These can be color-coded by category, reflecting current competencies and additional skills needed.

Figure 1. Competency Graphic

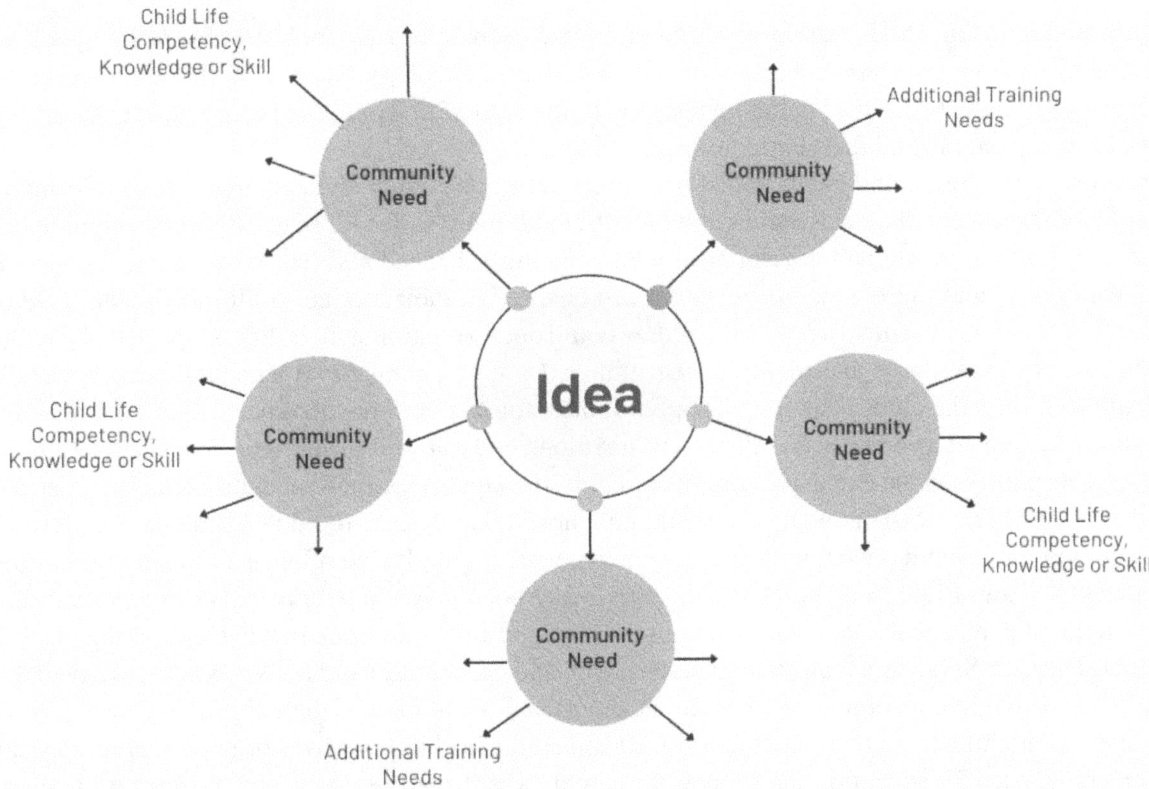

The third component of the needs assessment is personal drive and passion to move the project forward and sustain the nonprofit. One must think about the difference between traditional hospital-based work and providing child life services as a community-based organization. In addition to the child life competencies one demonstrates, it is essential also to evaluate whether an individual's personal attributes align with the unique needs of starting a nonprofit. Candidates must be honest with themselves and critically reflect on their desire to work in this nontraditional setting. Qualities such as autonomy, resourcefulness, efficiency, and maintaining healthy boundaries are all important to self-assess.

Often the child life specialist is working more independently. It is important to note that working in a community-based setting may be more professionally isolating than working within a hospital or larger organization. There are not multiple child life specialists within an office with whom to glean insights, share rewarding moments or express frustrations or even grief. This creates the professional necessity to seek out both formal and informal opportunities for supervision. Time for professional support, both in terms of peer support and professional supervision, must be made a high priority to maintain the efficacy and integrity of solid program delivery.

What this setting often does allow for is a flexible schedule. For some, this can be a great bonus. For others, it is hard to navigate as boundaries and accountability must be set both with clients and self. Often, hours can vary between weeks based on the needs of clients. Holidays are often not a work time, and this can be a great added bonus.

Case Example: Wonders and Worries Needs Assessment

The creation of Wonders & Worries came from the experiences of two Certified Child Life Specialists working in separate geographical locations within pediatric oncology settings. Within their work, they each recognized the benefits of child life tenets with the entire family unit and assessed a need for these services to expand beyond their current hospital settings.

Children understood and coped well when given developmentally and age-appropriate information regarding their cancer diagnosis and treatment. Offered opportunities for play, children, sought to continue their normal growth and development while gaining enhanced abilities to express and cope with their feelings related to the arduous treatment and changes in their routine. Additionally, the child life specialists witnessed the misperceptions children could obtain regarding their illness, specifically related to the causes of the illness and multiple other things if not given this developmentally appropriate information. Within the clinical setting, the opportunities for interaction with others experiencing similar situations facilitated awareness that they were not alone and allowed meaningful friendships to occur. The CCLSs witnessed the extensive benefits of child life support for these pediatric oncology patients.

Both child life specialists worked in children's hospitals adjacent to adult hospitals. Requests for consultation for an adult patient with cancer were received regularly, but often at a time of crisis or near the parent's death. Little to no guidance had previously been given to help parents through their diagnosis, treatment, and health care journey, nor how to support their children in what was taking place for parents. The CCLSs quickly realized that parents who had cancer often did not know what to say to their children and sought out support to navigate the emotional well-being of their children. Out of a desire to protect their children, parents and other significant adults in children's lives often said nothing. Thus, the emergent need for education and support for parents was strongly evident, and the need for guidance in their children's developmental and emotional well-being was clear. At the time of initial diagnosis, parents often did not know if or how they should communicate the cancer diagnosis. Parents and family members needed compassion, encouragement, and support. The need assessed was professional and trained guidance and support for parents. This includes how to explain illness and healthcare journeys to their children while supporting and maintaining a trusting relationship.

Parents' questions included: How will my child go on? Have I caused developmental damage that will impact my child for the rest of their life? The concern of what the child was wondering and worrying about frequently arose. These reflections and questions helped the child life specialists understand what it meant to be a parent with a serious and life-threatening illness. The need for comprehensive strength-based child life support for parents and families facing a cancer diagnosis and the children of these parents became clear and profoundly apparent to the CCLSs, which led to them founding the nonprofit Wonders & Worries. Further in-depth investigation revealed that little to no support existed in communities across the country for parents and children when it was the parent with a serious or life-threatening illness. The only community-based support that existed at the time of this inquiry was limited bereavement support after a parent died.

Simultaneously, during this time frame (the late 1990s to early 2000s), research was emerging to document the effects on children and teens of having a parent with cancer. The advancement of this research continued and began to show the detrimental effects of a parent with a serious illness and how to best meet the needs of children and teens in this family situation. Understanding the latest research further indicated that the stress within the family is higher prior to the death of a parent than following the death (Fann et al., 2008). When a parent has cancer, a child's earlier ways of thinking, including poor hypothesis testing and magical thinking, may reappear (Lewis, 2011). This means that the assumption that an adolescent can reason or problem-solve when a parent is diagnosed with cancer may be in error. There was also evidence that children may internalize their ill parent's behavior as them not being lovable or valued (Siegel et al., 1996). A child whose parent died due to a prolonged illness exhibited higher levels of maladaptive grief and posttraumatic stress symptoms than children who lost a caregiver to sudden death (Kaplow, Layne, and Howell, 2014).

With this emerging confirmation, both in professional experience and available research, three key variables emerged:

1. Providing developmental and age-appropriate information about a parent's illness.
2. Offering support with a specific focus on communication with parents, family members, and health professionals.
3. Creating an environment where children feel physically and emotionally safe to communicate all (positive and negative) emotions and have their experiences normalized among peers.
   Reflective Questions: Needs Assessment and Child Life Rationale
   - What is the unmet need?
   - Is the population currently being served in any way? If so, how? If not, why?
   - What research exists to confirm this need?
   - Are there evidence-based practices to meet this need?
   - Do child life specialists have the needed skills/experiences to serve that population?
   - Is additional training needed to become more qualified to meet the needs of the population?
   - What are the financial risks personally and professionally?
   - What community contacts and professional resources are known and available?

MISSION DEVELOPMENT

It is imperative to be thoughtful and strategic when establishing a clear and concise mission for the organization. The mission, as the public-facing aspect of the organization, is the cornerstone for marketing to potential funders, referral sources, clients, expansion, and development of all current and future programming for years to come.

Overall, the time spent developing the mission of the organization is essential. This will serve as the roadmap for the direction the organization takes and will be the touchstone when evaluating decisions. The mission statement will define the organization's purpose and the role it fills within the space it operates. Additionally, it defines the population that will be impacted. Creating a mission statement also requires balance. The statement should be broad enough not to limit the services or program but should be narrow enough to avoid ambiguity.

It is important over time to continually reassess the mission statement, especially when writing a strategic plan, to ensure it accurately reflects the current state of the organization and its priorities. Defining the unmet need and refining the mission to the population served is the crucial first step in program development. Thinking in terms of who is the primary client can often clarify programmatic and even business decisions within the organization at crucial times. This mission will drive the next phase of planning, the clinical and programmatic aspects of the organization.

It is wise to research professional organizations that align with the concept of program development. If financially feasible, joining the organization and attending in-person or virtual training and receiving communication such as electronic newsletters is beneficial. Networking with professionals either directly related to the mission or tangentially associated can augment and potentially enhance program ideas. Aspects of programming may be brought to light that is needed because of networking with diverse areas related to the area of focus. Conversely, awareness of program components that do not work or simply are not in the scope of the mission may be realized. Specific activities and materials are often shared between members, furthering the strength in developing an informed business and service delivery model. Valuable contacts may be made for referral sources or even potential funders. The list of assets gained from the right professional organizational memberships can be endless.

Case Example: Wonders and Worries Mission Development

Wonders & Worries began with a very broad mission and included children impacted by their own illness, a sibling, or another relative. It was quickly realized that this mission was too broad while addressing important psychosocial impacts. It created confusion within the community and had difficulty meeting all the needs of those distinct populations. The mission was then revised to reflect this change and has remained the focus of service delivery. The current mission of Wonders & Worries is:

"Wonders & Worries provides free, professional support for children and teenagers through a parent's serious illness so that they can reach their full potential. Our experts provide the foundation children, and teenagers need to reach their full potential even though their parent is ill. Through individual and group therapy sessions, kids and teens learn about illness and build coping and communication skills. Our comprehensive programming is the only one of its kind in the US." (www.wondersandworries.org)

Reflective Questions: Mission

- Who is the target population for support?
- What are the documented needs of this population?
- How will this organization meet those needs?
- Who would have a vested interest in partnering with you?
- What messages are conveyed in the mission statement?
- How might multiple audiences receive the message?

BUSINESS MODEL

There are two sides to a successful community-based nonprofit: clinical and business. The clinical side focuses on the delivery of a service that meets the need within the scope of a child life practice. Ideally, this offers an evidence-based practice that supports clients and allows the community to thrive as a result of the services provided. Balancing business practices with clinical ethics can occasionally create a conflict that must be addressed and resolved for a nonprofit to be sustainable. It is important to acknowledge this potential conflict and have a plan for addressing it for final decisions related to the clinical program and the organization.

Business skills are required to support a community-based nonprofit. It is important to identify gaps in knowledge to seek resources available to provide the needed education and consultation. These business skills are highlighted in Figure 2 below. Child life specialists should research the regulations that impact nonprofit organizations depending on the state and national governance policies and procedures in place. The nonprofit management and administration knowledge required must be sought out through additional courses or training from others with expertise in business practices and nonprofit management.

There are many resources to access and help build on these skills. Resources fall into three categories: national resources, local resources, and individual contacts. On a national basis, some entities exist to guide human service nonprofit organizations. While some resources may be specific, a good resource that offers a wide variety of tools and resources for nonprofits is the National Council of Nonprofits. Information on topics from governance and accountability to ethics and diversity can be found within this professional association. The actual formation of a nonprofit varies by state. For the development of a nonprofit business model, it is necessary to look at individual state laws. The filing of all needed paperwork and fees will vary between states, but all will most likely require filing articles of incorporation, bylaws, and a board of directors. In addition, marketing skills such as the creation of a logo and website are fundamental aspects of an organization. Having relationships with individuals that can guide this or make additional connections is a thoughtful way to begin in this area.

The importance of community connections and the establishment of community relationships are essential. Accessing opportunities and contacts within the community may lead to gaining skills and

Figure 2. Business Needs

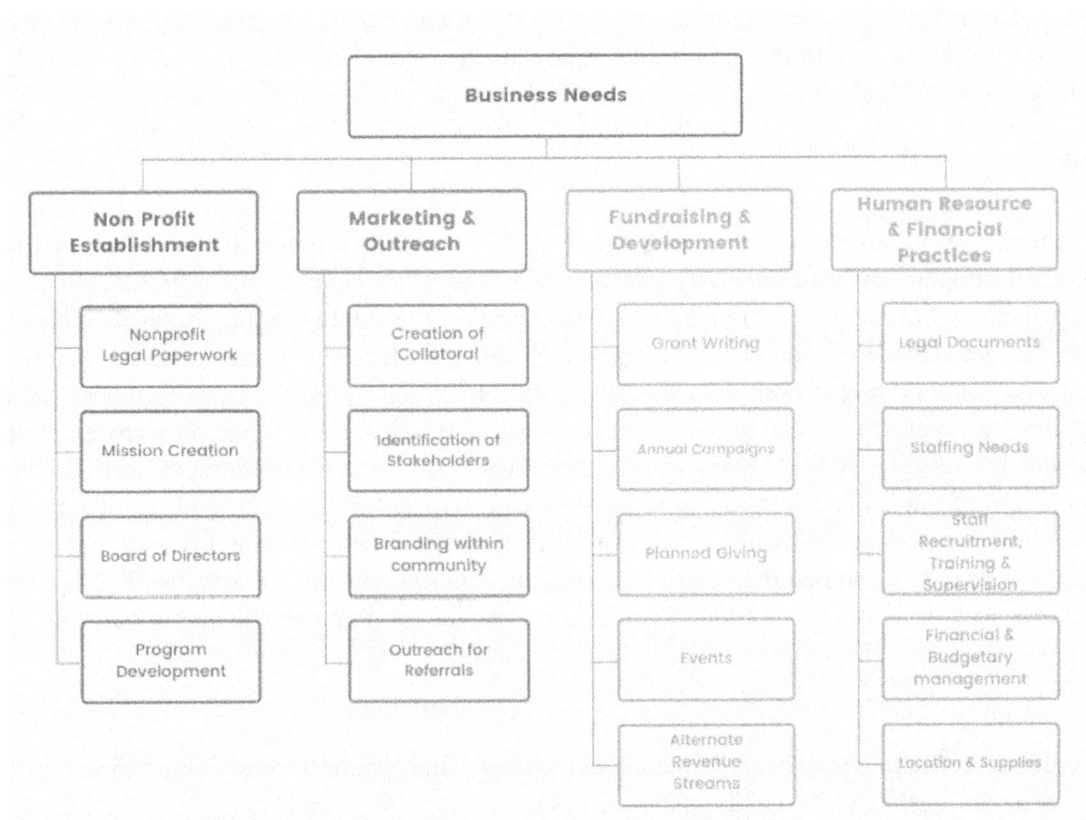

relationships beyond child life that enhance the creation of the business side of the nonprofit. These connections help to identify potential board members who connect with the mission and provide expertise and financial support to the organization.

Funding

Seek funders for advice and involvement in the organization to enhance their connection to the mission of the organization. This will endear them to the cause far more than 'telling them something' and promote a higher level of "buy-in" to what is being provided.

There are multiple sources to raise funds for the organization when the decision has been made to offer services free of charge, including not using a sliding fee. It is wise to diversify funding as much as possible. Diversity of funding lends to greater stability and a long-term sustainable financial picture for the organization.

Grants

One main source of funding to consider is grants, which may come from various sources. If just starting, a main source of grant funding may come from smaller family foundations. These are foundations that grant money, usually locally or in a few designated regions of the country. It has been successful for the founders of Wonders & Worries to look at the board of directors of various foundations that fund missions related to our mission and target population. Upon identifying these decision makers of the foundation, identify those to contact. Include board members in keeping them up to date on funding and processes. Think about circulating this list of potential funding partners to board members and others committed to assisting in finding funding sources. Ask if they would be willing to make an introduction to share your mission and services.

Events

Events are another funding source that occurs in the business world of nonprofits. Events have the benefit of increasing awareness of the entity among a wide variety of people. Often funding participation can vary, making it affordable to more people. There can be sponsorships at higher levels with varying benefits connected to these levels. This may appeal to businesses looking to gain awareness or align with the mission. Ticket pricing to events at lower levels can attract a supporter or interested person without as large a commitment. Silent and live auctions at the event and various other additional revenue streams can be added. There are a few notes of caution related to events. First, an event most likely will require a commitment of funds in advance. A strong budget with targeted goals specified is critical to making a profit on the event. An event is often a once-a-year activity that can create an influx of capital at one time of the year. There can be great dependence on an event that puts the organizational budget at risk when events such as a drop in the economy or a pandemic hit and that revenue do not come in.

Donors

Other options for funding may be individual donor giving. This generally comes about through the cultivation of a relationship with an individual over time. Strong strategic and evidence-based practices are associated with cultivating these types of relationships. The goal is to identify someone who relates to your mission and feels the need to support the organization and understand the motivation behind their reason for giving. These reasons may vary from personal experience with the mission to belief in you as a founder. Studying philanthropic giving provides insight into the reasons why people give. Some systems can be tapped to help grow these relationships and the resultant giving. Some donors may wish to be involved in giving circles where a group of people all contribute a designated yearly amount and enjoy special benefits such as a yearly update from the executive director or a gathering at an office to view programmatic-themed activities.

Marketing

Beyond a specific and strategic fundraising strategy, it is important to consider the marketing plan, including branding. Branding the initial business materials with your name, logo, website, mission statement, and other key documents, guidelines, and policies helps to establish recognition of your organization.

It is necessary to consider where clients come from in the community, who will be referring clients for services (i.e., the market segment), and the process for those referrals to be made. Identify the information the market segment needs to know. Create a clear message and pilot it with a small subgroup within the market. Questions to assess within this pilot include:

- What do consumers hear?
- How do consumers understand the service?
- Are there misperceptions?

You may need to experiment with the delivery means of the messaging, the timing of this messaging, and potentially adjust the content of the message.

When beginning to market services with referring providers, keep a database of these providers. Record contact information of email, phone number, the entity they are affiliated with, and their profession. This will allow planning for group messaging and maintaining solid professional relationships. Having an outreach or marketing calendar for the year will allow you to send out emails promptly and appropriately without overloading your referral sources with too many communications.

The use of a business plan template may prove very helpful and critical in framing thoughts and ensuring that all business aspects are addressed when developing a nonprofit agency. It establishes a stronger business model, and investors look to this when investing in companies, especially startups. These aspects will also be highlighted further in the chapter when discussing organizational development.

Finally, highlighting and telling a compelling story describing the community need and how the organization supports this need is an important tool in marketing. Using the data to tell a story will captivate the intended audience to support the organization's mission, make referrals, and use the services. Additionally, feedback from community members or potential clients and referral sources further illustrates the compelling need for the organization.

Reflective Questions to Consider for Business Model

- How much funding is needed to initiate services?
- How much funding will it take to serve each client for the services provided?
- How will data be shared with those who invest in you?

- ◦ How will you keep asking for additional funding?

PROGRAM DEVELOPMENT

Program development begins with a clear definition of program deliverables, Deliverables should be direct outcomes of the needs assessed and the therapeutic goals set in the nonprofit's mission. Therapeutic goals should be clear and use language that upholds health literacy, free of jargon to promote a high level of accessibility to any reader. These goals need to be evidence-based to support a foundation of intervention and practice delivery.

Staffing

After establishing the therapeutic goals, staffing the organization's programs should be considered. The importance of education and credentialing needed to deliver the programming is key. The staffing model lays the foundation for the recruitment of staff. Staffing considerations should include administrative, board of directors, and direct service staff.

Administrative

There are many skills necessary to run a nonprofit that often are not part of the training of the child life specialist. To be successful, a nonprofit requires staff with strong business skills that can provide important functions such as budgeting and accounting, management of human resources, and oversight of technology, as well as business systems and processes. Additionally, staff who are skilled in fundraising are necessary, which often encompasses grant writing, event management, and stewardship of donor relationships. Another set of unique skills important to the growth of a nonprofit includes public relations, marketing, and graphic design.

Board of Directors

Nonprofits are required to have a board of directors. However, the role and power of the board of directors vary based on how the nonprofit is structured. It is important to select people with complementary skills to the organization's needs and those committed to the mission and work of the nonprofit. Board members should not simply acquiesce to the founders but use their wisdom, opinions, influence, and resources to advance and sustain the organization.

Direct Service Staff

The delivery of services is provided by professional Certified Child Life Specialists. This staffing decision is a significant tenet of the Wonders & Worries service delivery model. This decision supports the overall program service delivery by established, credible team members who are well versed and highly proficient in child development and preventive concepts of support for stressful situations. Wonders & Worries does require education within the community as the general public is often less familiar with this profession until they encounter a need. The decision to always provide services by professionals as opposed to train volunteers is a distinguishing characteristic. Volunteers and practicum students are used to assist with group support and, in the case of practicum students, in a learning situation, for individual support. The focus on learning for the student and maintaining the recommended standards for student learning is upheld.

Location

Another aspect of program development to be considered is location. One must be thoughtful about location and consider the accessibility of services for clients. This can range from having adequate space for parents to wait to consider traffic concerns in the community. A central location that is accessible to families is essential. The consideration of home and school visits to aid in transportation struggles and meeting children and families where they are may be critical depending on the communities supported. There are additional aspects to process regarding these locations, such as comfort level, guidelines to establish entering private homes, and policies that schools may have related to outside professionals coming into the school.

Resources

A final logistical question in establishing program delivery relates to program resources and supplies. Identifying needed supplies and cost-effectively obtaining these is required. Identify how supplies will be obtained, organized, maintained, and stored when thinking about supplies.

Case Example: Wonders and Worries Program Development

One fundamental priority when establishing Wonders & Worries was the desire to provide services at no charge to families.

The following became the Wonders & Worries program deliverables:

1. Providing a developmentally appropriate understanding of illness, treatment, and side effects.
2. Facilitating communication of feelings related to changes within the family.
3. Identifying coping skills to help ease stress, sadness, anger, and fear.

These overarching program goals were embedded in a curriculum that consists of six sessions – the Wonders & Worries curriculum model. These sessions focused on the following themes:

First: Creating rapport and trust, assess understanding and concerns
Second and Third: Education of diagnosis, treatment, and side effects
Fourth: Feelings and emotional expression
Fifth: Identifying and expanding positive coping skills
Sixth: Catch-up and closure

The curriculum has been made flexible to meet the individual needs of those it serves. It can be delivered either in a group or individually, based on the child's or teen's developmental needs. It can be offered in person or virtually. Parent consultation is an additional crucial clinical service. This is offered in cases when the child is not able to attend sessions or if parents need some initial support and guidance regarding sharing information with their children prior to providing direct services to the children.

Through ongoing assessment, it was decided to offer individual support to children under five and limit virtual support to children six and above. Additionally, it is recognized that older children may choose individual support to continue their normal, developmentally appropriate routines, such as after-school sports and other extracurricular interests. Children with special needs are best served in an individual format.

Initially, the decision was made to offer support within the child's school if the child could not come to the Wonders & Worries office. Meeting with children in schools significantly impacted the organization in relation to staff time and expense due to travel from the office. The location of service delivery supported the vision of the organization for all children and families to have access to services. Refinement of how this is offered has occurred over time based on current circumstances in the community and for individual families. Due to traffic congestion, efforts were made to have multiple office sites to allow for easier access by families. Hours of services were also expanded with weekend therapeutic sessions becoming more extensive. This shift increased families' ability to reach an office for support. In addition, community partnerships were also in place to aid in delivering service for underserved families and are often found to have the most barriers to reaching designated Wonders & Worries offices.

It is also recognized that a recurrence may occur, new and different treatments may be required, or potentially the illness may shift to a more advanced stage. For these reasons, additional 'check-in' groups are offered as well as the opportunity to re-engage for individual support when needed. Thus, there is no limit to the length of time that a family remains a client within the scope of services for Wonders & Worries.

Families may access support at any time of the illness journey. While it is desired that families access Wonders & Worries support at the time of their diagnosis, it is recognized that some children may not express needs or concerns until a later time. Parents or family members may be too overwhelmed at the time of diagnosis or onset of treatment to seek support for their child. Furthermore, Wonders & Worries provides anticipatory grief support and initial bereavement support. This decision to limit the scope of Wonders & Worries is intended not to duplicate services that already exist in the community, focus on partnerships, and not compete for the same funding dollar.

Another program delivery challenge is meeting the needs of various populations of potential clients. It is well recognized that clients are most comfortable accessing services and revealing information about themselves and their families when speaking with someone 'like' them, someone they can identify with within their own identity. Establishing and recruiting Certified Child Life Specialists with similar racial, ethnic, and cultural identities, including meeting the language capabilities for the needs of your population, must be thought through. Using a cultural humility approach and recognizing potential barriers will help to reduce barriers and support access for children and their families. Designated funds for per diem (PRN) child life staff may be considered if the individual identified who can help meet this need within the organization cannot fully commit to being an employee of the organization. Other special needs of families should be considered when thinking through program delivery. For example, a parent who is deaf will have the right to have an interpreter present for intake and other communications. This can be an unexpected expense, and identifying a line item in the budget for access to the services offered is essential.

Reflective Questions to Consider for the Mission and Model of Support

- What service will be delivered?
- Is it supported by research and the CCLS skill set?
- What will be the model for program delivery?
- What are the short and long-term staff plans for the program and organization?
- Are the therapeutic goals for the program clearly articulated?
- Where will the program be offered?
- What are the supply needs and costs?

GROWTH AND SUSTAINABILITY

The intentional use of strategic planning and continual evaluation aids in the process of growth and refinement. Programmatic decisions are aligned to organizational values and the strategic plan. An organization must put adequate time and thought into meaningful strategic planning for the future sustainability of the organization. This ensures the organization continues to grow and sustain its focus aligned with the vision and mission.

Concerning organizational sustainability, a focus must be placed on the infrastructure of the organization. Allocating capital towards technology upgrades provides an organization with a strong foundation to deliver services and may result in financial savings.

Additionally, a focus on sustainability includes staff compensation and benefits. To be competitive within the job market, staff must be compensated fairly. Finally, a leadership transition plan must be made with the founders of an organization and all key organizational roles. Another point to address when pondering growth and sustainability is the organization's goals for replication or growth to other locations. This requires significant forethought and planning and should be included in any strategic planning initiatives.

Professional Responsibility and Clinical Supervision

Clinical supervision is an integral part of the professional responsibility of the program for both clinical staff and organizational leadership. Furthermore, continued assessment related to the scope of practice and functioning within that scope is imperative. A clear understanding of when referrals to outside services are necessary and having resources for those referrals allows this priority to be achieved. Special attention continues to be given to staff capacity for service delivery and policies necessary for staff retention. The organization and others making this child life staffing model choice should be keenly aware of their scope of practice.

Knowing when the scope of practice may be moving beyond appropriate professional guidelines can be challenging. For this reason and others, it is important to provide supervision for program staff and continue to uphold the integrity, ethics, and competencies of a Certified Child Life Specialist. Individual child life specialists meet with their direct supervisor, who offers individual focus both on specific therapeutic techniques for individual or group clients. Attention to the practitioner and what their thoughts, feelings, and needs are both for client support and the overall business workings of the organization is provided. This can be seen as taking away from staff productivity, reducing the number of clients seen, and thus increasing the cost to serve each client. Although it can be tempting to reduce or eliminate supervision to increase direct service delivery numbers, it is evidenced based practice to prioritize supervision of clinical staff.

Collaboration

Collaboration can take many forms and evolve over time. Initially, collaboration may focus on development aspects to acquire funding and professional collaboration to obtain referrals. Establishing community and academic partnerships is beneficial to facilitate research and provide additional services or opportunities for clients. One must ensure they are in partnership with organizations with similar values and priorities, and the collaboration offers the opportunity to be mutually beneficial.

Data Collection, Measurement, and Evaluation

Data collection, measurement, and evaluation is another important value. The commitment to evaluation and research is a significant strong point for the organization and contributes to its growth. The delivery of services begins with a grounding in current research that highlights best practices to meet the needs identified. It is unlikely that this need or best practice is static. Determining if the organization, academic establishment, or community will seek to participate in additional research is also a question to consider. Research is expensive, there may or may not be a budget for this depending on who partners in this research. It may require more standardization of program delivery than what currently exists within the organization. This can translate into tightening up the curriculum and training of staff to fully deliver the therapeutic sessions with as much consistency as possible. Research has multiple advantages; it offers the opportunity to promote the profession of child life in new ways within academia and the broader community. Research partnerships and advances appeal to many funders. This may resonate with a potential funder, giving the organization more credibility in meeting the need they are seeking to support. Another major benefit is that new best practices may be identified to serve clients more fully.

Case Example: Wonders and Worries Research

Wonders & Worries has contributed to this body of evidence-based practice through several research studies (Phillips, 2015; Phillips & Prezio, 2016; Phillips et al., 2022; Phillips et al., 2021). These studies provide additional data for others wishing to provide children of adult patients services within the community and support a data-informed approach to service delivery.

The first cross-sectional study of the impact of Wonders & Worries programming (Phillips & Prezio, 2016) found that among 156 families served, many reported amelioration of multiple children's issues, including improved communication skills (87%), reduced anxiety (84%), increased feeling of security at home (90%), and improved school performance (73%).

This multi-year sample of survey results was subsequently used to evaluate predictors of child psychosocial outcomes following their participation in the Wonders & Worries curriculum for families experiencing parental cancer (Phillips et al., 2021). Improvement in communication about the illness post-intervention was associated with improved sleep, feelings of security, and reduced anxiety. Families reporting financial difficulty were significantly more likely to report children's issues related to sleep, eating issues, feeling insecure at home, anxiety, and difficulty with the parent-child relationship. Results suggest variables such as a child's ability to communicate about the illness and the time since a parent's diagnosis affects outcomes. This study demonstrated that parents with cancer report their children to show improved psychological outcomes when participating in a child life intervention designed to address their worries and feelings.

The latest study was a randomized clinical trial focused on investigating the efficacy of the Wonders & Worries copyrighted, six-session curriculum (Phillips et al., 2022). The study enrolled 60 families with a parent diagnosed with early-stage cancer and their children. The intervention group significantly improved on parenting concerns, parenting self-efficacy, and family quality of life, while children in the intervention group had significantly lower emotional and behavioral problems and worries related to cancer compared to controls. The Wonders & Worries intervention was shown to promote positive adaptation for ill parents and their children in certain domains. This intervention is promising and warrants further refinement and testing with a larger, more diverse sample.

This body of research illustrates a solid foundation for building an evidence-based practice model for child life interventions supporting children of adult patients.

Innovation and Thought Leadership

A priority in growing and sustaining an organization should be related to innovation and thought leadership. In addition to providing excellent clinical service to clients, the organization must focus on program initiatives that will enhance and support clinical practice for the greater child life community. Webinars, continuing education courses, formalized training, and support programs are examples of how this can be accomplished.

Case Example: Wonders and Worries Growth and Sustainability

Financially, the budget of Wonders & Worries has grown from $120,000 per year to $1.5 million per year. A focus on diversified and targeted fundraising has allowed this growth. Additionally, seeking to add alternate revenue streams related to our mission is a focus. Within this category of revenue, the creation, publication, and sales of books and other products for professionals interested in continuing education and training have emerged.

Wonders & Worries has prioritized research not only to support our organization but also to add to the body of support for psychosocial services delivered by child life specialists and to the needs of children of adult patients. Research interests evolved from more general through the evaluative study of our services to more specific through the randomized clinical trial assessing our six-session illness education curriculum. The research agenda is a priority. Upon completion of the randomized clinical trial, a focus was placed on evaluating the advanced cancer curriculum and delivering virtual services. Longitudinal studies and anticipatory grief are also on the future research agenda.

Program initiatives created by Wonders & Worries have included virtual reality tours of a treatment center and funeral home to aid in preparation practices and application development to provide psychosocial support or resources to parents, teenagers, and professionals. Wonders & Worries has also committed to professional education through webinars and continuing education courses. Additionally, a formalized training and support program was created to provide education and resources to clinicians from around the world working with children of adult patients both in the community and in hospitals.

A helpline was created to further reach and support families outside of the Wonders & Worries offices. The helpline is staffed by Certified Child Life Specialists and provides support and consultation to both families and professionals. It was established to allow for family support and information to families when they need it most. For example, they may need to share their diagnosis with their children or have an immediate concern related to a child's behavior that can be addressed right away. This service is available to anyone, regardless of location. The focus is one-time consultation with referral to ongoing services if needed.

Reflective Questions to Consider for Organizational Growth and Sustainability

- What is the initial vision, and how has it evolved?
- What opportunities exist for growth?
- What values are lifelong and will stand the "test" of time?
- Do services need to reach beyond current capacity? If so, how will that happen?
- What is needed to sustain the organization into the future?
- What resources will be necessary, both financial and human?

EVALUATION AND DEFINING SUCCESS

Evaluation of both the clinical content of the program and the organization is imperative. This can be achieved by evaluative information gained from a variety of stakeholders. Having a trusted and outside consultant with expertise in the desired area of evaluation is best. An evaluation may be for the business components of the organization, such as a fundraising event or communication. It also must occur for the clinical delivery of services. This information must be continually assessed and calculated to sustain and promote strong programmatic changes. Both quantitative and qualitative information should be acquired for evaluation purposes and to refine program delivery or help establish research priorities. A plan for frequency and type of evaluation should be well laid out as often evaluation in the process of running a business can become an afterthought. It should remain a core value and practice to promote the program and organizational growth and sustainability.

Reflective Questions to Consider for Evaluation and Defining Success

- What does success look like, and how will it be shared?
- How will metrics be kept? (e.g., clients served per month, quarter and year)
- How will the quality of services be assessed? (e.g., progress of clients/satisfaction of clients)
- How will data and evaluation information be used to tell a compelling story for additional funding and referrals?
- How will lessons learned and challenges inform growth?

CONCLUSION AND FUTURE IMPLICATIONS

This chapter not only informs critical and reflective processes to begin the journey into the creation of a nonprofit but also seeks to inspire and motivate others to meet the many needs of children and families in the community. The vision to create a community-based nonprofit to support families coping with a variety of challenging life situations can be realized through dedication and passion for a project, program design, and the establishment of a program. Certified Child Life Specialists possess the clinical skills to deliver high-quality psychosocial programming in a variety of settings. This, coupled with additional information related to business development, creates the pathway for Certified Child Life Specialists to translate their skills into the community practice model. As more child life specialists have this interest and the needs of the community are evident, more nonprofits will be established by Certified Child Life Specialists, and more existing organizations will become aware of the value of adding child life services to their organization.

REFERENCES

Association of Child Life Professionals. (2018). *Position statement on child life practice for children of adult patients.* https://www.childlife.org/docs/default-source/aclp-official-documents/cbp-on-cl-practice-for-children-of-adult-patients_deireviewed.pdf?sfvrsn=4eb5834d_2

Association of Child Life Professionals. (2018). *Position statement on child life practice in community settings.* https://www.childlife.org/docs/default-source/aclp-official-documents/cbp-on-cl-practice-in-community-settings_deireviewed.pdf?sfvrsn=62b5834d_2

Association of Child Life Professionals. (2019). *Child life competencies.* https://www.childlife.org/docs/default-source/aclp-official-documents/child-life-competencies_november-2019-updates.pdf?sfvrsn=d33e8c4d_2

Association of Child Life Professionals. (2020). *The value of Certified Child Life Specialists: direct and downstream optimization of pediatric patient and family outcomes.* https://www.childlife.org/docs/default-source/aclp-official-documents/value-of-a-certified-child-life-specialist_full-report.pdf

Cooper, M., & Hicks, M. (2008). Nonprofits Providing Child Life Services. In M. Hicks (Ed.), *Child Life Beyond the Hospital* (pp. 169–193). Child Life Council.

Fann, J. R., Thomas-Rich, A. M., Katon, W. J., Cowley, D., Pepping, M., McGregor, B. A., & Gralow, J. (2008). Major depression after breast cancer: A review of epidemiology and treatment. *General Hospital Psychiatry, 30*(2), 112–126. doi:10.1016/j.genhosppsych.2007.10.008 PMID:18291293

Hicks, M. (Ed.). (2008). *Child Life Beyond the Hospital.* Child Life Council.

Hicks, M., & McCue, K. (2018). Child Life in the Community and in Other Non-traditional Roles. In *Thompson, R.) The handbook of child life: A guide for pediatric psychosocial care. 2nd Edition* (pp. 257–286). Charles C. Thomas.

Kaplow, J. B., Howell, K. H., & Layne, C. M. (2014). Do circumstances of the death matter? Identifying socioenvironmental risks for grief-related psychopathology in bereaved youth. *Journal of Traumatic Stress, 27*(1), 42–49. doi:10.1002/jts.21877 PMID:24478197

Lewis, F. M. (2011). Therapy for Parental Cancer and Dependent Children. In Handbook of Psychotherapy in Cancer Care (pp. 225-234). John Wiley & Sons, Ltd. doi:10.1002/9780470975176.ch19

Phillips, F. (2015). The experience of adolescents who have a parent with advanced cancer: A phenomenological inquiry. *Palliative & Supportive Care, 13*(4), 1057–1069. doi:10.1017/S1478951514001023 PMID:26165850

Phillips, F., & Prezio, E. (2016). *Wonders & Worries: Evaluation of a child centered psychosocial intervention for families who have a parent/primary caregiver with cancer* (Vol. 26). doi:10.1002/pon.4120

Phillips, F., Prezio, E. A., Currin-McCulloch, J., & Jones, B. (2022). Wonders & Worries Program Evaluation: A Randomized Clinical Trial of a Psychosocial Intervention for Children who have a Parent with Cancer. *Psycho-Oncology*. Advance online publication. doi:10.1002/pon.5943

Phillips, F., Prezio, E. A., Panisch, L. S., & Jones, B. L. (2021). Factors Affecting Outcomes Following a Psychosocial Intervention for Children When a Parent Has Cancer. *The Journal of Child Life: Psychosocial Theory and Practice.*

Siegel, K., Karus, D., & Raveis, V. H. (1996). Adjustment of children facing the death of a parent due to cancer. *Journal of the American Academy of Child and Adolescent Psychiatry, 35*(4), 442–450. doi:10.1097/00004583-199604000-00010 PMID:8919706

Wonders & Worries. (2022). *About Wonders & Worries.* Wonders & Worries https://wondersandworries.org/about/about-wonders-worries/

KEY TERMS AND DEFINITIONS

Deliverables: The goals of the program are defined by specific objectives.

Infrastructure: The business's hard items, technology systems, and processes utilized to conduct the mission objectives.

Stakeholders: Those people or institutions that have an invested interest in the success of the organization.

Thought Leadership: Possessing the capacity to look strategically at an issue or situation and initiating measured steps to achieve high-end goals.

Compilation of References

ACLP. (2019, November). *Child life competencies.* ACLP Official Documents. Retrieved April 11, 2022, from https://www.childlife.org/docs/default-source/aclp-official-documents/child-life-competencies_november-2019-updates.pdf?sfvrsn=d33e8c4d_2

ACLP. (2020, January). *Child life code of ethics.* ACLP Official Documents. Retrieved April 11, 2022, from https://www.childlife.org/docs/default-source/certification/child-life-code-of-ethics.pdf?sfvrsn=2

ACLP. (2020, November). *Community based standards and guidelines.* ACLP Official Documents. Retrieved April 11, 2022, from https://www.childlife.org/docs/default-source/aclp-official-documents/community-based-standards-and-guidelines_final-approved.pdf?sfvrsn=c7d1864d_2

Active Shooter Incidents 20-Year Review, 2000-2019. (2021). [File]. U.S. Department of Justice Federal Bureau of Investigation. https://www.fbi.gov/file-repository/active-shooter-incidents-20-year-review-2000-2019-060121.pdf/view

Adams, N. E. (2015). Bloom's taxonomy of cognitive learning objectives. *Journal of the Medical Library Association: JMLA, 103*(3), 152–153. doi:10.3163/1536-5050.103.3.010 PMID:26213509

Advantages of telemedicine for patients. (n.d.). Chiron Health. Retrieved August 8, 2022, from https://chironhealth.com/definitive-guide-to-telemedicine/telemedicine-info-patients/advantages-telemedicine-patients/

Ainsworth, M. D., Blehar, M. C., & Waters, E. (1978). *Patterns of attachment: A psychological study of the strange situation.* Lawrence Erlbaum.

Alberta Education. (2006). *Individualized program planning.* https://education.alberta.ca/media/384992/indidivualized-program-planning-2006.pdf

Albright, K., Greenbaum, J., Edwards, S. A., & Tsai, C. (2020). Systematic review of facilitators of barriers to, and recommendations for healthcare services for child survivors of human trafficking globally. *Child Abuse & Neglect, 100*, 104289. doi:10.1016/j.chiabu.2019.104289 PMID:31787336

Allen, K. E., Bell, J., Brown, C. D., Cross, J., Davitt, K., Desai, P. P., Fenn, L. D., Gaynard, L. L., Goldberger, J., Hicks, M., Hoffman, M., Hollon, E. C., Jessee, P. O., Johnson, B. H., Klinzing, D. G., Klinzing, D. R., McCue, K., McLeod, S. M., Mohl, A. L., . . . Wojtasik, S. (2009). The handbook of child life: A guide for pediatric psychosocial care. Academic Press.

Altindag, A., Ozen, S., & Sir, A. (2005). One-year follow-up study of post-traumatic stress disorder among earthquake survivors in Turkey. *Comprehensive Psychiatry, 46*(5), 328–333. doi:10.1016/j.comppsych.2005.01.005 PMID:16122532

Al-Yateem, N. B., Issa, W. B., & Rossiter, R. (2015). Childhood stress in health care settings: Awareness and suggested interventions. *Issues in Comprehensive Pediatric Nursing, 38*(2), 136–153. doi:10.3109/01460862.2015.1035465 PMID:25919580

Amar-Dolan, L. G., Horn, M. H., O'Connell, B., Parsons, S. K., Roussin, C. J., Weinstock, P. H., & Graham, R. J. (2020). "This is how hard it is". Family experience of hospital-to-home transition with a tracheostomy. *Annals of the American Thoracic Society*, *17*(7), 860–868. doi:10.1513/AnnalsATS.201910-780OC PMID:32267725

American Academy of Child and Adolescent Psychiatry. (2017). *Talking to kids about mental illnesses.* https://www.aacap.org/AACAP/Families_and_Youth/Facts_for_Families/FFF-Guide/Talking-To-Kids-About-Mental-Illnesses-084.aspx

American Academy of Child and Adolescent Psychiatry. (2022). *Ethical issues in clinical practice.* https://www.aacap.org/AACAP/Member_Resources/Ethics/Ethics_Committee/Ethical_Issues_in_Clinical_Practice.aspx

American Academy of Pediatrics. (2021). *Declaration of a national emergency in child and adolescent mental health.* https://www.aap.org/en/advocacy/child-and-adolescent-healthy-mental-development/aap-aacap-cha-declaration-of-a-national-emergency-in-child-and-adolescent-mental-health/

American Association of Post Acute Care Nursing. (2019, June 12) *Trauma-informed care. What it is and what and isn't.* https://www.aapacn.org/dns/trauma-informed-care-what-it-is-and-isnt/

American Federation of Teachers and New York Life Foundation. (2012). *Grief in the classroom.* https://www.newyorklife.com/assets/foundation/docs/pdfs/NYL-AFT-Bereavement-Survey.pdf

American Medical Association. (2020, August 7). *Why so many patients still can't connect to doctors via telehealth.* Retrieved October 10, 2022, from https://www.ama-assn.org/practice-management/digital/why-so-many-patients-still-can-t-connect-doctors-telehealth

American Medical Association. (n.d.). *CPT® overview and code approval.* Retrieved March 25, 2022, from https://www.ama-assn.org/practice-management/cpt/cpt-overview-and-code-approval

American Professional Society on the Abuse of Children. (2012). *Practice guidelines: Forensic interviewing in cases of suspected child abuse.* https://depts.washington.edu/uwhatc/PDF/guidelines/Forensic%20Interviewing%20in%20Cases%20of%20Suspected%20Child%20Abuse.pdf

American Psychiatric Association. (2013). *Diagnostic and statistical manual of mental disorders* (5th ed.). doi:10.1176/appi.books.9780890425596

American Psychiatric Association. (2017). Diagnostic and statistical manual of mental disorders: Dsm-5 (5th ed.). APA.

American Psychological Association. (2020). *Bias-free language.* https://apastyle.apa.org/style-grammar-guidelines/bias-free-language

American Psychological Association. (2022). *Resilience.* http://www.apa.org/topics/resilience

American Red Cross. (2022). *The Pillowcase Project.* https://www.redcross.org/get-help/how-to-prepare-for-emergencies/teaching-kids-about-emergency-preparedness/pillowcase-project.html

American School Counselor Association. (2019). *School Counselors Matter.* https://www.schoolcounselor.org/getmedia/b079d17d-6265-4166-a120-3b1f56077649/School-Counselors-Matter.pdf

American School Counselor Association. (2022). *School Counselor Roles and Ratios.* https://www.schoolcounselor.org/About-School-Counseling/School-Counselor-Roles-Ratios

American School Counselor Association. (n.d.). *Empirical Research Studies Supporting the Value of School Counseling.* https://www.schoolcounselor.org/getmedia/7d00dcff-40a6-4316-ab6c-8f3ffd7941c2/Effectiveness.pdf

Americans with Disabilities Act. (n.d.). *Information and technical assistance on the Americans with Disabilities Act.* https://www.ada.gov/ada_intro.htm

Ammerman, R. (1997). Physical abuse and childhood disability. *Journal of Aggression, Maltreatment & Trauma, 1*(1), 207–224. doi:10.1300/J146v01n01_11

Andrews, V. (2015). Interpreting silent cries. *Child Life Council Bulletin, 33*(4), 8–9.

Annie E. Casey Foundation. (2016). *A Shared Sentence: the devastating toll of parental incarceration on kids, families, and communities*. The Annie E. Casey Foundation.

AON. (2021). *2021 Weather, Climate, and Catastrophe Insight*. AON. https://www.aon.com/getmedia/1b516e4d-c5fa-4086-9393-5e6afb0eeded/20220125-2021-weather-climate-catastrophe-insight.pdf.aspx

Applying for a National Provider Identifier number. (2020). *Comphealth*. Retrieved March 25, 2022, from https://comphealth.com/resources/national-provider-identifier-npi/

ARC Family. (2020). *Child Life & ARC*. Retrieved August 4, 2022 from https://www.arcfamily.org/child-life-arc

Arnold, J. L., McKenzie, F., Miller, J. L., & Mancini, M. E. (2018). The many faces of patient-centered simulation: Implications for researchers. *Simulation in Healthcare: Journal of the Society for Simulation in Healthcare, 13*(3S), S51–S55. doi:10.1097/SIH.0000000000000312

Ashcraft, L. E., Asato, M., Houtrow, A. J., Kavalieratos, D., Miller, E., & Ray, K. N. (2019). Parent empowerment in pediatric healthcare settings: A systematic review of observational studies. *Patient, 12*(2), 199–212. doi:10.100740271-018-0336-2 PMID:30328069

Asnaani, A., & Hofmann, S. G. (2012). Collaboration in multicultural therapy: Establishing a strong therapeutic alliance across cultural lines. *Journal of Clinical Psychology, 68*(2), 187–197. doi:10.1002/jclp.21829 PMID:23616299

Association of Child Life Professionals. (2001). *Mission, values, vision and operating principles*. https://www.childlife.org/the-child-life-profession/values

Association of Child Life Professionals. (2001). *Mission, values, vision, and operating principles*. https://www.childlife.org/docs/default-source/the-child-life-profession/mission-vision-values.pdf

Association of Child Life Professionals. (2016). *Child life competencies*. https://www.childlife.org/docs/default-source/aclp-official-documents/child-life-competencies_november-2019-updates.pdf

Association of Child Life Professionals. (2016). *Child Life Competencies*. https://www.childlife.org/docs/default-source/the-child-life-profession/childlifecompetenciesjune2016.pdf?sfvrsn=2

Association of Child Life Professionals. (2018). *2018 ACLP member survey*. https://www.childlife.org/docs/default-source/default-document-library/aclp-2018-year-in-review.pdf?sfvrsn=454cb24d_4

Association of Child Life Professionals. (2018). *Association of child life professionals position statement on child life practice in community settings*. https://www.childlife.org/ docs/default-source/aclp-official-documents/cbp-on-cl-practice-in-community-settings_deireviewed.pdf?sfvrsn=62b5834d_2

Association of Child Life Professionals. (2018). *Association of Child Life Professionals position statement on child life practice in community settings*. https://www.childlife.org/docs/default-source/about-aclp/cbp-on-cl-practice-in-community-settings.pdf

Association of Child Life Professionals. (2018). *Position statement on child life practice for children of adult patients*. https://www.childlife.org/docs/default-source/aclp-official-documents/cbp-on-cl-practice-for-children-of-adult-patients_deireviewed.pdf?sfvrsn=4eb5834d_2

Association of Child Life Professionals. (2018). *Position statement on child life practice in community settings.* https://www.childlife.org/docs/default-source/about-aclp/cbp-on-cl-practice-in-community-settings.pdf

Association of Child Life Professionals. (2018). *Position statement on child life practice in community settings.* https://www.childlife.org/docs/default-source/aclp-official-documents/cbp-on-cl-practice-in-community-settings_deireviewed.pdf?sfvrsn=62b5834d_2

Association of Child Life Professionals. (2018). *Standards and guidelines for child life practice in community based & non-traditional settings.* https://www.childlife.org/docs/ default-source/aclp-official-documents/community-based-standards-and-guidelines_final-approved.pdf?sfvrsn=c7d1864d_2

Association of Child Life Professionals. (2019). Child life competencies. *ACLP Official Documents.* https://www.childlife.org/about-aclp/official-documents

Association of Child Life Professionals. (2019). *Child life competencies.* https://www.childlife.org/docs/default-source/aclp-official-documents/child-life-competencies_november-2019-updates.pdf?sfvrsn=d33e8c4d_2

Association of Child Life Professionals. (2019). *Child life competencies.* https://www.childlife.org/docs/default-source/the-child-life-profession/childlifecompetenciesjune2016.pdf?sfvrsn=2

Association of Child Life Professionals. (2019). *Eligibility Requirements effective 2019.* https://www.childlife.org/certification/becoming-certified/requirements-after-2019

Association of Child Life Professionals. (2020). *Association of Child Life Professionals position statement on child life in community settings.* https://childlife.org/docs/default-source/aclp-official-documents/updated-governance_position-statement-cl-practice-in-community-settings.pdf?sfvrsn=fa228c4d_10

Association of Child Life Professionals. (2020). Child life code of ethics. *ACLP Official Documents.* https://www.childlife.org/about-aclp/official-documents

Association of Child Life Professionals. (2020). *Child life code of ethics.* https://www.childlife.org/docs/default-source/aclp-official-documents/child-life-code-of-ethics4232ee9c90156ede9dafff00004f030f.pdf?sfvrsn=5327804d_2

Association of Child Life Professionals. (2020). *Child Life Code of Ethics.* https://www.childlife.org/docs/default-source/certification/child-life-code-of-ethics.pdf?sfvrsn=2

Association of Child Life Professionals. (2020). *Standards and guidelines for child life practice in community-based and non-traditional settings.* https://www.childlife.org/docs/default-source/aclp-official-documents/community-based-standards-and-guidelines_final-approved.pdf

Association of Child Life Professionals. (2020). *The value of Certified Child Life Specialists: direct and downstream optimization of pediatric patient and family outcomes.* https://www.childlife.org/docs/default-source/aclp-official-documents/value-of-a-certified-child-life-specialist_full-report.pdf

Association of Child Life Professionals. (2020). *The value of Certified Child Life Specialists: Direct and downstream optimization of pediatric patient and family outcomes.* https://www.childlife.org/docs/default-source/the-child-life-profession/value-of-cclss-full-report.pdf

Association of Child Life Professionals. (2020a). *Child Life Code of Ethics.* https://www.childlife.org/docs/default-source/aclp-official-documents/child-life-code-of-ethics4232ee9c90156ede9dafff00004f030f.pdf?sfvrsn=5327804d_2

Association of Child Life Professionals. (2020a). *Child life code of ethics.* https://www.childlife.org/docs/default-source/certification/child-life-code-of-ethics.pdf?sfvrsn=2

Association of Child Life Professionals. (2020b). *Position statement on diversity, equity, and inclusion.* https://www.childlife.org/docs/default-source/aclp-official-documents/statement-on-diversity-equity-and-inclusion.pdf?sfvrsn=c4d0864d_2

Association of Child Life Professionals. (2020b). *Standards of Clinical Practice.* https://www.childlife.org/docs/default-source/aclp-official-documents/4-standards-of-clinical-practice.pdf?sfvrsn=893e8c4d_4

Association of Child Life Professionals. (2021). *Child Life Professional Data Center.* https://www.childlife.org/resources/for-child-life-specialists/child-life-professional-data-center

Association of Child Life Professionals. (2021). *Position statement on child life practice in community settings.* ACLP Official Documents. https://www.childlife.org/docs/default-source/aclp-official-documents/cbp-on-cl-practice-

Association of Child Life Professionals. (2022). *ACLP Official Documents* Retrieved from https://education.childlife.org/aclp

Association of Child Life Professionals. (2022). *ACLP Official Documents.* https://www.childlife.org/the-child-life-profession/official-documents

Association of Child Life Professionals. (2022). *Standards of clinical practice.* Retrieved from: https://www.childlife.org/docs/default-source/aclp-official-documents/4-standards-of-clinical-practice.pdf?sfvrsn=893e8c4d_2

Association of Child Life Professionals. (2022, July 18). *Becoming certified: Academic requirements.* https://www.childlife.org/certification/becoming-certified

Association of Child Life Professionals. (2022a). *About Child Life.* https://www.childlife.org/the-child-life-profession

Association of Child Life Professionals. (2022b). *ACLP Official Documents.* https://www.childlife.org/the-child-life-profession/official-documents

Association of Child Life Professionals. (2022c). *Child Life Professional Certification Candidate Manual.* Association of Child Life Professionals. https://www.childlife.org/docs/default-source/certification/candidate-manual.pdf?sfvrsn=34

Association of Child Life Professionals. (n.d.). *Child life code of ethics.* https://www.childlife.org/docs/default-source/aclp-official-documents/child-life-code-of-ethics4232ee9c90156ede9dafff00004f030f.pdf?sfvrsn=5327804d_2

Association of Child Life Professionals. (n.d.). *Mission, Values, Vision, and Operating Principles.* https://www.childlife.org/docs/default-source/the-child-life-profession/mission-vision-values.pdf?sfvrsn=61b804d_2

Association of Child Life Professionals. (n.d.). *Position statement on diversity, equity, and inclusion.* https://www.childlife.org/docs/default-source/aclp-official-documents/statement-on-diversity-equity-and-inclusion.pdf

Atkins, M. S., Hoagwood, K. E., Kutash, K., & Seidman, E. (2010). Toward the integration of education and mental health in schools. *Administration and Policy in Mental Health, 37*(1-2), 40–47. doi:10.100710488-010-0299-7 PMID:20309623

Auerbach, M., Cheng, A., & Rudolph, J. W. (2018). Rapport management: Opening the door for effective debriefing. *Simulation in Healthcare: Journal of the Society for Simulation in Healthcare, 13*(1), 1–2. doi:10.1097/SIH.0000000000000266 PMID:29117095

Auerbach, M., Stone, K. P., & Patterson, M. D. (2016). The role of simulation in improving patient safety. In V. J. Grant & A. Cheng (Eds.), *Comprehensive healthcare simulation: Pediatrics* (pp. 55–65). Springer. doi:10.1007/978-3-319-24187-6_5

Bajaj, K., Meguerdichian, M., Thoma, B., Huang, S., Eppich, W., & Cheng, A. (2018). The PEARLS healthcare debriefing tool. *Academic Medicine, 93*(2), 336. doi:10.1097/ACM.0000000000002035 PMID:29381495

Ball, J., Bindler, R., & Cowen, K. (2014). *Child Health Nursing: Partnering with Children and Families*. Pearson.

Bandura, A. (1997). *Self-efficacy: The exercise of control*. Academic Press.

Bandyopadhyay, R. (2019). Volunteer tourism and "The White Man's Burden": Globalization of suffering, white savior complex, religion and modernity. *Journal of Sustainable Tourism*, *27*(3), 327–343. doi:10.1080/09669582.2019.1578361

Banks, D. M., & Weems, C. F. (2014). Family and peer social support and their links to psychological distress among hurricane-exposed minority youth. *The American Journal of Orthopsychiatry*, *84*(4), 341–352. doi:10.1037/ort0000006 PMID:24999520

Barker, J., Daniels, A., O'Neal, K., & Van Sell, S. L. (2017). Maternal-newborn bonding concept analysis. *International Journal of Nursing & Clinical Practices*, *4*(229). Advance online publication. doi:10.15344/2394-4978/2017/229

Barned, C., Dobson, J., Stintzi, A., Mack, D., & O'Doherty, K. C. (2018). Children's perspectives on the benefits and burdens of research participation. *AJOB Empirical Bioethics*, *9*(1), 19–28. doi:10.1080/23294515.2018.1430709 PMID:29369013

Barron, C., Beckett, A., Coussens, M., Desoete, A., Jones, N. C., Lynch, H., Prellwitz, M., & Salkeld, D. F. (2017). *Barriers to play for children and young persons*. De Gruyter Open Ltd.

Basaran, A., Karadavut, K. I., Uneri, S. O., Balbaloglu, O., & Atasoy, N. (2013). The effect of having children with cerebral palsy on quality of life, burn-out, depression and anxiety scores: A comparative study. *European Journal of Physical and Rehabilitation Medicine*, *49*(6), 815–822. PMID:24285025

Beaunoyer, E., Dupéré, S., & Guitton, M. (2020). COVID-19 and digital inequalities: Reciprocal impacts and mitigation strategies. *Computers in Human Behavior, 111*.

Becker-Blease, K. A., Turner, H. A., & Finkelhor, D. (2010). Disasters, victimization, and children's mental health. *Child Development*, *81*(4), 1040–1052. doi:10.1111/j.1467-8624.2010.01453.x PMID:20636681

Behar, S., & Cooper, J. (2015). Best practices in the emergency department management of children with special needs. *Pediatric Emergency Medicine Practice*, *12*(6). PMID:26118120

Behere, A. P., Basnet, P., & Campbell, P. (2017). Effects of family structure on mental health of children: A preliminary study. *Indian Journal of Psychological Medicine*, *39*(4), 457–463. doi:10.4103/0253-7176.211767 PMID:28852240

Bell, J. L., John, B. H., Desai, P. P., & McLeod, S. M. (2009). Family-centered care and the implications for child life practice. In R. H. Thompson (Ed.), *The Handbook of Child Life: A Guide for Pediatric Psychosocial Care* (pp. 95–115). Charles C. Thomas Publisher, Ltd.

Benard, B. (2006). Using strengths-based practice to tap the resilience of families. *The Strengths Perspective in Social Work Practice*, 197-220.

Bender, J. M. (2019). *My Daddy Is In Jail*. Youth Light Inc.

Benight, C. C., & Harper, M. L. (2002). Coping self-efficacy perceptions as a mediator between acute stress response and long-term distress following natural disasters. *Journal of Traumatic Stress*, *15*(3), 177–186. doi:10.1023/A:1015295025950 PMID:12092909

Benjamin, L., & Crawford-Browne, S. (2010). *The psychological impact of continuous traumatic stress–limitations of existing diagnostic frameworks* [Paper Presentation]. Continuous Traumatic Stress in South Africa Workshop, Department of Psychology, University of Cape Town, South Africa.

Benner, A. D., & Mistry, R. S. (2020). Child development during the COVID-19 pandemic through a life course theory lens. *Child Development Perspectives*, *14*(4), 236–243. doi:10.1111/cdep.12387 PMID:33230400

Berg, K., Shiu, C., Feinstein, R. T., Acharya, K., Medrano, J., & Small, M. E. (2019). Children with developmental disabilities experience higher levels of adversity. *Research in Developmental Disabilities*, *89*(1), 105–113. doi:10.1016/j.ridd.2019.03.011 PMID:30974258

Berg, S. H., Rortvelt, K., & Aase, K. (2017). Suicidal patients' experiences regarding their safety during psychiatric in-patient care: A systematic review of qualitative studies. *BMC Health Services Research*, *17*(73), 73. Advance online publication. doi:10.118612913-017-2023-8 PMID:28114936

Bergsund, H. B., Drozd, F., Hansen, M. B., & Jacobsen, H. (2018). Pre-adoption training: Experiences and recommendations from adoptive parents and course trainers. *Children and Youth Services Review*, *95*, 282–289. doi:10.1016/j.childyouth.2018.11.008

Berta, S., Blonsky, H., & Wogan, J. (2022). *Developing your school's student support teams: A practical guide for K-12 leaders, student services personnel, and mental health staff.* CRC Press. doi:10.4324/9781003240266

Bester, J., Cole, C. M., & Kodish, E. (2016). The limits of informed consent for an overwhelmed patient: Clinicians' role in protecting patients and preventing overwhelm. *AMA Journal of Ethics*, *18*(9), 869–886. doi:10.1001/journalofethics.2016.18.9.peer2-1609 PMID:27669132

Bethell, C. D., Kogan, M. D., Strickland, B. B., Schor, E. L., Robertson, J., & Newacheck, P. W. (2011). A national and state profile of leading health problems and health care quality for U.S. children: Key insurance disparities and across-state variations. *Academic Pediatrics*, *11*(3), S22–S33. doi:10.1016/j.acap.2010.08.011 PMID:21570014

Bethell, C. D., Solloway, M. R., Guinosso, S., Hassink, S., Srivastav, A., Ford, D., & Simpson, L. A. (2017). Prioritizing Possibilities for Child and Family Health: An Agenda to Address Adverse Childhood Experiences and Foster the Social and Emotional Roots of Well-being in Pediatrics. *Academic Pediatrics*, *17*(7, 7S), S36–S50. doi:10.1016/j.acap.2017.06.002 PMID:28865659

Bethell, C., Combojav, N., Solloway, M., & Wissow, L. (2016). Adverse childhood experiences, resilience and mindfulness-based approaches: Common denominator issues for children with emotional, mental, or behavioral problems. *Child and Adolescent Psychiatric Clinics of North America*, *25*(2), 139–156. doi:10.1016/j.chc.2015.12.001 PMID:26980120

Bethell, C., Newacheck, P., Hawes, E., & Halfton, N. (2014). Adverse childhood experiences: Assessing the impact on health and school engagement and the mitigating role of resilience. *Health Affairs*, *33*(12), 2106–2115. Advance online publication. doi:10.1377/hlthaff.2014.0914 PMID:25489028

Bhushan, B., & Sathya Kumar, J. (2009). Emotional Distress and Post-traumatic Stress in Children: The Impact of Direct Versus Indirect Exposure. *Journal of Loss and Trauma*, *14*(1), 35–45. doi:10.1080/15325020802537047

Biel, L., Peske, N., & Grandin, T. (2009). *Raising a sensory smart child: The definitive handbook for helping your child with sensory processing issues*. Penguin Books.

Biggs, E. E., & Carter, E. W. (2016). Supporting the social lives of students with intellectual disability. In *Handbook of research-based practices for educating students with intellectual disability* (pp. 243–262). Routledge.

Bishop, R. S. (1990). Mirrors, Windows, and Sliding Glass Doors. *Perspectives: Choosing and Using Books for Classroom, 6*(3), 1-2 https://scenicregional.org/wp-content/uploads/2017/08/Mirrors-Windows-and-Sliding-Glass-Doors.pdf

Blaze, J. T., & Shwalb, D. W. (2009). Resource loss and relocation: A follow-up study of adolescents two years after Hurricane Katrina. *Psychological Trauma: Theory, Research, Practice, and Policy*, *1*(4), 312–322. doi:10.1037/a0017834

Bodrova, E., & Leong, D. (2007). *Tools of the Mind: The Vygotskian approach to early childhood education*. Pearson/ Merrill Prentice Hall.

Boles, J. (2011, Fall). Creating a Culture of Research. *Child Life Bulletin*. https://www.childlife.org/docs/default-source/Publications/Bulletin/fall2011final.pdf?sfvrsn=2

Boles, J. C., Fraser, C., Bennett, K., Jones, M., Dunbar, J., Woodburn, A., Gill, M., Duplechain, A., Munn, E., & Hoskins, K. (2020). *The value of Certified Child Life Specialists: Direct and downstream optimization of pediatric patient and family outcomes* (Full report). https://www.childlife.org/docs/default-source/the-child-life-profession/value-of-cclss-full-report.pdf?sfvrsn=5e238d4d_2

Boles, J. C., Fraser, C., Bennett, K., Jones, M., Dunbar, J., Woodburn, A., Gill, M., Duplechain, A., Munn, E., & Hoskins, K. (2020, January). *The value of Certified Child Life Specialists: Direct and downstream optimization of pediatric patient and family outcomes* (Full report). Retrieved from: https://www.childlife.org/docs/default-source/the-child-life-profession/value-of-cclss-full-report.pdf?sfvrsn=5e238d4d_2

Boles, J., Fraser, C., Bennett, K., Jones, M., Dunbar, J., Woodburn, A., Gill, M. A., Duplechain, A., Munn, E. K., & Hoskins, K. (2020). *The value of certified child life specialists: Direct and downstream optimization of pediatric patient and family outcomes*. Association of Child Life Professionals. https://www.childlife.org/docs/default-source/aclp-official-documents/value-of-a-certified-child-life-specialist_full-report.pdf

Boles, J., Fraser, C., Bennett, K., Jones, M., Dunbar, J., Woodburn, A., Gill, M. A., Duplechain, A., Munn, E. K., & Hoskins, K. (2020). *The value of certified child life specialists: Direct and downstream optimization of pediatric patient and family outcomes*. Association of Child Life Professionals. https://www.childlife.org/docs/default-source/the-child-life-profession/value-of-cclss-full-report.pdf

Boles, J., Fraser, C., Bennett, K., Jones, M., Dunbar, J., Woodburn, A., Gill, M. A., Duplechain, A., Munn, E. K., & Hoskins, K. (2020). *The Value of Certified Child Life Specialists: Direct Downstream Optimization of Pediatric Patient and Family Outcomes*. Association of Child Life Professionals. https://www.childlife.org/the-child-life-profession/value-proposition-statement

Boles, J., Fraser, C., Bennett, K., Jones, M., Dunbar, J., Woodburn, A., Gill, M. A., Duplechain, A., Munn, E. K., & Hoskins, K. (2020, January). *The Value of Certified Child Life Specialists: Direct and Downstream Optimization of Pediatric Patient and Family Outcomes*. https://www.childlife.org/the-child-life-profession/value-proposition-statement#:~:text=The%20goal%20behind%20the%20Child,youth%2C%20families%2C%20and%20organizations

Boles, J., Fraser, C., Bennett, K., Jones, M., Dunbar, J., Woodburn, A., Gill, M. A., Duplechaine, A., Munn, E. K., & Hoskins, K. (2020). *The value of Certified Child Life Specialists: Direct and downstream optimization of pediatric patient and family outcomes*. https://www.childlife.org/docs/default-source/the-child-life-profession/value-of-cclss-full-report.pdf

Boles, J. (2018). Preparing children for healthcare encounters. In J. Rollins, R. Bolig, & C. Mahan (Eds.), *Meeting Children's Psychosocial Needs Across The Health-Care Continuum* (2nd ed.). PRO-ED.

Boles, J. C. (2017). Trauma-informed care: An intentional approach. *Pediatric Nursing*, *43*(5), 16–18.

Boles, J. C., & Daniels, S. R. (2019). Researching the experiences of children and youth with cancer: Considerations for practice. *Children (Basel, Switzerland)*, *6*(8), 93–104. doi:10.3390/children6080093 PMID:31426332

Boles, J. C., & Winsor, D. L. (2019). "My school is where my friends are": Interpreting the drawings of children with cancer. *Journal of Research in Childhood Education*, *33*(2), 225–241. doi:10.1080/02568543.2019.1577771

Boles, J., Turner, J., Rights, J., & Lu, R. (2021). Empirical evolution of child life. *The Journal of Child Life: Psychosocial Theory and Practice*, *2*(1), 4–14.

Bonanno, G. A., Brewin, C. R., Kaniasty, K., & Greca, A. M. L. (2010). Weighing the Costs of Disaster: Consequences, Risks, and Resilience in Individuals, Families, and Communities. *Psychological Science in the Public Interest, 11*(1), 1–49. doi:10.1177/1529100610387086 PMID:26168411

Bonanno, G. A., Neria, Y., Mancini, A., Coifman, K. G., Litz, B., & Insel, B. (2007). Is there more to complicated grief than depression and post-traumatic stress disorder? A test of incremental validity. *Journal of Abnormal Psychology, 116*(2), 342–351. doi:10.1037/0021-843X.116.2.342 PMID:17516766

Böök, M. L., & Mykkänen, J. (2014). Photo-narrative processes with children and young people. *International Journal of Child, Youth and Family Studies, 5*(4.1).

Botha, M., Hanlon, J., & Williams, G. L. (2021). Does language matter? Identity-first versus person-first language use in Autism research: A response to Vivanti. *Journal of Autism and Developmental Disorders*. Advance online publication. doi:10.100710803-020-04858-w PMID:33474662

Bowden, C. F., Worsley, D., Pettit, A. R., & Doupnik, S. K. (2022). Caregiver experiences during their child's acute medical hospitalization for a mental health crisis. *Journal of Child Health Care, 26*(1), 123–138. doi:10.1177/13674935211001222 PMID:33787342

Bowlby, J. (1969). Attachment and loss. Vol 1 Attachment. Pimlico: Basic Books.

Boyer, T. J., & Mitchell, S. A. (2021). Utilization of embedded simulation personnel in medical simulation. In *StatPearls*. StatPearls Publishing. https://www.ncbi.nlm.nih.gov/books/NBK562294/

Bray, B. (2019). *One school counselor per 455 students: Nationwide average improves.* Counseling Today. https://ct.counseling.org/2019/05/one-school-counselor-per-455-students-nationwide-average-improves/

Breau, L., & Burkitt, C. (2009). Assessing pain in children with intellectual disabilities. *Pain Research & Management, 14*(2), 116–120. doi:10.1155/2009/642352 PMID:19532853

Brewer, S., Gleditsch, S. L., Syblik, D., Tietjens, M. E., & Vacik, H. W. (2006). Pediatric anxiety: Child life intervention in day surgery. *Journal of Pediatric Nursing, 21*(1), 13–22. https://doi.org/10.1016/j.pedn.2005.06.004

Brill, S. A., Pepper, R., & Puttonen, M. (2011). *The transgender child: a handbook for families and professionals.* Post Hypnotic Press.

Brodzinsky, D., & Smith, S. L. (2014). Post-placement adjustment and the needs of birthmothers who place an infant for adoption. *Adoption Quarterly, 17*(3), 165–184. doi:10.1080/10926755.2014.891551

Bronfenbrenner, U. (1979). *The ecology of human development.* Harvard University Press.

Bronfenbrenner, U. (1981). *The Ecology of Human Development.* Harvard University Press. doi:10.2307/j.ctv26071r6

Bronfenbrenner, U. (1986). Ecology of the family as a context for human development: Research perspectives. *Developmental Psychology, 22*(6), 723–742. doi:10.1037/0012-1649.22.6.723

Brown, C. (2008). The School Setting. In Child life beyond the hospital (pp. 213-232). Child Life Council.

Brown, C., Mattera, G., Millar, T., Palm, S., & Rode, D. (2018). *Clinical Supervision Position Statement of the Child Life Council.* https://citeseerx.ist.psu.edu/viewdoc/download?doi=10.1.1.690.7183&rep=rep1&type=pdf

Brown, A. (2008). *The school setting. Child Life Beyond the Hospital.* Child Life Council, Inc.

Brown, C. (2009). Working with grieving children and families. In R. H. Thompson (Ed.), *The Handbook of Child Life: A Guide for Pediatric Psychosocial Care* (pp. 238–255). Charles C. Thomas Publisher, Ltd.

Browne-James, L., Litam, S. D. A., & McRae, L. (2021). Child sex trafficking: Strategies for identification, counseling, and advocacy. *International Journal for the Advancement of Counseling*, *43*(2), 113–125. doi:10.100710447-020-09420-y PMID:33432250

Burns, M., Griese, B., King, S., & Talmi, A. (2020). Childhood bereavement: Understanding prevalence and related adversity in the United States. *The American Journal of Orthopsychiatry*, *90*(4), 391–405. doi:10.1037/ort0000442 PMID:31999137

Burns-Nader, S. (2016). Examining children's healthcare experiences through drawings. *Early Child Development and Care*, *187*(11), 1809–1818. doi:10.1080/03004430.2016.1192616

Burns-Nader, S., Daniels, S., & Boles, J. (2021). Disseminating your study. In S. Daniels, S. Burns-Nader, & J. Boles (Eds.), *Research methods for child life specialists* (pp. 271–306). Cambridge Scholars Publishing.

Burns-Nader, S., & Hernandez-Reif, M. (2016). Facilitating play for hospitalized children through child life services. *Children's Health Care*, *45*(1), 1–21. https://doi.org/10.1080/02739615.2014.948161

Burns-Nader, S., Joe, L., & Pinion, K. (2017). Computer tablet distraction reduces pain and anxiety in pediatric burn patients undergoing hydrotherapy: A randomized trial. *Burns: Journal of the International Society for Burn Injuries*, *43*(6), 1203–1211. doi:10.1016/j.burns.2017.02.015 PMID:28318748

Cabaj, R. P. (2022). *Working with LGBTQ patients.* American Psychiatric Association. https://www.psychiatry.org/psychiatrists/cultural-competency/education/best-practice-highlights/working-with-lgbtq-patients

California Department of Education. (2019). *Designating Liaisons for Students Experiencing Homelessness.* https://www.cde.ca.gov/sp/hs/cy/documents/designatingliaisons.docx

Cardell, R., Bratcher, K. S., & Quinnett, P. (2009). Revisiting "suicide proofing" an inpatient unit through environmental safeguards: A review. *Perspectives in Psychiatric Care*, *45*(1), 36–44. doi:10.1111/j.1744-6163.2009.00198.x PMID:19154238

Carrington, J. (2020). *Kids these days: A game plan for (re)connecting with those we teach, lead & love.* IMPress Books.

Carstensen, K., Lou, S., Jensen, L. G., Nissen, N. K., Ortenblad, L., Pfau, M., & Ankerson, P. L. (2017). Psychiatric service users' experiences of emergency departments: A CERQual review of qualitative studies. *Nordic Journal of Psychiatry*, *71*(4), 315–323. doi:10.1080/08039488.2017.1288759 PMID:28413938

Case Western Reserve University. (2022). Plank, emma nuschi. In *The Encyclopedia of Cleveland History.* https://case.edu/ech/articles/p/plank-emma-nuschi

Casey, C. (2019). Management of aggressive patients: Results of an education program for nurses in non-psychiatric settings. *Medsurg Nursing*, *28*(1), 9–21.

Causey, D. L., McKay, M., Rosenthal, C., & Darnell, C. (1998). Assessment of hospital-related stress in children and adolescents admitted to a psychiatric inpatient unit. *Journal of Child and Adolescent Psychiatric Nursing*, *11*(4), 135–145. doi:10.1111/j.1744-6171.1998.tb00029.x PMID:10067477

Center on the Developing Child Harvard University. (n.d.). *Resilience* Retrieved March 15, 2022, from https://devhcdc.wpengine.com/science/key-concepts/resilience/

Centers for Disease Control and Prevention, National Center for Injury Prevention and Control, Division of Violence Prevention. (2022). *Preventing child abuse and neglect.* https://www.cdc.gov/violenceprevention/pdf/can/CAN-fact-sheet_2022.pdf

Centers for Disease Control and Prevention. (2020). *Disability and health overview.* https://www.cdc.gov/ncbddd/disabilityandhealth/disability.html

Centers for Disease Control and Prevention. (2021). *COVID-19 parental resources kit.* https://www.cdc.gov/mentalhealth/stress-coping/parental-resources/index.html

Centers for Disease Control and Prevention. (2021a). *Autism spectrum disorder.* https://www.cdc.gov/ncbddd/autism/index.html

Centers for Disease Control and Prevention. (2021b). *Developmental disabilities.* https://www.cdc.gov/ncbddd/developmentaldisabilities/facts.html

Centers for Disease Control and Prevention. (2021c). *What is children's mental health?* https://www.cdc.gov/childrensmentalhealth/basics.html

Centers for Disease Control and Prevention. (2022, January 24). *Chronic diseases in America.*https://www.cdc.gov/chronicdisease/resources/infographic/chronic-diseases.htm

Chang, T. P., Gerard, J., & Pusic, M. V. (2016). Screen-based simulation, virtual reality, and haptic simulators. In V. J. Grant & A. Cheng (Eds.), *Comprehensive healthcare simulation: Pediatrics* (pp. 105–114). Springer. doi:10.1007/978-3-319-24187-6_9

Chemtob, C. M., Nomura, Y., Rajendran, K., Yehuda, R., Schwartz, D., & Abramovitz, R. (2010). Impact of maternal post-traumatic stress disorder and depression following exposure to the September 11 attacks on preschool children's behavior. *Child Development*, *81*(4), 1129–1141. doi:10.1111/j.1467-8624.2010.01458.x PMID:20636686

Cheng, A., Auerbach, M., Calhoun, A., Mackinnon, R., Chang, T. P., Nadkarni, V., Hunt, E. A., Duval-Arnould, J., Peiris, N., Kessler, D., & INSPIRE Investigators (2018). Building a community of practice for researchers: The International Network for Simulation-Based Pediatric Innovation, Research and Education. *Simulation in Healthcare: Journal of the Society for Simulation in Healthcare, 13*(3S), S28–S34. doi:10.1097/SIH.0000000000000269

Chen, H. T. (2015). *Practical Program Evaluation: Theory-Driven Evaluation and the Integrated Evaluation Perspective* (2nd ed.). SAGE Publications, Inc.

Chen, S.-H., & Wu, Y.-C. (2006). Changes of PTSD Symptoms and School Reconstruction: A Two-year Prospective Study of Children and Adolescents after the Taiwan 921 Earthquake. *Natural Hazards*, *37*(1–2), 225–244. doi:10.100711069-005-4671-y

Chesak, S. S., Khalsa, T. K., Bhagra, A., Jenkins, S. M., Bauer, B. A., & Sood, A. (2019). Stress Management and Resiliency Training for public school teachers and staff: A novel intervention to enhance resilience and positively impact student interactions. *Complementary Therapies in Clinical Practice*, *37*, 32–38. doi:10.1016/j.ctcp.2019.08.001 PMID:31445365

Cheshire, A., Barlow, J. H., & Powell, L. A. (2010). The psychosocial well-being of parents of children with cerebral palsy: A comparison study. *Disability and Rehabilitation*, *32*(20), 1673–1677. doi:10.3109/09638281003649920 PMID:20178413

Child Life Certification Commission. (2020). *Child Life Code of Ethics.* Retrieved April 16, 2022, from https://www.childlife.org/docs/default-source/certification/child-life-code-of-ethics.pdf?sfvrsn=2

Child Life Council. (2006). *Guidelines for the development of child life programs in health care settings* (4th ed.). CLC.

Child Life Council. (2009). Preparing Children and Adolescents for Medical Procedures. *Child Life Council Evidenced-Based Practice Statement.* https://www.childlife.org/docs/default-source/research-ebp/ebp-statements.pdf?sfvrsn=6395bd4d_2

Child Life Council. (2014). *Child life services.* American Academy of Pediatrics. doi:10.1542/peds.2014-0556

Child Life Disaster Relief. (2022). *About us.* Child Life Disaster Relief. https://cldisasterrelief.org/about-us/

Child Mind Institute. (2021). *The impact of the COVID-19 pandemic on children's mental health: What we know so far.* https://childmind.org/wp-content/uploads/2021/10/CMHR-2021-FINAL.pdf

Childhelp. (n.d.). *Child abuse statistics.* https://www.childhelp.org/child-abuse-statistics/

Childlife.org. (n.d.a). Retrieved August 8, 2022, from https://www.childlife.org/docs/default-source/aclp-official-documents/child-life-code-of

Childlife.org. (n.d.b). Retrieved August 8, 2022, from https://www.childlife.org/docs/default-source/research-ebp/ebp-

Choudhury, R. G. (2020). Distinctive marketing strategies of different industries in India. *The Business & Management Review, 11*(2), 13–18. doi:10.24052/BMR/V11NU02/ART-02

Cicero, M. X., & Weiner, D. L. (2016). Simulation for pediatric disaster and multiple casualty incident training. In V. J. Grant & A. Cheng (Eds.), *Comprehensive healthcare simulation: Pediatrics* (pp. 253–264). Springer. doi:10.1007/978-3-319-24187-6_20

Cienfuegos, S. J. (2019, November 18). APD unveils soft interview rooms to ensure trauma-informed approach. *Hilltop Views.* https://www.hilltopviewsonline.com/20750/news/apd-unveils-soft-interview-rooms-to-ensure-trauma-informed-approach/

Cincinnati Children's Hospital Medical Center. (2013). *Psychosocial Risk Assessment in Pediatrics.* https://praptool.com/

Claridge, A. M., Hajec, L. P., Montgomery, L. P., & Knapp, B. M. (2020). Child and parent psychosocial experiences of hospitalization: An examination of the role of child life specialists. The Journal of Child Life, Psychosocial. *Theory into Practice, 1*(1).

Clutter, L. B. (2017). Open adoption placement by birth mothers in their twenties. *The American Journal of Maternal/Child Nursing, 42*(6), 345-351. doi:10.1097/NMC.0000000000000370

Clutter, L. B. (2020). Perceptions of birth fathers about their open adoption. *The American Journal of Maternal/Child Nursing, 45*(1), 26-32. doi:10.1097/NMC.0000000000000591

Clutter, L. B. (2014). Adult birth mothers who made open infant adoption placements after adolescent unplanned pregnancy. *JOGNN, 43*(2), 190–199. doi:10.1111/1552-6909.12280 PMID:24502258

Clutter, L. B. (2018). Spiritual *Needs in Children's Health Care Settings.* In R. Thompson (Ed.), *The Handbook of Child Life* (2nd ed., pp. 349–410). Charles C Thomas.

Cluver, L. D., Meinck, F., Steinert, J. I., Shenderovich, Y., Doubt, J., Romero, R. H., ... Gardner, F. (2018). Parenting for lifelong health: A pragmatic cluster randomised controlled trial of a non-commercialised parenting programme for adolescents and their families in South Africa. *BMJ Global Health, 3*(1), e000539. doi:10.1136/bmjgh-2017-000539 PMID:29564157

Cohen, D. H., Stern, V., Balaban, N., & Gropper, N. (2016). Recording children's behavior in dramatic play. In *Observing and recording the behavior of young children* (6th ed., pp. 66–90). Teachers College Press.

Cohen, J. A., Mannarino, A. P., & Deblinger, E. (2006). *Treating trauma and traumatic grief in children and adolescents.* The Guilford Press.

Cohen, J. A., Mannarino, A. P., Kliethermes, M., & Murray, L. A. (2012). Trauma-focused CBT for youth with complex trauma. *Child Abuse & Neglect, 36*(6), 528–541. doi:10.1016/j.chiabu.2012.03.007 PMID:22749612

Cole, L. P., Henechowicz, T. L., Kang, K., Pranjić, M., Richard, N. M., Tian, G. L. J., & Hurt-Thaut, C. (2021). Neurologic Music Therapy via telehealth: A survey of clinician experiences, trends, and recommendations during the COVID-19 pandemic. *Frontiers in Neuroscience*, *15*, 648489. doi:10.3389/fnins.2021.648489 PMID:33897362

Coleman, D. N., Hurley, M. L., March, K. S., Schommer, K. W., Curry, A. M., Gordon, M. D., & Hagan, J. L. (2021). Virtual reality as a form of interactive distraction for pediatric patients receiving immediate hypersensitivity skin tests: A randomized controlled trial. The Journal of Child Life, Psychosocial. *Theory into Practice*, *2*(2).

Cole, S. F., Eisner, A., Gregory, M., & Ristuccia, J. (2013). *Creating and advocating for trauma-sensitive schools*. Massachusetts Advocates for Children.

Collaborative for Academic, Social, and Emotional Learning. (n.d.). *What is the CASEL framework?* https://casel.org/fundamentals-of-sel/what-is-the-casel-framework/

Cooper, M., & Hicks, M. (2008). Nonprofits Providing Child Life Services. In M. Hicks (Ed.), *Child Life Beyond the Hospital* (pp. 169–193). Child Life Council.

Cornell University. (2021). *The therapeutic crisis intervention system* (7th ed.). Residential Child Care Project. https://rccp.cornell.edu/downloads/TCI_7_SYSTEM%20BULLETIN.pdf

Costa, N. M., Weems, C. F., & Pina, A. A. (2009). Hurricane Katrina and youth anxiety: The role of perceived attachment beliefs and parenting behaviors. *Journal of Anxiety Disorders*, *23*(7), 935–941. doi:10.1016/j.janxdis.2009.06.002 PMID:19577899

Couturier, J., Pindiprolu, B., Findlay, S., & Johnson, N. (2015). Anorexia nervosa and gender dysphoria in two adolescents. *International Journal of Eating Disorders*, *48*(1), 151–155. doi:10.1002/eat.22368 PMID:25421316

Cover, L. (2021, August 18). 7 statistics that prove the importance of social media marketing in business. *Sprout Social*. https://sproutsocial.com/insights/importance-of-social-media-marketing-in-business/

COVID-19 resources - telehealth considerations and resources. (n.d.). Retrieved August 7, 2022, from https://www.musictherapy.org/about/covid19_resources_telehealth_considerations_and_resources/

Craig, J. W. (2019). The neonatal intensive care unit (nicu): Self-efficacy of caregiving and the lived experience of parents post-nicu discharge. *Neonatology Today*, 25-31.

Crime Museum. (n.d.). *Types of Prisons*. Retrieved February 17, 2022, https://www.crimemuseum.org/crime-library/famous-prisons-incarceration/types-of-prisons/

Crisis Prevention Institute. (2019). *What is nonviolent crisis intervention training?* https://www.crisisprevention.com/What-We-Do

Crisis Prevention Institute. (2020). *CPI nonviolent crisis intervention training* (2nd ed.). [Participant workbook]. Author.

Crnjak, E., Kerns, M., Stevens, M., O'Connell, B., & Mednick, L. (2021, Sept. 19). *Child life at end of life: Enhancing psychosocial care through bereavement simulation training* [Poster presentation]. 13th International Pediatric Simulation Symposia and Workshops, IPSSV 2021: A Virtual Experience. https://www.eventscribe.net/2021/IPSSV2021/fsPopup.asp?efp=T05YTlpQQ1oxNTA1Nw&PosterID=427009&rnd=0.944971&mode=posterinfo

Cronholm, P. F., Forke, C. M., Wade, R., Bair-Merritt, M. H., Davis, M., Harkins-Schwarz, M., Pachter, L. M., & Fein, J. A. (2015). Adverse Childhood Experiences: Expanding the Concept of Adversity. *American Journal of Preventive Medicine*, *49*(3), 354–361. doi:10.1016/j.amepre.2015.02.001 PMID:26296440

Cryder, C. H., Kilmer, R. P., Tedeschi, R. G., & Calhoun, L. G. (2006). An exploratory study of post-traumatic growth in children following a natural disaster. *The American Journal of Orthopsychiatry*, *76*(1), 65–69. doi:10.1037/0002-9432.76.1.65 PMID:16569128

da Silva, I. M., & Sathiyaseelan, A. (2019). Emotional needs of women post-rescue from sex trafficking in India. *Cogent Psychology*, *6*(1), 1631584. doi:10.1080/23311908.2019.1631584

Dalla, R. L., & Kreimer, L. M. (2017). "After your honor is gone…": Exploration of developmental trajectories and life experiences of women working in Mumbai's red-light brothel districts. *Sexuality & Culture*, *21*(1), 163–186. doi:10.100712119-016-9388-4

Dalla, R. L., Panchal, T. J., Erwin, S., Peter, J., Roselius, K., Ranjan, R., Mischra, M., & Sahu, S. (2020). Structural vulnerabilities, personal agency, and caste: An exploration of child sex trafficking in rural India. *Violence and Victims*, *35*(3), 307–330. doi:10.1891/VV-D-19-00048 PMID:32606215

Daniels, S., & Toohey, S. J. (2019, September). *"Don't put your phone down!" Child life practice and the online worlds of hospitalized teens* [Conferences session]. 2nd Annual Southeastern Association of Child Life Professionals Regional Conference, Nashville, TN, United States.

Daniels, S., Burns-Nader, S., & Boles, J. (Eds.). (2021a). Research methods for child life specialists (edited collection). Cambridge Scholars Publishing.

Danielson, B. (2018, October). *Child life and psychiatry* [Conference presentation]. Great Lakes Association of Child Life Professionals, Cincinnati, OH, United States.

Danielson, B., McEwen, K., & Sullivan, K. (2019, April). *Please see me, I'm sick too: The journey through a mental health care admission* [Conference presentation]. Association of Child Life Professionals National Conference, Chicago, IL, United States.

Daniels, S. R., Yang, C., Toohey, S. J., & Willard, V. W. (2021b). Perspectives on social media from adolescents and young adults with cancer. *Journal of Pediatric Oncology Nursing*, *38*(4), 225–232. doi:10.1177/1043454221992319 PMID:33729902

Dargis, M., & Mitchell-Somoza, A. (2021). Challenges Associated with Parenting While Incarcerated: A Review. *International Journal of Environmental Research and Public Health*, *18*(9927), 1–16. doi:10.3390/ijerph18189927 PMID:34574849

De Claire, K., & Dixon, L. (2015). The Effects of Prison Visits From Family Members on Prisoners' Well-Being, Prison Rule Breaking, and Recidivism: A Review of Research Since 1991. *Trauma, Violence & Abuse*, *18*(2), 1–15. PMID:26330175

De Veaux, M. (2013). The Trauma of the Incarceration Experience. *Harvard Civil Rights-Civil Liberties Law Review*, *48*, 257–277.

Deaton, J. D., Ohrt, J. H., Linich, K., Wymer, B., Toomey, M., Leris, O., Guest, J. D., & Newton, T. (2022). Teachers' experiences with K-12 students' mental health. *Psychology in the Schools*, *59*(50), 932–949. doi:10.1002/pits.22658

DeFrain, J., & Asay, S. M. (2007). Strong families around the world: An introduction to the family strengths perspective. *Marriage & Family Review*, *41*(1-2), 1–10. doi:10.1300/J002v41n01_01

DeFrain, J., Asay, S., & Geggie, J. (2010). Family strengths: An international perspective. In F. Arney & D. Scott (Eds.), *Working with vulnerable families: A partnership approach* (pp. 29–48). Cambridge University Press. doi:10.1017/CBO9780511845376.004

Dehlin, M., & Lundh, L. G. (2018). Compassion fatigue and compassion satisfaction among psychologists: Can supervision and a reflective stance be of help? *Journal for Person-Oriented Research*, *4*(2), 95–107. doi:10.17505/jpor.2018.09 PMID:33569136

Demaria, S. Jr, Bryson, E. O., Mooney, T. J., Silverstein, J. H., Reich, D. L., Bodian, C., & Levine, A. I. (2010). Adding emotional stressors to training in simulated cardiopulmonary arrest enhances participant performance. *Medical Education*, *44*(10), 1006–1015. doi:10.1111/j.1365-2923.2010.03775.x PMID:20880370

DeWolfe, D. (2000). *Training manual for mental health and human services workers in major disasters* (2nd ed.). U.S. Department of Health and Human Services.

Diaz, M. C. G., Arnold, J. L., & Robinson, T. (2016). Simulation for patient- and family-centered care. In V. J. Grant & A. Cheng (Eds.), *Comprehensive healthcare simulation: Pediatrics* (pp. 329–340). Springer. doi:10.1007/978-3-319-24187-6_26

Dichter, H., Ruprecht, K., & Tomlin, A. (2020). Exploring Early Care and Education Policy for Young Children of Incarcerated Parents. *Zero to Three*, *40*(4), 51–58. https://hdl.handle.net/1805/28132

Dirik, A., Sandhu, S., Giacco, D., Barrett, K., Bennison, G., Collinson, S., & Priebe, S. (2017). Why involve families in acute mental health care? A collaborative conceptual review. *BMJ Open*, *7*(9), e017680. Advance online publication. doi:10.1136/bmjopen-2017-017680 PMID:28963308

Dirth, T., & Branscombe, N. (2017). Disability models affect disability policy support through awareness of structural discrimination. *The Journal of Social Issues*, *73*(2), 413–442. doi:10.1111/josi.12224

Dixey, R., & Woodall, J. (2012). The significance of "the visit" in an English category B prison: Views from prisoners, prisoners' families, and prison staff. *Community Work & Family*, *15*(1), 29–47. doi:10.1080/13668803.2011.580125

Dopheide, J. A. (2013). Recognizing and referring at-risk youth. *The Mental Health Clinician*, *2*(11), 353–361. doi:10.9740/mhc.n145475

Drake, J., Johnson, N., Stoneck, A. V., Martinez, D. M., & Massey, M. (2012). Evaluation of a coping kit for children with challenging behaviors in a pediatric hospital. *Pediatric Nursing*, *38*(4). PMID:22970487

Drewes, A. A., & Schaefer, C. E. (2015). *School-Based Play Therapy* (2nd ed.). John Wiley & Sons Inc.

Drigas, A. S., & Papoutsi, C. (2018). A new layered model on emotional intelligence. *Behavioral Sciences (Basel, Switzerland)*, *8*(5), 45. doi:10.3390/bs8050045 PMID:29724021

Drum, K. B., & Littleton, H. L. (2014). Therapeutic boundaries in telepsychology: Unique issues and best practice recommendations. *Professional Psychology, Research and Practice*, *45*(5), 309–315. https://doi.org/10.1037/a0036127

Duc, J. K., Herbert, A. R., & Heussler, H. S. (2017). Paediatric palliative care and intellectual disability- A unique context. *Journal of Applied Research in Intellectual Disabilities*, *30*(1), 1111–1124. doi:10.1111/jar.12389 PMID:28836319

Dummer, T. J., & Cook, I. G. (2008). Health in China and India: A cross-country comparison in a context of rapid globalization. *Social Science & Medicine*, *67*(4), 590–605. doi:10.1016/j.socscimed.2008.04.019 PMID:18554766

Dyregrov, A., Salloum, A., Kristensen, P., & Dyregrov, K. (2015). Grief and Traumatic Grief in Children in the Context of Mass Trauma. *Current Psychiatry Reports*, *17*(6), 48. Advance online publication. doi:10.100711920-015-0577-x PMID:25940038

Ebersöhn, L., Sefotho, M., Mampane, R., Loots, T., Omidire, F., Sherman, V., & Nxumalo-Tsebe, T. (2014). *Imbeleko report: Cultivating resourcefulness, not dependency*. Academic Press.

Edgar-Bailey, M., & Kress, V. E. (2010). Resolving child and adolescent traumatic grief: Creative techniques and interventions. *Journal of Creativity in Mental Health, 5*(2), 158–176. doi:10.1080/15401383.2010.485090

Edmondson, A. (1999). Psychological safety and learning behavior in work teams. *Administrative Science Quarterly, 44*(2), 350–383. doi:10.2307/2666999

Edmonton Catholic Schools. (2020). *Mental Health Strategic Plan.* https://sbecsdstor.blob.core.windows.net/docs/9115d70a-5ccc-4a1f-8273-a4176310f7a1_ECSMENTALHEALTHBROCH1920.pdf

Eijlers, R., Utens, E. M. W. J., Staals, L. M., de Nijs, P. F. A., Berghmans, J. M., Wijnen, R. M. H., Hillegers, M. H. J., Dierckx, B., & Legerstee, J. S. (2019). Systematic review and meta-analysis of virtual reality in pediatrics: Effects on pain and anxiety: Effects on pain and anxiety. *Anesthesia and Analgesia, 129*(5), 1344–1353. https://doi.org/10.1213/ANE.0000000000004165

Einfeld, S. L., & Tongue, B. L. (1996). Population prevalence of psychopathology in children and adolescents with intellectual disability, II: Epidemiological findings. *Journal of Intellectual Disability Research, 40*(2), 99–109. doi:10.1111/j.1365-2788.1996.tb00611.x PMID:8731467

Emergency Management in the United States. (n.d.). Federal Emergency Management Agency. Retrieved March 10, 2022, from https://training.fema.gov/emiweb/downloads/is111_unit%204.pdf

Eppich, W., & Cheng, A. (2015). Promoting excellence and reflective learning in simulation (PEARLS): Development and rationale for a blended approach to health care simulation debriefing. *Simulation in Healthcare: Journal of the Society for Simulation in Healthcare, 10*(2), 106–115. doi:10.1097/SIH.0000000000000072 PMID:25710312

Epstein, E. G., Arechiga, J., Dancy, M., Simon, J., Wilson, D., & Alhusen, J. L. (2017). Integrative review of technology to support communication with parents of infants in the NICU. *Journal of Obstetric, Gynecologic, and Neonatal Nursing, 46*(3), 357–366. doi:10.1016/j.jogn.2016.11.019

Erikson, E. (1950). *Childhood and Society*. W.W. Norton & Company.

Erin's Law. (n.d.). *What is Erin's Law?* https://www.erinslaw.org/erins-law/

Ertl, S., Bokor, B., Tuchman, L., Miller, E., Kappel, R., & Deye, K. (2020). Healthcare needs and utilization patterns of sex-trafficked youth: Missed opportunities at a children's hospital. *Child: Care, Health and Development, 46*(4), 422–428. doi:10.1111/cch.12759 PMID:32037615

Espe-Sherwindt, M. (2008). Family-centered practice: Collaboration, competency and evidence. *Support for Learning, 23*(3), 136–143. doi:10.1111/j.1467-9604.2008.00384.x

Every child deserves emotionally safe care. (2021, February 9). Emotional Safety Initiative. https://emotional-safety.org/

Fahrenwald, D., & Haley, J. (2021, September 10-12). *Piecing together autism, baker acts and community inequalities* [Conference presentation]. Florida Association of Child Life Professionals Annual Conference, Orlando, FL, United States.

Fallon, A. E., & Goldsmith, B. L. (2013). *Theoretical contributions to the understanding of parent-child bonding in adoption. In Working with adoptive parents: Research, theory, and therapeutic interventions*. Wiley.

Family Caregiver Alliance. (2012, September 21). *Caregiver isolation and loneliness*. https://www.caregiver.org/news/caregiver-isolation-and-loneliness/

Fann, J. R., Thomas-Rich, A. M., Katon, W. J., Cowley, D., Pepping, M., McGregor, B. A., & Gralow, J. (2008). Major depression after breast cancer: A review of epidemiology and treatment. *General Hospital Psychiatry, 30*(2), 112–126. doi:10.1016/j.genhosppsych.2007.10.008 PMID:18291293

Farrokhi, F., & Maytum, S. (2005, Winter). Why Research? *Child Life Bulletin.* https://www.childlife.org/docs/default-source/Publications/Bulletin/winter-2005-bulletin---final.pdf?sfvrsn=2

Felitti, V. J., Anda, R. F., Nordenberg, D., Williamson, D. F., Spitz, A. M., Edwards, V., Koss, M. P., & Marks, J. S. (1998). Relationship of childhood abuse and household dysfunction to many of the leading causes of death in adults. The Adverse Childhood Experiences (ACE) Study. *American Journal of Preventive Medicine, 14*(4), 245–258. doi:10.1016/S0749-3797(98)00017-8 PMID:9635069

Field, J., & Schubert, C. M. (2010). An examination of emergency department pediatric psychiatric services. *The Journal of Behavioral Health Services & Research, 37*(4), 412–426. doi:10.100711414-009-9189-8 PMID:19731041

Finkelhor, D. (2012). Characteristics of crimes against juveniles. Durham, NH: Crimes Against Children Research Center.

Flacking, R., Lehtonen, L., Thomson, G., Axelin, A., Ahlqvist, S., Moran, V. H., Ewald, U., & Dykes, F. (2012). Closeness and separation in neonatal intensive care. *Foundation Acta Pædiatrica, 101*(10), 1032–1037. doi:10.1111/j.1651-2227.2012.02787.x PMID:22812674

Foli, K. J., Schweitzer, R., & Wells, C. (2013). The personal and professional: Nurses' lived experiences of adoption. *The American Journal of Maternal/Child Nursing, 38*(2), 79-86. doi:10.1097/NMC.0b013e3182763446

Foli, K. J. (2012). Nursing care of the adoption triad. *Perspectives in Psychiatric Care, 48*(4), 208–217. doi:10.1111/j.1744-6163.2012.00327.x PMID:23005588

Forkey, H., Szilagyi, M., Kelly, E. T., Duffee, J., Springer, S. H., Fortin, K., Jones, V. F., Vaden Greiner, M. B., Ochs, T. J., Partap, A. N., Davidson Sagor, L., Allen Staat, M., Thackeray, J. D., Waite, D., & Weber Zetley, L. (2021). Trauma-informed care. *Pediatrics, 148*(2), e2021052580. doi:10.1542/peds.2021-052580 PMID:34312292

Foronda, C. (2020). A theory of cultural humility. *Journal of Transcultural Nursing, 31*(1), 7–12. doi:10.1177/1043659619875184 PMID:31516091

Fraatz, E., & Durand, T. M. (2021). Meeting the needs of children with autism spectrum disorder and their families in hospital settings: The perspectives of Certified Child Life Specialists and Nurses. *Journal of Child Life: Psychosocial Theory and Practice, 2*(2). Advance online publication. doi:10.55591/001c.27703

Francis, L., & Silvers, A. (2016). Perspectives on the meaning of "disability.". *American Medical Association Journal of Ethics, 18*(10), 1025–1033. doi:10.1001/journalofethics.2016.18.10.pfor2-1610 PMID:27780027

Franke, H. A. (2014). Toxic stress: Effects, prevention, and treatment. *Children (Basel, Switzerland), 1*(3), 390–402. doi:10.3390/children1030390 PMID:27417486

Franklin, M. B. (2000). The Meanings of Play in the Developmental-Interaction Tradition. In N. Nager & E. K. Shapiro (Eds.), *Revisiting a progressive pedagogy: The developmental interaction approach* (pp. 47–71). SUNY Press.

Fraser, C., CCLS, C., & Munn, E. K. (2020). *The Value of Certified Child Life Specialists: Direct and Downstream Optimization of Pediatric Patient and Family Outcomes.* Academic Press.

Freeman, J. C., Epston, D., & Lobovits, D. (1997). *Playful approaches to serious problems: Narrative therapy with children and their families.* WW Norton & Company.

Furr, J. M., Comer, J. S., Edmunds, J. M., & Kendall, P. C. (2010). Disasters and youth: A meta-analytic examination of post-traumatic stress. *Journal of Consulting and Clinical Psychology, 78*(6), 765–780. doi:10.1037/a0021482 PMID:21114340

Gaba, D. M. (2004). The future vision of simulation in health care. *Quality & Safety in Health Care, 13*(Suppl 1), i2–i10. doi:10.1136/qhc.13.suppl_1.i2

Gajarawala, S. N., & Pelkowski, J. N. (2021). Telehealth benefits and barriers. *The Journal for Nurse Practitioners: JNP, 17*(2), 218–221. https://doi.org/10.1016/j.nurpra.2020.09.013

Gallagher, K. A. S., Bujoreanu, L. S., Cheung, P., Choi, C., Golden, S., Brodziak, K., Andrare, G., & Ibeziako, P. (2017). Psychiatric boarding in the pediatric inpatient medical setting: A retrospective analysis. *Hospital Pediatrics*, *7*(8), 444–450. doi:10.1542/hpeds.2017-0005 PMID:28716803

Galvez, J., Eisenhower, M., England, W., Wartman, E., Simpao, A., Rehman, M., Lustig, R., & Hribar, M. (2019). An interactive virtual reality tour for adolescents receiving proton radiation therapy: Proof-of-concept study. *JMIR Perioperative Medicine*, *2*(1), e11259. doi:10.2196/11259 PMID:33393932

Gariépy, N., & Howe, N. (2003). The therapeutic power of play: Examining the play of young children with leukaemia. *Child: Care, Health and Development*, *29*(6), 523–537. doi:10.1046/j.1365-2214.2003.00372.x PMID:14616910

Gaynard, L., Hausslem, E., & Demarsh, J. P. (1989). Child life specialists: Report of an observational study. *Children's Health Care*, *18*(2), 75–81. doi:10.120715326888chc1802_3 PMID:10292919

Gaynard, L., Wolfer, J., Goldberger, J., Thompson, R., Redburn, L., & Laidley, L. (1998). *Psychosocial care of children in hospitals: A clinical practice manual from the ACCH child life research project*. Child Life Council, Inc.

Gaynard, L., Wolfer, J., Goldberger, J., Thompson, R., Redburn, L., & Laidley, L. (1998). *Psychosocial care of children in hospitals: A clinical practice manual from the acch child life research project*. Child Life Council.

Gaynard, L., Wolfer, J., Goldberger, J., Thompson, R., Redburn, L., & Laidley, L. (1998). *Psychosocial Care of Children in Hospitals: A clinical practice manual from the ACCH Child Life Research Project*. Child Life Council.

Gaynard, L., Wolfer, J., Goldgerger, J., Thompson, R., Redburn, L., & Laidley, L. (1990). *Psychosocial care of children in hospitals: A clinical practice manual for the ACCH child life research project*. Association for the Care of Children's Health.

Gibson, N. (2018). *Therapeutic photography: Enhancing self-esteem, self-efficacy and resilience*. Jessica Kingsley Publishers.

Ginsburg, K. R. (2007). The importance of play in promoting healthy child development and maintaining strong parent-child bonds. *Pediatrics*, *119*(1), 182–191. doi:10.1542/peds.2006-2697 PMID:17200287

Glasper, E. A. (2017). Optimizing the care of children with intellectual disabilities in hospitals. *Comprehensive Child and Adolescent Nursing*, *40*(2), 63–67. doi:10.1080/24694193.2017.1309827 PMID:29318949

Glesner, T. (2012). Addressing the Needs of Children of Incarcerated Parents. A Publication of the University of Vermont, James M. *Jeffords Center*, *2*(2), 2–4.

Gnana, S. R. (2018). Caste system, dalitization and its implications in contemporary India. *International Journal of Sociology and Anthropology*, *10*(7), 65–71. doi:10.5897/IJSA2017.0713

Goddard, A., Janicek, E., & Etcher, L. (2022). Trauma-informed care for the pediatric nurse. *Journal of Pediatric Nursing*, *62*, 1–9. https://doi.org/10.1016/j.pedn.2021.11.003

Goldberger, J., Lumbering Mohl, A., & Thompson, R. (2018). Psychological Preparation and Coping. In R. Thompson (Ed.), *The Handbook of Child Life* (2nd ed., pp. 268–312). Charles C Thomas.

Goldberger, J., Thompson, R. H., & Mohl, A. L. (2018). Psychological preparation and coping. In R. H. Thompson (Ed.), *The handbook of child life: A guide for pediatric psychosocial care* (2nd ed., pp. 268–316). Charles C. Thomas Pub. Ltd.

Gordon, J. (2021). Emotional safety in pediatrics. *Emotional Safety Initiative*. https://emotional-safety.org/emotional-safety-in-pediatrics/

Gordon, J., & Paisley, P. (2018). Trauma-Focused Medical Play. In L. Rubin (Ed.), Handbook of Medical Play Therapy and Child Life (pp. 154-172). Routledge.

Goshin, L. S., & Byrne, M. W. (2009). Converging Streams of Opportunity for Prison Nursery Programs in the United States. *Journal of Offender Rehabilitation*, *48*(4), 271–295. doi:10.1080/10509670902848972 PMID:19865610

Gould, C., & Ward, C. L. (2015). Positive parenting in South Africa: Why supporting families is key to development and violence prevention. *Institute for Security Studies. Policy Brief*, 77.

Grant, D. J., Grant, V. J., & Cheng, A. (2016). The future of pediatric simulation. In V. J. Grant & A. Cheng (Eds.), *Comprehensive healthcare simulation: Pediatrics* (pp. 401–410). Springer. doi:10.1007/978-3-319-24187-6_31

Greene, M. (1995). Chapter 11: Texts and Margins. In Releasing the Imagination: Essays on Education, the Arts, and Social Change. (3rd ed., 134–151). John Wiley & Sons

Greene, R. W. (2016). *Lost and found: Helping Behaviorally Challenging Students (and, While You're At It, All the Others)*. Jossey-Bass.

Greiner, C. M., Park, J., & Goldstein, S. E. (2022). Teacher trainees' experience with and beliefs about responding to students' challenging life events. *Teaching and Teacher Education, 111*, 103603. doi:10.1016/j.tate.2021.103603

Grissom, S., Boles, J., Bailey, K., Cantrell, K., Kennedy, A., Sykes, A., & Mandrell, B. N. (2016). Play-based procedural preparation and support intervention for cranial radiation. *Supportive Care in Cancer*, *24*(6), 2421–2427. doi:10.100700520-015-3040-y PMID:26634562

Grotberg, E. (1995). *A Guide to Promoting Resilience in Children: Strengthening the Human Spirit*. Bernard van Leer Foundation.

Gupta, N., Brown, C., Deneke, J., Maha, J., & Kong, M. (2019). Utilization of a novel pathway in a tertiary pediatric hospital to meet the sensory needs of acutely ill pediatric patients. *Frontier Pediatrics, 7*, 367. doi:10.3389/fped.2019.00367

Guss, C. E., Williams, D. N., Reisner, S. L., Austin, S. B., & Katz-Wise, S. L. (2016). Disordered weight management behaviors and non-prescription steroid use in massachusetts transgender youth. *The Journal of Adolescent Health*, *58*(2), S102–S103. Advance online publication. doi:10.1016/j.jadohealth.2015.10.217

Hairston, C. F. (1991). Family Ties During Imprisonment: Important to Whom and for What? *Journal of Sociology and Social Welfare*, *87*, 87–104.

Halpern, J., & Vermeulen, K. (2017). *Disaster mental health intervention: Core principles and practices*. Routledge. doi:10.4324/9781315623825

Halverson, K. K. (2018, March 6). *How infants grieve: A guide for new adoptive parents*. Adoption.com. https://adoption.com/how-infants-grieve-a-guide-for-new-adoptive-parents

Hamadi, L., & Fletcher, H. K. (2021). Are people with an intellectual disability at increased risk of attachment difficulties? A critical review. *Journal of Intellectual Disabilities*, *25*(1), 114–130. doi:10.1177/1744629519864772 PMID:31362566

Hanna, M. D., & Rogers, S. (2022). Real or imagined: Racial bias in family assessments. *Child Welfare*, *100*(2), 137–162.

Harrington, D. W., & Simon, L. V. (2021). Designing a simulation scenario. In *StatPearls*. StatPearls Publishing. https://www.ncbi.nlm.nih.gov/books/NBK547670/

Hart, L., Kelly, C., Kingston, A., Langlands, R., & Masselli, B. (2016). *Mental health first aid USA* [Workbook]. National Council for Behavioral Health.

Hawkins, R. (2009). Same as It Ever Was, Only Worse: Negative Life Events and Poverty Among New Orleans Katrina Survivors. *Families in Society*, *90*(4), 375–381. doi:10.1606/1044-3894.3922

Haynes, C., Eivors, A., & Crossley, J. (2011). 'Living in an alternative reality:' adolescents' experiences of psychiatric inpatient care. *Child and Adolescent Mental Health*, *16*(3), 150–157. doi:10.1111/j.1475-3588.2011.00598.x PMID:32847238

Hazen, E. P., & Prager, L. M. (2017). A quiet crisis: Pediatric patients waiting for inpatient psychiatric care. *Journal of the American Academy of Child and Adolescent Psychiatry*, *56*(8), 631–633. doi:10.1016/j.jaac.2017.03.022 PMID:28735689

Heffer, R. W., & Lowe, P. A. (2000). A review of school reintegration programs for children with cancer. *Journal of School Psychology*, *38*(5), 447–467. doi:10.1016/S0022-4405(00)00046-7

Heger, A., Ticson, L., Velasquez, O., & Bernier, R. (2002). Children referred for possible sexual abuse: Medical findings in 2384 children. *Child Abuse & Neglect*, *26*(6-7), 645–659.

Heiden-Rootes, K., Miller, B., & Moore, R. (2019). Cultural socialization in transracial adoption: Adoption support, multicultural experiences, perceptions of discrimination, and positive feelings toward racial minority groups. *Adoption Quarterly*, *22*(4), 247–264. doi:10.1080/10926755.2019.1627447

Herbert, J. L., Walsh, W., & Bromfield, L. (2018). A national survey of characteristics of child advocacy centers in the United States: Do the flagship models match those in broader practice? *Child Abuse & Neglect*, *76*, 583–595. https://doi.org/10.1016/j.chiabu.2017.09.030

Hicks, M. (Ed.). (2008). *Child Life Beyond the Hospital*. Child Life Council.

Hicks, M., & McCue, K. (2018). Child Life in the Community and in Other Non-traditional Roles. In *Thompson, R.) The handbook of child life: A guide for pediatric psychosocial care. 2nd Edition* (pp. 257–286). Charles C. Thomas.

Hobfoll, S. E., Watson, P., Bell, C. C., Bryant, R. A., Brymer, M. J., Friedman, M. J., Friedman, M., Gersons, B. P., De Jong, J. T., Layne, C. M., Maguen, S., Neria, Y., Norwood, A. E., Pynoos, R. S., Reissman, D., Ruzek, J. I., Shalev, A. Y., Solomon, Z., Steinberg, A. M., & Ursano, R. J. (2007). Five Essential Elements of Immediate and Mid–Term Mass Trauma Intervention: Empirical Evidence. *Psychiatry*, *70*(4), 283–315. doi:10.1521/psyc.2007.70.4.283 PMID:18181708

Hochschild, A. R. (2003). *The Managed Heart: Commercialization of Human Feeling*. University of California Press. doi:10.1525/9780520930414

Hoffenkamp, H. N., Tooten, A., Croon, M. A., Braeken, J., Winkel, F. W., Vingerhoets, A. J. J. M., & van Bakel, H. J. A. (2012). The impact of premature childbirth on parental bonding. *Evolutionary Psychology*, *10*(3), 542–2012. doi:10.1177/147470491201000311 PMID:22947677

Hoffmann, B. (2016). The role of expressive therapies in therapeutic interactions; art therapy - explanation of the concept. *Trakia Journal of Science*, *14*(3), 197–202. doi:10.15547/tjs.2016.03.001

Hollen, E., Clark, E., LeBlanc, C., & Skinner, L. (2018). Assessment and Documentation in Child Life. In R. Thompson (Ed.), *The Handbook of Child Life* (2nd ed., pp. 195–229). Charles C Thomas.

Hollins, W. Q. (2022). *Supporting Children of Incarcerated Parents in Schools Foregrounding Youth Voices to Improve Education Support*. Routledge.

Hollon, E., Clark, E., LeBlanc, C., & Skinner, L. (2018). Assessment and documentation in child life. In R. H. Thompson (Ed.), *The handbook of child life: A guide for pediatric psychosocial care* (2nd ed., pp. 195–229). Charles C. Thomas Pub. Ltd.

Honey, C. P., & Baker, J. A. (2011). Exploring the impact of journal clubs: A systematic review. *Nurse Education Today, 31*(8), 825–831. doi:10.1016/j.nedt.2010.12.020 PMID:21247668

Hornor, G., Davis, C., Sherfield, J., & Wilkinson, K. (2019). Trauma-informed care: Essential elements for pediatric health care. *Journal of Pediatric Health Care, 33*(2), 214–221. doi:10.1016/j.pedhc.2018.09.009 PMID:30777228

Housman, D. K. (2017). The importance of emotional competence and self-regulation from birth: A case for the evidence-based emotional cognitive social early learning approach. *International Journal of Child Care and Education Policy, 11*(1), 1–19. doi:10.118640723-017-0038-6

Houston, J. B., First, J., Spialek, M. L., Sorenson, M. E., & Koch, M. (2016). Public Disaster Communication and Child and Family Disaster Mental Health: A Review of Theoretical Frameworks and Empirical Evidence. *Current Psychiatry Reports, 18*(6), 54. Advance online publication. doi:10.100711920-016-0690-5 PMID:27086315

Hoven, C. W., Duarte, C. S., Lucas, C. P., Wu, P., Mandell, D. J., Goodwin, R. D., Cohen, M., Balaban, V., Woodruff, B. A., Bin, F., Musa, G. J., Mei, L., Cantor, P. A., Aber, J. L., Cohen, P., & Susser, E. (2005). Psychopathology among New York City public school children 6 months after September 11. *Archives of General Psychiatry, 62*(5), 545–551. doi:10.1001/archpsyc.62.5.545 PMID:15867108

Huang, Y.-M., Liang, T.-H., Su, Y.-N., & Chen, N.-S. (2012). Empowering personalized learning with an interactive e-book learning system for elementary school students. *Educational Technology Research and Development, 60*(4), 703–722. doi:10.1007/s11423-012-9237-6

Huang, L. (2018). Unmet needs and service satisfaction of victim support for the direct and indirect victims of serious violence: Results from a cross-sectional survey in Taiwan. *PLoS One, 13*(2), 1–16. doi:10.1371/journal.pone.0192905 PMID:29466463

Huang-Storms, L. (2018). *Autism parents seek help for behavioral crises.* Autism Speaks. https://www.autismspeaks.org/expert-opinion/autism-parents-seek-help-behavioral-crises

Hudson, L. (2022). Mental health of children and young people since the start of the pandemic. *Clinical Child Psychology and Psychiatry, 27*(1), 3–5. doi:10.1177/13591045211072721 PMID:35105247

Hugelius, K., Harada, N., & Marutani, M. (2021). Consequences of visiting restrictions during the COVID-19 pandemic: An integrative review. *International Journal of Nursing Studies, 121*(104000), 104000. https://doi.org/10.1016/j.ijnurstu.2021.104000

Hume, K., Regan, T., Megronigle, L., & Rhinehalt, C. (2015). Supporting students with autism spectrum disorder through grief and loss. *Teaching Exceptional Children, 48*(3), 128–136. doi:10.1177/0040059915618196

Hunter, N. C., Schaefer, M., Kurz, K., Prates, M. O., & Sinha, A. (2015). Individual and organizational predictors of pediatric psychiatric inpatient admission in Connecticut hospitals: A 6-month secondary analysis. *Administration and Policy in Mental Health, 42*(2), 176–185. doi:10.100710488-014-0558-0 PMID:24879633

Iacona, J., & Johnson, S. (2018). Neurobiology of trauma and mindfulness for children. *Journal of Trauma Nursing, 25*(3), 187–191. doi:10.1097/JTN.0000000000000365 PMID:29742631

Inova Newsroom. (2018, April 19). *Understanding sensory processing disorders.* Inova Newsroom. https://www.inovanewsroom.org/expert-commentary/2018/04/understanding-sensory-processing-disorders/

Institute for Patient and Family-Centered Care. (n.d.). Retrieved on April 5, 2022, from https://www.ipfcc.org/about/pfcc

International Association of Chiefs of Police. (2014). *Safeguarding Children of Arrested Parents*. The Bureau of Justice Assistance, U.S. Department of Justice.

International Network for Simulation-based Pediatric Innovation, Research & Education. (n.d.). *INSPIRE executive board*. Retrieved January 11, 2022, from https://inspiresim.org/what-is-inspire/executive-committee/

International Pediatric Simulation Society. (2021). *The 13th International Pediatric Simulation Symposia and Workshops - IPSSV2021: A virtual experience*. Retrieved January 11, 2022, from https://www.ipssglobal.org/ipssv2021-a-virtual-experience/

Internet/broadband fact sheet. (2021, April 7). Pew Research Center: Internet, Science & Tech. https://www.pewresearch.org/internet/fact-sheet/internet-broadband/?menuItem=3109350c-8dba-4b7f-ad52-a3e976ab8c8f

Ioverno, S., Belser, A. B., Baiocco, R., Grossman, A. H., & Russell, S. T. (2016). The protective role of gay–straight alliances for lesbian, gay, bisexual, and questioning students: A prospective analysis. *Psychology of Sexual Orientation and Gender Diversity*, *3*(4), 397–406. doi:10.1037gd0000193 PMID:28042585

Isikoglu Erdogan, N., Johnson, J. E., Dong, P. I., & Qiu, Z. (2018, May 28). Do Parents Prefer Digital Play? Examination of Parental Preferences and Beliefs in Four Nations. *Early Childhood Education Journal*, *47*(2), 131–142. https://doi.org/10.1007/s10643-018-0901-2

Jaaniste, T., Hayes, B., & von Baeyer, C. L. (2007). Providing children with information about forthcoming medical procedures: A review and synthesis. *Clinical Psychology: Science and Practice*, *14*(2), 124–143.

James, S. E., Herman, J. L., Rankin, S., Keisling, M., Mottet, L., & Anafi, M. (2016, December). *The report of the 2015 us transgender survey*. The National Center for Transgender Equality. Retrieved April 10, 2022, from https://transequality.org/sites/default/files/docs/usts/USTS-Full-Report-Dec17.pdf

Jensen, E. J., Geisthardt, C., & Sarigiani, P. A. (2020). Working with children with autism spectrum disorder in a medical setting: Insights from Certified Child Life Specialists. *Journal of Autism and Developmental Disorders*, *50*(1), 189–198. doi:10.100710803-019-04245-0 PMID:31583622

Jessee, P. O., & Gaynard, L. (2018). Paradigms of play. In R. H. Thompson (Ed.), *The handbook of child life: A guide for pediatric psychosocial care* (2nd ed., pp. 230–267). Charles C. Thomas Pub. Ltd.

Johns Hopkins Medicine. (2021). *Diagnosis education*. https://www.hopkinsallchildrens.org/Services/Child-Life/Patient-and-Family-Support/Diagnosis-Education

Johnson, B. (2019). *Psychotherapy: Understanding group therapy*. American Psychological Association. https://www.apa.org/topics/psychotherapy/group-therapy

Johnson, N., Lashley, J., Stonek, A. V., & Bonjour, A. (2012). Children with developmental disabilities at a pediatric hospital: Staff education to prevent and manage challenging behaviors. *Journal of Pediatric Nursing*, *27*(6), 742–749. doi:10.1016/j.pedn.2012.02.009 PMID:22465852

Jolly, A. (2012). Handle with care: Top ten tips a nurse should know before caring for a hospitalized child with autism spectrum disorder. *Pediatric Nursing*, *41*(1), 11–22. PMID:26281270

Kamptner, L. N. (2017). Evaluating the Efficacy of an Attachment-Informed Psychotherapeutic Program for Incarcerated Parents. *Journal of Prison Education and Reentry*, *4*(2), 62–81. doi:10.15845/jper.v4i2.1058

Kaplow, J. B., Howell, K. H., & Layne, C. M. (2014). Do circumstances of the death matter? Identifying socioenvironmental risks for grief-related psychopathology in bereaved youth. *Journal of Traumatic Stress*, *27*(1), 42–49. doi:10.1002/jts.21877 PMID:24478197

Kara, M., Foster, S., & Cantrell, K. (2022). Racial disparities in the provision of pediatric psychosocial end-of-life services: A systematic review. *Journal of Palliative Medicine*, *25*(10), 1510–1517. doi:10.1089/jpm.2021.0476 PMID:35588290

Karandikar, S. A., Gezinski, L. B., & Kaloga, M. E. P. (2015). *Health Care Among Sex-Trafficked Women and Girls in India*. Retrieved from: https://www.gahts.com/publications/ecjl9xjsxz95fhg-gns5a-7wc46-ksfe5-8pbkw-j7g9t-6pp2j-p6rf4-7xkhm-ssxlb-whxwr-7rd83-98ben-tawpp-3bhct-ww5eb-y7f5t-xs585-zaaff-m272e-96gr3-xxa77-pz4p4-4pse3-kzrd2-z67jx-ma9re-estlf

Kar, N., & Bastia, B. K. (2006). Post-traumatic stress disorder, depression and generalised anxiety disorder in adolescents after a natural disaster: A study of comorbidity. *Clinical Practice and Epidemiology in Mental Health*, *2*(1), 17. doi:10.1186/1745-0179-2-17 PMID:16869979

Kase, S. M., Waldman, E. D., & Weintraub, A. S. (2018). Compassion fatigue, burnout, and compassion satisfaction in pediatric palliative care (P.C.) providers in the U.S. *Pediatrics*, *142*(1). Advance online publication. doi:10.1542/peds.142.1MA7.672

Kazura, K., & Toth, K. (2004). Playrooms in Prison: Helping Offenders Connect with Their Children. *Corrections Today*, *66*(7), 128–130, 132.

Keller, H. (2018). Universality claim of attachment theory: Children's socioemotional development across cultures. *Proceedings of the National Academy of Sciences of the United States of America*, *115*(45), 11414–11419. doi:10.1073/pnas.1720325115 PMID:30397121

Kerrison, S. A., & Chapman, R. (2007). What general emergency nurses want to know about mental health patients presenting to their emergency department. *Accident and Emergency Nursing*, *16*(1), 48–55. doi:10.1016/j.aaen.2006.09.003 PMID:17198753

Kirmayer, L. J., & Gómez-Carrillo, A. (2019). *Culturally responsive clinical psychology and psychiatry: An ecosocial approach*. Hogrefe.

Knill, P. J., Levine, E. G., & Levine, S. K. (2005). *Principles and practice of expressive arts therapy: Toward a therapeutic aesthetics*. Jessica Kingsley Publishers.

Koh, E., Hanlon, R., Daughtery, L., & Linder, A. (2020). *Adoption by the numbers*. National Council for Adoption. https://adoptioncouncil.org/themencode-pdf-viewer-sc/?tnc_pvfw=ZmlsZT1odHRwczovL2Fkb3B0aW9uY291bmNpbC5vcmcvY29udGVudC91cGxvYWRzLzIwMjIvMDUvQWRvcHRpb24tYnktdGhlLU51bWJlcnMtTmF0aW9uYWwtQ291bmNpbC1Gb3ItQWRvcHRpb24tMjAyMi5wZGYmc2V0dGluZ3M9MTExMDEwMTExMDAxMDAxMDAwMCZsYW5nPWVuLVVT#page=&zoom=page-height&pagemode=thumbs

Kolb, E. (2019). 75,000 people per square mile? These are the most densely populated cities in the world. *USA Today*. Retrieved from: https://www.usatoday.com/story/news/world/2019/07/11/the-50-most-densely-populated-cities-in-the-world/39664259/

Kolb, A. Y., & Kolb, D. A. (2009). The learning way: Meta-cognitive aspects of experiential learning. *Simulation & Gaming*, *40*(3), 297–327. doi:10.1177/1046878108325713

Koller, D. (2007). Preparing children and adolescents for medical procedures. *Child Life Council Evidence-Based Practice Statement,* 1-13.

Koller, D. (2019). New ways of thinking and doing: A theoretical vision for child life. *ACLP Bulletin, 37*(4). https://www.childlife.org/membership/aclp-bulletin/fall-2019-table-of-contents/new-ways-of-thinking-and-doing-a-theoretical-vision-for-child-life/

Koller, D. (2008). *Child life assessment: Variables associated with a child's ability to cope with hospitalization*. Child Life Council.

Koschmann, E., Jacob, R., Robinson, J., Foster Friendman, M., Foster, A., Rodriguez-Quintana, N., Vichich, J., Smith, M., & Rajaram, H. (2022). Mental health needs in a large urban school district: Findings from a web-based survey. *Health Services Research, 57*(4), 830–841. Advance online publication. doi:10.1111/1475-6773.13924 PMID:35243624

Koukourikos, K., Tzeha, L., Pantelidoum, P., & Tsalogidou, A. (2015). The importance of play during hospitalization of children. *Journal of the Academy of Medical Sciences of Bosnia and Herzegovina, 27*(6), 438–441. doi:10.5455/msm.2015.27.438-441 PMID:26889107

Kraus, E. J., Nicosia, B., & Shalowitz, D. I. (2022). A qualitative study of patients' attitudes towards telemedicine for gynecologic cancer care. *Gynecologic Oncology, 165*(1), 155–159. https://doi.org/10.1016/j.ygyno.2022.01.035

Krebel, M., Clayton, C., & Graham, C. (1996). Child life programs in the pediatric emergency department. *Pediatric Emergency Care, 12*(1), 13–15. doi:10.1097/00006565-199602000-00004 PMID:8677171

Kuper, H., Monteath-van Dok, A., Wing, K., Danquah, L., Evans, J., Zuurmond, M., & Gallinetti, J. (2014). The impact of disability on the lives of children; cross-sectional data including 8900 children with disabilities and 898,834 children without disabilities across 30 countries. *PLoS One, 9*(9), 1–11. doi:10.1371/journal.pone.0107300 PMID:25202999

La Greca, A. M., & Silverman, W. K. (2009). Treatment and Prevention of Post-traumatic Stress Reactions in Children and Adolescents Exposed to Disasters and Terrorism: What Is the Evidence? *Child Development Perspectives, 3*(1), 4–10. doi:10.1111/j.1750-8606.2008.00069.x

La Greca, A. M., Silverman, W. K., Vernberg, E. M., & Prinstein, M. J. (1996). Symptoms of post-traumatic stress in children after Hurricane Andrew: A prospective study. *Journal of Consulting and Clinical Psychology, 64*(4), 712–723. doi:10.1037/0022-006X.64.4.712 PMID:8803361

Lambert, S. (2022, January 14). *Number of internet users in 2022/2023: Statistics, current trends, and predictions*. Retrieved September 23, 2022, from https://financesonline.com/number-of-internet-users/#:~:text=There%20are%20currently%20about%204.66,90%25%20as%20of%20January%202021

Landreth, G. L. (2012). *Play therapy: The art of the relationship* (3rd ed.). Routledge.

Landrethh, G. L., & Ray, D. C. (2019, September). Child-centered play therapy. *Play Therapy, 14*(3), 18–19.

Lateef, F. (2010). Simulation-based learning: Just like the real thing. *Journal of Emergencies, Trauma and Shock, 3*(4), 348–352. doi:10.4103/0974-2700.70743 PMID:21063557

Lazarus, R. S., & Folkman, S. (1984). *Stress, appraisal, and coping*. Springer Publishing Company.

Lerwick, J. (2019). An Exploration of the Roles of Certified Child Life Specialists & Registered Play Therapists in the United States. *International Journal of Pediatric Research, 5*, 49. doi:10.23937/2469-5769/1510049

Lerwick, J. L. (2016). Minimizing pediatric healthcare-induced anxiety and trauma. *World Journal of Clinical Pediatrics, 5*(2), 143–150. https://doi.org/10.5409/wjcp.v5.i2.143

Lewis, F. M. (2011). Therapy for Parental Cancer and Dependent Children. In Handbook of Psychotherapy in Cancer Care (pp. 225-234). John Wiley & Sons, Ltd. doi:10.1002/9780470975176.ch19

Lewis, T., Jones, K. D., Militello, M., & Meisenhelder, R. (2020). A Clear and Consistent Focus on Students: Principals' Perceptions of the Role of School Counselors. *Journal of School Leadership, 32*(1), 3–26. doi:10.1177/1052684620972067

Li, A. S. Y., Lang, Q., Cho, J., Nguyen, V. S., & Nandakumar, S. (2021). Cultural and structural humility and addressing systems of care disparities in mental health services for black, indigenous, and people of color. *Child and Adolescent Psychiatric Clinics of North America, 31*(2), 251–259. PMID:35361363

Liberman, D. B., Song, E., Radbill, L. M., Pham, P. K., & Derrington, S. F. (2016). Early introduction of palliative care and advanced care planning for children with complex chronic medical conditions: A pilot study. *Child: Care, Health and Development, 42*(3), 439–449. doi:10.1111/cch.12332 PMID:27028099

Liddle, M., Birkett, K., Bonjour, A., & Risma, K. (2018). A collaborative approach to improving health care for children with developmental disabilities. *Pediatrics, 142*(6), e20181136. doi:10.1542/peds.2018-1136 PMID:30385639

Liddle, M., & Sonnentag, T. L. (2021). Effectiveness of adaptive care plans for children with developmental disabilities during outpatient clinic appointments. *Journal of Autism and Developmental Disorders, 51*(9), 3028–3038. doi:10.100710803-020-04764-1 PMID:33118074

Lindley, L., Mack, J., & Bruce, D. (2016). Clusters of multiple complex chronic conditions: A latent class analysis of children at end of life. *Journal of Pain and Symptom Management, 51*(5), 868–874. doi:10.1016/j.jpainsymman.2015.12.310 PMID:26747723

Lindsey, L., Robertson, P., & Lindsey, B. (2018). Expressive arts and mindfulness: Aiding adolescents in understanding and managing their stress. *Journal of Creativity in Mental Health, 13*(3), 288–297. doi:10.1080/15401383.2018.1427167

Locke, R. A. (2010). *Rescued, rehabilitated, returned: Institutional approaches to the rehabilitation of survivors of sex trafficking in India and Nepal* (Doctoral dissertation, University of Denver). Retrieved from: https://digitalcommons.du.edu/cgi/viewcontent.cgi?article=1377&context=etd

Longbottom, S., & Slaughter, V. (2018). Sources of children's knowledge about death and dying. *Philosophical Transactions of the Royal Society B: Biological Sciences, 373*(1754). doi:10.1098/rstb.2017.0267

Lookabaugh, S., & Ballard, S. (2018). The Scope and Future Direction of Child Life. *Journal of Child and Family Studies, 27*(5), 1721–1731. doi:10.100710826-018-1031-6

Loo, M. E., Krishnasamy, C., & Lim, W. S. (2018). Considering face, rights, and goals: A critical review of rapport management in facilitator-guided simulation debriefing approaches. *Simulation in Healthcare: Journal of the Society for Simulation in Healthcare, 13*(1), 52–60. doi:10.1097/SIH.0000000000000258 PMID:29076968

Luijkx, J., van der Putten, A. J., & Vlaskamp, C. (2016). "I love my sister, but sometimes I don't": A qualitative study into the experiences of siblings of a child with profound intellectual and multiple disabilities. *Journal of Intellectual & Developmental Disability, 41*(4), 279–288. doi:10.3109/13668250.2016.1224333

Luther, K. (2015). Examining Social Support Among Adult Children of Incarcerated Parents. *Family Relations, 64*(4), 505–518. doi:10.1111/fare.12134

Maa, T., Heimberg, E., & Reid, J. R. (2016). In situ simulation. In V. J. Grant & A. Cheng (Eds.), *Comprehensive healthcare simulation: Pediatrics* (pp. 153–163). Springer. doi:10.1007/978-3-319-24187-6_12

Malchiodi, C. (2005). Using art activities to support trauma recovery in children. *Trauma & Loss: Research & Interventions, 5*(1), 8–11.

Ma, N., Roberts, R., Winfield, H., & Furber, G. (2015). The prevalence of psychopathology in siblings of children with mental health problems: A 20-year systematic review. *Child Psychiatry and Human Development*, *46*(1), 130–149. doi:10.100710578-014-0459-1 PMID:24652033

Marcon, T. D., Girz, L., Stillar, A., Tessier, C., & Lafrance, A. (2017). Parental involvement and child and adolescent eating disorders: Perspectives from residents in psychiatry, pediatrics, and family medicine. *Journal of the Canadian Academy of Child and Adolescent Psychiatry*, *26*(2), 78–85. PMID:28747930

Marks, J. (2020). *From The Desk of Zoe Washington*. Katherine Tegan Books.

Marks, S., Lamb, R., & Tzioumi, D. (2009). Do no more harm: The psychological stress of the medical examination for alleged child sexual abuse. *Journal of Paediatrics and Child Health*, *45*(3), 125–132. https://doi.org/10.1111/j.1440-1754.2008.01443.x

Marr, B. (2018). How much data do we create every day? The mind-blowing stats everyone should read. *Forbes*, *21*, 1–5.

Martínez-Monteagudo, M. C., Delgado, B., Díaz-Herrero, Á., & García-Fernández, J. M. (2020). Relationship between suicidal thinking, anxiety, depression and stress in university students who are victims of cyberbullying. *Psychiatry Research*, *286*, 112856. doi:10.1016/j.psychres.2020.112856 PMID:32062285

Maslow, A. H. (1943). A theory of human motivation. *Psychological Review*, *50*(4), 370–396. doi:10.1037/h0054346

Maslow, A. H. (1943). Dynamics of personality organization. *Psychological Review*, *50*(5), 514–539. doi:10.1037/h0062222

Maslow, A. H. (1954). *Motivation and Personality* (1st ed.). Harper.

Masten, A. S., & Narayan, A. J. (2012). Child Development in the Context of Disaster, War, and Terrorism: Pathways of Risk and Resilience. *Annual Review of Psychology*, *63*(1), 227–257. doi:10.1146/annurev-psych-120710-100356 PMID:21943168

McCarthy, J., & Boyd, J. (2002). Mental health services and young people with intellectual disability: Is it time to do better? *Journal of Intellectual Disability Research*, *46*(3), 250–256. doi:10.1046/j.1365-2788.2002.00401.x PMID:11896810

McDermott, B. M., & Cobham, V. E. (2012). Family functioning in the aftermath of a natural disaster. *BMC Psychiatry*, *12*(1), 55. doi:10.1186/1471-244X-12-55 PMID:22647086

McGee, K. (2003). The role of a child life specialist in a pediatric radiology department. *Pediatric Radiology*, *33*(7), 467–474. doi:10.100700247-003-0900-2 PMID:12819835

McGonigle, J. J., Venkat, A., Beresford, C., Campbell, T. P., & Gabriels, R. L. (2014, January). Management of agitation in individuals with autism spectrum disorders in the emergency department. *Child and Adolescent Psychiatric Clinics of North America*, *23*(1), 83–95. doi:10.1016/j.chc.2013.08.003 PMID:24231169

McGuire, S., & Meadan, H. (2022). Social inclusion of children with persistent challenging behaviors. *Early Childhood Education Journal*, *50*(61), 61–69. doi:10.100710643-020-01135-4

McLaughlin, A. M., Feehan, R., Coleman, H., & Reynolds, K. (2013). Negotiating openness a qualitative study of adoptive parents' experience of contact in open adoption. *Canadian Social Work Review*, *30*(1). https://www.researchgate.net/publication /260087431_Negotiating_openness_A_qualitative_study_of_adoptive_parents'_experien ce_of_contact_in_open_adoption

McLeod, S. (2007). Maslow's hierarchy of needs. *Simply Psychology*. https://www.simply psychology.org/maslow.html

McLeod, J. D., Uemura, R., & Rohrman, S. (2013). Adolescent mental health, behavior problems, and academic achievement. *Journal of Health and Social Behavior*, *53*(4), 482–497. doi:10.1177/0022146512462888 PMID:23197485

McManus, E., & Paul, S. (2019). Addressing the bereavement needs of children in school: An evaluation of bereavement training for school communities. *Improving Schools, 22*(1), 72–85. doi:10.1177/1365480219825540

McQuarrie, E. F. (2015). *The market research toolbox: A concise guide for beginners.* Sage Publications.

Mednick, L., O'Connell, B., Graber, K., Roussin, C., & Weinstock, P. (2021). "Ready SIM go": An adapted simulation "service line" for patients and caregivers. *Simulation in Healthcare: Journal of the Society for Simulation in Healthcare, 16*(2), 120–127. doi:10.1097/SIH.0000000000000448 PMID:32218091

Mental Health First Aid. (2022). *Mental health first aid for youth* [Workbook]. National Council for Mental Wellbeing. https://www.mentalhealthfirstaid.org/population-focused-modules/youth/

Meyer and Vadasy. (2008). *Sibshops: Workshops for siblings of children with special needs.* Paul H. Brookes Publishing Co.

Miron, O., Yu, K., Wilf-Miron, R., & Kohane, I. S. (2019). Suicide rates among adolescents and young adults in the United States 2000-2017. *Journal of the American Medical Association, 321*(23), 2362. Advance online publication. doi:10.1001/jama.2019.5054 PMID:31211337

Mkhwanazi, N., Makusha, T., Blackie, D., Manderson, L., Hall, K., & Huijbregts, M. (2018). Negotiating the care of children and support for caregivers. *Child Fam State, 70.*

Moon, J., Williford, A., & Mendenhall, A. (2017). Educators' perceptions of youth mental health: Implications for training and the promotion of mental health services in schools. *Children and Youth Services Review, 73,* 384-391. doi:10.1016/j.childyouth.2017.01.006

Morehouse, K. (2003, Spring). Research review: Children's psychological responses after critical illness and exposure to invasive technology. *Child Life Bulletin.* https://www.childlife.org/docs/default-source/Publications/Bulletin/2003---spring-bulletin.pdf?sfvrsn=69debe4d_2

Morgan-Mullane, A. (2018). Trauma-Focused Cognitive Behavioral Therapy with Children of Incarcerated Parents. *Clinical Social Work, 46*(3), 200–109. doi:10.100710615-017-0642-5 PMID:30100639

Morse, G., Salyers, M. P., Rollins, A. L., Monroe-DeVita, M. M., & Pfahler, C. (2011). Burnout in mental health services: A review of the problem and its remediation. *Administration and Policy in Mental Health, 39*(5), 341–352. doi:10.100710488-011-0352-1 PMID:21533847

Moslehi, S., Masoumi, G., & Barghi-Shirazi, F. (2022). Benefits of simulation-based education in hospital emergency departments: A systematic review. *Journal of Education and Health Promotion, 11*, 40. doi:10.4103/jehp.jehp_558_21 PMID:35281376

Murcia, J. (2020). *Child life specialists begin using telemedicine to reach hospitalized children during COVID-19.* Retrieved August 7, 2022, from https://connect.uclahealth.org/2020/04/03/child-life-specialists-begin-using-telemedicine-to-reach-hospitalized-children-during-covid-19/

Myers, J. E. B. & APSAC (American Professional Society on the Abuse of Children). (2010, June 16). *The APSAC Handbook on Child Maltreatment* (3rd ed.). SAGE Publications, Inc.

National Academies of Sciences, Engineering, and Medicine. (2018). *Opportunities for Improving Programs and Services for Children with Disabilities.* Washington, DC: The National Academies Press. . doi:10.17226/25028

National Alliance on Mental Illness. (2015). *Mental health facts: Children & teens* [Infogram]. https://www.nami.org/NAMI/media/NAMI-Media/Infographics/Children-MH-Facts-NAMI.pdf

National Alliance on Mental Illness. (2021a). *Identity and cultural dimensions.* https://www.nami.org/Your-Journey/Identity-and-Cultural-Dimensions/

National Alliance on Mental Illness. (2021b). *Letter to CDC director on child and adolescent mental health.* https://www.nami.org/getattachment/8b6d5549-1d83-431b-92d4-1acd226d720b/2021- Letter-to-CDC-Director-on-Child-Adolescent-Me

National Alliance on Mental Illness. (2021c). *Statement for the record on child and adolescent mental health.* https://www.nami.org/getattachment/7090292f-4cc0-4a54-94a6-bcadefc0620e/Statement-for- the-Record-on-Child-and-Adolescent-M

National Alliance on Mental Illness. (2022a). *How to talk to your child about their mental health.* https://www.nami.org/Your-Journey/Kids-Teens-and-Young-Adults/Kids/How-to-Talk-to-Your-Child-About-Their-Mental-Health

National Alliance on Mental Illness. (2022b). *LGBTQI.* https://www.nami.org/Your-Journey/Identity-and-Cultural-Dimensions/LGBTQI

National Alliance on Mental Illness. (2022c). *Mental health in schools.* https://nami.org/Advocacy/Policy-Priorities/Improving-Health/Mental-Health-in-Schools

National Center for Education Statistics. (2016). *Number and percentage of public schools by presence of counselors, psychologists and social workers on staff and selected school characteristics.* https://nces.ed.gov/surveys/ntps/tables/ntps1516_027_s1n_04.asp

National Center for Homeless Education. (n.d.). *The McKinney-Vento definition of homeless.* https://nche.ed.gov/mckinney-vento-definition/

National Center for School Crisis and Bereavement and the Coalition to Support Grieving Students. (2020). *Supporting grieving students in schools.* https://grievingstudents.org/wp-content/uploads/2020/06/TTM-Combined-May-31-2020.pptx

National Center on Disability and Journalism. (2021, August). *Disability language style guide.* https://ncdj.org/style-guide/

National Children's Alliance. (2017). *Standards for accredited members.* https://nationalchildrensalliance.org/wp-content/uploads/2015/06/NCA-Standards-for-Accredited-Members-2017.pdf

National Children's Alliance. (n.d.). *How the CAC model works & NCA's national standards of* accreditation. https://nationalchildrensalliance.org

National Commission on Children and Disasters. (2010). *2010 Report to the President and Congress.* Author.

National Education Association. (2022). *Poll results: Stress and burnout pose threat of educator shortages.* https://www.nea.org/sites/default/files/2022-02/NEA%20Member%20COVID-19%20Survey%20Summary.pdf

National Institute of Mental Health. (2009). *Treatment of children with mental illness: Frequently asked questions about the treatment of mental illness in children.* https://files.eric.ed.gov/fulltext/ED507899.pdf

National Institute of Mental Health. (2021). *Chronic illness and mental health: Recognizing and treating depression.* https://www.nimh.nih.gov/health/publications/chronic-illness-mental-health#part_6116

Nellis, A. (2021). *The Color of Justice: Racial and Ethnic Disparities in State Prisons.* The Sentencing Project.

Nestel, D., & Kneebone, R. (2010). Perspective: Authentic patient perspectives in simulations for procedural and surgical skills. *Academic Medicine, 85*(5), 889–893. doi:10.1097/ACM.0b013e3181d749ac PMID:20520046

NeuroClastic. (2021, August 14). *On Using NonSpeaking, Minimally Speaking, Or Unreliably Speaking Over "Non-Verbal": NonSpeakers Weigh In.* https://neuroclastic.com/on-using-nonspeaking-minimally-speaking-or-unreliably-speaking-over-non-verbal-nonspeakers-weigh-in/

New Jersey Department of Corrections, Divisions of Programs and Community Services, Office of Transitional Services. (2007). *"What About Me?" When a Parent Goes to Prison: A guide to discussing incarceration with your children.* Author.

New, A., Tucci, V. T., & Rios, J. (2017). A modern-day fight club? The stabilization and management of actively agitated patients in the emergency department. *The Psychiatric Clinics of North America, 40*(3), 397–410. doi:10.1016/j.psc.2017.05.002 PMID:28800797

Newman, K., Wang, A. H., Wang, A. Z. Y., & Hanna, D. (2019). The role of internet-based digital tools in reducing social isolation and addressing support needs among informal caregivers: A scoping review. *BMC Public Health, 19*(1), 1495. https://doi.org/10.1186/s12889-019-7837-3

Nieman, P., & Shea, S. (2004). Effective discipline for children. *Paediatrics & Child Health, 9*(1), 37–41. doi:10.1093/pch/9.1.37 PMID:19654979

Nkosi, B., & Daniels, P. (2007). Family Strengths. *Marriage & Family Review, 41*(1-2), 11–26.

Norris, F. H., Baker, C. K., Murphy, A. D., & Kaniasty, K. (2005). Social Support Mobilization and Deterioration after Mexico's 1999 Flood: Effects of Context, Gender, and Time. *American Journal of Community Psychology, 36*(1–2), 15–28. doi:10.100710464-005-6230-9 PMID:16134042

Norris, F. H., Friedman, M. J., Watson, P. J., Byrne, C. M., Diaz, E., & Kaniasty, K. (2002). 60,000 disaster victims speak: Part I. An empirical review of the empirical literature, 1981–2001. *Psychiatry, 65*(3), 207–239. doi:10.1521/psyc.65.3.207.20173 PMID:12405079

North, C. S., & Pfefferbaum, B. (2013). Mental Health Response to Community Disasters: A Systematic Review. *Journal of the American Medical Association, 310*(5), 507. doi:10.1001/jama.2013.107799 PMID:23925621

Nunez, A. (2018). Exploring communication differences: Complications children with developmental disabilities face in medical settings. *ACLP Bulletin, 36*(2).

Nunez, A. (2020). *My child needs to be admitted to the hospital. How can I help them cope with an inpatient stay? How can I explain their needs to the staff?* Autism Speaks. https://www.autismspeaks.org/expert-opinion/my-child-needs-be-admitted-hospital-how-can-i-help-them-cope-inpatient-stay-how-can

Olawale, O. A., Deih, A. D., & Yaadar, R. K. K. (2013). Psychological impact of cerebral palsy on families: The African perspective. *Journal ofNeurosciences in Rural Practice, 4*(2), 159–163. doi:10.4103/0976-3147.112752 PMID:23914092

Oliver, C. (2014). The Fundamentals of Strengths-Based Practice. *Relational Child & Youth Care Practice, 27*(3), 46–50. doi:10.1300/J002v41n01_02

Olsson, L., & Barbosa, H. (2019). *Land Degradation—Special Report on Climate Change and Land* (No. 4). Intergovernmental Panel on Climate Change. https://www.ipcc.ch/srccl/chapter/chapter-4/

Orgill, B. D., & Nolin, J. (2021). Learning taxonomies in medical simulation. In *StatPearls*. StatPearls Publishing. https://www.ncbi.nlm.nih.gov/books/NBK559109/

Ortiz, R. (2019, September-October). Building Resilience Against the Sequelae of Adverse Childhood Experiences: Rise Up, Change Your Life, and Reform Health Care. *American Journal of Lifestyle Medicine, 13*(5), 470–479. doi:10.1177/1559827619839997 PMID:31523212

Osborne, C. N. (2018). A child life perspective: The role of technology in preoperative preparation and distraction. The University of North Carolina at Charlotte.

Oulton, K., Sell, D., & Gibson, F. (2019). Hospitalized children with intellectual disability: Parents as partners in their care. *Journal of Applied Research in Intellectual Disabilities*, *33*(5), 917–926. doi:10.1111/jar.12713 PMID:32072753

Palaganas, J. C., Scott, E., Mancini, M. E., & Stryjewski, G. (2016). Interprofessional education. In V. J. Grant & A. Cheng (Eds.), *Comprehensive healthcare simulation: Pediatrics* (pp. 195–208). Springer. doi:10.1007/978-3-319-24187-6_15

Palmer, M., Saviet, M., & Tourish, J. (2016). Understanding and supporting grieving adolescents and young adults. *Pediatric Nursing*, *42*(6), 275–279. PMID:29406651

Pamplona, A. Y. M. C. (2000). Active participation of mothers during speech therapy improved language development of children with cleft palate. *Scandinavian Journal of Plastic and Reconstructive Surgery and Hand Surgery, 34*(3), 231–236. doi:10.1080/02844310050159800

Pappano, L. (2014). "Trauma-sensitive" schools: A new framework for reaching troubled students. *Harvard Education Letter*, *30*(3), 1–5.

Parker, S. G. (2001). *Establishing victim services within a law enforcement agency: The Austin experience.* Office for Victims of Crime. https://www.ncjrs.gov/ovc_archives/bulletins/evs_3_2001/welcome.html

PATHS Program LLC. (n.d.). *PATHS® curriculum research: Research-based with proven outcomes.* https://pathsprogram.com/paths-research

Patterson, S. (2020, Oct. 27). *Pioneering pediatric psychosocial education and the use of simulation based learning* [Conference session]. 12th International Pediatric Simulation Symposia and Workshops, IPSSV 2020: A Virtual Experience. https://www.eventscribe.com/2020/IPSSW2020/fsPopup.asp?Mode=presInfo&PresentationID=783321

Pearce, E., Launay, J., & Dunbar, R. I. M. (2015). The ice-breaker effect: Singing mediates fast social bonding. *Royal Society Open Science*, *2*(10), 150221. Advance online publication. doi:10.1098/rsos.150221 PMID:26587241

Pediatric Hospitalization. (n.d.). *Connecticut Hospital Association.* Retrieved March 6, 2022, from https://cthosp.org/advocacy/quality-and-patient-safety/patients-guide-to-quality-hospital-care/pediatric-hospitalization/

Perry, R. W. (2018). Defining Disaster: An Evolving Concept. In H. Rodríguez, W. Donner, & J. E. Trainor (Eds.), Handbook of Disaster Research (pp. 3–22). Springer International Publishing. doi:10.1007/978-3-319-63254-4_1

Perry, B. D., & Winfrey, O. (2021). *What happened to you? Conversations on trauma, resilience, and healing*. Melcher Media Inc.

Perry, B., & Szalavitz, M. (2008). *The boy who was raised as a dog and other stories from a child psychiatrist's notebook: What traumatized children can teach us about loss, love, and healing*. Basic Books.

Pershick, S. (2009). *Child Life Specialists' Perspective on Collaboration with Schools*. Ryerson University.

Petasis, A. (2019). Discrepancies of the medical, social, and biopsychosocial models of disability; A comprehensive theoretical framework. *The International Journal of Business Management and Technology*, *3*(4).

Pew Research Center. (2021). *Social media fact sheet.* https://www.pewresearch.org/internet/factsheet/social-media/

Pfefferbaum, B., Jacobs, A. K., Griffin, N., & Houston, J. B. (2015). Children's Disaster Reactions: The Influence of Exposure and Personal Characteristics. *Current Psychiatry Reports*, *17*(7), 56. Advance online publication. doi:10.100711920-015-0598-5 PMID:25980513

Pfefferbaum, B., Jacobs, A. K., Houston, J. B., & Griffin, N. (2015). Children's Disaster Reactions: The Influence of Family and Social Factors. *Current Psychiatry Reports*, *17*(7), 57. Advance online publication. doi:10.100711920-015-0597-6 PMID:25980512

Pfefferbaum, B., Noffsinger, M. A., Wind, L. H., & Allen, J. R. (2014). Children's Coping in the Context of Disasters and Terrorism. *Journal of Loss and Trauma*, *19*(1), 78–97. doi:10.1080/15325024.2013.791797 PMID:24683315

Phillips, F., & Prezio, E. (2016). *Wonders & Worries: Evaluation of a child centered psychosocial intervention for families who have a parent/primary caregiver with cancer* (Vol. 26). doi:10.1002/pon.4120

Phillips, F., Prezio, E. A., Panisch, L. S., & Jones, B. L. (2021). Factors Affecting Outcomes Following a Psychosocial Intervention for Children When a Parent Has Cancer. *The Journal of Child Life: Psychosocial Theory and Practice.*

Phillips, F. (2015). The experience of adolescents who have a parent with advanced cancer: A phenomenological inquiry. *Palliative & Supportive Care*, *13*(4), 1057–1069. doi:10.1017/S1478951514001023 PMID:26165850

Phillips, F., Prezio, E. A., Currin-McCulloch, J., & Jones, B. (2022). Wonders & Worries Program Evaluation: A Randomized Clinical Trial of a Psychosocial Intervention for Children who have a Parent with Cancer. *Psycho-Oncology*. Advance online publication. doi:10.1002/pon.5943

Phola. (2022). *Therapeutic approaches.* Phola – Healing the Nation. https://phola.org/therapeutic-approaches/

Pillai, R. L. I. (2020). We all need a little TLC: An argument for an increased role of child life services in patient care and medical education. *Hospital Pediatrics*, *10*(10), 913–917. doi:10.1542/hpeds.2020-0119 PMID:32887731

Pinquart, M. (2016). Systematic review: Bullying involvement of children with and without chronic physical illness and/or physical/sensory disability –a meta-analytic comparison with healthy/non-disabled peers. *Journal of Pediatric Psychology*, *42*(3), 245–259. doi:10.1093/jpepsy/jsw081 PMID:27784727

Pittesenbarger, Z. E., & Mannix, R. (2013). Trends in pediatric visits to the emergency department for psychiatric illnesses. *Academic Emergency Medicine*, *21*(1), 25–30. Advance online publication. doi:10.1111/acem.12282 PMID:24552521

Porter, L. S., Porter, B., McCoy, V., Bango Sanchez, V., Kissel, B., Williams, M., & Nunnewar, S. (2015). Massage–Parenting Enhancement Program on Recovering Substance-Abusing Mothers' Parenting Stress, Self-Esteem, Depression, Maternal Attachment, and Mother-Infant Interaction. *Asian Nursing Research*, *9*(4), 318–327. doi:10.1016/j.anr.2015.09.002 PMID:26724241

Potthoff, L. M., Glotzbecker, M. P., O'Connell, B., O'Neill, N. P., Graber, K. M., Byrne, C. A., Tremmel, J. M., Weinstock, P., & Mednick, L. (2021). SIMDiscovery: A simulation-based preparation program for adolescents undergoing spinal fusion surgery. *Spine Deformity*, *9*(5), 1363–1370. doi:10.100743390-021-00322-6 PMID:33689156

Prevent Child Abuse America. (n.d.). *Child sexual abuse prevention.* https://preventchildabuse.org/waht-we-do/child-sexual-abuse-prevention/

Purvis, K., Cross, D. R., & Sunshine, W. L. (2007). *The connected child: Bring hope and healing to your adoptive family*. McGraw Hill.

Pynoos, R., Schreiber, M., Steinberg, A., & Pfefferbaum, B. (2005). Impact of terrorism on children. In *Comprehensive textbook of psychiatry* (8th ed., pp. 3351–3564). Lippencott, Wiliams, and Wilkins.

Quinn, M., Gillooly, D., Kelly, S., Kolassa, J., Davis, E., & Jankowski, S. (2016). Evaluation of identified stressors in children and adolescents after Super Storm Sandy. *Pediatric Nursing*, *42*(5), 235. PMID:29406642

Rafferty, J. (2022, May 11). Gender Identity Development in Children. *Healthy Children.* Retrieved from https://www.healthychildren.org/English/ages-stages/gradeschool/Pages/Gender-Identity-and-Gender-Confusion-In-Children.aspx

Rafferty, J., Yogman, M., Baum, R., Gambon, T. B., Lavin, A., Mattson, G., Wissow, L. S., Breuner, C., Alderman, E. M., Grubb, L. K., Powers, M. E., Upadhya, K., Wallace, S. B., Hunt, L., Gearhart, A. T., Harris, C., Lowe, K. M., Rodgers, C. T., & Sherer, I. M. (2018). Ensuring comprehensive care and support for transgender and gender-diverse children and adolescents. *Pediatrics, 142*(4), e20182162. doi:10.1542/peds.2018-2162 PMID:30224363

Rai, R., & Rai, A. K. (2021). Nature of sex trafficking in India: A geographical perspective. *Children and Youth Services Review, 120,* 105739. doi:10.1016/j.childyouth.2020.105739

Ramachandra, G., Deutsch, E. S., & Nadkarni, V. M. (2020). A road map for simulation based medical students training in pediatrics: Preparing the next generation of doctors. *Indian Pediatrics, 57*(10), 950–956. doi:10.100713312-020-2001-9 PMID:33089810

Raphael, B. P., Takvorian-Bené, M., Gallotto, M., Tascione, C., McClelland, J., Rosa, C., Dinan, J., O'Connell, B., & Weinstock, P. (2021). Learning gaps and family experience, nurse-facilitated home parenteral nutrition simulation-based discharge training: Proof-of-concept study. *Nutrition in Clinical Practice: Official Publication of the American Society for Parenteral and Enteral Nutrition, 36*(2), 489–496. doi:10.1002/ncp.10421 PMID:31589007

Reavey, P., Poole, J., Corrigall, R., Zundel, T., Byford, S., Sarhane, M., Taylor, E., Ivens, J., & Ougrin, D. (2017). The ward as emotional ecology: Adolescent experiences of managing mental health and distress in psychiatric inpatient settings. *Health & Place, 46,* 210–218. doi:10.1016/j.healthplace.2017.05.008 PMID:28554098

Rezaei, S., Pastrana, L., Brown, K., & Lancaster, A. (2019). Openness in adoptions satisfaction and psychological outcomes among birth mothers. *Adoption Advocate, 133,* 1-8. www.adoptioncouncil.org

Ribbens, M. (2020). *Through Their Eyes: Photo Stories about Family Strengths in Johannesburg, South Africa* [Unpublished master's thesis]. University of Nebraska-Lincoln. https://digitalcommons.unl.edu/cehsdiss/374/

Rice, J. L., Tan, T. X., & Li, Y. (2021). In their voices: Experiences of adolescents during involuntary psychiatric hospitalization. *Children and Youth Services Review, 126,* 1–10. doi:10.1016/j.childyouth.2021.106045

Rogers, F. (n.d.). *He helped us with our feelings.* https://www.misterrogers.org/articles/he-helped-us-with-our-feelings/

Rollins, J. A. (2018). The Arts in Children's Healthcare Settings. In J. Rollins, R. Bolig, & C. Mahan (Eds.), *Meeting Children's Psychosocial Needs: Across the Health-Care Continuum* (2nd ed., pp. 119–165). PRO-ED.

Rollins, J. A., Bolig, R., & Mahan, C. C. (2005). *Meeting children's psychosocial needs across the health-care continuum.* Pro-ed.

Romito, B., Jewell, J., Jackson, M. (2021, January). AAP committee on hospital care, & association of child life professionals. Child Life Services. *American Academy of Pediatrics, 147*(1).

Romito, B., Jewell, J., Jackson, M., Ernst, K., Hill, V., Hsu, B., Lam, V., Mauro-Small, M., & Vinocur, C. (2021). Child Life Services. *Pediatrics, 147*(1), 1–10. doi:10.1542/peds.2020-040261 PMID:33372119

Roper Victim Assistance Academy of Maryland. (2019, September). *Certification.* https://www.rvaam.us/certification.html

Rosen, D. (2022). *GLSEN. Gender-neutral Bathrooms Are Radical, but Not How You Think.* Retrieved from https://www.glsen.org/blog/gender-neutral-bathrooms-are-radical-not-how-you-think

Rosenberg, A. R., Postier, A., Osenga, K., Kreicbergs, U., Neville, B., Dussel, V., & Wolfe, J. (2015). Long-term psychosocial outcomes among bereaved siblings of children with cancer. *Journal of Pain and Symptom Management*, *49*(1), 55–65. doi:10.1016/j.jpainsymman.2014.05.006 PMID:24880001

Röttger-Rössler, B., Scheidecker, G., & Lam, A. T. A. (2019). Narrating visualized feelings: Photovoice as a tool for researching affects and emotions among school students. In A. Kahl (Ed.), *Analyzing Affective Societies* (pp. 78–98). Routledge. doi:10.4324/9780429424366-5

Rudder, B. S., Boyd, S. L., Easley, S. A., Nusbaum, J. D., Sherman, A. K., Sommer, D. R., & Schremmer, R. D. (2019). Psychosocial simulation: A novel approach to interprofessional training. *Journal of Interprofessional Education & Practice*, *14*(1), 67–71. doi:10.1016/j.xjep.2018.12.004

Rudolph, J. W., Raemer, D. B., & Simon, R. (2014). Establishing a safe container for learning in simulation: The role of the presimulation briefing. *Simulation in Healthcare: Journal of the Society for Simulation in Healthcare*, *9*(6), 339–349. doi:10.1097/SIH.0000000000000047 PMID:25188485

Rudolph, J. W., Simon, R., Dufresne, R. L., & Raemer, D. B. (2006). There's no such thing as "nonjudgmental" debriefing: A theory and method for debriefing with good judgment. *Simulation in Healthcare: Journal of the Society for Simulation in Healthcare*, *1*(1), 49–55. doi:10.1097/01266021-200600110-00006 PMID:19088574

Rudolph, J. W., Simon, R., Raemer, D. B., & Eppich, W. J. (2008). Debriefing as formative assessment: Closing performance gaps in medical education. *Academic Emergency Medicine: Official Journal of the Society for Academic Emergency Medicine*, *15*(11), 1010–1016. doi:10.1111/j.1553-2712.2008.00248.x PMID:18945231

Russell, S. T., Pollitt, A. M., Li, G., & Grossman, A. H. (2018). Chosen name use is linked to reduced depressive symptoms, suicidal ideation, and suicidal behavior among transgender youth. *The Journal of Adolescent Health*, *63*(4), 503–505. doi:10.1016/j.jadohealth.2018.02.003 PMID:29609917

Russoniello, C., Skalko, T., O'Brien, K., McGee, S., Bingham-Alexander, D., & Beatley, J. (2002). Childhood Posttraumatic Stress Disorder and Efforts to Cope After Hurricane Floyd. *Behavioral Medicine (Washington, D.C.)*, *28*(2), 61–71. doi:10.1080/08964280209596399 PMID:12613287

Sackett, D., Rosenberg, W. C., Gray, J. A. M., Haynes, R. B., & Richardson, W. S. (1996). Evidence-based medicine: What it is and what it isn't. *BMJ (Clinical Research Ed.)*, *312*(7023), 71–72. doi:10.1136/bmj.312.7023.71 PMID:8555924

Sagalowsky, S. T., Agnant, J., Bailey, B., Woodward, H., Duncan, E., Grad, J., & Kessler, D. O. (2021a, Jan. 19). *Addressing inequity and structural competency through simulation: Transformative learning workshop* [Conference session]. International Meeting on Simulation in Healthcare, IMSH Delivers: Simulation - Bringing Learning to Life, Virtual. https://ssh.expoplanner.com/index.cfm?do=expomap.sess&event_id=12&session_id=5278

Sagalowsky, S. T., Kester, K., Woodward, H., Bailey, B., & Catallozzi, M. (2020). Lessons learnt from piloting paediatric patient-focused and family-focused simulation methodology in a clerkship objective structured clinical experience. *BMJ Simulation & Technology Enhanced Learning*, *6*(5), 306–307. doi:10.1136/bmjstel-2019-000532 PMID:35517386

Sagalowsky, S. T., Woodward, H., Evins, J., & Kessler, D. O. (2021b). Responding to microaggressions: Further frameworks from simulation debriefing. *Annals of Emergency Medicine*, *77*(3), 381–382. doi:10.1016/j.annemergmed.2020.10.006 PMID:33618815

Santiesteban, I., White, S., Cook, J., Gilbert, S. J., Heyes, C., & Bird, G. (2012). Training social cognition: From imitation to Theory of Mind. *Cognition*, *122*(2), 228–235. doi:10.1016/j.cognition.2011.11.004 PMID:22133627

Santoro, A. F., Shear, S. M., & Haber, A. (2018). Childhood adversity, health and quality of life in adults with intellectual and developmental disabilities. *Journal of Intellectual Disability Research, 62*(10), 854–863. doi:10.1111/jir.12540 PMID:30117608

Sasangohar, F., Dhala, A., Zheng, F., Ahmadi, N., Kash, B., & Masud, F. (2021). Use of telecritical care for family visitation to ICU during the COVID-19 pandemic: An interview study and sentiment analysis. *BMJ Quality & Safety, 30*(9), 715–721. https://doi.org/10.1136/bmjqs-2020-011604

Sawyer, W., & Wagner, P. (2022). *The Prison Policy Initiative*. Retrieved on February 17, 2022 day, from https://www.prisonpolicy.org/reports/pie2022.html

Sawyer, T., Fleegler, M. B., & Eppich, W. J. (2016). Essentials of debriefing and feedback. In V. J. Grant & A. Cheng (Eds.), *Comprehensive healthcare simulation: Pediatrics* (pp. 31–42). Springer. doi:10.1007/978-3-319-24187-6_3

Saywitz, K., & Camparo, L. (1998). Interviewing child witnesses: A developmental perspective. *Child Abuse & Neglect, 22*(8), 825–843. https://psycnet.apa.org/doi/10.1016/S0145-2134(98)00054-4

Schaeffer, P., Leventhal, J. M., & Asnes, A. G. (2011). Children's disclosures of sexual abuse: Learning from direct inquiry. *Child Abuse & Neglect, 35*, 343–352. https://dx.doi.org/10.1016/j.chiabu.2011.01.014

Schieve, L. A., Gonzalez, V., Boulet, S. L., Visser, S. N., Rice, C. E., Braun, K. N., & Boyle, C. A. (2012). Concurrent medical conditions and health care use and needs among children with learning and behavioral developmental disabilities., National Health Interview Survey, 2006-2010. *Research in Developmental Disabilities, 33*(2), 467–476. doi:10.1016/j.ridd.2011.10.008 PMID:22119694

Schniering, C., Einstein, D., Kirkman, J., & Rapee, R. (2022). Online treatment of adolescents with comorbid anxiety and depression: A randomized controlled trial. *Journal of Affective Disorders, 311*, 88–94.

Schonfeld, D. (2015). *Grieving children: An essential role for schools.* https://www.etr.org/blog/my-take-grievingchildren/

School Social Work Association of America. (n.d.). *Role of School Social Worker.* https://www.sswaa.org/school-social-work

Schott Foundation for Public Education. (2014). *Restorative practices: Fostering healthy relationships and promoting positive discipline in schools.* https://schottfoundation.org/sites/default/files/restorative-practices-guide.pdf

Schueller, S. M., Stiles-Shields, C., & Yarosh, L. (2017). Online treatment and virtual therapists in child and adolescent psychiatry. *Child and Adolescent Psychiatric Clinics of North America, 26*(1), 1–12. https://doi.org/10.1016/j.chc.2016.07.011

Scrimin, S., Moscardino, U., Capello, F., & Axia, G. (2009). Attention and Memory in School-Age Children Surviving the Terrorist Attack in Beslan, Russia. *Journal of Clinical Child and Adolescent Psychology, 38*(3), 402–414. doi:10.1080/15374410902851689 PMID:19437300

Seidemann, J. S., & Roxanna Barboza, R. (2021). *Rural imperatives in broadband adoption and digital inclusion.* Retrieved October 10, 2022, from https://www.ntca.org/sites/default/files/documents/2022-03/src-whitepaper-broadband-adoption-and-digital-inclusion.pdf

Shabiralyani, G., Hasan, K. S., Hamad, N., & Iqbal, N. (2015). Impact of Visual Aids in Enhancing the Learning Process Case Research: District Dera Ghazi Khan. *Journal of Education and Practice, 6*(16), 226–233. https://doi.org/https://eric.ed.gov/?id=EJ1079541

Shalev, A., & Freedman, S. (2005). PTSD following terrorist attacks: A prospective evaluation. *The American Journal of Psychiatry, 162*(6), 1188–1191. doi:10.1176/appi.ajp.162.6.1188 PMID:15930068

Sharfstein, S. S. (2009). Goals of inpatient treatment for psychiatric disorders. *Annual Review of Medicine*, *60*(1), 393–403. doi:10.1146/annurev.med.60.042607.080257 PMID:18729730

Sheridan, D., Spiro, D., Fu, R., Johnson, K., Sheridan, J. S., Oue, W. A., Van Nes, R., & Hansen, M. (2015). Mental health utilization in a pediatric emergency department. *Pediatric Emergency Care*, *31*(8), 555–559. doi:10.1097/PEC.0000000000000343 PMID:25834957

Sherred, L. (2019, August 31). *Does online speech therapy work as well as in-person therapy?* Expressable. Retrieved September 23, 2022, from https://www.expressable.com/learning-center/online-speech-therapy/does-online-speech-therapy-work-as-well-as-in-person-therapy

Shetty, R., & Nadkarni, V. (2016). Simulation in acute care pediatrics: New paradigms in care. *Journal of Pediatric Critical Care, 3*(3), 35-39. doi:10.21304/2016.0303.00136

Shirey, M. R., Hauck, S. L., Embree, J. L., Kinner, T. J., Schaar, G. L., Phillips, L. A., Ashby, S. R., Sweny, C. F., & McCool, I. A. (2011). Showcasing differences between quality improvement, evidence-based practice, and research. *Journal of Continuing Education in Nursing*, *42*(2), 57–68. doi:10.3928/00220124-20100701-01 PMID:20672761

Short, E. J., Schindler, R. C., Obeid, R., Noeder, M. M., Hlavaty, L. E., Gross, S. I., Lewis, B., Russ, S., & Manos, M. M. (2020). Examining the role of language in play among children with and without developmental disabilities. *Language, Speech, and Hearing Services in Schools*, *51*(3), 795–806. doi:10.1044/2020_LSHSS-19-00084 PMID:32402229

Shyman, E. (2016). The Reinforcement of Ableism: Normality, the Medical Model of Disability, and Humanism in Applied Behavior Analysis and ASD. *Intellectual and Developmental Disabilities*, *54*(5), 366–376. doi:10.1352/1934-9556-54.5.366 PMID:27673737

Siegel, M. (2018). *Help for children with autism and recurring behavioral crises: Part 2*. Autism Speaks. https://www.autismspeaks.org/expert-opinion/help-child-autism-recurring-behavioral-crises-part-2

Siegel, D. J. (2015). *Brainstorm: The power and purpose of the teenage brain*. Penguin.

Siegel, K., Karus, D., & Raveis, V. H. (1996). Adjustment of children facing the death of a parent due to cancer. *Journal of the American Academy of Child and Adolescent Psychiatry*, *35*(4), 442–450. doi:10.1097/00004583-199604000-00010 PMID:8919706

Simon, B. (2022, March 1). *Medical association statements supporting trans youth healthcare and against discriminatory bills*. GLAAD. Retrieved April 11, 2022, from https://www.glaad.org/blog/medical-association-statements-supporting-trans-youth-healthcare-and-against discriminatory

Singh, P. P., Kumar, V., & Sadeeq, M. (2018). Cyber bullying as an outcome of social media usage: A literature review. *Indian Journal of Public Health*, *9*(12).

Sisk, C., & Cantrell, K. (2021, Spring). How far have we come? *Child Life Bulletin*. https://www.childlife.org/membership/aclp-bulletin/spring-2021-table-of-contents/how-far-have-we-come

Sisk, C., & Daniels, S. (2021). Introduction. In S. Daniels, S. Burns-Nader, & J. Boles (Eds.), *Research methods for child life specialists* (pp. 1–11). Cambridge Scholars Publishing.

Society for Simulation in Healthcare. (n.d.a). *SIM center directory*. Retrieved January 10, 2022, from https://www.ssih.org/Home/SIM-Center-Directory

Society for Simulation in Healthcare. (n.d.b) *V2.0 addendum: Terms related to simulation at a distance*. Healthcare simulation dictionary. https://www.ssih.org/Dictionary

Southwick, S. M., Bonanno, G. A., Masten, A. S., Panter-Brick, C., & Yehuda, R. (2014). Resilience definitions, theory, and challenges: interdisciplinary perspectives. *European Journal of Psychotraumatology, 5*. doi:10.3402/ejpt.v5.25338

Spassiani, N. A., & Friedman, C. (2014). Stigma: Barriers to culture and identity for people with intellectual disability. *Inclusion*, *2*(4), 329–341. doi:10.1352/2326-6988-2.4.329

Staab, J. (2012, Winter). Unveiling a standard for knowledge translation: An evidence-based practice model for the child life profession. *Child Life Bulletin.* https://www.childlife.org/docs/default-source/Publications/Bulletin/clcbulletinwinter2012.pdf?sfvrsn

Standards of clinical practice chapter 4. (n.d.). Retrieved August 8, 2022, from https://www.childlife.org/docs/default-source/the-child-life-profession/standardsofclinicalpractice.pdf?sfvrsn=2

Staphorst, M. S., Hunfeld, J. A., van de Vathorst, S., Passchier, J., & van Goudoever, J. B. (2015). Children's self-reported discomforts as participants in clinical research. *Social Science & Medicine*, *142*, 154–162. doi:10.1016/j.socscimed.2015.08.019 PMID:26310591

Starr Commonwealth. (2019). *Children of Trauma and Resilience Guidebook*. www.starr.org

Statista. (2021, January 8). *Leading reasons for listening to podcasts in the U.S. 2019*. Retrieved October 10, 2022, from https://www.statista.com/statistics/610691/main-reasons-listening-to-podcasts-us/

Statista. (2022, February 23). *Number of podcast listeners in the United States 2017-2024*. Retrieved October 10, 2022, from https://www.statista.com/forecasts/1123105/statista-amo-podcast-reach-us

Stenman, K., Christofferson, J., Alderfer, M. A., Pierce, J., Kelly, C., Schifano, E., Klaff, S., Sciolla, J., Deatrick, J., & Kazak, A. E. (2019). Integrating play in trauma-informed care: Multidisciplinary pediatric healthcare provider perspectives. *Psychological Services*, *16*(1), 7–15. doi:10.1037er0000294 PMID:30431310

Stoerkel, M., & Sc, E. (2020). What is a strength-based approach? *On Positive Psychology*. Retrieved on March 23, 2022, from https://positivepsychology.com/strengths-based-interventions/

Stoneman, Z. (2005). Siblings of children with disabilities: Research themes. *Mental Retardation*, *43*, 339–350. PMID:16131231

Stunden, C., Stratton, K., Zakani, S., & Jacob, J. (2021). Comparing a virtual reality-based simulation app (VR-MRI) with a standard preparatory manual and child life program for improving success and reducing anxiety during pediatric medical imaging: Randomized clinical trial. *Journal of Medical Internet Research*, *23*(9), e22942. doi:10.2196/22942 PMID:34550072

Stygar, K., & Zadroga, J. (2021). *Infants have mental health needs, too*. Mayo Clinic Health System. https://www.mayoclinichealthsystem.org/hometown-health/speaking-of-health/infants-have-mental-health-needs-too

Substance Abuse and Mental Health Services Administration. (2014). Understanding the impact of trauma. In *Treatment improvement protocol: Trauma-informed care in behavioral health services*. https://www.ncbi.nlm.nih.gov/books/NBK207191/

Substance Abuse and Mental Health Services Administration. (2022). *Understanding child trauma*. https://www.samhsa.gov/child-trauma/understanding-child-trauma /

Sumner, K. E., & Brown, T. J. (2015). Neurodiversity and human resource management: Employer challenges for applicants and employees with learning disabilities. *The Psychologist Manager Journal*, *18*(2), 77–85. doi:10.1037/mgr0000031

Swartz, A., Brabender, V., Shorey, H. S., & Fallon, A. (2012). The maternal-bonding trajectory for mothers who adopt young, international children: A qualitative analysis. *Journal of Social Distress and the Homeless, 21*(3&4), 138–167. doi:10.1179/105307812805100171

Swick, K. J., & Williams, R. D. (2006). An analysis of Bronfenbrenner's bio-ecological perspective for early childhood educators: Implications for working with families experiencing stress. *Early Childhood Education Journal, 33*(5), 371–378. doi:10.100710643-006-0078-y

Szalavitz, M., & Perry, B. (2010). *Born for Love: Why empathy is essential and endangered.* Harper Collins.

Tally, M. (2011). Adolescents' perspectives about brief psychiatric hospitalization: What is helpful and what isn't helpful. *The Psychiatric Quarterly, 82*(2), 121–137. doi:10.100711126-010-9151-1 PMID:20824339

Taunt, H. M., & Hastings, R. P. (2002). Positive impact of children with developmental disabilities on their families: A preliminary study. *Education and Training in Mental Retardation and Developmental Disabilities, 37*, 410–420.

Tedeschi, R. G., & Calhoun, L. G. (1996). The post-traumatic growth inventory: Measuring the positive legacy of trauma. *Journal of Traumatic Stress, 9*(3), 455–471. doi:10.1002/jts.2490090305 PMID:8827649

Thayer, P. (2007, Summer). But is it a field? *Child Life Bulletin.* https://www.childlife.org/docs/default-source/Publications/Bulletin/summer-2007-bulletin---final.pdf

The Gender Unicorn. (2021, February 7). Trans Student Educational Resources. Retrieved April 10, 2022, from https://transstudent.org/gender/

The Trevor Project National Survey. (2021). The Trevor Project. Retrieved April 10, 2022, from https://www.thetrevorproject.org/survey-2021/

Theilen, U., Fraser, L., Jones, P., Leonard, P., & Simpson, D. (2017). Regular in-situ simulation training of paediatric Medical Emergency Team leads to sustained improvements in hospital response to deteriorating patients, improved outcomes in intensive care and financial savings. *Resuscitation, 115*, 61–67. doi:10.1016/j.resuscitation.2017.03.031 PMID:28359769

Theron, L. C., & Theron, A. M. (2010). A critical review of studies of South African youth resilience, 1990-2008. *South African Journal of Science, 106*(7), 1–8. doi:10.4102ajs.v106i7/8.252

Thomas, R. (2005). *Comparing theories of child development.* Wadsworth.

Thompson & Snow. (2009). Research in child life. In The Handbook of Child Life (pp. 36-56). Charles Thomas.

Thompson, R. (2018). *The handbook of child life: A guide for pediatric psychosocial care.* Charles C. Thomas.

Thompson, R. H., & Stanford, G. (1981). *Child life in hospitals: Theory and practice.* Charles C. Thomas.

Tsirogianni, S., & Andreouli, E. (2011). Beyond social cohesion: The role of 'fusion of horizons' in inter-group solidarities. *Papers on Social Representations, 20*(1), 5.1-5.25.

Tudor, M. E., & Lerner, M. D. (2015). Intervention and support for siblings of youth with developmental disabilities: A systematic review. *Clinical Child and Family Psychology Review, 18*(1), 1–23. doi:10.100710567-014-0175-1 PMID:25315924

Turner, J. (2009). Theoretical foundations of child life practice. In The Handbook of Child Life (pp. 23-35). Charles Thomas.

Turner, J. C. (2018). Theoretical foundations of child life practice. In R. H. Thompson (Ed.), *The Handbook of Child Life* (2nd ed., pp. 34–54). Charles C. Thomas Publishers.

Turner, J. C. (2018). Theoretical foundations of child life practice. In R. H. Thompson (Ed.), *The handbook of child life: A guide for pediatric psychosocial care* (2nd ed., pp. 34–54). Charles C. Thomas Pub. Ltd.

Turner, J. C., & Fralic, J. (2009). Making explicit the implicit: Child life specialists talk about their assessment process. *Child and Youth Care Forum, 38*(1), 39–54. https://doi.org/10.1007/s10566-009-9066-x

Turner, J., & Brown, C. (Eds.). (2014). *The Pips of Child Life: Early Play Programs in Hospitals*. Kendall Hunt Publishing.

Turner, J., & Brown, C. (Eds.). (2016). *The Pips of Child Life: The Middle Years of Play Programs in Hospitals*. Kendall Hunt Publishing.

Turney, K. (2019). Understanding the Needs of Children with Incarcerated Parents: What Educators Should Know. *American Educator, 43*(2), 22–28.

U. S. Department of Health and Human Services. Children's Bureau. (2022). *Child maltreatment* 2020. https://www.acf.hhs.gov/sites/default/files/documents/cb/cm2020.pdf

U. S. Department of Justice, Office for Victims of Crime. (n.d.). *Crime victims fund*. https://ovc.ojp.gov/about/crime-victims-fund

Unicef (2021, November 10). *Nearly 240 million children with disabilities around the world, UNICEF's most comprehensive statistical analysis finds*. https://www.unicef.org/press-releases/nearly-240-million-children-disabilities-around-world-unicefs-most-comprehensive

UNICEF. (2007). *The participation of children and young people in emergencies: A guide for relief aBOSTONgencies, based largely on experiences in the Asian tsunami response*. UNICEF East Asia and Pacific Regional Office.

United Nations Office on Drugs and Crime. (2000). *United Nations convention against transnational organized crime and the protocols thereto*. Retrieved from: https://www.unodc.org/documents/treaties/UNTOC/Publications/TOC%20Convention/TOCebook-e.pdf

United States Census Bureau. (2022). *Census—Geography Profile*. Retrieved April 10, 2022, from https://data.census.gov/cedsci/profile?q=United%20States&g=0100000US

University of Florida Health. (2022). *Baker act*. https://ufhealth.org/baker-act

Ursano, R. J. (Ed.). (2007). *Textbook of disaster psychiatry*. Cambridge University Press. doi:10.1017/CBO9780511544415

US Department of Education. (n.d.). *About IDEA, Individuals with Disabilities in Education Act. Section 300.8 Child with a disability*. https://sites.ed.gov/idea/regs/b/a/300.8

Vailshery, L. S. (2022, August 11). *Zoom daily meeting participants worldwide 2020*. Statista. Retrieved September 23, 2022, from https://www.statista.com/statistics/1253972/zoom-daily-meeting-participants-global/

Value Proposition Statement. (n.d.). *Default*. Retrieved August 8, 2022, from https://www.childlife.org/the-child-life-profession/value-proposition-statement

Van der Kolk, B. (2014). *The body keeps the score: Mind, brain and body in the transformation of trauma*. Penguin UK.

Van der Kolk, B. (2014). *The body keeps the score: Mind, brain and body in the transformation of trauma*. Penguin UK.

Van der Werf, H. M., Luttik, M. L. A., Francke, A. L., Roodbol, P. F., & Paans, W. (2019). Students growing up with a chronically ill family member; a survey on experienced consequences, background characteristics, and risk factors. *BMC Public Health, 19*(1), 1–8. doi:10.118612889-019-7834-6 PMID:31703664

Vance, S. R. Jr, & Rosenthal, S. M. (2018). A closer look at the psychosocial realities of LGBTQ youth. *Pediatrics, 141*(5), e20180361. doi:10.1542/peds.2018-0361 PMID:29661942

vanDiggele, C., Burgess, A., & Mellis, C. (2018). Journal clubs in health professional practice. *The Clinical Teacher, 16*(1), 13–18. PMID:29436113

Ventola, C. L. (2014). Social media and health care professionals: Benefits, risks, and best practices. *P&T, 39*(7), 491–499. https://www.ncbi.nlm.nih.gov/pmc/articles/PMC4103576/ PMID:25083128

Vernberg, E., & Vogel, J. (1993). Part 2: Interventions with children after disasters. *Journal of Clinical Child Psychology, 22*(4), 485–498. doi:10.120715374424jccp2204_8

Vohs, K. D., & Baumeister, R. F. (2016). *Handbook of self-regulation: Research, theory and applications* (3rd ed.). The Guilford Press.

Vora, S., Dahlen, B., Adler, M., Kessler, D. O., Jones, V. F., Kimble, S., & Calhoun, A. (2021). Recommendations and guidelines for the use of simulation to address structural racism and implicit bias. *Simulation in Healthcare: Journal of the Society for Simulation in Healthcare, 16*(4), 275–284. doi:10.1097/SIH.0000000000000591 PMID:34398114

Wagers, D. (2018). *What is the ONE VOICE approach?* OneVoice4Kids. https://www.onevoice4kids.com

Wagers, D. (2013). Speaking up for children undergoing procedures: The ONE VOICE approach. *Pediatric Nursing, 39*(5), 257. https://onevoice4kids.com/ PMID:24308094

Wagner, M., Jaki, C., Löllgen, R. M., Mileder, L., Eibensteiner, F., Ritschl, V., Steinbauer, P., Gottstein, M., Abulebda, K., Calhoun, A., & Gross, I. T. (2021). Readiness for and response to Coronavirus Disease 2019 among pediatric healthcare providers: The role of simulation for pandemics and other disasters. *Pediatric Critical Care Medicine: A Journal of the Society of Critical Care Medicine and the World Federation of Pediatric Intensive and Critical Care Societies, 22*(6), e333–e338. doi:10.1097/PCC.0000000000002649

Walker, S. L., Connery, C., Blackson, G. N., Divine, T. F., Walker, T. D., Williams, B., Finke, J. A., & Bartel, K. (2020). Developing Resilience in Youth with Incarcerated Parents: A Bibliotherapeutic Blueprint with Tween and Young Adult Literature Chapter Books. *Journal of Correctional Education, 71*(2), 37 56. https://www.jstor.org/stable/27042207

Walker, K., & Lippard, C. (2021). Adolescent cancer survivors' oncology camp experience. The Journal of Child Life, Psychosocial. *Theory into Practice*, 2(2).

Wang, A. L. (2022, February 10). *What is an LLC? Pros and cons of a limited liability company.* Nerdwallet. https://www.nerdwallet.com/article/small-business/starting-successful-llc#benefits-of-an-llc

Wang, K. W. K., & Barnard, A. (2004). Technology-dependent children and their families: A review. *Journal of Advanced Nursing, 45*(1), 36–46. doi:10.1046/j.1365-2648.2003.02858.x PMID:14675299

Webber, E. C., McMillen, B. D., & Willis, D. R. (2022). Health care disparities and access to video visits before and after the COVID-19 pandemic: Findings from a patient survey in primary care. *Telemedicine Journal and E-Health: The Official Journal of the American Telemedicine Association, 28*(5), 712–719. doi:10.1089/tmj.2021.0126

Weightman, S. (2017). Hinduism. In J. R. Hinnells (Ed.), *A New Handbook of Living Religions* (pp. 261–309). Wiley. doi:10.1002/9781405166614.ch5

Weiner, P. L., Hoffman, M., & Rosen, C. (2009). Child life and education issues: The child with a chronic illness or special healthcare needs. In R. H. Thompson (Ed.), *The Handbook of Child Life: A Guide for Pediatric Psychosocial Care* (pp. 310–326). Charles C Thomas.

Weiser, J. (2004). PhotoTherapy techniques in counselling and therapy—Using ordinary snapshots and photo-interactions to help clients heal their lives. *Canadian Art Therapy Association Journal*, *17*(2), 23–53. doi:10.1080/08322473.2004.11432263

Weller, M. R. (2019). "I Guess They're All Real Moms Then": Constructing Motherhood Through Language in the Adoption Community. *Adoption Quarterly*, *22*(4), 265–283. doi:10.1080/10926755.2019.1675836

Westphaln, K. K., Regoeczi, W., Masotya, M., Vazquez-Westphaln, B., Lounsbury, K., McDavid, L., Lee, H. N., Johnson, J., & Ronis, S. (2021). Outcomes and outputs affiliated with children's advocacy centers in the United States: A scoping review. *Child Abuse & Neglect*, *111*, 104828. https://doi.org/10.1016/j.chiabu.2020.104828

What is PFCC ? (n.d.). Retrieved August 8, 2022, from https://www.ipfcc.org/about/pfcc.html

Whitebread, D. (2017). Free play and children's mental health. *Lancet*, *1*, 167–169. PMID:30169163

Wigfield, A., Gladstone, J., & Turci, L. (2016). Beyond cognition: Reading motivation and reading comprehension. *Child Development Perspectives*, *10*(3), 190–195. https://doi.org/10.1111/cdep.12184

Wilkins, C. (2018). Play partners: Incorporating parents into medical play practices. In Handbook of Medical Play Therapy and Child Life: Interventions in Clinical and Medical Settings (pp. 277-295). Routledge.

William, L. I., Lopez, H. C., & Lee, V. (2007). Effects of preoperative therapeutic play on outcomes of school-age children undergoing day surgery. *Research in Nursing & Health*, *30*(3), 320–332.

Williams, A. M., Dawson, S., & Kristjanson, L. J. (2008). Exploring the relationship between personal control and the hospital environment. *Journal of Clinical Nursing*, *17*(12), 1601–1609. https://doi.org/10.1111/j.1365-2702.2007.02188.x

Wisner, B., Blaikie, P., Cannon, T., & Davis, I. (2004). *At Risk: Natural hazards, people's vulnerability and disasters.* Routledge.

Wittenberg, B., & Cantrell, K. (2021). Ethical research conduct. In S. Daniels, S. Burns-Nader, & J. Boles (Eds.), *Research methods for child life specialists* (pp. 91–125). Cambridge Scholars Publishing.

Wittenberg, E., Saada, A., & Prosser, L. A. (2013). How illness affects family members: A qualitative interview survey. *The Patient-Patient-Centered Outcomes Research*, *6*(4), 257–268. doi:10.100740271-013-0030-3 PMID:24142495

Wolfer, J., Gaynard, L., Goldberger, J., Laidley, L., & Thompson, R. (1988). An experimental evaluation of a model child life program. *Children's Health Care*, *16*(4), 244–254. doi:10.120715326888chc1604_1 PMID:10286751

Wonders & Worries. (2022). *About Wonders & Worries.* Wonders & Worries https://wondersandworries.org/about/about-wonders-worries/

Wood, M. (2020, December 16). *The advantages and disadvantages of sole proprietorship.* Nerdwallet. https://www.nerdwallet.com/article/small-business/advantages-of-a-sole-proprietorship

Woodward, H., & Ching, K. (2020, Oct. 26). *Impact of integrating child life specialists into simulation-based pediatric emergency medicine training* [Conference session]. 12th International Pediatric Simulation Symposia and Workshops, IPSSV 2020: A Virtual Experience. https://www.eventscribe.com/2020/IPSSW2020/fsPopup.asp?efp=Q0JUUERNQkk1Nzk4&PresentationID=782876&rnd=0.5213007&mode=presinfo

Woodward, H., & Patterson, S. (2020, Jan. 18). *Optimal technique to improve child life specialists' skills at cultivating emotional safety for families - A pilot study* [Oral presentation]. ALERT (Advanced Look Exploratory Research Template) presentation for INSPIRE (International Network of Simulation-based Innovation, Research & Education) meeting at 20th Annual International Meeting on Simulation in Healthcare, San Diego, CA, United States.

Woodward, H., Evins, J., O'Connell, B., & Diezel, K. (2018, May 5). *Simulation in child life practice: The next generation of preparation, education, and interprofessional collaboration* [Conference session]. Association of Child Life Professionals 36th Annual Conference, National Harbor, MD, United States. https://education.childlife.org/products/simulation-in-child-life-practice-the-next-generation-of-preparation-education-and-interprofessional-collaboration#tab-product_tab_overview

Woodward, H., Kessler, D. O., Fenster, D., Jamal, N., Evins, J., & Sagalowsky, S. T. (2017, June 3). *Stirring the pot: Blending medical, interprofessional & patient-centered objectives in simulation* [Conference session]. 9th International Pediatric Simulation Symposia and Workshops, Boston, MA, United States.

World Health Organization. (2019). *Burn-out an "occupational phenomenon": International classification of diseases.* https://www.who.int/news/item/28-05-2019-burn-out-an-occupational-phenomenon-international-classification-of-diseases

World Health Organization. (2021). *Adolescent mental health.* https://www.who.int/news-room/fact-sheets/detail/adolescent-mental-health

World Health Organization. (2021, November 21). *Disability and health.* World Health Organization. https://www.who.int/news-room/fact-sheets/detail/disability-and-health

World Population Review. (2022). *Mumbai Population 2022.* World Population Review. https://worldpopulationreview.com/world-cities/mumbai-population

Wu, J., Zhang, J., & Hong, Y. (2017). Quality of life of primary caregivers of children with cerebral palsy: A comparison between mother and grandmother caregivers in Anhui province of China. *Child: Care, Health and Development, 43*(5), 718–724. doi:10.1111/cch.12464 PMID:28497475

Yerkes, R. M., & Dodson, J. G. (1908). The relation of strength of stimulus to rapidity of habit-formation. *The Journal of Comparative Neurology and Psychology, 18*(5), 459–482. doi:10.1002/cne.920180503

Yinglin, M. E., Ruther, M. H., & Dubuque, E. M. (2022). Trends in geographic access to Board Certified Behavior Analysts among children with autism spectrum disorder, 2018-2021. *Journal of Autism and Developmental Disorders.* Advance online publication. doi:10.1007/10803-021-05402-0 PMID:34985719

Yogman, M., Garner, A., Hutchinson, J., Hirsh-Pasek, K., & Michnick Golinkoff, R. (2018). The Power of Play: A Pediatric Role in Enhancing Development in Young Children. *Pediatrics, 142*(3), e20182058. doi:10.1542/peds.2018-2058 PMID:30126932

Young, R. (2013). The importance of bonding volume. *The International Journal of Childbirth Education, 28*(3), 11–16.

Yule, W. (2006). Theory, training and timing: Psychosocial interventions in complex emergencies. *International Review of Psychiatry (Abingdon, England), 18*(3), 259–264. doi:10.1080/09540260600656134 PMID:16753663

Ziemer, R., & Tomlinson, A. (2017). *Helping kids discover their a-PILL-ities.* https://www.childlife.org/docs/default-source/professional-development/conference/2017-posters/helping-kids-discover-their-a-pill-ities2.pdf?sfvrsn=

About the Contributors

Genevieve Lowry has been a Certified Child Life Specialist since 1990, working both in clinical settings and private practice. She is currently faculty at Bank Street College of Education in the Child Life Program and teaches the course; The Role of the Child Life Specialist Beyond the Hospital: A local, national and global view. Her interest in child life practice in the community led to the facilitation of a parenting discussion group at a local jail. Additionally, she provides consulting to a wide array of organizations, schools, and nonprofits, providing workshops, educational training, and online materials. She is trained as a Reiki Teacher and in guided imagery and is a certified educator of infant massage, family trauma, and an end-of-life doula. She is the founder of the Convenient Classroom providing online learning opportunities for child life specialists, co-host of the podcast Coping Kits for Everyday Life and provides clinical supervision to child life specialists working in community settings. She received her undergraduate degree from Wheelock College and her Masters's from Fordham University.

Lindsey Murphy, PhD, CCLS, is an Assistant Professor and Graduate Child Life Studies Program Director at Missouri State University in Springfield, MO, USA. She got her doctoral degree from University of Missouri, where she studied the experiences of first responders working with children during emergency events. She co-founded the nonprofit organization, Child Life Disaster Relief (CLDR), in 2016. She served on the CLDR Board of Directors from 2016-2020, and led a team of Certified Child Life Specialists nationwide that worked to integrate child life specialists into their communities during crises. She has been a Certified Child Life Specialist since 2009, she began her career in the level 1 Pediatric Trauma and Emergency Department and continued her clinical work later in the Division of Developmental and Behavioral Pediatrics. She is on the Founding Council for the Child Life Academic Society and currently serves on the Association of Child Life Professionals Community-Based Practice Committee.

Cara Smith received her BA in Psychology from Graceland University (2003) and her MA from University of Missouri – Columbia in Human Development and Family Studies – Child Life (2005). Cara worked as a Certified Child Life Specialist at Children's Mercy Hospital in Kansas City, MO for 8 years before moving in to an academic role as a child life clinical instructor at Missouri State University for 9 years. During her time in academia, Cara continued her clinical work as a CCLS with the Wellness and Resiliency program of the Kansas City Police Athletic League and through volunteer and professional work with Child Life Disaster Relief. Cara has worked around the globe to advocate for the psychosocial needs of children facing challenging experiences. She is currently employed as a full time CCLS in a hospital in Doha, Qatar. Cara integrates her trainings in mindfulness, resiliency building, self-regulation, interpersonal neurobiology, Trust Based Relational Interventions (TBRI), and yoga (RTY-200) into her clinical practice and teachings. She is passionate about the healing powers of connection and play in building resiliency.

* * *

Samantha Ainsworth MA, CCLS, CIMI, has been a Certified Child Life Specialist since 2015. She received her MA in Human Development and Family Science from the University of Missouri. In addition to her clinical role with the child abuse population, she is an adjunct professor at Southern Connecticut State University teaching a therapeutic play course. She is also a certified educator of infant massage. Her interest in child life practice and the community setting has led to collaborative educational efforts focused on child trafficking safety and prevention.

Vanessa Andrews, MA, CCLS, ATR-BC, LCAT, RPT is a Certified Child Life Specialist, Board Certified and Licensed Art Therapist, and Registered Play Therapist and has spent over 17 years working as a child life specialist, leader, and consultant at Elizabeth Seton Children's Center in Yonkers, NY, specializing in medically fragile children and their families. Vanessa also runs a private practice in Westchester, NY called Imagine Me Shine. Her background in trauma, play, child development, and art therapy allows her to develop a strong rapport with children and families, partnering with them to help build resilience and overcome adversity. Vanessa is also an adjunct professor at Bank Street College of Education and University of California Santa Barbara Extension, teaching courses on child development, community, and leadership. She serves on various committees and boards, including the current Treasurer for Child Life of Greater New York and a member of the Association of Child Life Professionals' Community-Based Practice Committee.

Jessika Boles, PhD, CCLS, is an assistant professor of practice in the psychology and human development department at Vanderbilt University in Nashville, TN, USA. She continues to work clinically as a Certified Child Life Specialist, having accumulated nearly fifteen years of experience across pediatric oncology, critical care, and bereavement. She has authored many peer-reviewed academic journal articles, book chapters, and professional pieces about the impact of child life services on patient and family perceptions, experiences, and outcomes.

Shawn Brasher, MS, CCLS, has over 25 years of experience working in the child life profession. He is currently employed by St. Jude Children's Research Hospital in Memphis, Tennessee where he serves as director of the child life program. Clinically, he is part of the patient activity team and is a co-handler for one of St. Jude's facility dogs, CC. These work efforts allow him the opportunity to provide the patient/family interventions that drew him into the profession. Administratively, he loves to see the child life and music therapy staff understand their purpose, find their work worthwhile, and acknowledge how they make a meaningful difference with patients, families, and staff. Shawn has worked in various positions and hospitals over the span of his career. He earned his Bachelor of Science in Family Infancy and Early Childhood Education and a Master of Science in Family and Child Development from Louisiana Tech University, in Ruston, Louisiana. Shawn is married to wife, Christy and they have a wonderful daughter, Bailey.

Meredith Cooper, former executive director and co-founder, envisioned, launched, and grew Wonders & Worries from its beginnings in 2001. Following 15 years of success, Meredith stepped into a founder role in 2017, where she continues providing strategic direction for national growth and programmatic initiatives. Meredith has a bachelor's and a master's degree in Child Development. She is a Certified Child Life Specialist and a Licensed Professional Counselor who has been involved with children's healthcare in the Austin community for more than 25 years, including being the first pediatric oncology child life specialist for Austin. In 2010 Meredith received the Helping Hand Home's Champion for Children Award and the Girl Scout Woman of Distinction Award in 2013. Meredith is married with one son, two daughters and four grandsons and three granddaughters.

Sarah Daniels, PhD, CCLS, (pronouns she/her/hers) is a Certified Child Life Specialist working in a remote research role for St. Jude Children's Research Hospital in Memphis, Tennessee. She also works as an adjunct instructor teaching Research Methods for Child Life Specialists at Bank Street College and Loss and Bereavement at the University of Alabama. Sarah received her bachelor's degree in Psychology from Rhodes College, and both master's and doctoral degrees in Educational Psychology and Research from the University of Memphis. Sarah's research and quality improvement interests include projects that evaluate the feasibility, efficacy, and role of child life services in the hospital setting. More specifically, Sarah enjoys exploring trends in technology use and youth development, psychosocial aspects of adolescent and young adult oncology, and mixed methods research design. Sarah volunteers for the ACLP Journal Committee as a member of the Review Board for the Journal of Child Life: Psychosocial Theory and Practice.

Bridgette Danielson, MA, CCLS II received both her BS in Child and Family Development with a Psychology Minor and her MA in Family and Consumer Sciences with a child life concentration from Western Michigan University. She has been a Certified Child Life Specialist since 2017 in inpatient pediatric psychiatry. In 2020, she received her clinical advancement to CCLS II. Bridgette has presented to several conferences, collegiate programs, and child life departments regarding the topic of child life and psychiatry. She is trained in Therapeutic Crisis Intervention (TCI) and as a Child Life Disaster Relief Responder.

Danielle Eaves Hernandez is a Certified Child Life Specialist, Therapeutic Recreation Specialist and certified in Public Health in Jacksonville, Florida. Danielle has worked at Community Hospice & Palliative Care since her graduation from University of Florida in 2008. Danielle received her Master in Public Health from University of North Florida in 2017. She works with pediatric hospice and palliative patients in the community-based setting and formerly supported children and grandchildren of adult patients. Danielle was president of the Florida Association of Child Life Professionals in 2015. She currently serves on behalf of the Association of Child Life Professionals on the Pediatric Palliative Care Taskforce for the National Hospice and Palliative Care Organization. Her mission is to raise awareness of the role child life specialists serve in palliative and hospice care both as an integral member of the interdisciplinary palliative team as well as the importance of the child life specialty profession outside the hospital walls.

Jessica Foster earned her BS degree in Family and Human Services and her MS degree in Child Life, Administration, and Family Collaboration from Towson University. She has worked as a Certified Child Life Specialist for over seven years. Jessica spent the first four years of her career working in a pediatric hospital setting and two years working in a hospice setting. After providing child life services to patients and families in surgery centers, on inpatient units, and in the homes of patients on hospice, Jessica sought an opportunity to deliver child life services outside of the medical setting. Jessica began working as a Victim/Witness Services Coordinator with law enforcement where the knowledge and skills of a Certified Child Life Specialist are highly valuable in supporting victims of crime and law enforcement professionals. Jessica continues to serve in her role with the Charles County Sheriff's Office in Charles County, Maryland.

Christy French is A Certified Child Life Specialist at Cohen Children's Medical Center (CCMC), the largest provider of pediatric health services in New York state. CCMC is a part of Northwell Health, New York State's largest health care provider and private employer. Ms. French resides in Locust Valley, NY. She has three children. Her daughter, who will enter her first year of college this Fall 2022, was gender non-conforming/gender expansive until the age of 10. Consequently, Ms. French is passionate about supporting LGBTQ+ youth and families. She believes gender is a infinite spectrum of expressions, all of which should be honored and respected.

Melissa Hicks has been a child life specialist for over 30 years. She is co-founder of Wonders & Worries a community-based nonprofit supporting children impacted by parental illness. She has worked at the Johns Hopkins Children's Center and the AFLAC Cancer Center at Children's Healthcare of Atlanta. Additionally, Melissa has served as a psychosocial program director for Camp Sunshine (Atlanta), a private practice clinician and a school counselor at a charter elementary school. Melissa has been the President and Director of the Association for Child Life Professionals and the Child Life Certification Chairperson. She was honored to receive the Child Life Council Distinguished Service Award in 2010. She publishes and speaks on the topics of children impacted by cancer, coping with chronic illness and child life practice in non-traditional settings. Melissa is a certified Child Life Specialist, a licensed clinical mental health counselor and a Registered Play Therapist.

Audra Holst-VanNoord received her BS in Psychology from Grand Valley State University and her Masters of Public Health with an emphasis in Leadership, Management, and Policy from the University of Cincinnati. She worked as a Certified Child Life Specialist at Cincinnati Children's Hospital and then Helen DeVos Children's Hospital, doing clinical work for 9 years. She then moved to the nonprofit sector before taking her child life experience to the school systems in 2018. She worked as a School Child Life Specialist and currently works as a Coordinator of Student Supports - Child Life Specialist at Lowell Area Middle School in Michigan and presents on trauma-informed care and building resilience.

Catherine J. Howe, MS, CCLS worked as a child life specialist at The Children's Hospital of Oklahoma for eight and a half years. She then continued her career as a Certified Child Life Specialist working as an infant adoption specialist in the adoption field and has served biological families, adoptive families, and children over the past sixteen years. She is currently an Adoptive Parent Supervisor at a Southern adoption agency.

Victoria Isaacson, MA, CCLS, NCC received a graduate degree in Counseling from The College of New Jersey. She began her child life career in 2005, and has been working with the child abuse population within the context of a child advocacy center for the last 12 years. Victoria is co-coordinator for the child life student internship program at the hospital where she is currently employed and has been adjunct faculty at Southern Connecticut State University since 2019. She is also currently serving in the role of director on the Association of Child Life Professionals Board of Directors.

Korie Leigh, Ph.D., CCLS, CT, holds a doctorate in psychology, master's in public health and thanatology, and bachelor's in child development and child life. Korie is a practicing Certified Thanatologist and Certified Child Life Specialist and has spent over 17 years working in pediatric palliative and hospice care providing psychosocial and grief support to children and their families. Currently, Korie is an Associate Professor and Program Director for the Thanatology department at Marian University and is the Director of Family Services at Hero's Path Palliative in New Mexico. She works individually with children and families in her private practice. To learn more visit her website at www.korieleighphd.com.

Jessica Lewin received her BS in Psychology from Indiana Wesleyan University in 2014. In 2015, she was hired as a Certified Child Life Specialist (CCLS) at Beacon Children's Hospital in South Bend, Indiana. In 2016, she proposed and implemented a position in the outpatient surgery center to create meaningful change for patients undergoing unfamiliar procedures. She also pursued her passion for walking alongside child life students as the practicum coordinator for five years. In 2021, Jessica proposed a position as a CCLS in the school setting and was hired at River Valley Middle-High School. Jessica continues to teach and engage students and specialists through her blog, Child Life Wild Life, and her podcast, the Child Life Wild Life Podcast.

Briana McDonald received her M.S. in Child Life from Azusa Pacific University in 2020. In 2021 she was hired as Blue Monarch's first ever Child Life Specialist where she serves children of mothers recovering from addiction in a long term rehabilitation facility. She is particularly interested in child life work in residential rehabilitation facilities.

Cheryl Murray Miyamasu, MA, owns a health and wellness business and works as a health coach in Cincinnati, Ohio. She worked as a Certified Child Life Specialist both in the US across pediatric specialty clinics, critical and emergency care, and bereavement, and India, with survivors of human trafficking.

Angeles Nunez, MS, CCLS, CPMT received her Bachelor's degree in Early Care and Education with a Psychology minor from Florida Atlantic University and her MS in Human Development with a concentration in Developmental Differences from the University of Rochester. She has been a Certified Child Life Specialist since 2016 with experience working in psychiatry, rehabilitation and intensive care. Angeles has additional experience working with children and families in the fields of special education and applied behavior analysis and she is trained in pediatric massage, kids yoga and as a Child Life Disaster Relief Responder.

Adrianna Ortega received her BA in Religious Studies in 2003 and her BS in Human Development and Family Sciences in 2007 from the University of Texas at Austin. In 2007 she was hired as a child life specialist at the Children's Hospital of Austin which later became Dell Children's Medical Center of Texas. She started working as a bilingual child life specialist at Wonders & Worries in late 2007 and continues to support children and families there. She has two children of which one is cisgender, and one is transgender. Her journey as a mother led her to start Caterpillar Child Life, her private practice, where she has supported children who are transgender and gender expansive since 2019.

Alli Reilly received her Bachelor of Science degree in Rehabilitation Services from Penn State University and her Master of Science degree in Educational Psychology from the University of Pittsburgh. She has been a Certified Child Life Specialist since 2008, holding clinical child life positions at St. Jude Children's Research Hospital in Memphis, TN and Johns Hopkins Children's Center in Baltimore, MD. Additionally, she worked with the Association of Child Life Professionals (formerly Child Life Council, Inc.) as the Manager of Professional Resources and Services, has senior-level supervisory experience, and taught a combined undergraduate and graduate level course on supporting hospitalized children at Towson University. She transitioned out of traditional child life work in 2019 and currently supports the families of organ, tissue, and eye donors at The Living Legacy Foundation of Maryland while working with a dedicated team of professionals with a shared goal of honoring the legacies of those who save and enhance the lives of others.

Megan Ribbens has a bachelors in elementary education from Dordt University, an M.S. in International Family Studies from University of Nebraska, a PgC in therapeutic photography from Robert Gordon University, and is a Certified Child Life Specialist. Megan worked at Helen DeVos Children's Hospital in Grand Rapids, MI for 3 years and has been doing child life work in community settings in Nigeria and South Africa since 2007.

Courtney Rosborough received her MS in Child Life and Pediatric Psychosocial Care from the Health Sciences department at McMaster University in 2017. She has been a Certified Child Life Specialist since 2014 and was initially hired as a child life specialist at the Stollery Children's Hospital in Edmonton, Alberta, Canada. Since then, she has taken child life out into the community in non-traditional settings such as the non-profit organization Kids with Cancer Society and private specialized services company Kids Uncomplicated. For the past six years, she has worked in an elementary/junior high school within the Edmonton Catholic School District as an Emotional Behavioural Specialist. Courtney is passionate about collaborative communication, the power of play, and advocating for child life beyond the hospital walls.

Amelia Ryan has worked as a Certified Child Life Specialist for over fifteen years. Amelia spent the first twelve years of her career working in a pediatric hospital setting. After providing child life services specifically to patients and families in the emergency department setting, Amelia discovered the need for child life in the communities surrounding hospitals. Amelia sought out the opportunity to work with youth and families in urban community settings. Amelia currently works with Kansas City youth who attend programming at the Police Athletic League of Kansas City, Missouri.

Katie Taylor is the CEO of Child Life On Call. She is a Certified Child Life Specialist with over 10 years of experience working in various pediatric healthcare settings. Katie has written children's books, and presented on the topics of child life and entrepreneurship, psychosocial care in the hospital, and supporting caregivers in the NICU setting both nationally and internationally. She is also the creator and host of the Child Life On Call Podcast which focuses on the integration of child life, virtual settings, and empowering caregivers at and beyond the bedside.

Magellan Taylor-Brickey received her Master's degree in Human Development and Family Studies, with an emphasis in child life, from The University of Missouri in 2013. She is a Certified Child Life Specialist with ten years of experience in the palliative care and hospice settings. Magellan is currently a Certified Child Life Specialist for The University of Texas Southwestern Medical Center, where she is developing their child life program for children of adult patients. Magellan also holds a Child and Adolescent Grief Counseling Certification, which lends well to her focus on child life services for children and families facing serious, life-threatening or life-limiting illness. Magellan has published multiple professional articles, co-led Association of Child Life Professionals (ACLP) webinars and conference presentations, and presented for the National Alliance for Children's Grief.

Shani Thornton is a Certified Child Life Specialist in private practice in the Sacramento region of Northern California. She supports families coping with life's challenges of illness, trauma, loss, and transitions. Through therapeutic play, creative arts, education, and emotional support, she helps children process these challenges and create a coping plan to best support their needs. She offers in-home visits, phone/virtual consultations, caregiver workshops, and support to community programs and schools. She is also a Registered Wonders & Worries Provider, serving children who have a loved one with a medical diagnosis. To learn more about her services, check out her website at Childlifemommy.com or follow her on social media @ChildLifeMommy.

Emmalee Tresnan, MSW, CCLS, is a Certified Child Life Specialist in the community-based hospice and palliative care setting. Emmalee has completed her master's degree in social work. Emmalee has been certified and practicing in the child life community for over six years. Currently, Emmalee serves the pediatric hospice and adult hospice/palliative population to provide child life services and psychosocial support to patients enrolled at Community Hospice in northeast Florida. Emmalee has been part of the Association of Child Life Professionals, Florida Association of Child Life Professionals, Red Cross volunteers and a Child Life Disaster Relief member. Outside of Emmalee's work in hospice she focuses on volunteering her services to children affected by disasters and children enrolled in a community bereavement camp. Emmalee has focused on presenting at a variety of conferences to educate and advocate for children facing their own death, the death of a loved one, or parent/guardian.

Laura Weber received her MS from Missouri State University in Child Life Studies in 2022 and served as the graduate assistant for the child life program. Laura completed a clinical internship and a child life internship in an alternative setting. She continues to meld her passions for environmentalism, travel, and child life as she begins her career.

Hilary Woodward, MS, CCLS, is a child life specialist in the Pediatric Emergency Department at NewYork-Presbyterian Morgan Stanley Children's Hospital at Columbia University Irving Medical Center. She is also an adjunct faculty member at Bank Street College of Education and Director of Child Life for BASE Camp, a simulation-based training program in pediatric emergency medicine for physician fellows, nurses, and child life specialists. In 2021, she was elected to the Executive Board of International Network for Simulation-based Pediatric Innovation, Research, & Education (INSPIRE). Hilary presents nationally and internationally on interprofessional education and simulation.

Index

H

I

J

K

L

M

N

O

P

Q

R

S

T

U

V

W

Y

www.ingramcontent.com/pod-product-compliance
Lightning Source LLC
LaVergne TN
LVHW060353300926
849162LV00006B/1254